Anticoagulation and Hemostasis in Neurosurgery

Christopher M. Loftus
Editor

Anticoagulation and Hemostasis in Neurosurgery

Springer

Editor
Christopher M. Loftus
Stritch School of Medicine
Loyola University
Maywood, IL, USA

ISBN 978-3-319-27325-9 ISBN 978-3-319-27327-3 (eBook)
DOI 10.1007/978-3-319-27327-3

Library of Congress Control Number: 2016937979

Printed on acid-free paper

This Springer imprint is published by Springer Nature
The registered company is Springer International Publishing AG Switzerland

This book is dedicated to my daughter Mary Catherine Loftus, a violinist, who brings light and beauty to our world.

Preface

The book I offer here is intended to be a comprehensive treatment of hemostasis and anticoagulation issues that apply to neurosurgical and neurocritical care practice. I designed it so that in any clinical encounter where a practicing physician encountered a difficult situation, the answer could be found in this single reference. This meant that I had to review my own experience with such complex patients and design a table of contents that addressed any and all areas where the troublesome conflict between need for anticoagulation and the otherwise best surgical care of the patient interfaced. This was not intended to be an easy read or an easy book. The information is detailed, complex, and involves many areas of physiology that neurosurgeons knew in medical school, reviewed assiduously for their written board examination, and have been most likely gradually losing touch with since then.

It should be no surprise that the chapters overlap in scope frequently, but I do not believe this is a detriment to the overall design or value of the book. As I reviewed the chapters to send them off to Springer, I resisted the temptation to add cross-references to other chapters, since any effort to do so would have been mostly incomplete. Realistically, few readers will probably go cover to cover in a book of this scope, so my purpose was to design the table of contents, and the global design, to be comprehensive but also to allow each chapter to stand alone as a reference for the majority of readers who are looking for the one answer to their question. The best way to find such an answer is in the Table of Contents itself, and the design of that is where the true effort in conceptualizing a book like this takes place. Any experienced editor will agree with this no doubt.

The field of therapeutic anticoagulation is moving quickly, and improvements come frequently. The arrival of the TSOAC agents changed our practices, with good evidence that they reduce stroke risk and complication risk for appropriate patients. As this book was in preparation, the first DTI inhibitor reversal agent, Praxbind (idarucizumab), was approved by the FDA for clinical release, and the appropriate chapters, by Jeske and Ardelt, have been amended to reflect this late-breaking news. We suspect that Factor Xa inhibitor reversal agents (also discussed eloquently by Jeske), such as andexanet alfa, may well be approved before the book is actually published.

The chapter contributions come from authors both within and without the neurosurgical world. I am appreciative of the outstanding work they submitted, for the most part on time, and hope that the reader finds this book to be useful and informative, as was my intention from the beginning of the project.

We give special thanks to the hemostasis group at Loyola led by Dr. Jawed Fareed, who was instrumental in developing the framework of the book, and whose colleagues and faculty have made so many seminal contributions to the final product. Finally, we must express our deepest gratitude to our Springer colleagues, Richard Hruska, Sverre Klemp, and Brian Halm, who shepherded the process efficiently and elegantly. As always, I welcome any reader feedback or criticism that would allow us to refine and enhance future works.

Maywood, IL, USA Christopher M. Loftus, MD, Dr. hc (Hon), FAANS

Contents

Part 1

General Principles

1 Physiology of Hemostasis

Jawed Fareed and Omer Iqbal

The Hemostatic System

Overview

Cardiovascular disease, including intravascular clot formation, represents the primary cause of death in the Western world. Blood coagulation is essential to our health; however, when it proceeds abnormally, myocardial infarction (heart attack), stroke, or pulmonary embolism can result. Pharmacologic interventions to control and correct these thromboembolic disorders have recently made much progress as the mechanisms of blood clotting have become better understood. This chapter will review the components of the hemostatic system and the process of blood coagulation. The anticoagulant and antiplatelet drugs used to treat thrombotic conditions as well as research trends will be reviewed.

To maintain blood in a fluid state is vital in order to deliver oxygen, nutrients, and physiological messengers throughout the body. When vascular damage occurs the body reacts with an immediate response to preserve normal physiology. The hemostatic system achieves this balance between the fluid and solid states of blood. The components of the hemostatic system include blood flow, blood vessels, platelets, the coagulation system, and the fibrinolytic system (Table 1.1) [1, 2].

When the integrity of the vascular system has been compromised, the blood clots to preserve the continuity of the vasculature and the blood supply (Fig. 1.1). The initial response is the formation of the platelet aggregate. Platelets in the flowing blood rapidly adhere to the exposed subendothelial vessel wall matrix and become activated at the site where the endothelial cells have been damaged. During this activation process, products from the platelets are released causing further platelet activation and platelet aggregation. The platelet plug initially arrests the loss of blood. This, however, is not a permanent block. Negatively charged phospholipids on the outer membrane of activated platelets create a procoagulant surface on which coagulation activation takes place. The formation of a fibrin clot stabilizes the platelet plug. Subsequently, additional recruitment of other cellular components of blood contributes to the composition of this lesion, resulting in a stable thrombus.

J. Fareed, Ph.D.
Departments of Pathology and Pharmacology, Loyola University Health System, Maywood, IL 60153, USA
e-mail: jfareed@luc.edu

O. Iqbal, M.D. (✉)
Departments of Pathology and Ophthalmology, Loyola University Health System, Maywood, IL 60153, USA
e-mail: oiqbal@luc.edu

C.M. Loftus (ed.), *Anticoagulation and Hemostasis in Neurosurgery*,
DOI 10.1007/978-3-319-27327-3_1

Table 1.1 Components of the hemostatic system

The function of the hemostatic system is to maintain blood flow throughout the body and to react immediately to repair vascular damage to avoid blood loss. This is accomplished by an integrated balance between several cellular and plasma-based components
• Cellular elements
– Blood vessel
– Endothelial cells
– Platelets
– Leukocytes
– Erythrocytes
• Plasma-based elements
– Coagulation system
Activators
Cofactors
Inhibitors
– Fibrinolytic system
Activators
Inhibitors
• Blood flow/viscosity

Therefore, thrombosis is a multifactorial pathophysiologic process. Various pharmacologic processes can be used to target these sites.

The coagulation system is a network of coagulation factors, their activators and inhibitors that work together to ultimately form fibrin, the physical structure of the blood clot (Fig. 1.2). Traditionally coagulation has been viewed as having two distinct branches, the intrinsic and the extrinsic pathways depending on the initiating source of activation. However, interdependence of the different proteases is known to amplify the action of proteases which contribute to the eventual formation of thrombin.

The extent to which each component of the hemostatic system contributes to the final clot is dependent upon where in the circulation the clot is formed. In the venous circulation, where blood flow is relatively sluggish, clots contain a higher proportion of fibrin and fewer trapped blood cells. In the arterial circulation, where flow rates

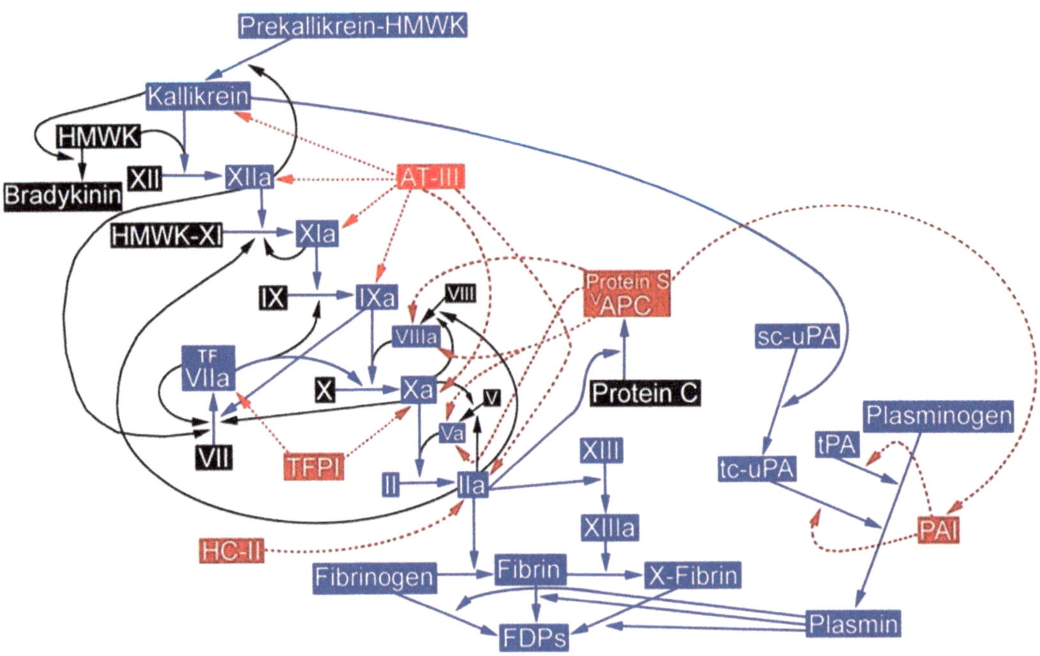

Fig. 1.1 The coagulation network represents a complex process in which proenzyme, enzymes, inhibitors and their activators contribute to the regulation of the hemostatic process. The intrinsic and extrinsic processes lead to the activation of factor X to Xa and subsequent processes result in the generation of thrombin eventually leading to the formation of fibrin clot. The fibrin clot formation can take place in the hemostatic process to stop bleeding and in the thrombotic processes to generate endogenous fibrin which may include the vasculature. The fibrinolytic processes and independent proteolytic processes resulting in the formation of dissolved clots. Several inhibitors, mainly serine protease inhibitors such as antithrombin and antiplasmin regulate the proteolytic functions of thrombin and plasmin

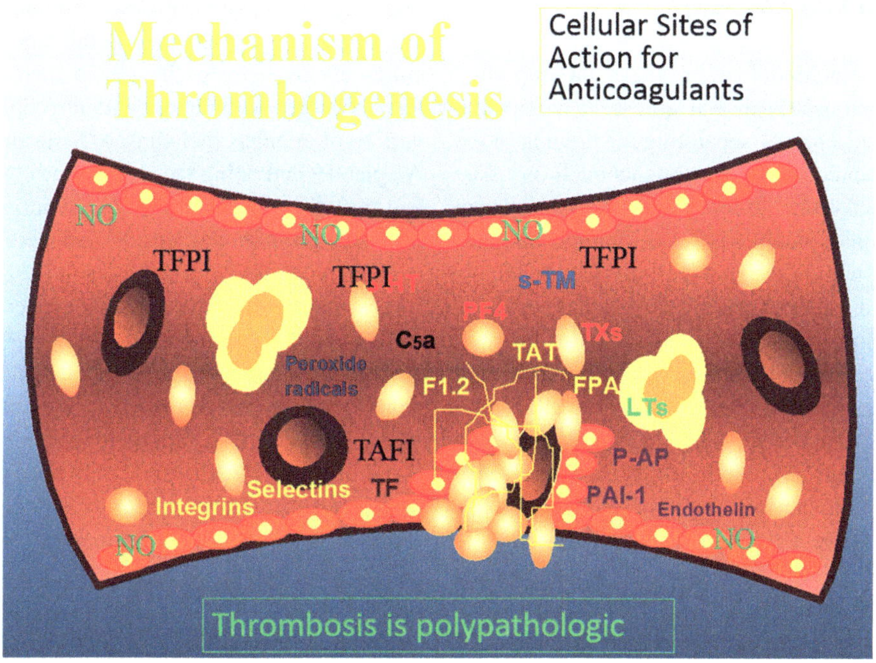

Fig. 1.2 Illustration of the cellular components of the hemostatic system: endothelial cells on the blood vessel wall, platelets (quiescent and activated), leukocytes and erythrocytes. These cells normally express surface mediators that regulate coagulation, fibrinolysis and platelet activation. Upon activation the cells express and/or release substances that modulate the physiological responses of cells and proteins in their environment and cause cell–cell interactions. These dynamic reactions take place under the physical conditions of flowing blood with vasoconstriction and relaxation of the blood vessel wall

Table 1.2 Risk factors of thrombosis (partial list)

Congenital deficiencies/abnormalities of the hemostatic components
(e.g., Factor V Leiden, prothrombin 20210, mutations of the AT molecule)
Antiphospholipid antibodies/Lupus anticoagulant
Hyper-homocysteinemia
Heparin-induced thrombocytopenia
Heart failure
Malignancy
Burn
Previous thrombosis
Smoking
Oral contraceptives
Obesity
Age
Surgery
Physical inactivity/Stasis/Immobilization

Usually two or more risk factors need to be present for thrombosis to occur.

are higher and the presence of a stenosis leading to areas of high shear stress is more likely, clots tend to be richer in platelets. When a blood clot is no longer needed, it is broken down (lysed) by activated components of the fibrinolytic system.

Both the coagulation system and the fibrinolytic system are composed of several activators and inhibitors that provide for efficient physiological checks and balances. If any one component is over- or under-activated due to congenital or acquired abnormalities, pathologic blood clotting (thrombosis) occurs. As the components of hemostasis are many, there are multiple targets for therapeutic intervention. Targeting the mechanism that initiated the cardiovascular disorder will enhance the efficacy of the antithrombotic treatment. Bleeding complications can arise if the balance is pushed to the other extreme with drug treatment or due to physiologic abnormalities (Table 1.2).

Vascular Endothelium

The vascular endothelium plays an important role in hemostasis in that quiescent endothelial cells act as a barrier separating the flowing blood from subendothelial components such as tissue factor (activation of coagulation) and collagen (activation of platelets) (Fig. 1.1). More than just a passive barrier, the endothelium also produces a variety of substances that modulate platelet, coagulation, fibrinolytic, and vascular contraction processes (Figs. 1.1 and 1.2). Endothelial cells play a regulatory role to balance cellular and plasmatic reactions. The functional interactions of endothelial cells can be either procoagulant or anticoagulant in nature, as summarized in the following. These actions can lead to either maintenance of normal hemostasis or to pathologic occlusive disorders (stenosis, thrombosis).

Antithrombotic actions of endothelium:

1. Release of prostaglandin derivatives to control platelet activation
2. Synthesis and release of TFPI to control coagulation activation
3. Regulation of thrombin function through thrombomodulin
4. Release of fibrinolytic mediators to regulate the fibrinolytic system
5. Release of nitric oxide to promote vascular dilatation
6. Presence of antithrombotic glycosaminoglycans (heparin-like molecules)

Prothrombotic actions of endothelium:

1. Release of tissue factor to initiate the clotting process
2. Release of PAI-1 to inhibit the fibrinolytic response
3. Generation of procoagulant proteins
4. Expression of von Willebrand factor to promote platelet adhesion

Platelets

Platelets are disc-shaped, anuclear cells that contain a contractile system, storage granules, and cell surface receptors. Platelets normally circulate in a non-activated state in the blood but are extremely reactive to changes in their environment. Platelet membranes contain receptors for a variety of agonists including ADP, thromboxane A_2, platelet activating factor, immune complexes, and thrombin. Serotonin and epinephrine synergistically promote aggregation induced by other agents.

Upon **activation** the expression of cell receptors and procoagulant phospholipids on the platelet surface is upregulated (Figs. 1.1 and 1.2). A number of glycoproteins (GP) present on the membrane serve as receptors for collagen (GPIa/IIa), fibrinogen (GPIIb/IIIa), and von Willebrand factor (GPIb). These receptors belong to the superfamily of adhesive protein receptors known as integrins as they integrate cell–cell and cell–matrix interactions. Stimulation of these processes allows for bidirectional signaling between the intracellular and extracellular compartments of the platelet. Of the platelet-associated integrins, GPIIb/IIIa is the most abundant. Lack of GPIIb/IIIa receptors leads to the congenital bleeding disorder known as Glanzmann's thrombasthenia. Platelet GPIb binding to von Willebrand factor, which acts as a bridge to collagen binding in the blood vessel, is important as it serves to anchor the platelets to the blood vessel. Lack of the GPIb receptor leads to the congenital bleeding disorder known as Bernard–Soulier syndrome.

Platelet aggregation is another of the fundamental platelet functions. Fibrin(ogen) binding to platelet GPIIb/IIIa receptors is important as it serves as a bridge that links individual platelets together to form a large platelet aggregate. During the activation process, there is a morphologic shape change in the overall platelet structure as pseudopods are formed. This facilitates the platelet aggregation process. Platelet aggregates serve to plug the damage to the vascular wall and their granule release products aid to vasoconstrict the blood vessel. In normal pathology, this decreases blood loss; in abnormal pathology, this causes stenosis of a blood vessel that can result in downstream tissue ischemia.

An increase in cytosolic calcium levels leads to activation of internal platelet enzymes with the subsequent **release of platelet granule contents**. The α storage granules contain platelet factor 4 (PF4), β-thromboglobulin, platelet-derived growth factor, fibrinogen, factor V, von Willebrand factor, and plasminogen activator inhibitor-1 (PAI-1). The dense or β-granules contain ATP, ADP, and serotonin. The release of platelet granule contents leads to further platelet activation and aggregation as well as coagulation activation.

Platelet activation also leads to the formation of **platelet-derived microparticles**. These are small fragments of the platelet membrane cleaved off from the platelet surface. Platelet microparticles promote activation of the coagulation system and further platelet activation (Figs. 1.1 and 1.2). The role of platelets bound to leukocytes in coagulation activation is under study.

Of particular interest in the study of thrombosis and antithrombotic drugs is the acute coronary syndrome (ACS) which encompasses unstable angina, non-ST segment myocardial infarction (MI), and acute ST elevation (transmural) myocardial infarction (AMI). ACS stems from rupture of atherosclerotic plaque, leading to intravascular thrombosis. Disruption of the protective cap exposes procoagulant materials (tissue factor, thrombin) that activate platelets and coagulation (factor Xa and thrombin generation). The role of platelets in ACS, in addition to the role of thrombin and the coagulation system, has been the focus of extensive drug development.

The Coagulation System

The plasma proteins that comprise the coagulation system are referred to as coagulation factors. Most coagulation proteins are zymogens (non-activated enzymes) that upon activation are converted into active serine proteases. A schematic of the coagulation cascade is depicted in Fig. 1.2. Several of the coagulation factors are dependent on vitamin K for structural formation required for activity.

In the **intrinsic pathway of the coagulation system**, activation occurs when the complex of factor XII, factor XI, prekallikrein, and high molecular weight kininogen come together on a negatively charged surface. This is referred to as contact activation. Factor XII is converted to its active form, factor XIIa, which in turn converts prekallikrein to kallikrein. Kallikrein can convert factor XII to its active form, thereby setting up a positive feedback loop that amplifies the activation of the coagulation system.

Factor XIIa converts factor XI to factor XIa, which, in turn, activates factor IX. Factor IXa bound to the negatively charged phospholipid (on activated platelet membranes) along with its cofactor factor VIIIa and calcium ions form the "tenase" complex. Through this complex, factor X is converted to factor Xa initiating activation of the common pathway of the coagulation system.

The **extrinsic pathway of coagulation** is activated when circulating factor VII comes into contact with tissue factor. Tissue factor is a transmembrane glycoprotein that is expressed by subendothelial cells that surround the blood vessel. Tissue factor expression can also be induced on activated monocytes and activated endothelial cells.

Factor VII exhibits a weak procoagulant activity on its own, typically accounting for about 1–2 % of the total factor VII/VIIa activity. Upon binding to tissue factor, a 10,000,000-fold increase in factor VIIa enzymatic activity occurs. Both factor VII and factor VIIa bind to tissue factor with equal affinity. The factor VIIa–tissue factor complex can then activate factor X. The tissue factor–factor VIIa complex also activates factor IX to factor IXa.

The small amounts of factor Xa initially generated are sufficient to cleave prothrombin and generate a small amount of thrombin. In a feedback loop, thrombin activates factors V, VIII, and possibly XI, thereby sustaining continued activation of the coagulation cascade. Factors V and VIII are activated through direct proteolytic cleavage by factor Xa or thrombin; they are not active proteases as are the other coagulation factors.

The majority of factor Xa joins with its cofactor factor Va, calcium ions and phospholipid (on surface membranes of activated platelets) to form the "prothrombinase" complex. The prothrombinase complex acts to convert prothrombin (factor II) into the active enzyme thrombin (**the common pathway of coagulation**). Thrombin (factor IIa) serves many functions in coagulation as well as in various physiological processes. In the coagulation cascade, thrombin holds the key position in that it cleaves soluble fibrinogen to generate an insoluble fibrin clot (thrombus).

Fibrinogen circulates as a disulfide-linked dimer containing two A-α chains, two B-β chains and two γ chains. Cleavage of fibrinogen by thrombin results in the release of fibrinopeptides A and B and the exposure of charged domains at opposite ends of the molecule. Exposure of these charged domains leads to polymerization of the fibrin monomers. These monomers are cross-linked by the transaminase factor XIIIa and calcium to form the physical meshwork of the fibrin clot.

Thrombin augments its own generation through several feedback loops in the coagulation cascade activating factors XII, XI, VIII, and V. Thrombin also activates platelets, it activates the coagulation inhibitor protein C through binding with thrombomodulin, and it stimulates activated endothelial cells to release the profibrinolytic enzyme tissue plasminogen activator (see Figs. 1.1 and 1.2).

The outcome of activation of the various factors that comprise the coagulation system is to generate thrombin. Excessive **thrombin generation** (a **hypercoagulable state**) results in unwanted blood clots that cause tissue ischemia. Depending on the location of the thrombus, skeletal muscle, heart, lung, brain, or other organs are affected. There are several anticoagulant drugs that target one or another of the coagulation factors to reduce thrombin generation. Inhibition of one or more of the coagulation factors that excessively reduces thrombin generation, such as by a congenital factor deficiency or overdose of anticoagulant treatment, may result in bleeding.

Natural Inhibitors of Coagulation

Antithrombin (AT) is a single chain glycoprotein with a molecular weight of approximately 58,000 Da. Normal plasma levels of AT are approximately 2–3 μM. AT is the primary inhibitor of coagulation and targets most coagulation factors as well as trypsin, plasmin, and kallikrein (Fig. 1.2). Inhibition takes place when a stoichiometric complex between the active site serine of the enzyme and the Arg393–Ser394 bond of AT forms.

The efficient inhibition of proteases by AT requires heparin as a cofactor. In the presence of heparin, the inhibition rate constants for thrombin and factor Xa have been estimated to be accelerated 1000-fold to 3×10^7 and 4×10^6 L/mol s^{-1}, respectively. Deficiency of AT due to low protein levels or to functionally abnormal molecules predisposes an individual to thrombotic complications.

Heparin cofactor II (HCII) is another plasma inhibitor that resembles AT in that it is activatable by glycosaminoglycan binding. HCII has a molecular weight of about 68,000 Da. The normal plasma level of HCII is approximately 1.0–1.4 μM. Two patients to date have been described as having HCII deficiency related to thrombosis.

HCII has a higher protease specificity than AT. Of the coagulation enzymes, it only inhibits thrombin (Fig. 1.2). However, it has also been shown to inhibit chymotrypsin and leukocyte cathepsin G. Like AT, HCII inhibits proteases by forming a 1:1 stoichiometric complex with the enzyme. Whereas AT contains an Arg–Ser bond as its active site, HCII is unique in containing a Leu–Ser bond, suggesting that another portion of the HCII molecule may be required for protease binding.

Although the inhibition of protease activity by HCII is promoted by glycosaminoglycan binding, it can be activated by a wide variety of agents unlike AT which is dependent on the presence of a specific heparin chain sequence. Heparins, heparans, and dermatan sulfate all bind to HCII and promote thrombin inhibition. Agents with relatively little sulfation such as chondroitin 4-O- or

6-O-sulfate, keratan sulfate, or hyaluronic acid do not activate HCII.

Tissue factor pathway inhibitor (TFPI) is a 42 kDa inhibitor that contains three Kunitz domains tandemly linked between a negatively charged amino terminus and a positively charged carboxy-terminus. It serves an important function to control coagulation activation. The active site of the first Kunitz domain binds to the active site of the VIIa-tissue factor complex; the active site of the second Kunitz domain binds to the active site of factor Xa. The second domain appears to facilitate the inhibitory action of the first domain, and the carboxy-terminus appears to facilitate the action of the second domain. The third Kunitz domain has been shown to contain a heparin-binding site. Mutation of the active site of the third Kunitz domain has no effect on the inhibition of either factor VIIa or factor Xa.

TFPI is produced by megakaryocytes and the endothelium (Fig. 1.1). Small amounts of TFPI are stored in platelets (less than 2.5 %) and can be released upon platelet activation. Plasma TFPI accounts for 10–50 % of the total pool. Most plasma TFPI is bound to lipoproteins, only about 5 % of the plasma pool of TFPI circulates in the free form. Lipoprotein bound TFPI is of relatively low inhibitory activity. The largest pool of TFPI is bound to the endothelial surface. TFPI bound to the endothelium can be released into the plasma by heparin and low molecular weight heparin treatment.

Protein C is another important natural anticoagulant. Circulating thrombin can bind to a high affinity receptor on the endothelium known as thrombomodulin (Fig. 1.1). The complex of thrombin bound to thrombomodulin is a 20,000 fold better activator of protein C than is free thrombin. Thrombomodulin-bound thrombin no longer cleaves fibrinogen, is not able to activate other coagulation proteases such as factors V and VIII and does not activate platelets.

Protein C is a vitamin K-dependent zymogen. It is made up of disulfide linked heavy and light chains and has a molecular weight of approximately 62,000 Da. Protein C derives its anticoagulant properties from its ability to cleave and inactivate membrane bound forms of factors Va and VIIIa. Protein C requires two cofactors to express its anticoagulant activity, protein S and factor V.

The Fibrinolytic System

The fibrinolytic system keeps the formation of blood clots in check. Like the coagulation cascade, this system consists of a number of serine protease activators and inhibitors (Fig. 1.2). The zymogen **plasminogen** normally circulates in the blood in micromolar concentrations.

Two endogenous activators of plasminogen, **tissue-type plasminogen activator** (tPA) and **urokinase-type plasminogen activator** (uPA), are produced primarily by the endothelium and circulate in sub-picomolar amounts. tPA and uPA convert plasminogen to the active fibrinolytic enzyme **plasmin**. Plasmin ultimately cleaves fibrin into smaller fibrin degradation products.

Regulation of the fibrinolytic pathway occurs at the level of several inhibitors. **Plasminogen activator inhibitor-1** (PAI-1) inhibits the enzymatic activity of the activators tPA and uPA. PAI-1 covalently binds to the active site of these plasminogen activators, thereby preventing the generation of plasmin. Activated platelets are an important source of PAI-1. Secondly, plasmin can be directly inhibited by the serine protease inhibitor **α_2-antiplasmin**.

Thrombin activatable fibrinolytic inhibitor (TAFI) is a third recently identified inhibitor that has a different type of inhibitory function. TAFI is a procarboxypeptidase that is activated by the thrombin–thrombomodulin complex. Activated TAFI (TAFIa) catalyzes the cleavage of carboxy-terminal basic amino acids (such as arginine and lysine) from fibrin, plasmin, and other proteins. Without these end structures plasmin loses it ability to digest fibrin. Thus, fibrinolytic activity is suppressed leaving procoagulant activity to proceed unopposed. New studies have revealed that certain antithrombotic drugs in addition have a pro-fibrinolytic effect mediated by the drug's interaction with and blockade of TAFI.

Leukocytes

Recent studies suggest more and more that the line between coagulation and inflammation is less distinct [3]. Studies have indicated that leukocytes, alone or bound to platelets, play a role in coagulation activation (Fig. 1.1). Cytokines elicit the expression of tissue factor (extrinsic coagulation system activator) on mononuclear cells, and procoagulant activity associated with leukocytes is not limited to the expression of tissue factor (Fig. 1.2). Several monocyte/macrophage derived procoagulant activities have been characterized including factor VII, factor XIII, factor V/Va, and binding sites for factor X and for the factor IXa–VIII complex. Prothrombin can be activated on the cell surface of monocytes and lymphocytes. Monocyte procoagulant activity is also induced by endotoxin, complement and prostaglandins.

Coagulation that takes place on the surface of endothelial cells is affected by inflammatory process. Cytokines released from activated leukocytes, such as interleukin-1 (IL-1), IL-6, and tumor necrosis factor (TNF), upregulate the procoagulant and downregulate the fibrinolytic nature of endothelial cells.

In addition, products of the coagulation process such as thrombin, fibrinopeptides, and fibrin degradation products have chemotactic and mitogenic properties.

Autonomic Nervous System

Although limited research has been undertaken in this area, there is supportive evidence that the autonomic nervous system may impart control on the regulation of hemostasis and activation mechanisms leading to thrombogenesis. Circadian variations with peak incidences of coronary events in the morning hours have been known. This has been shown to be associated with an increase in blood pressure, heart rate, platelet aggregability, and a decrease in fibrinolytic activity. These physiological responses reflect sympathetic activity largely induced by increased levels of plasma noradrenaline [4, 5]. In combination with an increase in sympathetic mediated vasoconstriction, these factors can lead to atherosclerotic plaque rupture. During hemorrhage the hemostatic mechanisms controlling hemostasis are also partly controlled by the autonomic nervous system [6, 7].

Theories of Blood Coagulation

Hemostasis is a dynamic equilibrium between coagulation and fibrinolysis. It serves as a host defense mechanism to stop the blood loss after an injury. This is regulated by vascular wall, platelets and the coagulation cascade. Historically, the coagulation process was familiar to Hippocrates, Aristotle, Celsius, and Galen who knew that freshly drawn blood clots within minutes. Jean-Louis Petit, a French surgeon in 1720s noted that hemostasis after amputation of the limb was caused by clots which were formed in the blood vessels. A Swiss Physician, Fredrich Hopf in 1820 noted that the familial bleeding tendency later recognized as hemophilia was associated with prolonged hypocoagulability [8]. Later, Rudolph Virchow in 1860 described clots and their tendency to embolize [8]. Based on these developments, Paul Morawitz in 1905 proposed the classic theory of coagulation in which prothrombin by calcium activation caused the generation of thrombin which transformed fibrinogen to fibrin [9].

1. **The Coagulation/Waterfall Cascade Hypothesis**: The modern concept of coagulation started in 1940s, when Paul Owen in 1947 noted that a bleeding diathesis in a young woman could not be explained by the four factor hypothesis proposed by Morawitz [10]. By 1957, several factors such as von Willebrand Factor (vWF), Factor V, FVII, FVIII, FIX, FXI, and FX were described [10–19]. Although several coagulation factors were discovered, how they interacted to convert fibrinogen to fibrin was not clearly understood. In 1964, Macfarlane proposed the "cascade" model [20] and Davie and Ratnoff proposed the "waterfall" model [21] that described each clotting factor as a proenzyme which could be converted to an active enzyme, and activation of each clotting factor led to the activation of another resulting in thrombin generation. Thus, coagulation was

understood to be initiated by the "intrinsic pathway" (so named because all the components were present in the blood), or by an "extrinsic pathway," in which the subendothelial tissue factor was required in addition to the components present in the blood. The initiation of the intrinsic and extrinsic pathways resulted in the activation of Factor X which transformed the fibrinogen to fibrin via the common pathway [22] (Figs. 1.1 and 1.2).

2. **Cell Based Model of Coagulation**: The concept that evolved over the last two decades is that the exposure of blood to cells that expressed tissue factor on their surface is both necessary and sufficient to initiate blood coagulation in vivo. It is believed that the contact pathway or the intrinsic pathway does not have a true physiological role in hemostasis [23] and that although FXII deficiency does not result in bleeding problems, the absence of FXII does not protect against pathological thrombosis [24]. Based on this model it is believed that hemostasis requires the formation of a platelet and fibrin plug at the site of vessel injury and that the procoagulant substances activated in this process remain localized to the site of injury. The blood coagulation is initiated by exposure of blood to tissue factor present on circulating cellular microparticles derived from white blood cells, endothelium, and platelets, resulting in pathological hemostasis or thrombosis [25]. The coagulation process in this system is described in phases rather than in pathways. The various phases include, a phase of initiation, amplification, propagation, and termination.

Initiation Phase: The initiation phase, localized to the cells that express tissue factor, involves the interaction of plasma-derived FVIIa with tissue factor following perturbation of the vascular endothelium and circulating blood cells.

Amplification Phase: The thrombin generated on the tissue factor-bearing cells serves to activate the platelets exposing receptors and binding sites for activated clotting factors releasing partially activated forms of FV onto their surfaces. Thrombin also serves to activate FV and FVIII on the platelet surface, dissociating FVIII–vWF complex and allowing vWF to mediate more platelet adhesion and aggregation at the site of injury.

Propagation Phase: The propagation phase occurring on the surface of activated platelets generates more thrombin and forming a more stable platelet plug to stop the blood loss.

Termination Phase: The termination phase limits the clotting process to avoid thrombotic occlusion in surrounding normal areas.

While in the cell based model of coagulation the intrinsic pathway may only serve as an amplification loop initiated by the extrinsic tissue factor pathway, recent studies provide a reappraisal of the intrinsic coagulation pathway and indicate that it is activated more or less in parallel with the extrinsic pathway. Three physiological triggers of activation of the intrinsic pathway include collagen [26], the linear phosphate polymers, termed polyphosphates [27], and neutrophil extracellular traps (NETs) [28]. The intrinsic pathway is activated by cell- and platelet-derived polyphosphates binding to and activating FXII leading to downstream activation of plasma kallikrein, FIX, and other coagulation factors [29]. However, FXII deficiency does not affect hemostasis in vivo [30]. The platelet-derived polyphosphates play a role in clot stability as platelets are abundantly present at the site of injury [20, 31]. This explains why increased levels of FXII are associated with thrombosis but FXII deficiency leads to an unstable clot that promotes embolization [32]. Polyphosphates have recently been shown to act as a cofactor for thrombin-mediated activation of FV and FXI [33] and that it inhibits clot fibrinolysis through activation of thrombin activatable fibrinolytic inhibitor (TAFI) [34]. While the shorter chain polyphosphates secreted by platelets are known to be more active in FV conversion, the longer chain polyphosphates cause FXII activation [34]. Extracellular DNA is another phosphate source which has been recently shown to stimulate activation of FXII and FXI during thrombosis, rather than in hemostasis [35]. NETs also lead to activation of FXII [28].

Polyphosphates and Activation of Contact Pathway

Inorganic polyphosphate (PolyP), linear negatively charged polymer of phosphates held together by high-energy phosphoanhydride bonds, is present in many infectious organisms and is secreted by mast cells and platelets. Polyp has recently been shown to accelerate blood clotting and slow fibrinolysis in a manner which is very much dependent on polymer length [36]. Very long chain polyphosphates activate the intrinsic or contact pathway, enhance the proinflammatory properties of histones and may participate in host responses to pathogens [36]. Furthermore, polyphosphate inhibit complement and may have a role in inflammation and innate immunity [36]. Shorter polyphosphate accelerates factor V activation, opposes anticoagulant properties of TFPI, modulates fibrin clot structure and promote FXI activation, may have a role in controlling bleeding and may act as an anticoagulant [36]. PolyP containing approximately 60–100 phosphate units at high concentrations are stored in dense granules of platelets and are released upon platelet activation [37, 38]. PolyP containing 70 and 700 units can elicit proinflammatory responses to vascular endothelial cells [39] by interacting with the receptor for advanced glycation end products (RAGE) and purinergic receptor (P2Y1) [40], thereby activating NF-κB, promoting expression of cell adhesion molecules and inducing barrier-disruptive effects in endothelial cells [39]. Recently, PolyP has been shown to elicit proinflammatory responses through activation of mammalian target of rapamycin complexes 1 and 2 in vascular endothelial cells [41].

Role of Extracellular DNA and Histones in Activation of Contact Pathway

In response to bacterial products, neutrophils release NETs which comprise DNA, histones, neutrophil granule enzymes, and bactericidal molecules [42]. NETs promote thrombus formation through the activation of platelets and clotting factors. Cell free DNA (cfDNA) and histones are key components of NETs and aid in the host response to infection and inflammation [43]. Cell-free DNA and histones may trigger coagulation, inflammation and cell death by impairing fibrinolysis [43]. cfDNA and histones may have a role in macrovascular and microvascular thrombosis, including venous thromboembolism, cancer, sepsis, and trauma [43]. cfDNA and histones, released into the circulation through NETosis, a newly described form of active cell death [44]. NETosis can be triggered by microorganisms as well as lipopolysaccharides (LPS), inflammatory cytokines such as TNF-α, IL-8, high-mobility group protein B1 (HMGB1), monosodium urate crystals, immune complexes, and autoantibodies [44–49]. The cfDNA trigger the contact pathway of coagulation by catalyzing the autoactivation of FXII to FXIIa [43]. The histones bind to protein C and impair thrombomodulin-dependent protein C activation [43]. Furthermore, histones activate inflammation and cell death pathways by direct interaction with the cell membrane or indirectly via TLR2, TLR-4, and TLR-9 signaling pathways [43]. Histones either alone or as a complex with DNA activate platelets, causing aggregation and increased cell surface expression of phosphatidyl serine (PS), P-selectin, and FV/FVa [43]. Activated platelets through release of polyphosphates could further potentiate coagulation by activating FXII, accelerating FXI activation by thrombin and enhancing FV activation [43]. Intercalating into fibrin clots NETs suppress fibrinolysis and make thicker fibers which are more stable and resistant to shear forces [43]. Fibrinolysis is also suppressed by DNA through inactivation of tPA by PAI1 and through competing with fibrin for plasmin [43]. While DNA can be degraded by DNase 1 or neutralized by synthetic nucleic acid-binding polymers, histones are inhibited by activated protein C, C-reactive protein, and heparin [43].

Innate Immunity and Coagulation: During evolution coagulation was an integral part of the innate immune response [50]. The immune responses which fight infection are also known to initiate coagulation. To check excessive coagulation due to infection the natural anticoagulant system in the body helps to limit the host damage initiated by the innate immune response. The natural anticoagulant systems include thrombomodulin, the protein C system, antithrombin, and heparin-like proteoglycans on the vascular surface and tissue factor pathway inhibitor (TFPI) that inhibits factor Va and VIIIa, the serine proteases, factor IXa, Xa and thrombin and the TF–FVIIa complexes [51]. Thrombomodulin, which lines the blood vessels, binds with thrombin when formed and then activates the protein C into activated protein C, a natural anticoagulant that in the presence of protein S degrades factors Va and VIIa [52, 53]. Thrombomodulin downregulates HMGB1 released from dead cells [54] that can increase cytokine levels [55–57]. Furthermore thrombomodulin inhibits complement through accelerating the inactivation of complement C3b [58] and through activation of TAFI [59]. Activated TAFI is known to potently remove the C terminal Arg residues from complement C5a and C3a resulting in inactivation of these anaphylatoxins [60–62]. Toll-like receptors are known to play a role in innate immune response [63]. The toll-like receptor 4 (TLR-4) on platelet surface can enhance the expression of NETs [64]. The NETs generated can then trigger platelet activation, red cell accumulation, and thrombosis [65, 66]. Immunothrombosis, if unregulated, may lead to thrombotic disorders including deep vein thrombosis (DVT) [43].

Role of Hemostasis in Wound Repair and Endothelial Barrier Function

Proteases of the coagulation cascade cleave and activate the family of protease activated receptors (PARs). Each of the four isomers of PARs is specific for a particular coagulation protease. PAR 1 is primarily activated by thrombin [67]. PAR 2 is not activated by thrombin but by FXa, TF/VIIa, trypsin, and mast cell tryptase [68–70]. Activation of PAR2 by TF/FVIIa or FIXa is currently thought to play an important role in wound healing, angiogenesis, and tissue remodeling as a result of proliferation and migration of epithelial cells into wound [71]. TF/FVIIa signaling via PAR2 may also play a role in cutaneous wound healing since PAR2 are abundant in squamous epithelial cells [72]. However, the APC is known to promote endothelial barrier function via signaling pathways dependent on Rac activation and cortical actin rearrangements [73].

Newer concepts are constantly evolving to enable better understanding of Hemostasis that helps close off damaged blood vessels, keep blood in a fluid state, and dissolve blood clots following restoration of vascular integrity. Hemostasis is now known to be involved in wound healing and endothelial barrier protection. NETs are now known to have a role in fibrinolysis. DNA and histones that are components of NETs are released at the site of infection and intravascular thrombi. Combinations of DNA and histones play an important role in delaying fibrinolysis [74]. Large fibrin degradation products (FDP) bound to DNA and histones may stabilize lysing clots and hence there is a rationale for using DNAse as adjuncts to thrombolytic therapy [75].

Current Understanding of the Molecular Mechanisms Involved in the Regulation of Hemostasis

Traditionally, a coagulation process focusing on the formation of fibrin through the action of thrombin was considered to be the foundation of hemostatic process. This process is primarily regulated by plasma proteins acting as proenzymes, activators, and inhibitors regulating the complex protease network. The protease cleavage products during the conversion of proenzyme to enzyme and other proteolytic fragments are also known to contribute to the activation and inhibition of hemostasis. Additionally endothelial regulators including Von Willebrand factor also contribute to the hemostatic process. The role of blood cellular components and endothelial cells is continually being elucidated in the regulation of hemostasis in both health and disease states. Other molecular mechanisms including protein polymorphism also contribute to the individual hemostatic responses. Similarly surgical intervention resulting in the generation of tissue factor, microparticles, and other mediators also play an important role. More recently, the role of inflammation in the regulation of hemostasis and pathophysiologic transitions leading to thrombogenesis and hemorrhagic complications has also been elucidated.

References

1. Colman RW, Hirsh J, Marder VJ, Salzman EW. Hemostasis and thrombosis. Basic principles and clinical practice. 3rd ed. Philadelphia, PA: J.B. Lippincott; 1994.
2. Loscalzo J, Schafer AI. Thrombosis and hemorrhage. 2nd ed. Baltimore: Williams and Wilkins; 1998.
3. Celi A, Lorenzet R, Furie B, Furie BC. Semin Hematol. 1997;34(4):327–35.
4. Kiowski W, Osswald S. J Cardiovasc Pharmacol. 1993;21 Suppl 2:S45–8.
5. Kawahara J, Sano H, Fukuzaki H, Saito K, Hirouchi H. Am J Hypertens. 1989;2(9):724–6.
6. DiPasquale G, Andreoli A, Lusa AM, Urbinati S, Biancoli S, Cere E, Borgatti ML, Pinelli G. J Neurosurg Sci. 1998;42 Suppl 1:33–6.
7. Svigelj V, Grad A, Kiauta T. Acta Neurol Scand. 1996;94(2):120–6.
8. Nichols WL, Bowie EJ, editors. A history of blood coagulation: Charles A Owen, Jr. Rochester, MN: Mayo Foundation for Medical Education and Research; 2001.
9. Morawitz P. The chemistry of blood coagulation [Die Chemie der Blutgerinnung] (R Hartman & PF Guenter, Trans.). Springfield, IL: Charles C Thomas; 1958.
10. Owen PA. The coagulation of blood: investigations on a new clotting factor. Acta Medica Scandinavia. 1947;194:521–49.
11. Von Willebrand EA. Uber hereditare pseudohemophilie [On hereditary pseudohemophilia]. Acta Med Scand. 1931;76:521–49.
12. Alexander V, Goldstein R, Landwehr G, Cook C. Coagulation serum prothrombin conversion accelerator (SPCA) deficiency: a hitherto unrecognized coagulation defect with hemorrhage rectified by serum and serum fraction. J Clin Invest. 1951;30:596–608.
13. Patek J, Stetson RH. Hemophilia: 1. The abnormal coagulation of blood and its relation to the blood platelets. J Clin Invest. 1936;15:531–42.
14. Aggrelor PM, White SJ, Gladenning MB, et al. Plasma thromboplastin component (PTC) deficiency: a new disease resembling hemophilia. Proc Soc Exp Biol Med. 1952;79:692–4.
15. Briggs R, Douglas AS, Macfarlane RG, et al. Christmas disease: a condition previously mistaken for hemophilia. Br Med J. 1952;2:1378–82.
16. Schulman I, Smith CH. Hemorrhagic disease in an infant due to deficiency of a previously undescribed clotting factor. Blood. 1952;7:794–807.
17. Rosenthal RL, Dreskinoff OH, Rosenthal N. New hemophilia-like disease caused by a deficiency of a third plasma thromboplastin factor. Proc Soc Exp Biol Med. 1953;82:171–4.
18. Hougie C, Barrow EM, Graham JB. Segregation of an hereditary hemorrhagic state from the heterogenous group heretofore called 'stable factor' (SPCA) proconvertin, factor VII deficiency. J Clin Invest. 1977;36:485–96.
19. Telfer TR, Denson KW, Wright DR. A "new" coagulation defect. Semin Hematol. 1956;6:479–93.
20. Macfarlane RG. An enzyme cascade in the blood clotting mechanism, and its function as a biological amplifier. Nature. 1964;202:498–9.
21. Davie EW, Ratnoff OD. Waterfall sequence for intrinsic blood clotting. Science. 1964;145:1310–2.
22. Luchtman-Jones L, Broze J. The current status of coagulation. Ann Med. 1995;27(1):47–52.
23. Hoffbrand VA. In: Catovsky D, Tuddenham E, editors. Postgraduate hematology. 5th ed. Malden, MA: Blackwell; 2005.
24. Kleischnitz C, Stoll G, Bendszus M, Schuh K, et al. Targeting coagulation factor XII provides protection from pathological thrombosis in cerebral ischemia without interfering with hemostasis. J Exp Med. 2006;203(3):513–8.
25. Osterud B, Bjorklid E. Sources of tissue factor. Semin Thromb Hemost. 2006;32:11–23.
26. van den Meijden PE, Munnix IC, Auger JM, et al. Dual role of collagen in factor XII-dependent thrombus formation. Blood. 2009;114:881–90.
27. Renne T, Gailani D. Role of Factor XII in hemostasis and thrombosis: clinical implications. Expert Rev Cardiovasc Ther. 2007;5:733–41.
28. Von Bruhl ML, Stark K, Steinhart A, et al. Monocytes, neutrophils and platelets cooperate to initiate and propagate venous thrombosis in mice in vivo. J Exp Med. 2012;209:819–35.
29. Muller I, Mutch NJ, Schenk WA, et al. Platelet polyphosphates are proinflammatory and procoagulant mediators in vivo. Cell. 2009;139:1143–56.
30. Pauer HU, Renne T, Hemmerlein B, et al. Targeted deletion of murine coagulation factor XII gene – a model for contact phase activation in vivo. Thromb Haemost. 2004;92:503–8.
31. Ratnoff OD, Colopy JE. A familial hemorrhagic trait associated with a deficiency of a clot promoting fraction of plasma. J Clin Invest. 1955;34:602–13.
32. Versteeg HH, Heemskerk JWM, Levi M, Reitsma PH. New fundamentals in hemostasis. Physiol Rev. 2013;93:327–58.
33. Choi SH, Smith SA, Morrissey JH. Polyphosphates is a cofactor for the activation of factor XI by thrombin. Blood. 2011;118:6963–70.

34. Smith SA, Choi SH, Davis-Harrison R, et al. Polyphosphate esters differential effects on blood clotting, depending on polymer size. Blood. 2010;116:4353–9.
35. Kannenmeier C, Shibamiya A, Nakazawa F, et al. Extracellular RNA constitutes a natural procoagulant cofactor in blood coagulation. Proc Natl Acad Sci U S A. 2007;104:6388–93.
36. Morrissey JH, Smith SA. Polyphosphate as modulator of hemostasis, thrombosis and inflammation. Thromb Haemost. 2015;13 suppl 1:S92–7.
37. Ruiz FA, Lea CR, Oldfield E, et al. Human platelet dense granules contain polyphosphates and are similar to acidocalconomes of bacteria and unicellular eukaryotes. J Biol Chem. 2004;279:44250–442557.
38. Morrissey JH, Choi SH, Smith SA. Polyphosphate: an ancient molecule that links platelets, coagulation and inflammation. Blood. 2012;119:5972–9.
39. Dinarvand P, Hassanian SM, Qureshi SH, et al. Polyphosphate amplifies proinflammatory responses of nuclear proteins through interaction with receptor for advanced glycation end products and P2Y1 purinergic receptor. Blood. 2014;123:935–45.
40. Holmstrom KM, Marina N, Baev AY, et al. Signaling properties of inorganic polyphosphate in the mammalian brain. Nat Commun. 2013;4:1362.
41. Hassanian SM, Dinarvand P, Smith SA, Rezaie AR. Inorganic polyphosphate has elicits proinflammatory responses through activation of mammalian target of rapamycin complexes 1 and 2 in vascular endothelial cells. J Thromb Haemost. 2015;13:800–71.
42. Brinkmann V, Reichard U, Goosman C, et al. Neutrophil extracellular traps kill bacteria. Science. 2004;303:1532–5.
43. Gould TJ, Lysov Z, Liaw PC. Extracellular DNA and histones: double-edged swords in immunothrombosis. J Thromb Haemost. 2015;13 Suppl 1:882–91.
44. Kaplan MJ, Radic M. Neutrophil extracellular traps: double-edged swords of innate immunity. J Immunol. 2012;189:2689–95.
45. Tadie JM, Bae HB, Jiang S, et al. HMGB1 promotes neutrophil extracellular trap formation through interaction with toll-like receptor 4. Am J Physiol Lung Cell Mol Physiol. 2013;304:L342–9.
46. Maugeri N, Campana L, Gavina M, et al. Activated platelets present high mobility group box 1 to neutrophils, including autophagy and promoting the extrusion of neutrophil extracellular traps. J Thromb Haemost. 2014;12:2074–88.
47. Schorn C, Janko C, Latzko M, et al. Monosodium urate crystals induce extracellular DNA traps in neutrophils, eosinophils and basophils but not in mononuclear cells. Front Immunol. 2012;3:277.
48. Mitroulis I, Kambas K, Chrysanthapoulou A, et al. Neutrophil extracellular trap formation is associated with IL-1beta and autophagy-related signaling in goat. PLoS One. 2011;6:e29318.
49. Schauer C, Janko C, Munoz LE, et al. Aggregated neutrophil extracellular traps limit inflammation by degrading cytokines and chemokines. Nat Med. 2014;20:511–7.
50. Esmon CT, Xu J, Lupu F. Innate immunity and coagulation. J Thromb Haemost. 2011;9 Suppl 1:182–8.
51. Esmon CT. Coagulation. In: Fink MP, Abraham E, Vincent J-L, Kochanek PM, editors. Textbook of critical care. 5th ed. Philadelphia: Elsevier Saunders; 2005. p. 165–72.
52. Esmon CT, Owen WG. Identification of an endothelial cell cofactor for thrombin-catalyzed activation of protein C. Proc Natl Acad Sci U S A. 1981; 78:2249–52.
53. Walker FJ. Regulation of activated protein C by a new protein: a role for bovine protein S. J Biol Chem. 1980;255:5521–4.
54. Abeyama K, Stern DM, Ito Y, et al. The N-t domain of thrombomodulin sequesters high mobility group-B1 protein, a novel anti-inflammatory mechanism. J Clin Invest. 2005;115:1267–74.
55. Tracey KJ. The inflammatory reflex. Nature. 2002;420:853–9.
56. Cohen MJ, Brohi K, Calfee CS, et al. Early release of high mobility group box nuclear protein 1 after severe trauma in humans: role of injury severity and tissue hypoperfusion. Crit Care. 2009;13:R174.
57. Wang H, Bloom O, Zhang M, et al. HMG-1 as a late mediator of endotoxin lethality in mice. Science. 1999;285:248–51.
58. Delvaeye M, Noris M, De Vriese A, Esmon T, et al. Thrombomodulin mutations in atypical hemolytic uremic syndrome. N Engl J Med. 2009;361:345–57.
59. Bajar L, Morser J, Nesheim M. TAFI, or plasma procarboxypeptidase B, couples the coagulation and fibrinolytic cascades through the thrombin-thrombomodulin complex. J Biol Chem. 1996;271:16603–8.
60. Campbell WD, Lazoura E, Okada N, et al. Inactivation of C3a and C5a octapeptides by carboxypeptidase R and carboxypeptidase N. Microbiol Immunol. 2002;46:131–4.
61. Myles T, Nishimura T, Yun TH, et al. Thrombin activatable fibrinolysis inhibitor: a potential regulator of vascular inflammation. J Biol Chem. 2003;278:51059–67.
62. Li Y, Karlin A, Loike JD, et al. A critical concentration of neutrophils is required for effective bacterial killing in suspension. Proc Natl Acad Sci U S A. 2002;99:8289–94.
63. West AP, Koblanky AA, Ghosh S. Recognition and signaling by Toll-like receptors. Annu Rev Cell Dev Biol. 2006;22:409–37.
64. Clark SR, Ma AC, Tavener SA, et al. Platelet TLR4 activates neutrophil extracellular traps to ensure bacteria in septic blood. Nat Med. 2007;13:463–9.
65. Fuchs TA, Brill A, Duerschmied D, et al. Extracellular DNA traps promote thrombosis. Proc Natl Acad Sci U S A. 2010;107:15880–5.

66. Massberg S, Grahl L, von Bruehl M-L, et al. Reciprocal coupling of coagulation and innate immunity via neutrophil serine proteases. Nat Med. 2010;16:887–97.
67. Liu LW, Vu TKH, Esmon CT, et al. The region of the thrombin receptor resembling hirudin binds to thrombin and alters enzyme specificity. J Biol Chem. 1991;266:16977–80.
68. Carnerer E, Gjernes E, Wiger M, et al. Binding of factor VIIa to tissue factor on keratinocytes induces gene expression. J Biol Chem. 2000;275:6580–5.
69. Nysteadt S, Emillson K, Wahlstedt C, et al. Molecular cloning of a potential proteinase activated receptor. Proc Natl Acad Sci U S A. 1994;91:9208–12.
70. Riewald M, Ruf W. Mechanistic coupling of proteinase signaling and initiation of coagulation by tissue factor. Proc Natl Acad Sci U S A. 2001;98:7742–7.
71. Hoffman M, Monroe DM. The multiple roles of tissue factor in wound healing. Front Biosci. 2012;4: 713–21.
72. Santuli RJ, Derian CK, Darrow AL, et al. Evidence for the presence of proteinase-activated receptor distinct from the thrombin receptor in human keratinocytes. Proc Natl Acad Sci U S A. 1995;92:9151–5.
73. Finigan JH, Dudek SM, Singleton PA, et al. Activated protein C mediates novel lung endothelial barrier enhancement: role of sphingosine 1-phosphate receptor transactivation. J Biol Chem. 2005;280:17286–93.
74. Martinod K, Wagner DD. Thrombosis: tangled up in NETs. Blood. 2014;123:2768–76.
75. Longstaff C, Varju I, Sotonyi P, et al. Mechanical stability and fibrinolytic resistance of clots containing fibrin. DNA and histones. J Biol Chem. 2013; 288:6946–56.

Laboratory Assessment of Physiologic and Pathologic Hemostasis

2

Jeanine M. Walenga

Introduction

Hemostasis is a complex physiologic process that involves the interaction of blood vessels, vascular endothelium, platelets, coagulation enzyme activation, and control systems throughout these pathway [1].

Tests performed in the coagulation laboratory are used to investigate a hemostasis disorder indicated by either patient history or physical examination (Table 2.1). Screening tests are used to place the defect in one of several broad categories with definitive diagnosis subsequently established using more specialized testing [2–11]. For thrombotic disorders, because there is no screening test available a panel of various tests is typically performed. However, due to the cost of these a stepwise testing approach based on patient medical history and population frequency of the known disorders is prudent.

The high volume testing performed in a hemostasis laboratory centers on assays that use clot formation as the assay endpoint (Table 2.2). These **clot-based tests** include the prothrombin time (PT), partial thromboplastin time (PTT), fibrinogen test, factor assays and other tests. All clot-based tests need special considerations when interpreting results. There are many pre-analytical variables and interfering substances in patient specimens that affect coagulation function, plus the integrity of the entire coagulation cascade is relevant to the final test result. Thus, these assays are not highly specific.

Many of the newer tests that quantitate specific enzymes and inhibitors such as antithrombin and plasminogen are **chromogenic substrate based tests**. The advantage of this type of assay is the better specificity as they do not rely on the cascade but rather are single analyte specific; they have the ability to measure proteins that do not clot; and they are less affected by the many interfering substances that affect clotting assays.

There are two categories of tests in the hemostasis laboratory, **functional** and **non-functional**. Assays that measure the function of an analyte are the clot-based and chromogenic assays, as well as platelet function assays. **Immunoassays** measure the presence of a protein but do not evaluate its function. Both types of assays provide

J.M. Walenga, Ph.D. (✉)
Department of Thoracic and Cardiovascular Surgery, Loyola University Medical Center, Maywood, IL, USA

Department of Pathology, Loyola University Medical Center, Maywood, IL, USA

Cardiovascular Institute,
Loyola University Chicago,
Stritch School of Medicine, CTRE Room 434, 2160 S. First Avenue, Maywood, IL 60153, USA
e-mail: jwaleng@luc.edu

C.M. Loftus (ed.), *Anticoagulation and Hemostasis in Neurosurgery*,
DOI 10.1007/978-3-319-27327-3_2

Table 2.1 Available hemostatic tests

Assays	Comment
Platelet function tests	Bleeding time, aggregation, PFA-100
Von Willebrand disease testing	VWD is diagnosed and monitored through selected platelet-based tests
Platelet assays relevant to bleeding	Antiplatelet antibodies
Platelet assays relevant to thrombosis	HIT antibodies, platelet release proteins, thromboxane metabolites, sticky platelets
Screening tests for coagulation deficiencies	Clot-based tests include the PT, PTT, TCT, TEG/ROTEM
Specific tests for coagulation deficiencies	Fibrinogen, factor assays, factor inhibitors, FXIII
Mixing study	Differentiates between factor deficiencies and lupus anticoagulant/factor inhibitors
Tests for a hypercoagulable state	See Table 2.4, TEG/ROTEM
Tests for fibrinolysis	D-dimer, plasminogen, tPA, PAI-1, TAFI

Table 2.2 Types of assay principles used in the hemostasis laboratory

Functional hemostatic assays	
Clot-based assays	Results are dependent on normal levels of factors and fibrinogen; results affected by numerous pre-analytical variables (see Table 2.3)
Chromogenic assays	More specific and less affected by pre-analytical variables than clot-based assays; results not dependent on normal coagulation cascade; able to measure proteins that do not clot
Platelet aggregation, platelet-based assays	Requires special blood collection procedure and handling
Non-functional hemostatic assays	
Immunoassays	Measure protein levels; useful to identify type of deficiency

information that is useful for the diagnosis of bleeding or thrombotic disorders.

The results of all hemostatic tests results are highly dependent on the **appropriateness and integrity of the specimen**. Proper specimen collection, transport, storage, and centrifugation ensure a valid test result.

Hemostasis Specimens

Integrity of the patient's blood specimen for hemostasis testing is critical for obtaining accurate laboratory results (Table 2.3). Protocols for specimen collection and management must be followed to avoid pre-analytical variables that affect coagulation test results invalidating the results. More than for any other clinical laboratory testing, coagulation test results are highly dependent on how specimens are collected and handled. Certain special hemostasis tests require even more detailed special handling procedures. What may seem trivial to a non-laboratorian can have a profound effect on test results.

Hemostasis Specimen Collection

For hemostasis blood sample collection, patients need not fast but should avoid vigorous activities and should rest quietly 30 min prior to collection. There are numerous drugs that affect the outcome of coagulation tests. Aspirin suppresses most platelet function, anticoagulants prolong all clot-based tests (PT, PTT, factor assays, etc.), antibiotics and other drugs also can affect hemostatic parameters. Patients should be instructed to discontinue drugs that may interfere with coagulation test results before specimen collection.

Most hemostasis laboratory tests are performed on venous whole blood. The bore of the needle should be sufficient to prevent hemolysis and activation of platelets and plasma procoagulants. Blood is collected in plastic blue-capped sterile evacuated blood collection tubes containing a specified volume of 3.2 % sodium citrate anticoagulant. Tubes of uncoated glass are unsuitable because their negative surface charge activates platelets and plasma procoagulants. Special hemostasis assays may require syringe collection and initial "discard tubes."

Table 2.3 Pre-analytical variables in hemostasis testing: the need for specimen integrity

Issue	Comment
Short draw	Blood volume less than the required volume in the blue top tube will cause false prolongation of all clot-based assays
Blood collection	Specific instructions must be followed to avoid mishandling of blood; instructions vary by test
Clot in specimen	Even a small clot in the specimen invalidates the result of all assays
Visible hemolysis	Hemolysis indicates activation of platelets and coagulation leading to unreliable results
Lipemia or icterus	Certain instruments cannot measure clot formation on these samples
Prolonged tourniquet application	Stasis elevates the concentration of von Willebrand factor and factor VIII; falsely decreases fibrinolytic parameters; and falsely shortens clot-based test results
Specimen storage at 1–6 °C	refrigerator temperature precipitates large von Willebrand factor multimers, activates factor VII, destroys platelet integrity
Specimen storage at >25 °C	Storage above room temperature causes deterioration of factors V and VIII
Specimen age	Specimens must be tested within 4 h of collection
Interfering substances	Clot-based assays are affected by fibrin degradation products, high factor VIII, high fibrinogen, lupus anticoagulant
Activated platelets	Invalidates heparin levels; affects functional hemostatic assays
Lupus anticoagulant	PT result is invalid; use chromogenic factor X assay instead of PT
Anticoagulant therapy	Presence of an anticoagulant will inhibit the coagulation test reaction and falsify the result
Aspirin, antiplatelet drugs	For platelet function tests these drugs must be discontinued 7–10 days prior to testing (unless testing is being used to monitor therapy)

Blood specimens may be drawn from heparin or saline locks, ports in intravenous lines, peripherally inserted central catheters (PICC lines) or central venous catheters. Before blood is collected, the line must be flushed with 5 mL of saline and the first 5 mL of blood, or six times the volume of the tube, must be collected and discarded. The line is not to be flushed with heparin. Blood is collected into a syringe and transferred to a blue-top collection tube.

Less commonly other anticoagulants are used for hemostasis specimens, and certain tests require further handling precautions. The laboratory will provide guidance for proper collection to assure that validated specimens are used.

Hemostasis Specimen Management

The citrated specimen once collected is maintained as well-mixed, whole blood, sealed and at 18–24 °C. Storage at 1–6 °C activates factor VII, destroys platelet activity and causes cryoprecipitation of large VWF multimers. Specimens should never be stored at temperatures >24 °C because heat causes deterioration of coagulation factors V and VIII. Typically, specimens are to be tested within 4 h of the time of collection.

Platelet Function Tests

Platelet function tests are designed to detect qualitative (functional) platelet abnormalities.

Qualitative platelet abnormalities are suspected when bleeding symptoms are present and the platelet count exceeds 50,000/μL. Hereditary platelet function disorders are rare, but acquired defects are common being associated with liver disease, renal disease, myeloproliferative neoplasms, myelodysplastic syndromes, myeloma, uremia, autoimmune disorders, anemias, and drug therapy. Platelet morphology can provide useful information. The presence of large platelets on the blood film associated with elevated mean platelet volume often indicates rapid platelet turnover, such as in immune thrombocytopenic purpura.

Bleeding Time Test for Platelet Function

The bleeding time test is the original test of platelet function. Using a blood pressure cuff inflated to 40 mmHg, a controlled puncture wound is made with a calibrated spring-loaded lancet triggered on the volar surface of the forearm, and the resulting wound is blotted every 30 s until bleeding stops.

A prolonged bleeding time signals a functional platelet disorder such as von Willebrand disease (VWD), a vascular disorder such as vasculitis, or therapy with aspirin and other nonsteroidal anti-inflammatory drugs (NSAIDs).

Because the bleeding time test is affected by non-platelet variables (intra-capillary pressure, skin thickness, size and depth of the wound), and it has inadequate predictive value, it has been largely discontinued. Although not exactly the same, some institutions have replaced the bleeding time test with the PFA-100 (Siemens, Deerfield, IL), the Multiplate (DiaPharma, West Chester, OH) platelet aggregometer or the ROTEM.

Platelet Aggregometry

Functional platelets *adhere* to subendothelial collagen, *aggregate* with each other, and *secrete* the contents of their alpha- and dense-granules. Normal adhesion requires intact platelet membranes and functional plasma von Willebrand factor (VWF). Normal aggregation requires that platelet membranes and platelet activation pathways are intact, that the plasma fibrinogen concentration is normal, and that normal secretions are released from platelet granules. Platelet adhesion, aggregation, and secretion are assessed using platelet aggregometry, a complex test requiring a skilled, experienced operator. Also special blood collection and handling procedures are required and testing must be completed within 4 h of specimen collection.

To test for abnormalities of membrane binding sites and the eicosanoid pathway, the agonists used to activate platelets are thrombin or synthetic thrombin receptor-activating peptide (TRAP), adenosine diphosphate (ADP), epinephrine, collagen, arachidonic acid, and ristocetin. Antiplatelet and other drugs that affect platelet function must be discontinued at least 1 week before blood is collected for aggregometry, unless aggregometry is ordered to monitor the effects of these drugs.

TRAP cleaves two platelet membrane protease-activatable receptors (PARs), PAR-1 and PAR-2, both members of the seven-transmembrane repeat platelet receptor family. TRAP also cleaves glycoprotein (GP) 1bα and GP V. Internal platelet activation is effected by membrane-associated G proteins and both the eicosanoid and the diacylglycerol pathways. Thrombin-induced activation results in full secretion and aggregation. Secretion is absent in storage pool deficiency.

ADP binds platelet membrane receptors $P2Y_1$ and $P2Y_{12}$, also members of the seven-transmembrane repeat receptor family. ADP-induced platelet activation relies on the response of membrane-associated G protein and the eicosanoid synthesis pathway. The end product of eicosanoid synthesis, thromboxane A_2, raises cytosolic free calcium, which mediates platelet activation and induces secretion of ADP stored in dense-granules. The secreted ADP activates neighboring platelets.

The ADP concentration can be adjusted to detect platelet granule release. At ADP concentrations near 1 μmol/L, platelets achieve only primary aggregation, followed by disaggregation in 1–2 min. Primary aggregation involves shape change with formation of microaggregates, both reversible. Secondary aggregation is the formation of full platelet aggregates after release of platelet dense granule ADP. At agonist ADP concentrations near 10 μmol/L, there is simultaneous irreversible shape change, secretion, and formation of aggregates. Secretion in response to ADP at 5 μmol/L is diminished in platelet membrane disorders, eicosanoid synthesis pathway enzyme deficiencies, or aspirin, NSAID or clopidogrel therapy. Secretion is absent in storage pool deficiency.

Epinephrine binds platelet α-adrenergic receptors and activates the platelet through the same metabolic pathways as reagent ADP. The results of epinephrine-induced aggregation match those of ADP except that epinephrine cannot induce aggregation in storage pool disorder or eicosanoid synthesis pathway defects no matter how high its concentration.

Collagen binds GP Ia/IIa and GP VI, but induces no primary aggregation. Aggregation induced by collagen at 5 μg/mL requires intact membrane receptors, functional membrane G proteins and normal eicosanoid pathway function. Loss of collagen-induced aggregation may indicate a membrane abnormality, storage pool disorder, release defect, or the presence of aspirin.

Arachidonic acid assesses the viability of the eicosanoid synthesis pathway. Aggregation is independent of membrane integrity. Deficiencies in eicosanoid pathway enzymes, including deficient or aspirin-suppressed cyclooxygenase result in reduced aggregation and secretion.

Platelets may become either dysfunctional or hyperactive in **acquired disorders**. These disorders should be considered where aggregation is abnormal and no other explanation is available. Platelet aggregometry results may predict the risk of bleeding or thrombosis in the patient with acquired platelet functional disorders.

Platelet Function Analyzer

The PFA-100 Platelet Function Analyzer (Siemens, Deerfield, IL) is an automated instrument that detects quantitative and qualitative platelet abnormalities. Test cartridges contain membranes coated with collagen/epinephrine or collagen/ADP to stimulate platelet adhesion/aggregation. Whole blood is aspirated under controlled flow conditions through a microscopic aperture in the membrane. The time required for a platelet plug to occlude the aperture is an indication of platelet function. The PFA-100 system is sensitive to VWD and aspirin therapy.

Tests for von Willebrand Disease

The **ristocetin-induced platelet aggregation (RIPA) test** uses platelet aggregation to detect platelet agglutination induced by the ristocetin reagent. A normal RIPA result may imply that normal concentrations of functional VWF are present and that the platelets possess a functional VWF receptor, GP Ib/IX/V. Specimens from patients with VWD, except for subtype 2B VWD, produce a reduced or absent reaction, although all other agonists (above) generate normal tracings. Addition of VWF to the test system restores a normal RIPA reaction, confirming the diagnosis. In patients with Bernard-Soulier syndrome, a congenital abnormality of the GP Ib or IX portion of the GP Ib/IX/V receptor results in a diminished RIPA reaction that is not corrected by the addition of VWF.

In VWD subtype 2B, a VWF gain-of-function mutation, aggregation occurs even when reduced ristocetin concentrations (1 mg/mL) are added. This illustrates the increased affinity of large VWF multimers for the platelet receptors.

The RIPA test is qualitative, diagnostic in only about 70 % of cases, and has poor predictive value with considerable variation in results. Comprehensive testing must include the ristocetin cofactor test, **the VWF antigen immunoassay** and the **coagulation factor VIII activity assay**. Many laboratories also offer the VWF activity immunoassay and the VWF collagen-binding assay. Ultimate confirmation and characterization of VWD is based on **gel immunoelectrophoresis** to characterize VWF monomers.

Ristocetin Cofactor Assay for VWF activity substitutes formalin-fixed or lyophilized normal "reagent" platelets for the patient's platelets. Patient's platelet-poor plasma is mixed with reagent platelets and ristocetin induced aggregation is determined. Comparison of patient results against standard dilutions of normal plasma permits a quantitative expression of the VWF activity level. This test suffers from poor precision.

The **VWF activity immunoassay** employs a monoclonal antibody specific for an *active* VWF epitope and the **VWF collagen binding assay** mimics the collagen adhesion property of VWF. Both reflect VWF activity rather than concentration and offer improved precision when compared to the ristocetin cofactor assay.

Tests for Antiplatelet Antibodies

Antiplatelet antibodies are numerous and can be assessed by flow cytometric assays using specific monoclonal antibodies. These tests are performed by experts in reference laboratories.

Another antibody mediated platelet function defect is **heparin-induced thrombocytopenia** (HIT). An immunoassay, which detects antibodies to the PF4–heparin complex, is the first line of testing. If positive, a platelet function assay is performed to confirm that the antibodies produce a heparin-dependent activation of platelets. Platelet function tests include the serotonin release assay (^{14}C-SRA) and platelet aggregation based assays.

Other Platelet Activation Assays

Upon activation platelets secrete **β-thromboglobulin** (β-TG) and **platelet factor 4** (PF4). The plasma levels of these two platelet specific proteins are elevated in thrombotic stroke and coronary thrombosis. Both proteins can be measured, but special blood collection techniques are necessary and assays are performed by a reference lab.

Thromboxane B_2, a stable metabolite of the platelet eicosanoid pathway, can be measured by immunoassay. **Urine 11-dehydrothromboxane B_2** levels can also be used to characterize platelet activation, monitor aspirin therapy and identify aspirin therapy failure.

A less commonly used assay, but one that has shown relevance to a hypercoagulable state, is the test for '**sticky platelets**'. This test uses platelet aggregation and low concentrations of ADP and epinephrine agonists to determine if platelets are hyperactivated.

There are several applications of platelet specific activation markers using **flow cytometry**; however, these are research use only at this time.

Clot-Based Coagulation Tests

The result endpoint of the clot-based coagulation screening tests, prothrombin time (PT), partial thromboplastin time (PTT) and fibrinogen assay use the principle where a prolonged time to form a standard clot indicates a coagulation deficiency. Specialized tests, such as coagulation factor assays, inhibitor assays, and lupus anticoagulant testing also use this same assay principle. Patient citrated plasma (centrifuged to remove all cells) is used. Clots formed in the test system are detected by optical or electromechanical sensors.

Clot-Based Assay Limitations

Great care should be taken to minimize preanalytical variables of the patient specimen (Table 2.3). Proper blood collection and handling as discussed above is essential. Clotted, hemolyzed, icteric, or lipemic specimens are rejected because they give unreliable results. The antithrombotic effects of heparin and other therapeutic anticoagulants, FDP levels >100 µg/mL, presence of a lupus anticoagulant, high fibrinogen and high factor VIII levels prolong the time to clot formation leading to false results. Factor VII activation occurs during refrigeration of plasma at 4–10 °C. The specificity of any assay that uses a clotting endpoint is compromised when factor deficiencies, low fibrinogen levels, or any of the above is present.

Prothrombin Time

PT reagents are prepared from recombinant or affinity-purified tissue factor suspended in phospholipids. Reagents from different manufacturers have differing sensitivities to various factors, warfarin, heparin, and the lupus anticoagulant. When mixed with citrated plasma, the PT reagent plus calcium triggers fibrin polymerization by activating factor VII. The test is most sensitive to factor VII deficiencies, moderately sensitive to factor V and X deficiencies, sensitive to severe fibrinogen and prothrombin deficiencies, and insensitive to deficiencies of factors VIII and IX. Any suspected single-factor deficiency is confirmed with a factor assay.

No clinical data support the use of the PT as a general screening test for individuals at low risk of bleeding. Preoperative PT screening of asymptomatic surgical patients to predict intra-operative hemorrhage is not supported by prevalence studies, unless the patient known to be at high-risk for bleeding.

Acquired multiple deficiencies such as disseminated intravascular coagulation (DIC) and vitamin K deficiency affect factor VII activity and are detected through prolonged PT results. The PT is particularly sensitive to liver disease, which causes factor VII levels to become rapidly diminished. Vitamin K deficiency is seen in severe malnutrition, during use of broad-spectrum antibiotics that destroy gut flora, with parenteral nutrition, and in malabsorption syndromes. Vitamin K levels are low in newborns as bacterial colonization of the gut has not begun. Both factor V and factor VII are reduced in liver disease; only factor VII is reduced in vitamin K deficiency.

Partial Thromboplastin Time

The PTT (also called the activated partial thromboplastin time, APTT) is prolonged in all congenital and acquired procoagulant deficiencies except for deficiencies of factors VII and XIII. Most PTT reagents are designed so that the test is prolonged when the plasma has <30 % of factors VIII, IX, or XI. The PTT is also performed to detect lupus anticoagulants, specific factor inhibitors (e.g., anti-factor VIII antibodies) and to monitor heparin therapy. DIC prolongs the PTT but vitamin K deficiency does not.

No clinical data support the use of the PTT as a general screening test for individuals at low risk of bleeding.

The PTT reagent contains phospholipid and a negatively charged particulate activator such as silica, kaolin or celite in suspension. The activator provides a surface that mediates a conformational change in factor XII that results in its activation. Factor XIIa initiates clot formation through the intrinsic pathway. Calcium and phospholipid supplied in the reagent catalyze the conversion of factor X to Xa and prothrombin to thrombin. Thrombin catalyzes the polymerization of fibrinogen and the formation of the fibrin clot endpoint of the assay.

Thrombin Clotting Time

Commercially prepared bovine thrombin cleaves fibrinopeptides A and B from fibrinogen to form a detectable fibrin polymer in patient plasma. The thrombin clotting time (TCT) is prolonged when the fibrinogen level is <100 mg/dL (hypofibrinogenemia) or in the presence of antithrombotic substances such as FDPs, paraproteins or heparin. Afibrinogenemia (absence of fibrinogen) and dysfibrinogenemia (biochemically abnormal and nonfunctional fibrinogen) also prolonged the TCT.

Global Coagulation Assays

The **thromboelastograph (TEG)** (Haemonetics, Braintree, MA) and the **ROTEM** (Tem, Durham, NC) analyzers assess the entire (global) process of the evolving clot formation in whole blood. The aspects of the dynamic process reveal the interaction between platelets, plasma proteins, inhibitors, cofactors, and antithrombotic drugs if present. The generation of thrombin that initiates the blood clot formation, initial fibrin formation induced by thrombin-activated platelets, speed of full fibrin formation and polymerization, strength and stability of the clot from the combined effects of platelet function, fibrinogen concentration, fibrin–platelet interactions and factor XIII, as well as the fibrinolytic clot breakdown activity are demonstrated in this assay and can be quantitated.

Bleeding or thrombotic risk in hepatic disease, liver transplant surgery, cardiac surgery, obstetrics, and trauma has been shown. This assay aids in determining the need for clotting factor administration, platelet transfusion, fibrinolytic therapy, and/or antiplatelet therapy.

Specific Tests Using Clot-Based Assays

Fibrinogen Assay

A modification of the TCT using known calibrators is the procedure for quantitating a functional fibrinogen level.

Single-Factor Assays

If the PTT is prolonged and the PT and TCT are normal, and heparin therapy, lupus anticoagulant or a factor-specific inhibitor are not present, a congenital single-factor deficiency such as factor VIII, IX, and XI deficiency may be suspected. A specific factor level can also be used to monitor supportive therapy during bleeding episodes or invasive procedures in patients with a known factor deficiency.

If, on the other hand, the PTT and the PT are both prolonged, the TCT is normal, and liver disease, vitamin K deficiency, DIC, or warfarin therapy are not present, a congenital single-factor deficiency of the common pathway such as prothrombin, factor V or X deficiency may be suspected.

If the PT is prolonged and all other test results are normal, factor VII deficiency is suspected.

To diagnose a congenital single-factor deficiency a factor assay is performed. A modification of the PT or PTT is used, incorporating commercial plasma depleted of the factor in question (but with normal activity of all other coagulation factors). Results of various dilutions of patient's plasma compared to a calibration curve allow quantitating the level of the coagulation factor in the patient's plasma.

Coagulation Factor Inhibitors

Acquired inhibitors are IgG immunoglobulins directed against individual coagulation factors. Anti-factor VIII, the most common, and anti-factor IX inhibitors develop during factor concentrate treatment. Autoantibodies to factor VIII may occasionally arise in individuals without hemophilia, usually in young women where they are associated with a postpartum bleeding or in older patients with autoimmune disorders. Mixing studies, factor assays, and Bethesda titers to confirm the presence of and quantitate the inhibitor can be performed.

Other Coagulation Tests

Factor XIII Assay

Coagulation factor XIII is a transglutaminase that catalyzes covalent cross-links between α and γ chains of the fibrin polymer, strengthening the fibrin clot and rendering it resistant to proteases. This is essential for normal hemostasis and wound healing. Slowly resolving hematomas, recurrent spontaneous abortion and posttraumatic hemorrhage are associated with factor XIII deficiency. Inherited factor XIII deficiency (rare) and acquired factor XIII inhibitors from certain drugs have been described. Factor XIII activity is determined by a functional assay. Immunoassays for factor XIII are also available.

Thrombophilia Tests

Laboratory screening for thrombophilia, or a hypercoagulable state, is appropriate for individuals whose medical or family history suggests the presence of an underlying predisposition to

Table 2.4 Panel of hemostatic tests ordered to test for a hypercoagulable state

Hypercoagulable panel	Comment
Antiphospholipid antibodies: lupus anticoagulant, anticardiolipin antibodies, anti-β2GPI antibodies	
Free Protein S antigen	Prefer the antigen as the first line test since it is less susceptible to pre-analytical variables
Protein C activity	
Antithrombin activity	
FV Leiden (gene mutation)	Other option is to screen with the clot-based activated protein C resistance test then, if positive, reflex to the gene mutation test
Prothrombin gene mutation	
Homocysteine	Reflex to methylene tetrahydrofolate reductase mutation testing if homocysteine level very high
C-reactive protein	
Lipoprotein (a)	
The following are second line tests:	
FVIII clotting activity	
Fibrinogen clotting activity	
Plasminogen activity	
Plasminogen activator inhibitor (PAI-1) antigen	
Tissue plasminogen activator (tPA) antigen	

Functional activity assays are typically the preferred first line test

For all tests, avoid testing during the acute phase of thrombosis or anticoagulant therapy for accurate results

clot development. There is no global assay available to evaluate for thrombophilia. For this reason panels of assays must be performed (Table 2.4). It is preferable to use functional assays in the first line assessment of hypercoagulability. Current anticoagulant therapy and ongoing or recent thrombotic events interfere with the interpretation of many of these tests.

Lupus Anticoagulant Testing

Lupus anticoagulants (LA) are immunoglobulins with affinity for phospholipid-bound proteins. Because they have a variety of target antigens LAs are nonspecific inhibitors. LA testing is part of every thrombophilia profile. An unexpectedly prolonged screening PTT may also trigger an LA investigation. Rarely the PT assay is unexpectedly prolonged.

The first step to identify a LA is to perform a **mixing study** to distinguish inhibitors from factor deficiencies. To work-up a prolonged screening PTT, patient plasma (1 part) is mixed with normal plasma (1 part) and the PTT is repeated. If the mixture corrects the PTT to within 10 % of the normal control PTT a factor deficiency is presumed. If the mixture PTT fails to correct, LA is suspected. Some LAs are time- and temperature-dependent, requiring incubation for detection.

Due to the variety of LA characteristics, two test systems are required to confirm a LA. The two most commonly recommended test systems are the **dilute Russell viper venom time** (DRVVT) and the **silica-based partial thromboplastin time** (PTT), both formulated with low phospholipid concentrations to be LA sensitive.

Antiphospholipid Antibodies

Antiphospholipid (APL) antibodies are a family of immunoglobulins that bind protein–phospholipid complexes. APL antibodies include LAs, detected by clot-based assays, **anticardiolipin** (ACL) antibodies and **anti-β_2-glycoprotein I** (anti-β_2-GPI) antibodies detected by immunoassay for IgM and IgG isotypes. Any APL assay yielding positive results is repeated on a new specimen collected after 12 weeks to distinguish a transient alloantibody from a chronic autoantibody.

For cases in which an APL antibody is suspected but the LA, ACL, and anti-β_2-GPI assay results are negative, the immunoassay for

anti-phosphatidylserine antibodies can be tested. Annexin V and prothrombin have also been implicated as targets.

Activated Protein C Resistance and Factor V Leiden Mutation

The activated protein C (APC) in complex with protein S inactivates activated factors V and VIII. A mutation in the factor V gene substitutes glutamine for arginine at position 506 of the factor V molecule (FV R506Q; FV Leiden). The arginine molecule is a normal cleavage site for APC; the substitution slows or resists APC hydrolysis. The resistant factor Va remains active and raises the production of thrombin, leading to thrombosis.

The **APC resistance clot-based assay** is used to screen for FV Leiden. This is a PTT-based assay that incorporates factor V-depleted plasma and APC. A ratio of PTT results between an aliquot with or without APC determines if there is abnormal factor V activity (APC resistance). LA affects the test system adversely; if present, the molecular test for FV Leiden is indicated.

The APC resistance diagnosis is confirmed using the **molecular FV Leiden mutation test**. The determination of zygosity is important to predict the risk for thrombosis and establish a treatment regimen.

Prothrombin G20210A

A guanine-to-adenine mutation at base 20210 of the 3′ untranslated region of the prothrombin (factor II) gene has been identified. The increased risk of thrombosis in those with the mutation seems to be related to mildly elevated prothrombin activity (levels averaging 130 %). There is a molecular test for this mutation.

Methylene Tetrahydrofolate Reductase

Although elevated homocysteine levels contribute to the risk of cardiovascular disease and thrombosis, a direct link has not been established. MTHFR mutations, detected by a polymerase chain reaction molecular assay, are associated with elevated plasma levels of homocysteine. Typically this test is only ordered as a follow-up in patients with known elevated levels of homocysteine.

Antithrombin

Antithrombin (AT) is a serine protease inhibitor (SERPIN) that neutralizes factors IIa (thrombin), IXa, Xa, XIa, and XIIa. Antithrombin activity is enhanced by binding to heparin. About 90 % of cases of antithrombin deficiency are quantitative (reduced production; type I); the remainder is caused by mutations creating structural abnormalities in the antithrombin protease binding site or the heparin binding site. The latter type II mutations do not reduce antithrombin production but the molecules are nonfunctional.

The chromogenic substrate test for plasma antithrombin activity is quantitative and detects mutations affecting the proteolytic site, but not the heparin binding site. A clot-based assay is also available but less commonly used because of stability and reproducibility issues. However, the clot-based antithrombin assay detects mutations in both the proteolytic and heparin binding sites. AT concentration can also be measured by immunoassay.

Protein C and Protein S

When thrombin binds endothelial cell membrane thrombomodulin it becomes an anticoagulant. The thrombin–thrombomodulin complex activates plasma protein C, and activated protein C (APC) binds free plasma protein S. The stabilized APC–protein S complex hydrolyzes factors Va and VIIIa to slow thrombin generation and fibrin formation. Protein S circulates either free or covalently bound to the complement binding protein C4bBP. Bound protein S cannot participate in the protein C anticoagulant pathway; only free plasma protein S is available to serve as the APC cofactor.

Functional assays detect both quantitative and qualitative protein C deficiencies. Chromogenic and clot-based protein C activity assays are available. The chromogenic assay detects abnormalities that affect the molecule's proteolytic properties (active serine protease site), but misses those that affect protein C's phospholipid binding site or protein S binding site. A clot-based protein C assay will detect abnormalities at these additional sites on the molecule.

Enzyme immunoassay is used to measure protein C antigen when the functional activity is low. The protein C antigen assay detects most deficiencies but it does not detect qualitative abnormalities, which is why it is used only in response to an abnormally reduced protein C functional assay result.

For protein S deficiency testing by a functional assay, a clot-based assay is performed (no chromogenic assay is available). When there is a low protein S activity level, an enzyme immunoassay is performed. Assays are available to measure either free or total protein S. The concentration of plasma C4bBP, measured with an immunoassay, is available for research use only.

For screening purposes, recommended assays are the chromogenic protein C functional and free protein S antigen to avoid as many preanalytical variables as possible.

Other Assays

The **fibrinogen** level has often been included in risk assessment profiles for a hypercoagulable state/thrombosis; however, no clinical trial has yet confirmed its role. Elevated fibrinogen supports coagulation and activates platelets by binding to their GP IIb/IIIa membrane receptors, and becomes integrated into atherothrombotic lesions. Statin therapy, smoking cessation, and exercise lower fibrinogen levels.

Dysfibrinogenemia and elevated levels of **factor VIII, IX, and XI** activity contribute to thrombin generation and may increase the risk of thrombosis.

Tissue factor pathway inhibitor (TFPI) is an important control protein against tissue factor (TF) activation. It inhibits the factor VIIa–TF complex and factor Xa. Assays are available for research use only at this time.

Tests of Fibrinolysis

D-Dimer

During coagulation, fibrin polymers become cross-linked by factor XIIIa and simultaneously bind plasma plasminogen and tissue plasminogen activator (tPA). Over several hours, bound tPA activates nearby plasminogen to form plasmin. The bound plasmin cleaves fibrin and yields the fibrin degradation products (FDP) D, E, X, and Y and D-dimer. The FDPs represent fibrinogen domains; D-dimers are covalently linked fibrin D domains reflecting the cross-linking effect of factor XIIIa and thrombosis.

Assays for FDPs and D-dimer detect active fibrinolysis. There are numerous plasma D-dimer immunoassays. Sensitivity varies depending on the avidity of the monoclonal anti-D-dimer and the detection method.

The quantitative D-dimer assay is used to rule-out ischemic stroke, acute myocardial infarction, or venous thromboembolic disease in patients with low pretest probability, and is required for detecting and monitoring DIC. D-dimer assays have negative predictive values of 90–95 %. Chronic or acute inflammation is accompanied by elevated D-dimer concentrations.

Plasminogen

Plasminogen is the precursor to plasmin, the active enzyme of the fibrinolytic system. Excessive increase in circulating plasmin has the potential to cause hemorrhage. On the other hand, a deficiency of plasminogen activity (although rare) can cause thrombosis. Plasminogen rises in inflammation and during pregnancy.

Chromogenic assays are available to determine plasma plasminogen levels.

Tissue Plasminogen Activator and Plasminogen Activator Inhibitor-1

The two physiologic plasminogen activators are tPA and urokinase. tPA is the primary mediator of fibrinolysis. PAI-1, secreted from endothelial cells, covalently binds to and inactivates both activators.

tPA activity exhibits diurnal variation and rises upon exercise. Special blood specimen collection and handling is required because tPA is unstable and it rapidly binds PAI-1. Plasma concentration of tPA can be determined by enzyme immunoassay and activity is measured by a chromogenic assay; kits are for research use only.

Elevated PAI-1 is associated with venous thrombosis and may be a cardiovascular risk factor. A few cases of PAI-1 deficiency have been reported; however, hemorrhage apparently occurs only in the complete absence of PAI-1. Special blood specimen collection and handling is required. Several immunoassays and chromogenic substrate methods are available for PAI-1, which are for research use only.

Thrombin Activatable Fibrinolytic Inhibitor

Activated TAFI functions as an antifibrinolytic enzyme by preventing the binding of tPA and plasminogen to fibrin, thus blocking the formation of plasmin. Thrombin is required for activation of TAFI. Decreased levels of TAFIa result in increased fibrinolysis and bleeding. Conversely, increased levels of TAFIa result in decreased fibrinolysis and thrombosis. Assays for TAFIa are available for research use only at this time.

Table 2.5 Assays to monitor or assess the efficacy and safety of antiplatelet and antithrombotic drugs

Drug	Assay for monitoring or simple assessment
Antiplatelet drugs	
Aspirin	Platelet aggregation, Verify Now
$P2Y_{12}$ receptor inhibitors	Platelet aggregation, Verify Now
GP IIb/IIIa receptor inhibitors	Platelet aggregation, Verify Now
Heparins	
Unfractionated heparin	PTT, anti-FXa; ACT for high doses
LMW heparins	Anti-FXa
Fondaparinux	Anti-FXa
Thrombin inhibitors (intravenous)	
Argatroban	PTT; ACT for high doses
Bivalirudin	PTT; ACT for high doses
Warfarin	
Coumadin, others	PT/INR; chromogenic FX if lupus anticoagulant present
New oral anticoagulants	
Dabigatran	TCT, PTT; diluted TCT with calibrators is preferred
Rivaroxaban	PT; anti-FXa with calibrators is preferred
Apixaban	Anti-FXa with calibrators
Edoxaban	Anti-FXa with calibrators
Thrombolytic therapy	
Reteplase, alteplase, tenecteplase	Fibrinogen levels

Antithrombotic Drug Monitoring

Table 2.5 summarizes the assays available for assessing the activity of antiplatelet and anticoagulant drugs.

Antiplatelet Drugs

Antiplatelet drugs such as the nonsteroidal anti-inflammatory drugs (NSAIDs) aspirin, ibuprofen, indomethacin, and sulfinpyrazone permanently inactivate or temporarily inhibit cyclooxygenase. The thienopyridine antiplatelet drugs clopidogrel and prasugrel, and the nucleoside ticagrelor irreversibly occupy the ADP receptor $P2Y_{12}$. **Platelet aggregometry** can be employed to monitor response to these drugs. The NSAIDs limit or eliminate the aggregation and secretion responses to arachidonic acid and collagen. Thienopyridines suppress aggregation and secretion responses to ADP.

The Accumetrics **VerifyNow System** (San Diego, CA) measures platelet activity by agglutination of fibrinogen-coated microbeads. Response to aspirin therapy is determined using arachidonic acid as the test reagent; response to $P2Y_{12}$ inhibitor treatment is determined using ADP as the test reagent; and response to GP IIb/IIIa inhibitor treatment (abciximab, tirofiban, eptifibatide) is determined using TRAP as the test reagent.

Heparins

The **PTT** has long been the standard method for monitoring heparin therapy. It is important that platelets in the blood specimen are not activated since released PF4 will inactivate heparin. A heparin therapeutic range is established by the local laboratory. The newer **chromogenic anti-factor Xa assay** determines the inhibition of activated factor X (Xa) by heparin bound to AT. Since it is not affected by variables that affect clot-based tests such as high factor VIII and fibrinogen, lupus anticoagulant or any coagulation factor deficiency/inhibitor, the anti-factor Xa assay provides a more reliable determination of heparin levels and has become the recommended method over the PTT.

LMW heparins (enoxaparin, dalteparin, tinzaparin) selectively catalyze the neutralization of factor Xa more so than the neutralization of thrombin, and fondaparinux only inhibits factor Xa. The effect of these drugs cannot be measured by the PTT, but the chromogenic anti-factor Xa heparin assay can be used.

Appropriate sample handling is critical for accurate results of heparin levels. In particular, in mishandled specimens platelets release PF4 (a heparin-neutralizing protein), which falsely decreases the heparin level.

The activated clotting time (ACT) utilizes a particulate clot activator such as celite or kaolin in a prefilled test tube to which patient whole blood is added. The ACT is widely used as a point-of-care assay to monitor high dosage heparin as used in percutaneous intervention (cardiac catheterization) and coronary artery bypass graft surgery.

Argatroban and Bivalirudin

These thrombin inhibitors used for patients with heparin-induced thrombocytopenia can be monitored with the same PTT assay as used for monitoring heparin. The target therapeutic range is 1.5–3.0 fold higher than the laboratory normal, but not more than 90 s. The ACT is employed during cardiac catheterization or cardiac surgery; drug dosing and ACT assessment protocols from the manufacturers should be followed.

Warfarin

The PT with international normalized ratio (INR) calculation effectively monitors warfarin therapy because it is sensitive to reductions of factors II, VII, and X. The PT begins to prolong within 6–8 h of treatment due to decreasing factor VII activity levels; however, anticoagulation becomes therapeutic only when the activities of factors II and X decrease to less than 50 % of normal, in approximately 5 days. The activity of the anticoagulant protein C also reduces during the initial phase of warfarin treatment so the patient actually incurs the risk of thrombosis (not detected by the PT assay). For this reason, warfarin is covered by heparin therapy for at least 5 days and the patient is monitored by both PT/INR and PTT.

The INR is used to compensate for the inherent variations among thromboplastin reagents and allows all laboratories to report nearly the same results for patients who have reached a stable response to warfarin therapy. During the first week of warfarin therapy, however, the PT results in seconds should be used to monitor therapy. The INR is *only* validated for stable phase warfarin monitoring and should not be used when evaluating a patient for coagulopathies.

The chromogenic factor X assay (not to be confused with the chromogenic anti-factor Xa heparin assay) can be useful when the PT is compromised by lupus anticoagulant, a factor inhibitor, or a coagulation factor deficiency. The warfarin therapeutic range is typically close to 20–40 % of normal factor X activity.

The intravenously administered thrombin inhibitors argatroban and bivalirudin prolong the PT/INR. In switching to warfarin therapy, the combination of a thrombin inhibitor and warfarin can nearly double the PT. The chromogenic factor X assay is one means for monitoring warfarin dosage during the cross-over period if the thrombin inhibitor anticoagulant effect is excessively high.

New Oral Anticoagulants

Four new oral anticoagulants have been FDA approved. These include dabigatran (thrombin inhibitor), rivaroxaban, apixaban, and edoxaban (factor Xa inhibitors). At the time of their release, no laboratory assay was recommended to assess drug levels. Clinical practice, however, has clarified the importance for drug assessment in certain clinical settings. FDA approved assays and associated therapeutic ranges for each drug are not yet definitive.

The thrombin clotting time is very sensitive to **dabigatran**. A normal TCT indicates no dabigatran is present; a prolonged TCT indicates that dabigatran is present but does not indicate the plasma concentration. The PTT response to dabigatran is unreliable and there is considerable variability in sensitivity to dabigatran among PTT reagents. A modification of the TCT, the plasma-diluted TCT (Hemoclot Direct Thrombin Inhibitor Assay, Aniara Hyphen, West Chester, OH), provides a quantitative measure of dabigatran when used with calibrators but is currently restricted to research use only.

Rivaroxaban slightly prolongs the PT, but to a lesser extent than warfarin and this effect is highly reagent dependent. **Apixaban and edoxaban** have no effect on the PT or PTT. The new factor Xa inhibitor drugs are better assessed using the chromogenic anti-factor Xa assay modified with specific calibrators for rivaroxaban, apixaban, or edoxaban. The use of the anti-factor Xa assay for this purpose is currently restricted to research use only.

Thrombolytic Therapy

Thrombolytic therapy, which employs recombinant forms of tPA (reteplase, alteplase, tenecteplase), raises the risk of hemorrhage, particularly intracranial hemorrhage. Treatment is typically not measured by laboratory tests; however, fibrinogen levels can be used to assure effective hemostatic levels are present.

Conclusion

This chapter describes all the commonly used and the newly developed hemostasis tests available for the clinical laboratory. There are other known analytes of the hemostatic system and biomarkers of activation but laboratory tests are not FDA approved for clinical use. As research continues into the mechanisms of hemostasis and thrombosis, and clinical trials prove the validity of the clinical assessment of the newly identified analytes, improved clinical laboratory testing will be developed.

References

1. Fritsma MG, Fritsma GA. Normal hemostasis and coagulation, Chapter 37. In: Keohane EM, Smith LJ, Walenga JM, editors. Rodak's hematology. Clinical principles and applications. 5th ed. St. Louis, MO: Elsevier; 2016.
2. Fristma GA. Hemorrhagic disorders and laboratory assessment, Chapter 38. In: Keohane EM, Smith LJ, Walenga JM, editors. Rodak's hematology: clinical principles and applications. 5th ed. St. Louis, MO: Elsevier; 2016.

3. Fristma GA. Thrombotic disorders and laboratory assessment. Chapter 39. In: Keohane EM, Smith LJ, Walenga JM, editors. Rodak's hematology: clinical principles and applications. 5th ed. St. Louis, MO: Elsevier; 2016.
4. Fristma GA. Laboratory evaluation of hemostasis, Chapter 42. In: Keohane EM, Smith LJ, Walenga JM, editors. Rodak's hematology: clinical principles and applications. 5th ed. St. Louis, MO: Elsevier; 2016.
5. Kitchens CS, Konkle BA, Kessler CM, editors. Consultative hemostasis and thrombosis. Philadelphia, PA: Elsevier; 2013.
6. Rodgers GM. Testing for inherited and acquired thrombotic disorders, Chapter 9. In: Bennett ST, Lehman CM, Rodgers GM, editors. Laboratory hemostasis. A practical guide for pathologists. New York, NY: Springer Science+Business Media; 2007. p. 143–66.
7. practical-hemostasis.com. Accessed 4 Mar 2015.
8. labtestsonline.org. Accessed 4 Mar 2015.
9. www.esoterix.com (Dorothy Adcock, MD). Accessed 4 Mar 2015.
10. clevelandcliniclabs.com (Kandice Kottke-Marchant, MD, PhD). Accessed 4 Mar 2015.
11. mghlabtest.partners.org (Elizabeth M. Van Cott, MD and Michael Laposata, MD, PhD). Accessed 4 Mar 2015.

Current Anticoagulation Drugs and Mechanisms of Action

3

Tarik F. Ibrahim, Sean Maxwell, and Omer Iqbal

Introduction

The era of advanced medical treatment has resulted in an increasingly elderly population that is faced with multiple, complex disease processes. Many neurosurgical patients are therefore on anticoagulation at the time of both elective and emergent presentation. It is an issue with which all neurosurgical practitioners should be well versed as anticoagulants are increasingly being used in the patient population seen both in the clinic and the emergency department. These medications can make an already dangerous neurologic condition such as intracranial hemorrhage (ICH) even more precarious.

While vitamin K antagonists like warfarin have been used for many years, its use is limited by genetic polymorphisms, drug–drug interactions, and food–drug interactions [1, 2]. It is because of these lifestyle and pharmacologic limitations that target specific oral anticoagulants (TSOACs) were developed.

It is important to know the mechanisms of action, pharmacology, and methods of reversal of VKAs, heparin and low-molecular weight heparin (LMWH), and TSOACs such as direct thrombin inhibitors (DTIs) and factor X inhibitors (FTIs) (Fig. 3.1).

T.F. Ibrahim, M.D. (✉)
Department of Neurosurgery, Loyola University Medical Center,
2160 S. First Avenue, Bldg 105, Room 1900,
Maywood, IL 60153, USA
e-mail: Tarik.ibrahim@gmail.com;
tibrahim@lumc.edu

S. Maxwell, B.S., M.A.
Department of Neurosurgery, Loyola University Stritch School of Medicine,
2160 South First Avenue, Bldg 105 Room 1900,
Maywood, IL 60153, USA
e-mail: smaxwell@luc.edu

O. Iqbal, M.D., F.A.C.C., F.E.S.C.
Department of Pathology & Ophthalmology,
Loyola University Health System,
2160 S. First Avenue, Building 102, Room 2646,
Maywood, IL 60153, USA
e-mail: oiqbal@luc.edu

Vitamin K Antagonists

Drugs: Warfarin (Coumadin, Jantoven), Acenocoumarol (Sintrom), Phenprocoumon (Marcoumar), Fluindione (Previscan)

Mechanism of Action

The most commonly used VKA is warfarin (Figs. 3.2 and 3.3). These drugs exert their effect by antagonizing vitamin K in the synthesis of clotting factors II, VII, IX, X as well as the regulatory factors protein C, protein S, and protein Z [3]. These members of the clotting cascade require

C.M. Loftus (ed.), *Anticoagulation and Hemostasis in Neurosurgery*,
DOI 10.1007/978-3-319-27327-3_3

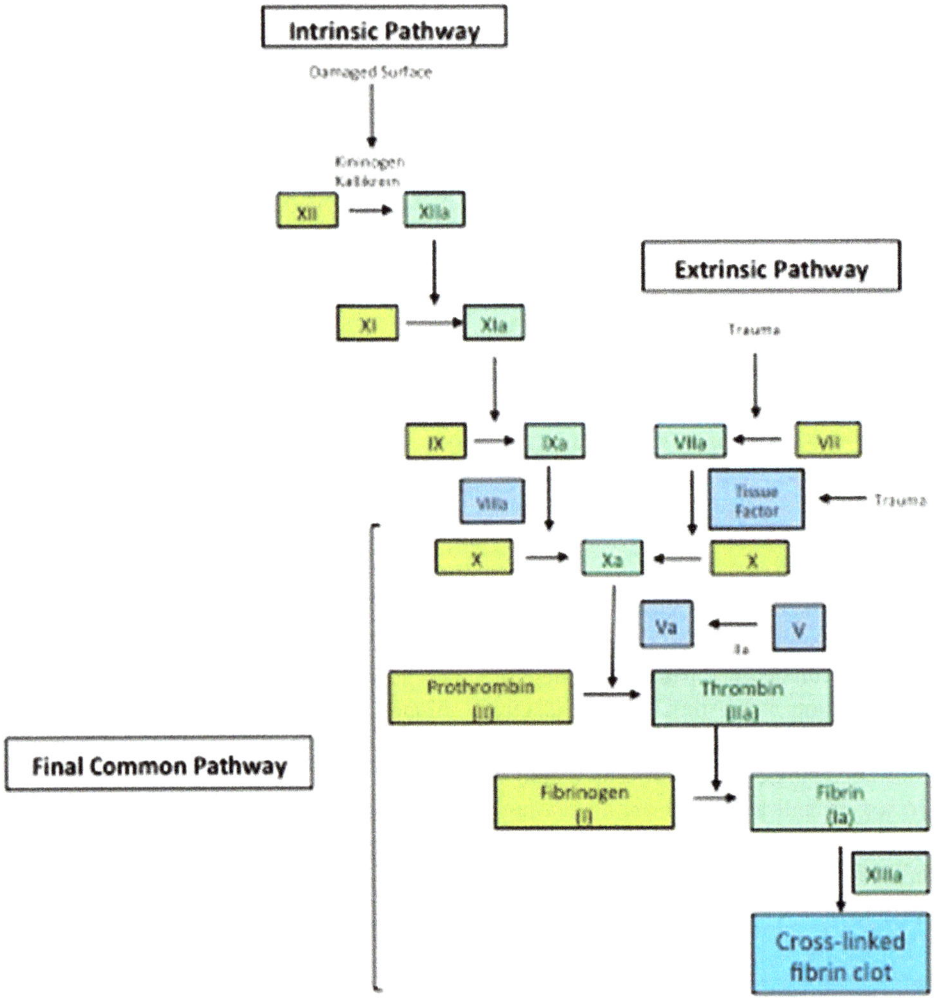

Fig. 3.1 Coagulation cascade. The physiologic clotting cascade consists of the intrinsic and extrinsic pathways that eventually converge on the common pathway of blood coagulation

carboxylation of their glutamic acid residues to bind to the phospholipid surface of the vascular endothelium. The enzyme that carries out the carboxylation, gamma-glutamyl carboxylase (GGC), can only function if it can concurrently convert vitamin K hydroquinone to vitamin K epoxide. The vitamin K epoxide is in turn recycled back to vitamin K and vitamin K hydroquinone by vitamin K epoxide reductase (VKOR) and vitamin k Reductase (VKR) respectively [4]. Warfarin is a racemic mixture of S and R enantiomers; the former inhibits VKOR thereby much more significantly than the latter inhibits VKR. This diminishes the availability of vitamin K to be used by GGC and effectively halting the synthesis of biologically active molecules.

The blood-thinning effect of VKAs takes days to realize; however, due to the long half-lives of already circulating clotting factors, patients may in fact become slightly hypercoagulable during that time as proteins C and S become depleted first [5]. As such, it is common practice to use either intravenous (IV) heparin or low molecular weight heparin (LMWH) as bridge therapy until the patient is therapeutic on their Coumadin.

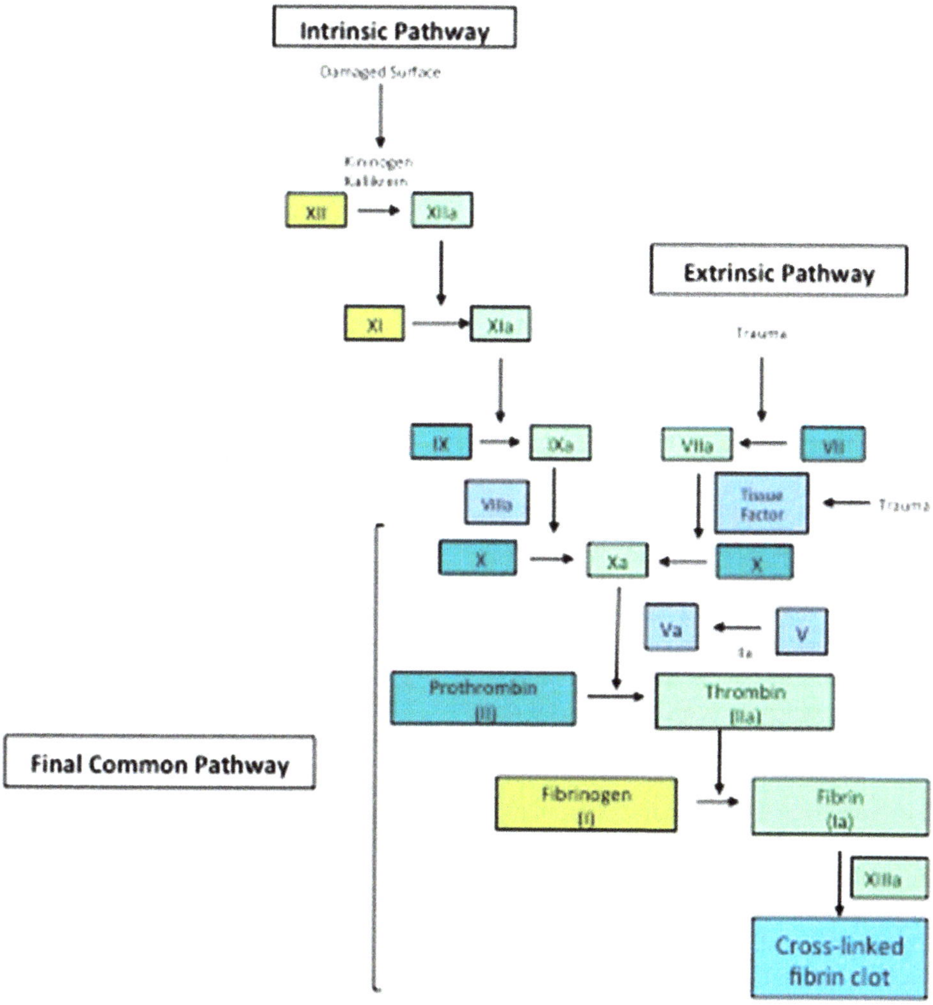

Fig. 3.2 Warfarin effect. Clotting factors II, VII, IX, and X are all affected by ingestion of warfarin. By inhibiting the liver's ability to carboxylate the inactive proteins, there are fewer active proteins available for coagulation

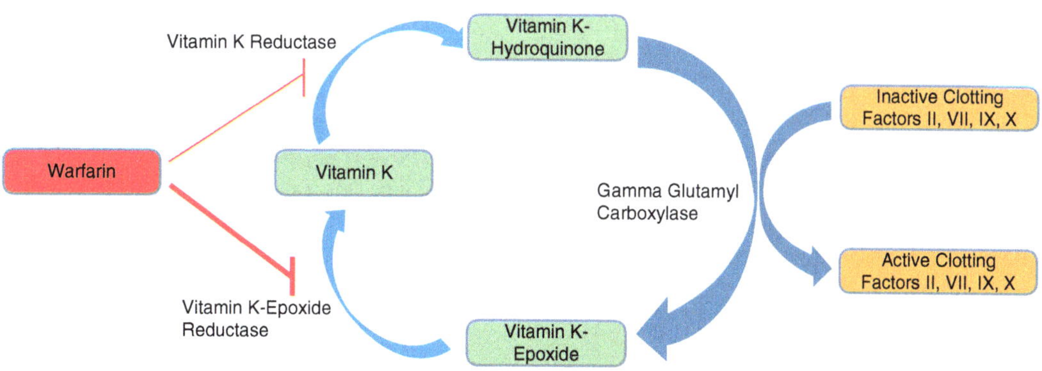

Fig. 3.3 Warfarin mechanism of action. Warfarin inhibits VKOR and VKR (the former much more significantly than the latter). This decreases the amount of reduced vitamin K (Vitamin K hydroquinone) available to be simultaneously recycled by GGC in the carboxylation process of clotting factors II, VII, IX, and X

Pharmacology and Surveillance

- Half-life: 1–2 days for warfarin [6]
- Metabolism: CYP2C9 is the most important liver enzyme in metabolizing warfarin [7, 8]. There is significant inter-patient variability that is partly responsible for the difficulty in achieving the desired steady-state at times.
- Clearance: Renal
- Monitoring: Prothrombin time (PT) and the international normalized ratio (INR)

Adverse Effects

It is estimated that more than 65,000 patients are treated in US Emergency Departments every year with a warfarin-associated hemorrhage [9]. The most notable complication is spontaneous ICH that occurs secondary to hypoprothrombinemia. Other side-effects include ecchymosis, purpura, and hematuria. Patients can also experience skin necrosis secondary to the depletion of protein C and S mentioned earlier; this leads to thrombosis of vessels supplying the skin in the extremities.

Long-term users of VKAs have an annual major hemorrhage rate of 1.5–5.2 % [10] according to a recent meta-analysis with an annual incidence of all major bleeding events estimated at 3.36 % [11]. Mortality from all major hemorrhagic events while on VKAs is 13 % [12]; ICH accounts for 8.7 % of these events [10]. When patients present with ICH while on VKAs, the mortality rate is estimated to reach 46–55 % [13, 14] with significant long-term disability in those that do survive [15, 16].

Reversal

There are several methods to reverse warfarin; some take time for their effects while others are much more rapid. These are detailed below in the order of increasing rate of reversal.

1. Vitamin K
   (a) Promotes synthesis of factors II, VII, IX, and X. Reversal takes time as clotting ability is dependent on synthesis of enzymes by the liver. This is often given in conjunction with other reversal agents listed below to prevent a rebound of anticoagulation.
   (b) *Route*: Oral or IV administration (the latter is more effective)
   (c) *Time to maximum effect*: New synthesis begins in 1–3 h and maximum effect is reached after 24–36 h.
   (d) *Half-life*: Effect lasts until INR within therapeutic range again
   (e) *Benefits*: Relatively safe
   (f) *Risks*: Reversal is slow hence utility in emergent situations is very limited
2. Fresh frozen plasma (FFP)
   (a) Contains factors II, VII, IX, and X as well as fibrinogen, von Willebrand factor, and antithrombin
   (b) *Route*: IV administration
   (c) *Time to maximum effect*: Requires thawing and full reversal is variable; one study evaluating time to full INR reversal in PCC and FFP found the latter was 11.8 h [17].
   (d) *Half-life*: 1.5–2 days [6]
   (e) *Benefits*: If the patient is hypovolemic, FFP can augment the intravascular compartment.
   (f) *Risks*: Infection/transfusion related acute lung injury (TRALI) [18], volume overload, time consuming
3. Prothrombin complex concentrate (PCC)
   (a) Contains activated factors II, VII, IX, X and protein C and S in a concentration approximately 25 times that of FFP
   (b) *Route*: IV administration
   (c) *Time to maximum effect*: The same study as above revealed full reversal with PCC in 5.7 h. This is partly due to the fact that PCC does not require thawing and has a higher concentration of factors [17, 19, 20].
   (d) *Half-life*: 6–8 h [6]
   (e) *Benefits*: Rapid and more efficient reversal [6], limited volume, virus inactivated
   (f) *Risks*: Thromboembolic risk may be overestimated in small case series but there is a risk. It is possibly related to preparations

of PCC with higher concentrations of factors and those that include procoagulants (factors C and S) [19].

4. Recombinant Factor VIIa
   (a) Contains factor VIIa
   (b) *Route*: IV administration
   (c) *Time to maximum effect*: Less than 10 min
   (d) *Half-life*: Less than 60 min
   (e) *Benefits*: Rapid reversal
   (f) *Risks*: Thromboembolic complications [21]

Heparin and LMWH

Drugs: Unfractionated heparin (UFH). LMWHs: Dalteparin (Fragmin), Tinzaparin (Innohep), Enoxaparin (Lovenox), Ardeparin (Normiflo), Danaparoid (Orgaran), Nadroparin (Fraxiparine), Certoparin (Embolex) (Fig. 3.4)

Mechanism of Action

Antithrombin (AT, previously known as antithrombin III), is a serine-protease inhibitor that regulates many of the enzymes activated during coagulation, particularly Xa and IIa (thrombin) [22, 23]. AT preferentially targets free enzymes over those that are part of prothrombinase complex. AT's role is to limit the coagulation cascade to areas of vascular injury and thus protect the remainder of the circulation from undesired thrombotic events [22]. AT is an inefficient inhibitor but UFH and LMWH significantly potentiate its effect by binding and inducing a conformational change in the shape of the AT molecule that increases by over a 100-fold the rate at which each proteinase can be inhibited [24]. UFH binding to AT causes a decrease in Xa and IIa activity in a 1:1 ratio [23]. LMWH ulti-

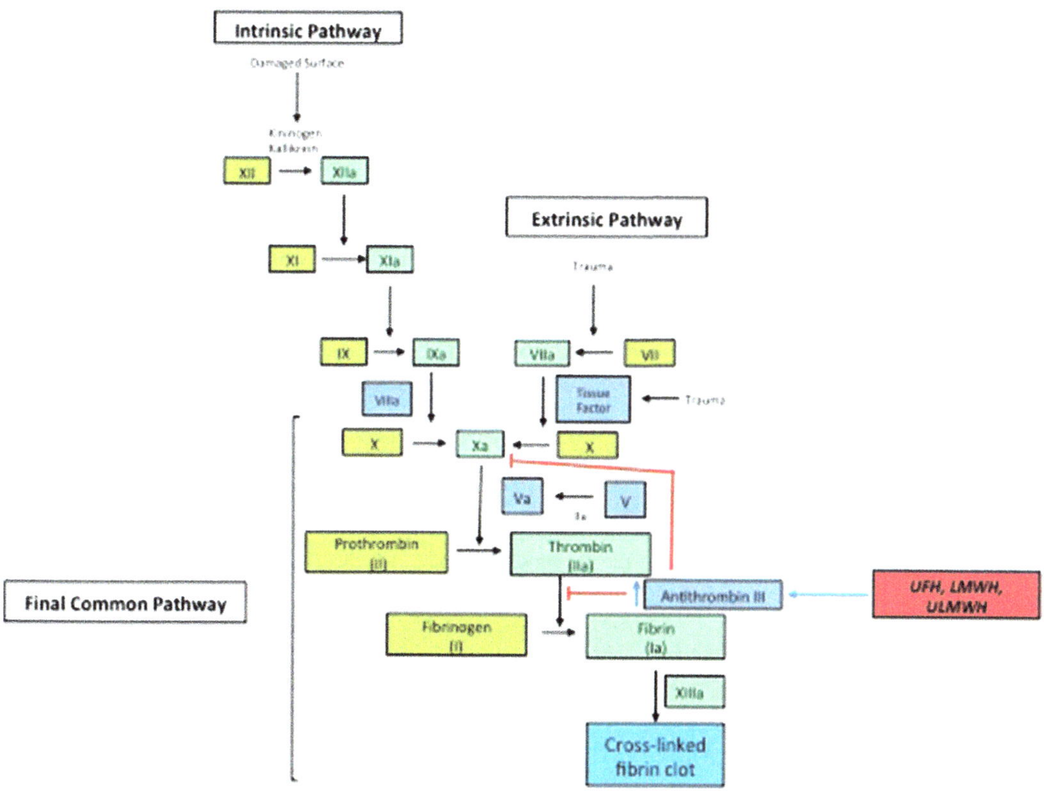

Fig. 3.4 Heparin and LMWH effect. AT is a natural, but inefficient inhibitor of factors Xa and IIa. Heparin and LMWH both increase the ability of AT to bind and inactivate these proteins. Heparin causes AT to affect Xa and IIa in an even fashion ratio while LMWH ultimately has a more significant impact on Xa

mately has the same effect as UFH but affects Xa and IIa in a 3:1 or 2:1 ratio [23, 25].

UFH is a heterogeneous anticoagulant composed of heparin molecules with different lengths—all of which have at least 18 saccharide units [26]. Larger saccharide chains are cleared more quickly than smaller ones making heparin molecules with smaller chains more bioavailable [27]. Due to its multiple amino acid chains, not all of which are involved in anticoagulation, UFH also binds other plasma proteins and cells thus further complicating attempts to predict the anticoagulant response. The anticoagulant effect is nonlinear and increases disproportionately as the dose increases [27]. This variability is one of the reasons that UFH requires monitoring and dose adjustment based on the activated partial thromboplastin time (aPTT).

LMWH is derived from UFH to produce molecules that are one-third the molecular weight of UFH [27]. LMWHs and their smaller chains do not bind other plasma proteins as significantly as UFH thus making their pharmacokinetics much more predictable and thereby eliminating the need for routine monitoring in most situations [27]. The decreased binding of non-AT molecules also confers less risk of heparin-induced thrombocytopenia (HIT) and less bone loss. It is also associated with an increased ratio of Xa to IIa inhibition (see Table 3.1) that confers upon LMWH the ability to inhibit thrombosis without producing significant anticoagulant activity [27–29]. This has been correlated with lower levels of bleeding [30].

Ultra-LMWH (ULMWH) a newer class of drugs structurally similar, but smaller version of LMWHs that is currently in development. They are sparsely used compared to LMWH and none are approved for use within the USA. The hope for ULMWHs is that because they have an even larger Xa to IIa inhibitory ratio that they will be associated with lower risk of bleeding and HIT.

Pharmacology and Surveillance

See Table 3.1 for details.

Adverse Effects

UFH is responsible for non-hemorrhagic side-effects as well as significant bleeding complications. HIT and osteoporosis are the main non-hemorrhagic side effects. HIT occurs when platelet-activating IgG antibodies bind to the epitope platelet factor 4 (PF4) while it is bound to heparin. The PF4-heparin complex normally occurs as a manner of heparin inactivation but clearly does not always lead to HIT. This causes activation of platelets that leads to arterial or venous thrombosis (venous is more common [31]) as well as thrombocytopenia. HIT is defined as a platelet count $<150 \times 10^9$/L and occurs in 85–90 % of HIT patients [32]. Some clinicians also use a broader definition in which the platelet count falls 30–50 %; this is seen in 90–95 % of HIT cases [32]. HIT type I

Table 3.1 Heparins pharmacology and surveillance

Agent (class)	Anti-Xa to anti-IIa ratio	Elimination half-life (h)	Time to peak activity	Laboratory monitoring
Heparin (UFH)	1.1:1	0.5–2.5; dose-dependent	Varies with dose and route	aPTT
Enoxaparin (LMWH)	2.8:1	4.5	~3–5 h	None
Dalteparin (LMWH)	2.3:1	2.0–2.3	~3–5 h	None
Tinzaparin (LMWH)	2.8:1	3.4	~3–5 h	None
Nadroparin (LMWH)	3.5:1	3.5	~3–5 h	None
Certoparin (LMWH)	2.0–2.2:1	4.6–4.7	~3–5 h	None
Semuloparin (ULMWH)	80:1	16–20	~1–2 h	None
Bemiparin (ULMWH)	8:1	5.3	~2–3 h	None

The different drugs and their pharmacology are depicted here [26, 27]. Heparin has a 1:1 ratio of Xa to IIa inhibition while LMWH inhibits Xa more strongly than IIa

(HIT1) is mild and occurs in the first 4 days of heparin administration [33]. The platelet count is often between 100 and 150×10^9/L. HIT1 is not associated with bleeding or thrombosis [33]. It is often difficult to distinguish HIT1 from postoperative hemodilution in patients who recently had surgery. The typical onset for HIT type II (HIT2) is 5–10 days after initiation of heparin [34]. "Rapid-onset HIT" can occur in patients who have circulating HIT antibodies due to exposure to heparin usually within the last month although exposure could be as long as 100 days prior [32]. HIT2 is more pronounced with a median nadir of 60×10^9/L [33]. HIT2 is associated with potential bleeding and thrombosis. Osteoporosis occurs secondary to heparin binding to osteoblasts that then release factors to activate osteoclasts [32].

HIT occurs three times less with LMWH as compared to UFH [35]. While LMWH can form complexes with PF4, the interaction is chain length-dependent and thus occurs with much less frequency. There is still a risk for osteoporosis/osteopenia with LMWHs although it is not as significant as with UFH due to a lesser affinity for osteoblast/osteoclast activation [27].

Reversal

If there is excessive anticoagulant action of heparin, initial treatment is immediate discontinuation of the drug. If bleeding is present, administration of protamine sulfate can neutralize heparin [36]. Administration of 1 mg Protamine Sulfate per 100 units UFH will neutralize the anticoagulant effect. This same effect does not hold true with LMWH. Administration of protamine sulfate is only partially effective at reversing LMWH. For example, 1 mg protamine sulfate may be used to partially reverse 1 mg of enoxaparin [36, 37].

Direct Thrombin Inhibitors

Drugs: Bivalirudin (Angiomax), Argatroban (Acova), Dabigatran (Pradaxa), Desirudin (Iprivask), Lepirudin (Refludan), Hirudin (Thrombexx), Melagatran (Ximelagatran) (Fig. 3.5)

Mechanism of Action

As opposed to UFH and LMWH that indirectly antagonize thrombin by catalyzing AT, DTIs directly bind to thrombin and block its enzymatic activity. Thrombin is essential to the clotting process as it serves several roles. Thrombin converts fibrinogen to fibrin, activates clotting factors V, VIII, and IX, thus generating more thrombin and stimulates platelets. Thrombin is also responsible for activation of factor XIII that cross-links fibrin bonds and stabilizes clots (Fig. 3.6).

Thrombin possesses one active (catalytic) site and two exosites. DTIs can bind to any of these domains to block thrombin action. Univalent DTIs (Argatroban, Melagatran, Dabigatran) only bind the thrombin active site whereas bivalent DTIs (Hirudin, Bivalirudin, Lepirudin, Desirudin) bind exosite 1 and the active site. Heparin binds exosite 2.

One advantage of this direct thrombin antagonism over UFH and LMWH is that DTIs can inhibit thrombin already bound to fibrin or fibrin degradation products to prevent further fibrin deposition and cross-linking [38–40]. The AT-UFH/LMWH complex is not able to bind thrombin that is already bound to fibrin, which can be problematic as bound thrombin continues to have enzymatic activity that causes thrombus growth. Other advantages of thrombin over UFH are its lack of binding to other plasma proteins and the fact that it is not inactivated by PF4. This results in a more predictable response than UFH and likely LMWH [41]. Additionally, by directly inhibiting thrombin, DTIs slow the positive feedback loop that activates more thrombin and also prevents platelet activation.

Pharmacology and Surveillance

The difficulty in monitoring TSOACs is one of their drawbacks. PT/INR are not affected by DTIs. There is a nonlinear relationship between the DTI dose and rise of aPTT. This means that aPTT can confirm that a patient is indeed anticoagulated but cannot assess how coagulopathic the patient is [42]. Thrombin time (TT) and ecarin

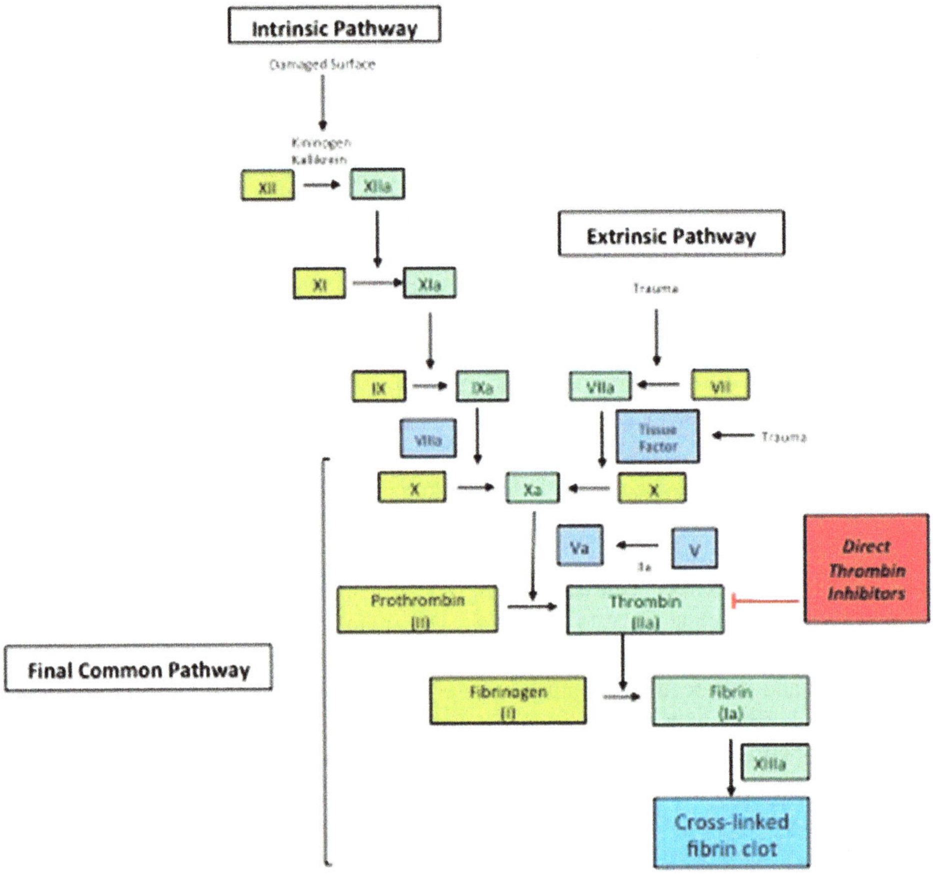

Fig. 3.5 Direct thrombin inhibitor effect. Both soluble and bound thrombins are inactivated by DTIs. These drugs directly bind to thrombin without AT and block its subsequent effects

clotting time (ECT) are more quantitative for DTI activity but the former is oversensitive and the latter is not often available in many hospitals in the USA [42]. See Table 3.2 for further details.

Adverse Effects

As with other forms of anticoagulation, major bleeding is the most serious side-effect of DTIs. The RE-LY study [11] evaluated over 18,000 patients to assess the effects of Dabigatran compared to warfarin in patients with atrial fibrillation (AF) with the authors assessing stroke, systemic embolism, and hemorrhage rates at an average follow-up of 2 years. The rate of ICH was statistically less in the Dabigatran group (0.23 % and 0.3 % per year for the 110 mg and 150 mg groups, respectively) compared to warfarin.

Reversal

There is no specific reversal agent for DTIs and evidence-based recommendations for other methods are lacking. Discontinuation of the drug is the first step and patients who have taken a DTI dose in the 1–2 h prior to presentation can also be given oral activated charcoal to remove the drug. PCC may attenuate bleeding, but this is based on low quality evidence and can be

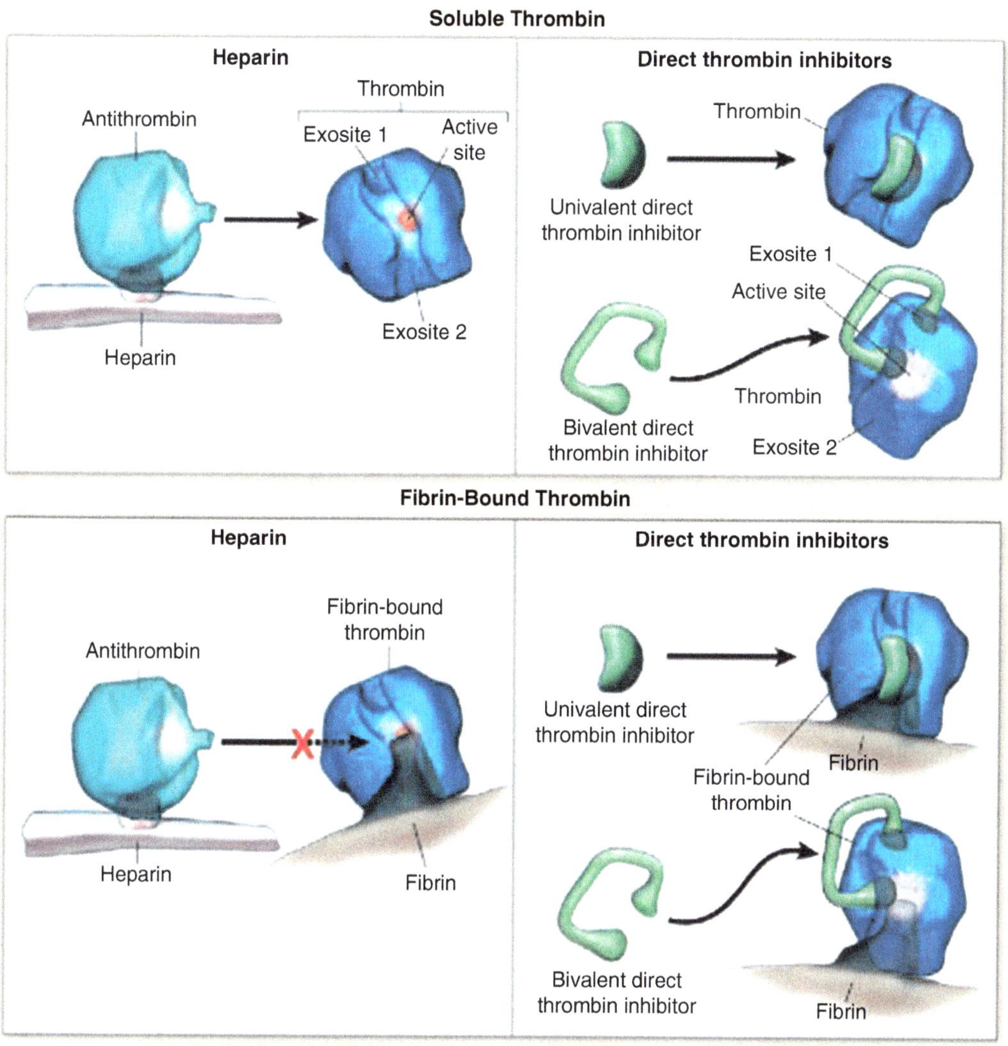

Fig. 3.6 Direct thrombin inhibitor mechanism of action. Used with permission from NEJM

Table 3.2 Direct thrombin inhibitors pharmacology and surveillance [36, 37, 41]

Drug	Half-life (h)	Time to peak activity (h)	Clearance (primary)	Laboratory monitoring
Dabigatran	Oral: 12	1–2	Renal	TT or ECT
Ximelagatran/Melagatran	IV/SQ: 2–3 Oral: 3–5	2–3	Renal	TT or ECT
Recombinant Hirudins (desirudin, lepirudin)	IV: 1 SQ: 2	4–5	Renal	TT or ECT
Bivalirudin	IV: 0.25	Immediate	Renal, hepatic	TT or ECT
Argatroban	IV: 0.75	1–3	Hepatic	TT or ECT

associated with thrombotic complications [43–47]. If PCC is used, aPTT, ECT, and TT are not necessarily expected to normalize [48]. In emergent situations, dialysis can be used to remove DTIs [49]. Other agents that have been considered are antifibrinolytic agents (tranexamic acid, ε-aminocaproic acid). Patients who have taken a DTI dose in the 1–2 h prior to presentation can also be given oral activated charcoal to remove the drug.

Factor Xa Inhibitors

Drugs: *Indirect*—Fondaparinux (Arixtra) (Fig. 3.7)

Direct—Rivaroxaban (Xarelto), Apixaban (Eliquis), Edoxaban (Savaysa)

Mechanism of Action

Factor Xa inhibitors are another class of TSOACs that affect the common coagulation pathway. Whereas DTIs bind and inhibit thrombin, all FTIs except for Fondaparinux directly inhibit factor Xa, the enzyme responsible for activation of thrombin. FTIs competitively bind the active site Xa in its soluble form and while it is contained within a clot [50]. One theorized advantage of targeting factor Xa as opposed to thrombin directly is that it prevents thrombin amplification thereby necessitation smaller doses of FTI [1, 51] (Fig. 3.8).

Fondaparinux is the only FTI that inactivates factor Xa indirectly. It binds AT and causes a conformational change at the active site that increases its reactivity with Xa; once AT and Xa are bound together, Fondaparinux dissociates and can bind other AT molecules [52].

Pharmacology and Surveillance

Similar to DTIs, agents that inhibit factor Xa do not have a designated test to monitor degree of anticoagulation. There is a FTI assay but it is neither readily available at many hospitals nor is it rapid in providing a result. The PT can be used to confirm a patient has been taking Rivaroxaban but not how much. A modified aPTT may provide the same information about apixaban that PT does for rivaroxaban [53]. See Table 3.3 for further details.

Adverse Effects

The ROCKET AF trial [54] randomized patients to rivaroxaban or warfarin and also found significantly less ICH in the former group (0.5 % and 0.7 % per year respectively) [54, 55]. The ARISTOTLE trial [56] compared apixaban and warfarin and found significantly less major bleeding episodes including ICH. Interestingly, a meta-analysis of all RCTs of TSOACs (DTI and FTI) found them to have a lower rate of fatal hemorrhage than VKAs even though no antidote was available in these clinic trials [10].

Reversal

As with DTIs, there is no specific antidote in reversing factor Xa inhibitors nor is there a gold standard in management. Immediate discontinuation of the drug is the first step in management. As with DTIs, activated charcoal can be given if the patient has taken a dose just prior to presentation. Unlike DTIs, FTIs are largely bound to plasma proteins and therefore dialysis is ineffective in removing the anticoagulant [53]. PCC has been found to completely restore normal levels of PTT in healthy patients who were given rivaroxaban, but it has not been evaluated in human subjects taking apixaban.

Conclusion

The topic of whether to use VKAs, LMWH, DTIs, or FTIs is one that is currently being heavily studied in the literature. All anticoagulants possess a risk–benefit profile and some offer advantages over the others in one area while

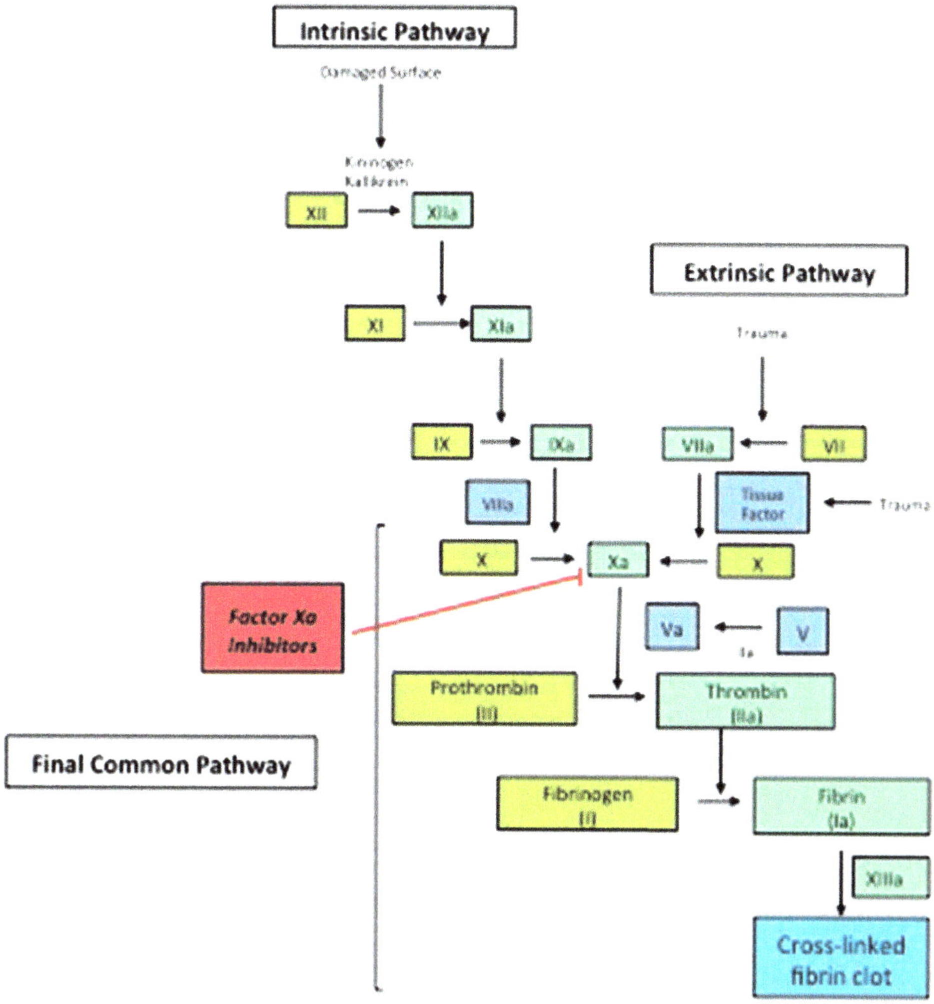

Fig. 3.7 Factor Xa inhibitor effect. Fondaparinux is the only indirect Xa inhibitor that binds and uses AT to actually cause Xa to be nonfunctional. The other drugs directly bind factor Xa

being more problematic in others. As an example, TSOACs such as DTIs and FTIs are more predictable pharmacologically, easier to use and cause less ICH than warfarin in multiple randomized controlled trials (RCT). However, when an ICH occurs, TSOACs do not have an easy method of reversal like warfarin does.

Chai-Adisaksopha et al. found in their meta-analysis that TSOACs were associated with less major bleeding, fatal bleeding, intracranial bleeding, clinically relevant non-major bleeding, and total bleeding when compared to VKAs with an INR target of 2.0–3.0 [10].

In the event of ICH, rapid reversal is often necessary to slow bleeding and facilitate surgery if needed. The neurosurgical team should be familiar with how to reverse different anticoagulants to expedite treatment. In less emergent situations where it is still necessary to reverse or halt anticoagulation, it is often prudent to involve the prescribing service or physician to assess patient risk while off the offending medication. These practitioners' input will also be needed when resuming anticoagulation once it is safe to do so from a neurosurgical perspective (Fig. 3.9).

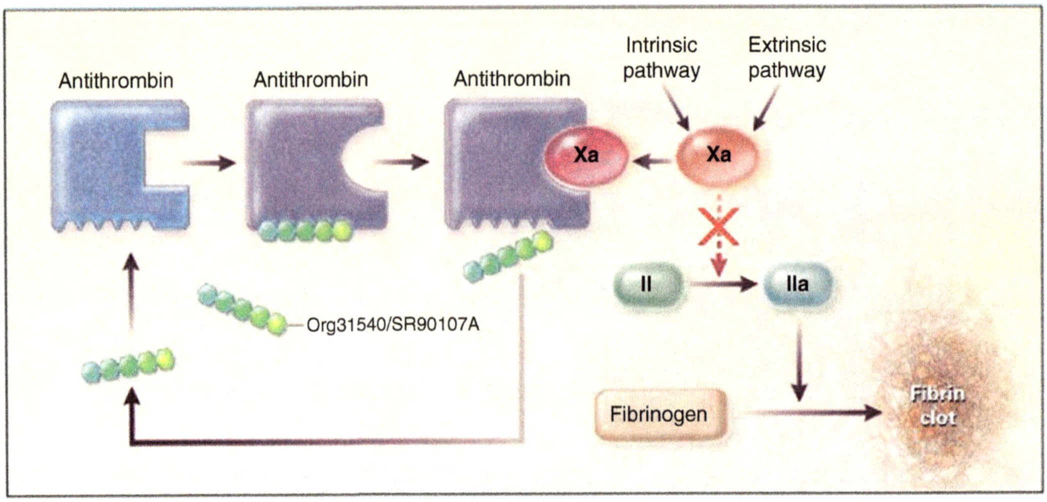

Fig. 3.8 Fondaparinux inhibitor mechanism of action. As the only indirect Factor Xa Inhibitor, Fondaparinux binds AT to inhibit the activation of clotting factor IIa

Table 3.3 Factor Xa inhibitor pharmacology and surveillance [51–53]

Drug	Half-life (h)	Time to peak activity (h)	Clearance (primary)	Laboratory monitoring
Apixaban	12	3–4	Hepatobiliary	Anti-factor Xa
Edoxaban	10–14	1–2	Renal	Anti-factor Xa
Fondaparinux	17–20	2	Renal	Anti-factor Xa
Rivaroxaban	7–11	1–4	Renal	Anti-factor Xa

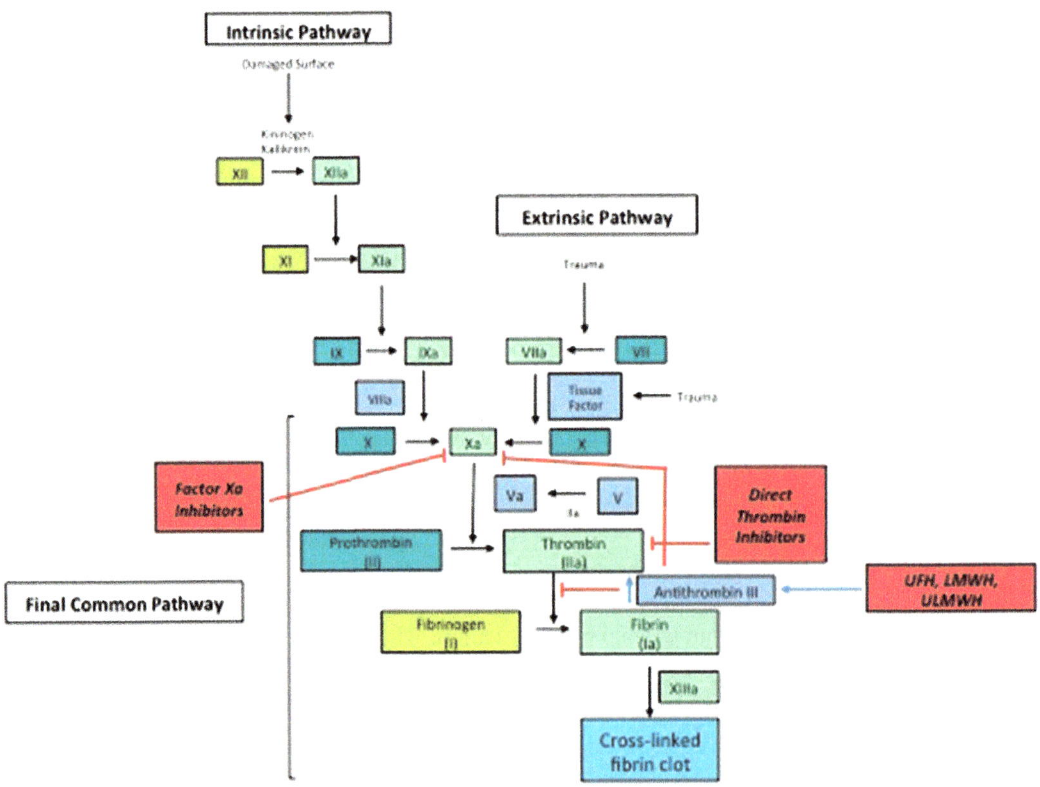

Fig. 3.9 Summary of current anticoagulants. All the different classes and their effect on the clotting cascade are depicted

References

1. Eriksson BI, Borris LC, Friedman RJ, et al. Rivaroxaban versus enoxaparin for thromboprophylaxis after hip arthroplasty. N Engl J Med. 2008;358(26):2765–75.
2. Aguilar MI, Hart RG, Kase CS, et al. Treatment of warfarin-associated intracerebral hemorrhage: literature review and expert opinion. Mayo Clin Proc. 2007;82(1):82–92.
3. Choi Q, Kim JE, Hyun J, Han KS, Kim HK. Contributions of procoagulants and anticoagulants to the international normalized ratio and thrombin generation assay in patients treated with warfarin: potential role of protein Z as a powerful determinant of coagulation assays. Thromb Res. 2013;132(1):e70–5.
4. Li T, Chang CY, Jin DY, Lin PJ, Khvorova A, Stafford DW. Identification of the gene for vitamin K epoxide reductase. Nature. 2004;427(6974):541–4.
5. Guyatt GH, Eikelboom JW, Gould MK, et al. Approach to outcome measurement in the prevention of thrombosis in surgical and medical patients: Antithrombotic therapy and prevention of thrombosis, 9th ed: American College of Chest Physicians Evidence-Based Clinical Practice Guidelines. Chest. 2012;141(2 Suppl):e185S–94.
6. Vang ML, Hvas AM, Ravn HB. Urgent reversal of vitamin K antagonist therapy. Acta Anaesthesiol Scand. 2011;55(5):507–16.
7. Wadelius M, Chen LY, Eriksson N, et al. Association of warfarin dose with genes involved in its action and metabolism. Hum Genet. 2007;121(1):23–34.
8. Takahashi H, Echizen H. Pharmacogenetics of warfarin elimination and its clinical implications. Clin Pharmacokinet. 2001;40(8):587–603.
9. Shehab N, Sperling LS, Kegler SR, Budnitz DS. National estimates of emergency department visits for hemorrhage-related adverse events from clopidogrel plus aspirin and from warfarin. Arch Intern Med. 2010;170(21):1926–33.
10. Chai-Adisaksopha C, Crowther M, Isayama T, Lim W. The impact of bleeding complications in patients receiving target-specific oral anticoagulants: a systematic review and meta-analysis. Blood. 2014; 124(15):2450–8.
11. Connolly SJ, Ezekowitz MD, Yusuf S, et al. Dabigatran versus warfarin in patients with atrial fibrillation. N Engl J Med. 2009;361(12):1139–51.
12. Pisters R, Lane DA, Nieuwlaat R, de Vos CB, Crijns HJ, Lip GY. A novel user-friendly score (HAS-BLED) to assess 1-year risk of major bleeding in patients with atrial fibrillation: the Euro Heart Survey. Chest. 2010;138(5):1093–100.
13. Linkins LA, Choi PT, Douketis JD. Clinical impact of bleeding in patients taking oral anticoagulant therapy for venous thromboembolism: a meta-analysis. Ann Intern Med. 2003;139(11):893–900.
14. Fang MC, Go AS, Chang Y, et al. Death and disability from warfarin-associated intracranial and extracranial hemorrhages. Am J Med. 2007;120(8):700–5.
15. Alonso A, Bengtson LG, MacLehose RF, Lutsey PL, Chen LY, Lakshminarayan K. Intracranial hemorrhage mortality in atrial fibrillation patients treated with dabigatran or warfarin. Stroke. 2014;45(8): 2286–91.
16. Sacco S, Marini C, Toni D, Olivieri L, Carolei A. Incidence and 10-year survival of intracerebral hemorrhage in a population-based registry. Stroke. 2009;40(2):394–9.
17. Hickey M, Gatien M, Taljaard M, Aujnarain A, Giulivi A, Perry JJ. Outcomes of urgent warfarin reversal with frozen plasma versus prothrombin complex concentrate in the emergency department. Circulation. 2013;128(4):360–4.
18. Benson AB, Moss M, Silliman CC. Transfusion-related acute lung injury (TRALI): a clinical review with emphasis on the critically ill. Br J Haematol. 2009;147(4):431–43.
19. Bershad EM, Suarez JI. Prothrombin complex concentrates for oral anticoagulant therapy-related intracranial hemorrhage: a review of the literature. Neurocrit Care. 2010;12(3):403–13.
20. Ansell J, Hirsh J, Hylek E, et al. Pharmacology and management of the vitamin K antagonists: American College of Chest Physicians evidence-based clinical practice guidelines (8th Edition). Chest. 2008;133(6 Suppl):160S–98.
21. Diringer MN, Skolnick BE, Mayer SA, et al. Thromboembolic events with recombinant activated factor VII in spontaneous intracerebral hemorrhage: results from the Factor Seven for Acute Hemorrhagic Stroke (FAST) trial. Stroke. 2010;41(1):48–53.
22. Dahlback B. Blood coagulation. Lancet. 2000;355(9215):1627–32.
23. Weitz JI. Blood coagulation and anticoagulant, fibrinolytic, and antiplatelet drugs. In: Brunton LL, editor. Goodman & Gilman's the pharmacological basis of therapeutics, vol. 211. 12th ed. New York: McGraw Hill Medical; 2011. p. 848–76.
24. Olson ST, Richard B, Izaguirre G, Schedin-Weiss S, Gettins PG. Molecular mechanisms of antithrombin-heparin regulation of blood clotting proteinases. A paradigm for understanding proteinase regulation by serpin family protein proteinase inhibitors. Biochimie. 2010;92(11):1587–96.
25. Gresham C, Levine M, Ruha AM. Case files of the Medical Toxicology Fellowship at Banner Good Samaritan Medical Center in Phoenix, AZ: a non-warfarin anticoagulant overdose. J Med Toxicol. 2009;5(4):242–9.
26. Walenga JM, Lyman GH. Evolution of heparin anticoagulants to ultra-low-molecular-weight heparins: a review of pharmacologic and clinical differences and applications in patients with cancer. Crit Rev Oncol Hematol. 2013;88(1):1–18.

27. Garcia DA, Baglin TP, Weitz JI, Samama MM, American College of Chest Physicians. Parenteral anticoagulants: Antithrombotic therapy and prevention of thrombosis, 9th ed: American College of Chest Physicians evidence-based clinical practice guidelines. Chest. 2012;141(2 Suppl):e24S–43.
28. Young E, Wells P, Holloway S, Weitz J, Hirsh J. Ex-vivo and in-vitro evidence that low molecular weight heparins exhibit less binding to plasma proteins than unfractionated heparin. Thromb Haemost. 1994;71(3):300–4.
29. Holmer E, Kurachi K, Soderstrom G. The molecular-weight dependence of the rate-enhancing effect of heparin on the inhibition of thrombin, factor Xa, factor IXa, factor XIa, factor XIIa and kallikrein by antithrombin. Biochem J. 1981;193(2):395–400.
30. Carter CJ, Kelton JG, Hirsh J, Cerskus A, Santos AV, Gent M. The relationship between the hemorrhagic and antithrombotic properties of low molecular weight heparin in rabbits. Blood. 1982;59(6):1239–45.
31. Warkentin TE, Kelton JG. A 14-year study of heparin-induced thrombocytopenia. Am J Med. 1996;101(5):502–7.
32. Linkins LA, Dans AL, Moores LK, et al. Treatment and prevention of heparin-induced thrombocytopenia: Antithrombotic therapy and prevention of thrombosis, 9th ed: American College of Chest Physicians evidence-based clinical practice guidelines. Chest. 2012;141(2 Suppl):e495S–530.
33. Michelson AD. Platelets. 3rd ed. Oxford: Elsevier; 2013.
34. Warkentin TE, Kelton JG. Temporal aspects of heparin-induced thrombocytopenia. N Engl J Med. 2001;344(17):1286–92.
35. Warkentin TE, Levine MN, Hirsh J, et al. Heparin-induced thrombocytopenia in patients treated with low-molecular-weight heparin or unfractionated heparin. N Engl J Med. 1995;332(20):1330–5.
36. Katzung B, Masters S, Revor A, editors. Basic and clinical pharmacology 12/E. New York: McGraw-Hill Professional; 2012.
37. Harter K, Levine M, Henderson SO. Anticoagulation drug therapy: a review. West J Emerg Med. 2015; 16(1):11–7.
38. Bates SM, Weitz JI. The mechanism of action of thrombin inhibitors. J Invasive Cardiol. 2000;12(Suppl F):27F–32.
39. Weitz JI, Hudoba M, Massel D, Maraganore J, Hirsh J. Clot-bound thrombin is protected from inhibition by heparin-antithrombin III but is susceptible to inactivation by antithrombin III-independent inhibitors. J Clin Invest. 1990;86(2):385–91.
40. Weitz JI, Leslie B, Hudoba M. Thrombin binds to soluble fibrin degradation products where it is protected from inhibition by heparin-antithrombin but susceptible to inactivation by antithrombin-independent inhibitors. Circulation. 1998;97(6):544–52.
41. Di Nisio M, Middeldorp S, Buller HR. Direct thrombin inhibitors. N Engl J Med. 2005;353(10):1028–40.
42. Eriksson BI, Quinlan DJ, Weitz JI. Comparative pharmacodynamics and pharmacokinetics of oral direct thrombin and factor Xa inhibitors in development. Clin Pharmacokinet. 2009;48(1):1–22.
43. Marlu R, Hodaj E, Paris A, Albaladejo P, Cracowski JL, Pernod G. Effect of non-specific reversal agents on anticoagulant activity of dabigatran and rivaroxaban: a randomised crossover ex vivo study in healthy volunteers. Thromb Haemost. 2012;108(2):217–24.
44. Wong H, Keeling D. Activated prothrombin complex concentrate for the prevention of dabigatran-associated bleeding. Br J Haematol. 2014;166(1):152–3.
45. Ross B, Miller MA, Ditch K, Tran M. Clinical experience of life-threatening dabigatran-related bleeding at a large, tertiary care, academic medical center: a case series. J Med Toxicol. 2014;10(2):223–8.
46. Dager WE, Gosselin RC, Roberts AJ. Reversing dabigatran in life-threatening bleeding occurring during cardiac ablation with factor eight inhibitor bypassing activity. Crit Care Med. 2013;41(5):e42–6.
47. Dumkow LE, Voss JR, Peters M, Jennings DL. Reversal of dabigatran-induced bleeding with a prothrombin complex concentrate and fresh frozen plasma. Am J Health Syst Pharm. 2012;69(19):1646–50.
48. Eerenberg ES, Kamphuisen PW, Sijpkens MK, Meijers JC, Buller HR, Levi M. Reversal of rivaroxaban and dabigatran by prothrombin complex concentrate: a randomized, placebo-controlled, crossover study in healthy subjects. Circulation. 2011;124(14):1573–9.
49. Chang DN, Dager WE, Chin AI. Removal of dabigatran by hemodialysis. Am J Kidney Dis. 2013;61(3):487–9.
50. Cabral KP, Ansell JE. The role of factor Xa inhibitors in venous thromboembolism treatment. Vasc Health Risk Manag. 2015;11:117–23.
51. Alexander JH, Singh KP. Inhibition of factor Xa: a potential target for the development of new anticoagulants. Am J Cardiovasc Drugs. 2005;5(5):279–90.
52. Boneu B, Necciari J, Cariou R, et al. Pharmacokinetics and tolerance of the natural pentasaccharide (SR90107/Org31540) with high affinity to antithrombin III in man. Thromb Haemost. 1995;74(6):1468–73.
53. Fawole A, Daw HA, Crowther MA. Practical management of bleeding due to the anticoagulants dabigatran, rivaroxaban, and apixaban. Cleve Clin J Med. 2013;80(7):443–51.
54. Patel MR, Mahaffey KW, Garg J, et al. Rivaroxaban versus warfarin in nonvalvular atrial fibrillation. N Engl J Med. 2011;365(10):883–91.
55. Piccini JP, Garg J, Patel MR, et al. Management of major bleeding events in patients treated with rivaroxaban vs. warfarin: results from the ROCKET AF trial. Eur Heart J. 2014;35(28):1873–80.
56. Granger CB, Alexander JH, McMurray JJ, et al. Apixaban versus warfarin in patients with atrial fibrillation. N Engl J Med. 2011;365(11):981–92.

Reversal of Target-Specific Oral Anticoagulants

4

Walter Jeske

Introduction

Anticoagulation is used to prevent thromboembolism following orthopedic surgery, in patients with atrial fibrillation and to treat acute venous thromboembolism. Short-term anticoagulation has traditionally been provided by the administration of heparin (or low molecular weight heparin), while long-term anticoagulation has been achieved through the administration of a vitamin K antagonist such as warfarin. Both heparin and warfarin produce their anticoagulant effects through the inhibition of multiple coagulation factors. Heparin, by binding to antithrombin, inhibits thrombin, factor Xa, factor IXa and, to a lesser extent, other intrinsic pathway factors while warfarin, by antagonizing vitamin K, prevents the formation of active forms of coagulation factors II, VII, IX, and X.

In recent years, several target-specific oral anticoagulants (TSOAC) have been introduced to clinical practice as alternatives to the use of warfarin. These drugs include the factor Xa inhibitors apixaban (Eliquis, Bristol-Myers Squibb, Princeton, NJ-Pfizer, New York, NY), rivaroxaban (Xarelto, Bayer Healthcare, Leverkusen, Germany), and edoxaban (Savaysa, Daiichi Sankyo, Tokyo, Japan) and the thrombin inhibitor dabigatran etexilate mesylate (Pradaxa, Boehringer-Ingelheim, Ridgefield, CT). Another factor Xa inhibitor, betrixaban (Portola, South San Francisco, CA), is in development. These target-specific oral anticoagulants offer advantages over warfarin in that their onset of action is much faster, typically ranging from 1 to 4 h post-dose, the half-life of drug action is shorter, ranging from 5 to 9 h for rivaroxaban to approximately 13 h for dabigatran and no food or drug interactions have been reported. These properties translate clinically into more reliable plasma drug concentrations that do not need to be routinely monitored. These agents have shown favorable efficacy profiles in comparison to standard warfarin therapy in a variety of clinical conditions including the prevention of stroke in patients with non-valvular atrial fibrillation.

The major side-effect associated with the use of anticoagulation is an increase in the occurrence or intensity of bleeding that can range from nuisance value to life threatening. Such enhanced bleeding can occur in response to injury or trauma; or when anticoagulation is supratherapeutic bleeding can occur spontaneously. Although clinical trials have shown that the safety of these new drugs in terms of the incidence of major hemorrhage is similar or better than that observed with conventional therapies, major hemorrhage can still occur.

W. Jeske, Ph.D. (✉)
Cardiovascular Institute, Loyola University Chicago
Health Sciences Division,
2160 S First Ave, Maywood, IL 60153, USA
e-mail: wjeske@luc.edu

C.M. Loftus (ed.), *Anticoagulation and Hemostasis in Neurosurgery*,
DOI 10.1007/978-3-319-27327-3_4

Increased levels of anticoagulation with warfarin, as measured by an International Normalized Ratio (INR) greater than 4.0, are associated with an increased risk of developing an intracerebral hemorrhage (ICH) [1] and warfarinized patients have an increased risk of hematoma expansion compared to patients with ICH who are not anticoagulated [2]. It is estimated that approximately 50 % of warfarin-treated ICH patients will experience hematoma expansion and of these, nearly half will experience a fatal outcome.

Each of the target-specific oral anticoagulants has been tested versus warfarin for their ability to prevent stroke and/or systemic embolism in patients with atrial fibrillation. In each study, the tested dose of TSOAC was associated with a lower rate of ICH compared to warfarin. In the RE-LY study, intracranial hemorrhage was observed in 0.32 %/year of patients treated with dabigatran compared to 0.76 %/year in warfarin-treated patients [3]. In the ROCKET-AF study, the rates of ICH were 0.8 and 1.2 %/year, respectively, for rivaroxaban and warfarin-treated patients [4]. In the ARISTOTLE study, the rates of ICH were 0.33 and 0.8 %/year, respectively, for apixaban and warfarin-treated patients [5]. In the ENGAGE-AF study, the rates of ICH were 0.39 and 0.85 %/year, respectively, for edoxaban and warfarin-treated patients [6].

To minimize the chances of hematoma expansion, it is necessary to reverse the anticoagulation. Lowering the INR to ≤1.3 within 2 h has been shown to have beneficial preventative effects on hematoma expansion. While anticoagulation due to warfarin can be reversed by the administration of vitamin K, this effect takes some time as new coagulation factors are being synthesized. In cases where emergent reversal is necessary, the administration of prothrombin complex concentrates to replace active coagulation factors can be used.

Agent-specific or mechanism-specific reversal agents are not currently available for the target-specific oral anticoagulants leading to concern about what can be done in cases of overdose or in medical emergencies. A variety of approaches to reverse anticoagulant activity or hemorrhage have been tested using in vitro systems, ex vivo using blood samples from anticoagulated subjects, and in vivo using animal models and healthy individuals.

Activated Charcoal

In cases of purposeful or accidental overdose, or when an adverse event occurs shortly after TSOAC administration, it may be desirable to prevent the anticoagulant from reaching the circulation. In an in vitro study, addition of **activated charcoal** to solutions of dabigatran resulted in a reduction in the concentration of free dabigatran in solution [7], suggesting that administration of activated charcoal may be effective in preventing dabigatran absorption in the case of overdose. Although reports of its effectiveness in patients are not available, the administration of activated charcoal has been recommended for treatment of TSOAC overdose, if the anticoagulant was administered within the previous 2–3 h.

Hemodialysis

Dialysis can be used to remove excess concentrations of some drugs from the circulation. While this would be ineffective for reducing circulating plasma concentrations of rivaroxaban and apixaban, owing to their high levels of protein binding (95 and 87 %, respectively), there is some evidence to suggest its benefit for removing dabigatran, which exhibits a much lower level of protein binding. In patients with ESRD given a single 50 mg dose of dabigatran, hemodialysis was shown to reduce plasma dabigatran concentrations by 60–70 % after 2–4 h of dialysis [8]. Similar reductions was observed following high-flux intermittent dialysis in a series of patients receiving the standard twice daily 150 mg dose of dabigatran who were admitted to hospital due to life-threatening bleeding [9]. Mean clearance of dabigatran by veno-venous hemodiafiltration in a patient presenting with dabigatran overdose was estimated to be 32–58 ml/h [10]. A concern with using dialysis to remove dabigatran is the potential for dabigatran levels to rebound after completion of dialysis as drug redistributes to the plasma compartment. This has led to a recommendation to use prolonged intermittent dialysis or intermittent dialysis followed by continuous renal replacement therapy.

Nonspecific Reversal Agents

Since the TSOACs do not yet have specific reversal agents, reversal of their activity has focused on the off-label use of prothrombin complex concentrates (**PCC**) as factor replacement therapy and the use of pro-hemostatic agents such as rFVIIa in a variety of experimental paradigms. PCCs are a family of human plasma-derived products that have been used to treat hemophilia and more recently for warfarin reversal. PCCs contain varying amounts of coagulation factors and are divided into the categories of three factor products (containing factors II, IX and X), four factor products (containing factors II, VII, IX, and X) and activated PCC (containing factors II, VIIa, IX and X). In addition to having varying relative levels of these factors, some products may also contain anticoagulant substances such as Protein C, Protein S, Protein Z, antithrombin, or added heparin. **Recombinant FVIIa** (NovoSeven, Novo Nordisk, Bagsvaerd, Denmark) is used clinically to treat and prevent bleeding in hemophilic patients and has also been tested as a potential reversing agent for target-specific oral anticoagulants.

Evidence to demonstrate that nonspecific reversal agents can reverse anticoagulation produced by TSOACs exists on several levels. In the simplest system, addition of activated PCC to dabigatran- and rivaroxaban-supplemented plasmas has been shown to reverse the inhibition of thrombin generation. Supplementation of activated PCC was also shown to be more effective than PCC or rFVIIa at reversing apixaban-induced alterations in thrombin generation and fibrin clot structure [11].

Animal Studies

Animal models that are utilized to assess the relative hemorrhagic potential of anticoagulant drugs involve making a standardized wound in treated animals and measuring the bleeding time or quantitating the amount of blood lost. Such models have been applied to the question of how to reverse TSOAC-induced bleeding. In a mouse tail transection model, aPCC or a combination of PCC + rFVIIa shortened the dabigatran-induced prolongation of bleeding time, but did not reduce the total amount of blood lost [12]. Similarly, in rats, dabigatran etexilate resulted in a prolongation of bleeding time that was reversed by the subsequent administration of three factor PCCs, four factor PCCs, activated PCC and rFVIIa [13, 14]. FVIIa effectively reduced rivaroxaban-induced bleeding time but not blood loss in a rabbit model [15]. Four-factor PCC has been shown to be effective in reducing bleeding following liver laceration in dabigatran-treated animals and following kidney laceration in rivaroxaban-treated animals [16]. Animal studies have also pointed out that stoppage of bleeding following administration of PCC or rFVIIa did not necessarily correlate with a complete reversal of plasma clotting time prolongation.

Intracerebral hemorrhage has been modeled in mice by intrastriatal injection of collagenase. In this model, anticoagulation with either rivaroxaban or dabigatran increased the hematoma volume compared to that seen in non-anticoagulated mice [17, 18]. In rivaroxaban-treated mice, PCC, rFVIIa, and fresh frozen plasma administered 30 min after collagenase treatment prevented excess intracerebral hematoma formation. In dabigatran-treated animals, PCC was more effective than fresh frozen plasma and rFVIIa was observed to be ineffective at preventing hematoma expansion.

Humans: Healthy Volunteers

Several studies using healthy human volunteers have been carried out which demonstrate the ability of PCCs or rFVIIa to reverse anticoagulant effects of dabigatran and rivaroxaban. In one study, blood samples were drawn from volunteers 2 h after they had received a single dose of either rivaroxaban or dabigatran [19]. Rivaroxaban was observed to prolong the time until initiation of thrombin generation and reduce the total amount of thrombin formed while dabigatran only prolonged the time until thrombin generation began. Supplementation of activated PCC or rFVIIa to the plasma samples normalized the lag time to thrombin generation initiation. Supplementation of either four-factor or activated PCC normalized the amount of thrombin generated.

In a randomized double-blind placebo controlled study in 12 healthy volunteers, repeated dosing of rivaroxaban or dabigatran prolonged clotting time and inhibited thrombin generation [20]. Following the fifth dose of anticoagulant, a single bolus dose (50 IU/kg) of a four-factor PCC was infused over 15 min. Serial blood samples were collected to measure a variety of coagulation parameters. Rivaroxaban significantly prolonged the prothrombin time and inhibited thrombin generation. Both effects were rapidly reversed upon administration of PCC. The anticoagulant effect of dabigatran was observed as prolongations of the aPTT, thrombin time and ecarin clotting time. Administration of four-factor PCC did not reverse any of the prolongations of clotting time. Administration of a lower dose of PCC (37.4 IU/kg) was subsequently shown to significantly increase thrombin generation in healthy volunteers treated with rivaroxaban [21].

One study has been carried out in healthy volunteers using bleeding as an endpoint [22]. In this randomized, double-blind, placebo controlled phase I study, volunteers were anticoagulated with a single oral dose of the factor Xa inhibitor edoxaban followed 2 h later by an infusion of one of three doses of four-factor PCC. Thirty minutes after completion of PCC infusion, a punch biopsy was performed. Four-factor PCC dose-dependently reversed the effects of edoxaban on bleeding duration, bleeding volume, thrombin generation and prothrombin time with a complete reversal of the prolongation of bleeding duration, the increase in bleeding volume, and the inhibition of thrombin generation observed at the highest dose of PCC tested (50 IU/kg).

Humans: Case Reports

Currently lacking in the literature are clinical studies to demonstrate the effectiveness of PCCs or rFVIIa to reverse hemorrhagic effects in patients treated with TSOACs. A variety of case studies, however, have been reported, which demonstrate variable effectiveness of the reversal therapies. The usefulness of aPCC (administered at doses ranging from 42 to 100 IU/kg) or PCC (2000 IU) to treat patients with potentially life-threatening bleeding brought about by dabigatran administration has been suggested [23, 24].

Guidelines

With a lack of clinical trial data to guide the usage of nonspecific reversal agents, a number of authors and professional societies have developed algorithms for dealing with bleeding brought on by the use of TSOACs [25–28]. Each of these strategies incorporates risk stratification to target the appropriate intervention. For minor to moderate bleeding, these guidelines suggest stopping anticoagulation if the perceived benefit of stopping outweighs the risk of continuing and using local compression and transfusion of blood components as necessary. Treatment with nonspecific prohemostatic agents (PCCs and rFVIIa) or removal of the drug by the administration of activated charcoal or the use of hemodialysis should be reserved for those patients with severe or life-threatening bleeding.

Future Agents

Efforts are being made to develop agents that will prevent TSOACs from expressing anticoagulant activity rather than trying to overcome the anti-coagulation as is done with the PCCs and rFVIIa. Several more specific antagonists are currently under development. One of these is a modified form of factor Xa (PRT064445; **Andexanet alfa**; Portola Pharmaceuticals) which is catalytically inactive due to a mutation of the serine residue at the active site and also lacks a membrane-binding γ-carboxyglutamic acid domain [29]. This factor Xa variant retains its ability to bind to factor Xa inhibitors and acts as a decoy by binding direct Factor Xa inhibitors or heparin-activated anti-thrombin and allowing native factor Xa to express its hemostatic function.

Andexanet alfa

In in vitro assays, supplementation of andex-anet alfa was shown to inhibit anti-factor Xa activity induced by a variety of direct factor Xa inhibitors. Administration of andexanet alfa to animals anticoagulated with direct factor Xa inhibitors (betrixaban, rivaroxaban, apixaban) or antithrombin-dependent factor Xa inhibitors (enoxaparin, fondaparinux) was shown to reverse the anticoagulant effects measured ex vivo, and to reduce blood loss caused by standardized wounds.

Phase III, randomized, double-blind, placebo controlled trials are being conducted to assess the ability of andexanet alfa to reverse antico-agulation with rivaroxaban (ANNEXA-R study) or apixaban (ANNEXA-A study). The primary outcome for these studies is the reversal of anti-coagulation as assessed by the percent change in anti-Factor Xa activity from baseline to nadir, with secondary endpoints being plasma levels of unbound rivaroxaban or apixaban and the change in thrombin generation. Both studies have shown the effectiveness of a single bolus of andexanet alfa to rapidly and significantly reverse anticoagulant activity. An additional arm in each study to evaluate bolus plus infusion dosing of andexanet alfa are ongoing. A phase 4 open-label study in patients anticoagulated with apixaban, rivaroxaban or enoxaparin who present with an acute major bleed is being initiated.

Idarucizumab

Idarucizumab (BI655075, Boehringer Ingelheim) is a humanized antibody fragment that is being developed as an antidote for dabigatran. This antibody fragment has been shown to reverse dabigatran-induced anticoagulant activity when added in vitro to dabigatran-supplemented plasma and when infused to dabigatran anticoagulated rats [30]. Correlating with this decrease in anticoagulant activity was a decrease in rat tail bleeding time. Similarly in a porcine model of blunt hepatic trauma, anti-dabigatran Fab was shown to reverse dabigatran anticoagulation [31].

A number of human studies using idarucizumab to reverse dabigatran have been carried out or are ongoing. A phase 1 study has indicated that onset of action of idarucizumab can be detected immediately following a 5 min infusion. Administration of idarucizumab to dabigatran-treated healthy volunteers restores wound site fibrin formation. Safety, tolerability and PK/PD of idarucizumab has been investigated in a randomized double-blind, placebo-controlled cross over study in healthy subjects and patients with mild/moderate renal impairment who were treated with dabigatran (220 mg bid or 150 mg bid, respectively) for 4 days to achieve steady-state anticoagulation. Complete reversal of anti-coagulation was observed at the end of the infusion period. The RE-VERSE AD trial (NCT 02104947), a Phase 3 case series clinical study, will determine the effectiveness of idarucizumab to reverse anticoagulation in dabigatran-treated patients who present with uncontrolled bleeding or who require emergency surgery or procedures. The primary endpoint is the maximum reversal of anticoagulant effect measured by dilute thrombin time or ecarin clotting time within 4 h of infusion. Secondary endpoints include reversal of other anticoagulant parameters, the occurrence of intraoperative or 24 h postoperative major bleeding in patients undergoing surgery and the time to cessation of bleeding in patients presenting with overt hemorrhage. The study is expected to be completed in early 2017.[1]

Per977

Per977 (aripazine, Perosphere, Danbury, CT) is a synthetic, positively charged, small molecule that has been shown to bind with heparins and a wide variety of direct oral anticoagulants including rivaroxaban, apixaban, dabigatran and edoxaban via hydrogen bonding or charge-based interactions. When administered to animals anticoagulated with enoxaparin, dabigatran, rivaroxaban or apixaban, PER977 was observed to inhibit anticoagulant activity as measured by a variety of assays (thromboelastography, aPTT, anti-Xa) and also reduce the amount of blood lost from standardized wounds. The ability of PER977 to reverse the anticoagulant effect of edoxaban was tested in a phase I clinical study involving 80 healthy volunteers [32]. When PER977 (100 or 300 mg) was administered 3 h after edoxaban (60 mg), whole blood clotting time was reduced to within 10 % of baseline within 10 min. A phase 2 study to evaluate the impact of PER977 treatment on re-anticoagulation with edoxaban is ongoing.

Summary

The TSOACs provide interesting alternatives to the use of the conventional anticoagulants heparin and warfarin. While clinical studies have shown TSOACs to be at least comparable, and sometimes better, in efficacy, they achieve this with some practical benefits including fixed dosing and no need for routine monitoring of drug levels. Although meta-analyses suggest a lower risk for bleeding with TSOAC therapy and similar levels of total bleeding, there will be times when it is desirable or necessary to reverse the anticoagulation produced by TSOACs such as with overdose, traumatic emergencies, or the need for urgent surgery.

Heparin and warfarin target multiple sites in the hemostatic cascade and offer the benefit of specific antagonists—protamine for heparins and vitamin K for warfarin. For the time being, the pendulum has swung in the opposite direction in that while the newer oral anticoagulants are single targeting, the means of reversing their activity has largely encompassed the off-label use of nonspecific pro-hemostatic agents such as PCCs and rFVIIa.

The usefulness of PCCs and rFVIIa at reversing the anticoagulant and/or hemorrhagic effects of TSOAC treatment has been shown on a number of levels. Addition of PCCs to plasma that has been supplemented in vitro with TSOACs reverses the anticoagulant activity. Similar reversals in anticoagulant activity have been observed when blood from animals or healthy humans, who have been anticoagulated with TSOACs, is supplemented ex vivo with PCCs or rFVIIa. The ability of nonspecific reversal agents to reduce hemorrhage has been shown in a variety of animal models that incorporate standardized wounds and in specific models of ICH. One important point to take away from these studies is that reversal of the hemorrhagic effects does not necessarily correlate with reversal of ex vivo anticoagulant activity. In that regard, the mechanism behind the PCC effect is not clear. Several possibilities have been suggested including an enhancement of prothrombinase complex on the platelet surface and an increase in the velocity of thrombin generation [33]. A recent study has demonstrated differential effects of PCC, aPCC, and rFVIIa on clot structure and the rate of fibrin polymerization [11] which may explain some of the differences in the effectiveness of TSOAC reversal that have been observed in earlier studies.

Much less is known about the effectiveness of PCCs and rFVIIa in stopping bleeding in patients

1 Editor's note—Subsequent to the initial preparation of this chapter, Praxbind® (idarucizumab), was approved by the FDA in October 2015 for reversal of dabigatran effect.

treated with TSOACs. Here, the evidence is currently limited to case reports describing experience with a single patient or a small series of patients. Although guidelines have been developed recommending the usage of PCCs and rFVIIa to maintain hemostasis in TSOAC-treated patients presenting with serious or life-threatening bleeding, the variability in outcomes reported in the literature preclude identifying an optimal dosing regimen in terms of which product to use or the dose to treat with. In the reported case studies, the patients described present with different levels of anticoagulation, different comorbid conditions and adjunctive medications and different dosing regimens for the reversal agent(s) used.

The use of the nonspecific reversal agents is also complicated by the need to not tip the hemostatic balance too far in the opposite direction and place the patient in a prothrombotic state, particularly with the use of rFVIIa. Data from animal studies suggests the possibility of "over-correcting" thrombin generation beyond baseline with the use of high doses of PCC, though the impact of such an over-correction on patients has not been defined.

The urgent need for effective TSOAC antagonists is highlighted by the FDA's designation of idarucizumab and andexanet alfa as Breakthrough Therapies. Such a designation is intended to expedite the development and review of drugs for serious or life-threatening conditions. Promising therapies such as these coupled with an enhanced understanding of how PCCs reverse TSOAC-induced anticoagulation are expected to allow for effective treatment of TSOAC-induced hemorrhagic episodes.

References

1. Fang MC, Chang Y, Hylek EM, et al. Advanced age, anticoagulation intensity, and risk for intracranial hemorrhage among patients taking warfarin for atrial fibrillation. Ann Intern Med. 2004;141:745–52.
2. Flibitte JJ, Hagan N, O'Donnell J, et al. Warfarin, hematoma expansion, and outcome of intracerebral hemorrhage. Neurology. 2004;63:1059–64.
3. Connolly SJ, Ezekowitz MD, Yusuf S, et al. Dabigatran versus warfarin in patients with atrial fibrillation. N Engl J Med. 2009;361(12):1139–51.
4. Patel MR, Mahaffey KW, Garg J, et al. Rivaroxaban versus warfarin in nonvalvular atrial fibrillation. N Engl J Med. 2011;365(10):883–91.
5. Granger CB, Alexander JH, McMurray JJV, et al. Apixaban versus warfarin in patients with atrial fibrillation. N Engl J Med. 2011;365(11):981–92.
6. Giugliano RP, Ruff CT, Braunwald E, et al. Edoxaban versus warfarin in patients with atrial fibrillation. N Engl J Med. 2013;369:2093–104.
7. Van Ryn J, Stangier J, Haertter S, et al. Dabigatran etexilate—a novel, reversible, oral direct thrombin inhibitor: interpretation of coagulation assays and reversal of anticoagulant activity. Thromb Haemost. 2010;103:1116–27.
8. Stangier J, Rathgen K, Stahle H, et al. Influence of renal impairment on the pharmacokinetics and pharmacodynamics of oral dabigatran etexilate: an open label, parallel-group, single-centre study. Clin Pharmacokinet. 2010;49:259–68.
9. Singh T, Maw TT, Henry BL, et al. Extracorporeal therapy for dabigatran removal in the treatment of acute bleeding: a single center experience. Clin J Am Soc Nephrol. 2013;8(9):1533–9.
10. Chiew AL, Khamoudes D, Chan BS. Use of continuous veno-venous haemodiafiltration therapy in dabigatran overdose. Clin Toxicol. 2014;52(4):283–7.
11. Martin AC, Gouin-Thibault I, Siguret V, et al. Multimodal assessment of non-specific hemostatic agents for apixaban reversal. J Thromb Haemost. 2015;13:426–36.
12. Lambourne MD, Eltringham-Smith LJ, Gataiance S, et al. Prothrombin complex concentrates reduce blood loss in murine coagulopathy induce by warfarin, but not in that induced by dabigatran etexilate. J Thromb Haemost. 2012;10:1830–40.
13. Van Ryn J, Schurer J, Kink-Eiband M, et al. Reversal of dabigatran-induced bleeding by coagulation factor concentrates in a rat-tail bleeding model and lack of effect on assays of coagulation. Anesthesiology. 2014;120:1429–40.
14. van Ryn J, Ruehl D, Priepke H, et al. Reversibility of the anticoagulant effect of high doses of the direct thrombin inhibitor dabigatran, by recombinant factor VIIa or activated prothrombin complex concentrate. 13th Congress of the European Hematology Association. Copenhagen, Denmark; 2008. p. 148.
15. Godier A, Miclot A, Le Bonniec B, et al. Evaluation of prothrombin complex concentrate and recombinant activated factor VII to reverse rivaroxaban in a rabbit model. Anesthesiology. 2012;116:94–102.
16. Herzog E, Kaspereit F, Krege W, et al. Correlation of coagulation markers and 4F-PCC-mediated reversal of rivaroxaban in a rabbit model of acute bleeding. Thromb Res. 2015;135:554–60.
17. Zhou W, Schwarting S, Illanes S, et al. Hemostatic therapy in experimental intracerebral hemorrhage associated with the direct thrombin inhibitor dabigatran. Stroke. 2011;42:3594–9.

18. Zhou W, Zorn M, Nawroth P, et al. Hemostatic therapy in experimental intracerebral hemorrhage associated with rivaroxaban. Stroke. 2013;44:771–8.
19. Marlu R, Hodaj E, Paris A, et al. Effect of non-specific reversal agents on anticoagulant activity of dabigatran and rivaroxaban: a randomized crossover ex vivo study in healthy volunteers. Thromb Haemost. 2012;108:217–24.
20. Eerenberg ES, Kamphuisen PW, Sijpkens MK, et al. Reversal of rivaroxaban and dabigatran by prothrombin complex concentrate: a randomized, placebo-controlled, crossover study in healthy subjects. Circulation. 2011;124:1573–9.
21. Cheung W, Barco S, Coppens M, et al. In vivo reversal of the anticoagulant effect of rivaroxaban with 4-factor prothrombin complex concentrate. J Am Coll Cardiol. 2014;63(12):A334.
22. Zahir H, Brown KS, Vandell AG, et al. Edoxaban effects on bleeding following punch biopsy and reversal by a 4-factor prothrombin complex concentrate. Circulation. 2015;131:82–90.
23. Schulman S, Ritchie B, Goy JK, et al. Activated prothrombin complex concentrate for dabigatran-associated bleeding. Br J Haematol. 2014;164:308–10.
24. Dumkow LE, Voss JR, Peters M, et al. Reversal of dabigatran-induced bleeding with a prothrombin complex concentrate and fresh frozen plasma. Am J Health Syst Pharm. 2012;69(19):1646–50.
25. Vilchez JA, Gallego P, Lip GYH. Safety of new oral anticoagulant drugs: a perspective. Ther Adv Drug Saf. 2014;5(1):8–20.
26. Siegal DM, Garcia DA, Crowther MA. How I treat target-specific oral anticoagulant-associated bleeding. Blood. 2014;123(8):1152–8.
27. Fawole A, Daw HA, Crowther MA. Practical management of bleeding due to the anticoagulants dabigatran, rivaroxaban, and apixaban. Cleve Clin J Med. 2013;80(7):443–51.
28. Steiner T, Bohm M, Dichgans M, et al. Recommendations for the emergency management of complications associated with the new direct oral anticoagulants (DOACs), apixaban, dabigatran and rivaroxaban. Clin Res Cardiol. 2013;102: 399–412.
29. Lu G, DeGuzman FR, Hollenbach SJ, et al. A specific antidote for reversal of anticoagulation by direct and indirect inhibitors of coagulation factor Xa. Nat Med. 2013;19:446–51.
30. Schiele F, van Ryn J, Canada K, et al. A specific antidote for dabigatran: functional and structural characterization. Blood. 2013;121:3554–62.
31. Grottke O, Honickel M, van Ryn J, et al. A specific antidote to dabigatran reduces blood loss in dabigatran- and trauma-induced bleeding in pigs. J Am Coll Cardiol. 2014;63(12):A295.
32. Ansell JE, Bakhru SH, Laulicht BE, et al. Use of PER977 to reverse the anticoagulant effect of edoxaban. N Engl J Med. 2014;371:2141–2.
33. Hoffman M, Dargaud Y. Mechanisms and monitoring of bypassing agent activity. J Thromb Haemost. 2012;10:1478–85.

Overview, Measurement and Point-of-Care Testing of Platelet Function

5

Daphne Li, Wael Hassaneen-Mostafa, and Asterios Tsimpas

Overview of Platelet Function

Platelets are small cells without a nucleus that have an average life span of 5–9 days. They play a crucial role in monitoring the integrity of the vascular endothelium. Vascular injury initiates a series of events that result in rapid protection against bleeding, as well as formation of stable blood clots via the coagulation cascade. These events are: platelet adherence, activation and secretion, aggregation, and interaction with coagulation factors.

Under normal circumstances, the vascular endothelium provides a non-adhesive surface for platelets via secretion of prostaglandin I_2 and nitric oxide. Disruption of the endothelium exposes highly thrombogenic, subendothelial collagen fibers. These fibers bind glycoprotein (GP) Ib-IX-V and GP VI receptors on the platelet surface via von Willebrand factor (vWF) at sites of vascular injury. Platelet interaction with these collagen fibers serves as a surface for platelet adhesion, as well as a stimulus for platelet activation. Endothelial disruption also exposes tissue factor (TF), which interacts with activated factor VIIa to promote local coagulation and generate thrombin.

At the site of vascular injury, activated platelets produce local platelet activating factors (PAF), such as adenosine diphosphate (ADP), thromboxane A2 (TXA2), serotonin, and thrombin. TXA2 is produced via conversion of arachidonic acid by cyclooxygenase-1 (COX-1) and thromboxane synthase. Its release promotes vasoconstriction and platelet aggregation. Serotonin, which is released by platelet dense granules, typically causes vasodilation, but will induce vasoconstriction in the setting of dysfunctional endothelium. The effects of ADP are mediated through binding of P2Y1 and P2Y12 platelet surface receptors. Release of ADP from activated platelets contributes to platelet recruitment, platelet conformation change via calcium ion influx leading to increased surface area, increased expression of pro-inflammatory molecules, and activation of GP IIb/IIIa receptors. GP IIb/IIIa receptors are the most abundant receptor on the platelet surface. Upon activation, GP IIb/IIIa receptors mediate platelet aggregation by binding to vWF and fibrinogen. Fibrinogen is released from platelet alpha granules and forms bridges between activated platelets, leading to thrombus stabilization and formation of a "white clot" [1–3].

D. Li, M.D. • A. Tsimpas, M.D., M.Sc. (✉)
• W. Hassaneen-Mostafa, M.D., Ph.D.
Department of Neurological Surgery,
Loyola University Medical Center, 2160 South
1st Avenue, Maywood, IL 60153, USA
e-mail: daphne.li@lumc.edu;
atsimpas@lumc.edu;
whassaneen@lumc.edu

C.M. Loftus (ed.), *Anticoagulation and Hemostasis in Neurosurgery*,
DOI 10.1007/978-3-319-27327-3_5

Thrombin (activated factor IIa) is arguably the most potent activator of platelets. It activates platelets by binding to PAR-1 receptors and forms fibrin through cleavage of fibrinogen. Activation of PAR-1 receptors leads to platelet shape change, aggregation, and granule secretion. Progression through the coagulation cascade leads to formation of a fibrin-rich red clot superimposed on the initial white thrombus.

Measuring Platelet Function

The assessment of platelet function in patients on or off antiplatelet therapy provides physicians with an idea of hemostatic effectiveness. It can help determine whether or not emergent reversal may be required in the setting of hemorrhage or emergent surgery. Early means of assessing platelet function were limited to a small number of unreliable tests with difficulties in simulating hemostasis in vitro. However, since the late 1980s, advances in laboratory platelet analysis have created newer and more reliable methods of evaluating platelet function.

Bleeding Time

Bleeding time, first proposed by Duke in 1910, is the first in vivo test of platelet function [4]. It can be used to detect qualitative defects in platelets, vascular defects, von Willebrand's disease, or thrombocytopenia. This test has limited clinical application due to poor sensitivity and its invasive nature [5–7]. As well, it is impractical to use serially and requires experienced operators to judge the subjective endpoint of the test. Thus, it is rarely used in preoperative assessments of platelet function [8].

Platelet Count

Although Platelet count does not provide a direct assessment of platelet function, it is still used as a first line assessment of a patient's risk for hemorrhagic complications. A goal of at least 80–100,000/μL is used a threshold to proceed with a safe intervention [9]. Although several automated methods have been developed to count platelets, the manual count, using phase contrast microscopy, is still recognized as the gold standard. However, the manual count is imprecise, with coefficients of variation (CV) in the range of 15–25 % [10].

Automated cell counters, although more rapid, precise, and reproducible, do have their flaws. These cell counters tend to overestimate the platelet count in samples containing cellular debris. As well, they tend to underestimate platelet count in patients with large platelets, such as in immune thrombocytopenia [11]. The development of optical and flow cytometric methods have greatly improved the accuracy of counting methods. Optical cell counters identify platelets based on their light scattering properties or via fluorescence following addition of a suitable dye. Flow cytometry counters derive the platelet count by labeling platelets with a fluorescent monoclonal antibody, dividing that number with the number of red blood cell events and multiplying this ratio by the red blood cell count. These derived platelet counts are much more accurate, with CVs of less than 5 % [10].

Platelet Aggregometry

Light transmission aggregometry (LTA), developed in the 1960s, is the classic aggregometry platelet function test [12]. This test involves shining a light through platelet-rich plasma while platelet agonists are added. The platelet agonists, such as ADP, increase light transmission secondary to decreased turbidity of the plasma due to induced platelet aggregation. Various platelet agonists may be introduced at various concentrations and paired with the appropriate antiplatelet agents in order to test resistance (i.e., aspirin correlates with ADP/arachidonic acid/collagen, clopidogrel correlates with ADP, GP IIb/IIIa inhibitors correlate with ADP/thrombin receptor agonists). Although this test is the gold standard, it is a labor-intensive, requires technical expertise, its performance is not standardized and it is not widely available. The test itself often underestimates the degree of GP IIb/IIIa inhibitors [13] and is not sensitive to test microaggregates [14]. This translates into relative insensitivity for detecting preexisting aggregates or monitoring of the early phases of aggregation, which may be essential in studying patients with hyperfunctioning platelets.

Whole blood aggregometry is less labor-intensive than LTA. The *Multiplate analyzer* (*Roche Diagnostics International, Rotkreuz, Switzerland*) allows platelet aggregation to be measured after addition of commonly used agonists. The assay involves stirring whole blood samples, anticoagulated with hirudin, between two platinum electrodes. This will cause platelets to adhere to the electrodes upon the addition of agonists, resulting in changes in impedance of the circuit. This method is widely used in Europe for diagnosing platelet defects, and monitoring aspirin and clopidogrel. Unfortunately, this assay has poor sensitivity to microaggregates [15].

Flow cytometry can be used, not only to count platelets, but also to assess platelet function via particle size analysis. Using this method, the formation of aggregates of all sizes, including micro-aggregates, during the early platelet aggregation phase can be detected with high accuracy. Unfortunately, this method is expensive and requires some expertise, since disaggregation may occur during dilution procedures, if the samples are not appropriately handled [6].

Laser platelet aggregometry is a highly accurate method of detecting small microaggregates, involving light scattering. This method can detect aggregates as small as two to three platelets, and is capable of continuously monitoring aggregate formation [16, 17]. Unfortunately, there is little widespread experience with the use of this method [6].

Point-of-Care (POC) Function Assays

Therapies inhibiting platelet function are commonly used to prevent thrombotic complications in patients, such as stent occlusion and/or stroke. Three classes of potent antiplatelet agents, which will be addressed in another chapter, include P2Y12 inhibitors, GP IIb/IIIa inhibitors and salicylates. Variation in an individual's response to therapy may be due to genetic variation, drug-to-drug interactions, poor general health status or noncompliance. Due to this variability in response, as well as a need to achieve adequate inhibition of normal platelet function in certain clinical settings, POC function assays have been developed. The goal of POC assays is to assess a patient's response to antiplatelet therapy with the potential for guiding dosing or choice of therapeutic agent in the setting of lower or nonresponsiveness.

Platelet Counting

ICHOR Point of Care Hematology Counter, or Plateletworks (*Helena Laboratories, Beaumont, TX*) (Fig. 5.1), functions as an indirect measurement of platelet function. The assay stimulates platelets within anticoagulated whole blood samples using platelet agonists to induce aggregation. The ratio between platelet counts in the control versus activated sample is calculated as a measure of platelet functionality. This assay is easy to use, requiring no sample preparation, and has wide availability in clinical laboratories, since the only equipment needed is a cell counter [6]. Although clinical experience is limited, Plateletworks has been shown to correlate with

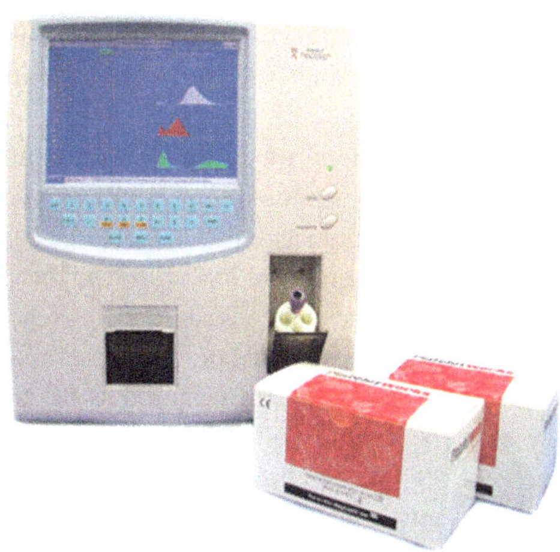

Fig. 5.1 ICHOR Point of Care Hematology Counter, or Plateletworks (Helena Laboratories, Beaumont, Texas)

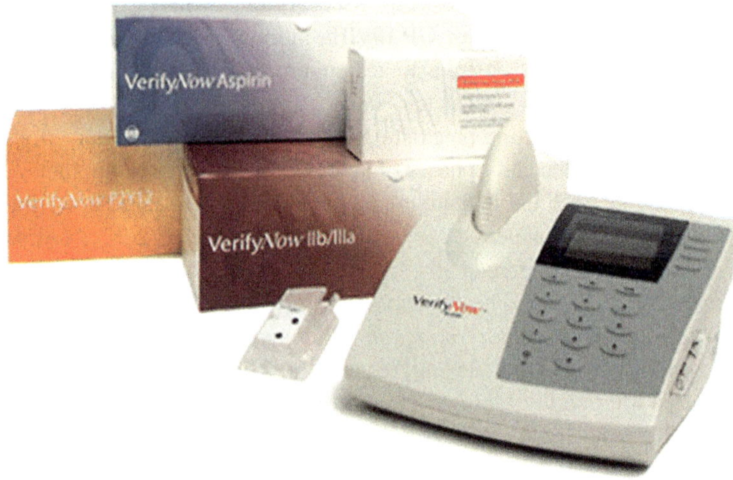

Fig. 5.2 Verify*Now* System (Accumetrics, San Diego, California)

adverse cardiovascular events in patients requiring dual antiplatelet therapy with aspirin and clopidogrel [18].

Aggregometry

VerifyNow (*Accumetrics, San Diego, CA*), previously known as the Ultegra Rapid Platelet Function assay, is an assay that provides rapid measurement of platelet responsiveness of antiplatelet therapies (Fig. 5.2). It measures increases in light transmittance in platelet containing whole blood or plasma secondary to platelet aggregation, much like the LTA. In fact, results of VerifyNow have been shown to correlate well with LTA results [19]. Different platelet agonists are employed depending on which agent is being tested. Arachidonic acid is the agonist for aspirin, clopidogrel is tested with an ADP activator, and GP IIb/IIIa inhibitors are tested with thrombin receptor activating peptides (iso-TRAP). Administration of these agonists induces platelet aggregation on fibrinogen-coated polystyrene beads, leading to increased light transmittance. Results of these assays indicate what percentage of platelet receptors are successfully inhibited by antiplatelet therapy, with the premise that in order to achieve significant clinical efficacy with antiplatelet agents, greater than or equal to 80 % platelet receptors need to be blocked [20].

The aspirin test measures platelet aggregation in aspirin reaction units (ARUs). ARU values less than 550 are consistent with aspirin-induced inhibition of platelet function, while values greater than 550 are inconsistent. The PRU test is a whole blood test used to measure P2Y12 receptor blockade. Not only does this test employ an ADP agonist to activate platelets, but it also uses prostaglandin E1 (PGE1) to increase intraplatelet cyclo-adenosine monophosphate (cAMP) and decrease the activation of P2Y1 receptors, making the test more specific. PRUs less than 194, the lower limit of the reference rage (194–418), are highly specific for a P2Y12 inhibitor effect. Documentation of at least a 30 % change in reactivity is often recommended prior to intracranial stent placement. Very low levels of P2Y12 reaction units (PRUs) may be associated with increased risk of bleeding.

It should be noted that GPIIb/IIIa inhibitors might interfere with the aspirin and the PRU test, because the activation of GPIIb/IIIa receptors is required for fibrinogen-coated microparticles to bind platelets and form aggregates. Therefore, investigators should wait for platelet function to be restored prior to measuring platelet function inhibition using the aspirin or PRU test (Accumetrics, San Diego, CA). Of note, the FDA has recalled the IIb/IIIa test in 2014 due to concerns in reporting of erroneous platelet aggregation unit results [9]. Regardless, VerifyNow can provide useful clinical information with its use prior to initiation of antiplatelet therapy and immediately prior to a planned endovascular procedure.

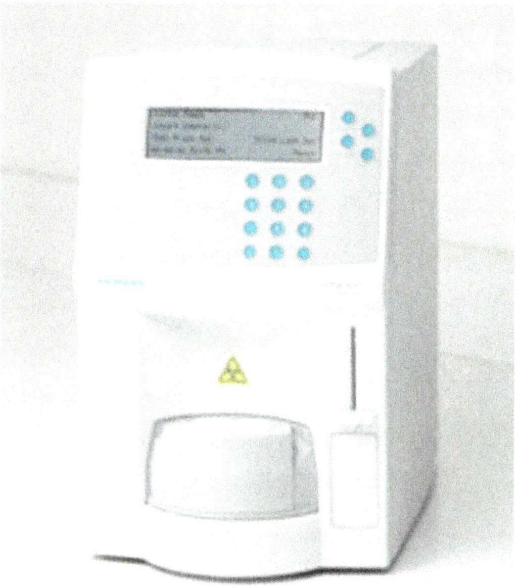

Fig. 5.3 Platelet Function Analyzer (PFA-100; Siemens Healthcare Diagnostics, Deerfield, Illinois)

Simulating Platelet Function In Vitro

The *Platelet Function Analyzer (PFA-100; Siemens Healthcare Diagnostics, Deerfield, IL)* simulates hemostasis in a blood vessel by exposing platelets, in whole blood, to shear stress while in a platelet-agonist coated capillary (Fig. 5.3). Epinephrine is used as the platelet agonist for aspirin therapy and ADP is used as the agonist for monitoring P2Y12 receptor inhibition. As platelets are activated and adhere/aggregate on the capillary walls, time to closure of the central aperture (diameter 100 μm) is measured and reported as a parameter called closing time (CT). These assays serve as simulations of in vivo platelet physiology, with many of them mimicking vessel wall damage and focusing on shear-induced platelet activation. The PFA-100 has almost completely replaced in vivo bleeding time as a global assessment of hemostasis [21] (Fig. 5.3).

This global test of platelet function is simple, fast and does not require specialist training. The CT may be affected by absolute platelet count, levels of von Willebrand factor (vWF) and hematocrit. In fact, PFA-100 has also been used as a screening tool for vWD and verifying the effects of desmopressin in presurgical patients [22]. It has numerous clinical applications, in addition to screening for vWD, including identification of inherited and acquired platelet defects, monitoring antiplatelet therapy, assessing surgical bleeding risk and assessing thrombotic risk [23]. The PFA-100 has a high negative predictive value. However, due to its lack of specificity, any platelet function defects detected by prolonged CT will need to be confirmed by more specific test.

The *Clot Signature Analyzer (Xylum, Scarsdale, NY)* assesses the ability of flowing, non-anticoagulated blood to form hemostatic plugs via fibrin formation. The device, a hemostatometer, is a closed pressurized tubing system through which blood is perfused under physiologic conditions. Two holes are punched in the tube to initiate the coagulation cascade while the pressure is closely monitored. A measure of bleeding time equivalent is the time it takes for a platelet and fibrin clot to plug the holes and recover initial pressure. The activated-clotting time equivalent is the time it takes for the clot to occlude the tube, resulting in a drop in distal pressure. The whole blood is passed through another tube containing collagen fibrils with a time measured for collagen-induced thrombus formation sufficient to occlude the tube or result in a 50 % drop in pressure [24]. This assay is not sensitive enough to discriminate platelet function under conditions of GP IIa/IIIb inhibition. However, it is able to detect abnormalities in primary hemostasis and coagulation.

The *thrombotic status analyzer (TSA)* test involves drawing a whole blood sample through a capillary tube, which induces platelet activation and capillary tube occlusion. This assay allows measurement of thrombotic and thrombolytic activities in non-anticoagulated blood [25]. It can assess defective or excessive platelet function and monitor antiplatelet and thrombolytic therapy.

Impact (Diamed, Cressier, Switzerland) involves rotation of a cone filled with whole blood in order to create a high shear stress mimicking the intra-arterial environment. Platelet adhesion and aggregation on an extracellular matrix are then analyzed. This can be used to

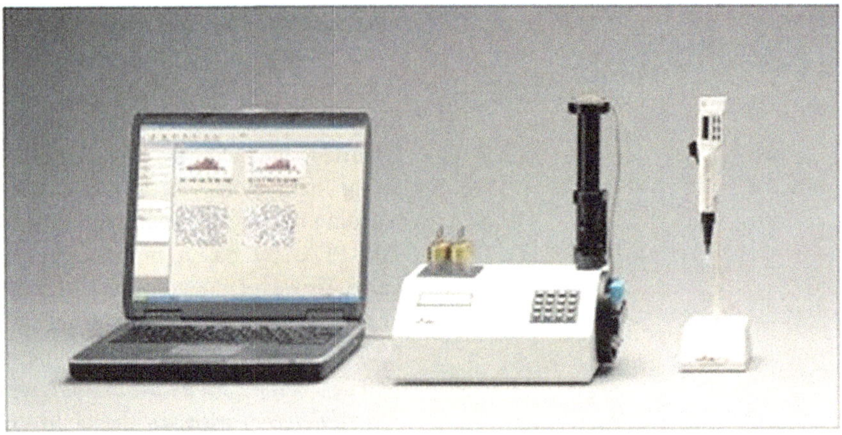

Fig. 5.4 Impact-R (Diamed, Cressier, Switzerland)

assess platelet function in patients with diabetes, thrombocytopenia, vWD and thrombotic thrombocytopenic purpura [26]. *Impact-R (Diamed)* involves the incubation of a platelet agonist with the whole blood sample prior to addition of antiplatelet agents in order to measure changes in surface coverage (Fig. 5.4). There was modest correlation found between this method and LTA. This assay is dependent on hematocrit and platelet levels [27], and clinical experience with device is limited.

Platelet Mediated Thrombin Generation

Activated clotting time (ACT) is a parameter of global platelet function that has been used to monitor heparin anticoagulation. Various systems and tests have been developed, including the *HMS Plus Hemostasis Management System (Medtronic USA, Minneapolis, MN)* (Fig. 5.5), the *Hemochron series (Keller medical, Bad Sodenam Taunus, Germany)* (Fig. 5.6) *and i-STAT Kaolin ACT (Abbott Point of Care, Abbott Park, IL)* (Fig. 5.7). These tests generally operate based on the mixing of a whole blood sample with a particulate activator, such as kaolin, silica, glass or celite. Complete activation is indicated when clots form as activated thrombin converts fibrinogen to fibrin. The type of activator used and the dose of heparin given will affect the degree of ACT prolongation [21]. ACT is also influenced by thrombocytopenia, impaired platelet function, hemodilution, low fibrinogen, coagulation factor deficiencies, and temperature [21].

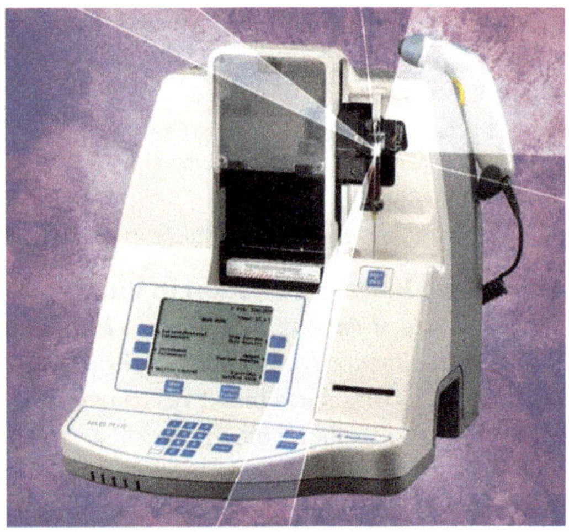

Fig. 5.5 HMS Plus Hemostasis Management System (Medtronic USA, Minneapolis, MN)

HemoSTATUS is a test that exploits the ability of PAF to accelerate the clot formation of the kaolin-ACT [28]. This test is performed on the *HMS plus* system with various cartridges preloaded with increasing concentrations of PAF. A clot ratio (CR) is determined for each individual patient based on the PAF-accelerated ACT compared to the standard ACT. The patient's CR is compared to the maximal CR, determined from a group of normal volunteers, to provide a relative measure of platelet function. In the setting of platelet dysfunction, higher concentrations of

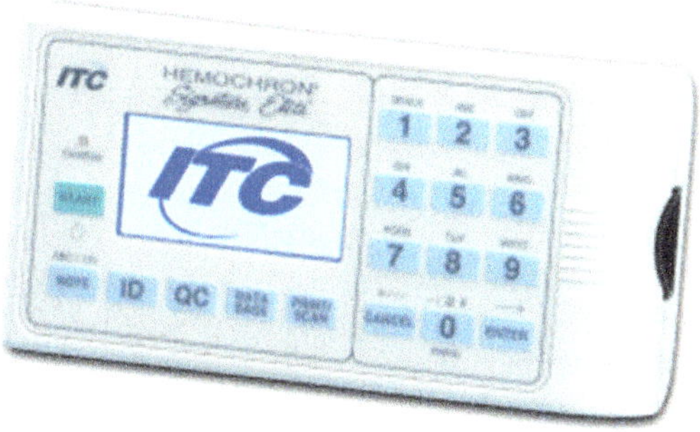

Fig. 5.6 Hemochron Signature Elite—whole blood microcoagulation system (Keller medical, Bad Sodenam Tannus, Germany)

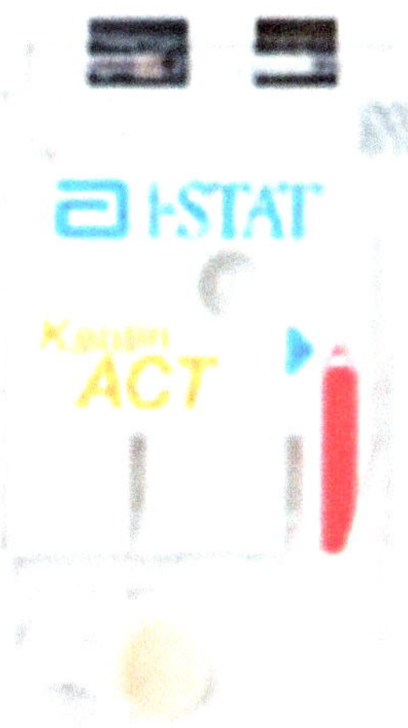

Fig. 5.7 i-STAT Kaolin ACT (Abbott Point of Care, Abbott Park, IL)

PAF are required to achieve a comparable PAF-accelerated ACT. As well, the maximal CR improved after desmopressin and platelet administration. This test is insensitive to aspirin and GP Ib function, but may be useful for monitoring GP IIb/IIIa inhibitors [29].

Thromboelastography (*TEG*) (Fig. 5.8) *or rotational thromboelastometry* (*ROTEM*) (Fig. 5.9) are another set of tests measuring the efficiency of blood coagulation (platelet function, clot strength and fibrinolysis) by triggering clot formation, followed by computerized coagulation analysis [30]. As blood clots in an oscillating cup, the torque of the cup is transmitted to the immersed pin. The computer produces a tracing in which the reaction time represents the rate of

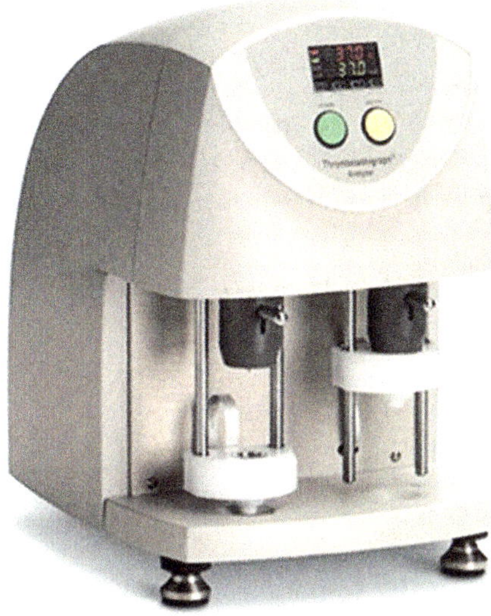

Fig. 5.8 TEG® 5000 Thrombelastograph® Hemostasis Analyzer system (Haemonetics Corporation, Braintree, MA)

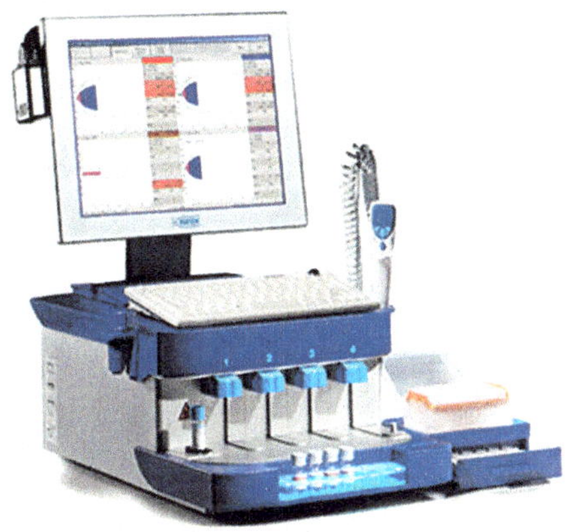

Fig. 5.9 Rotational)thromboelastometry (ROTEM) point-of-care diagnostics system (Tem International GmbH, Munich, Germany)

initial fibrin formation, and the maximal amplitude correlates with the absolute strength of the clot (Fig. 5.10a, b). TEG and ROTEM are less-specific platelet function tests, generally used to determine the risk of bleeding and to guide transfusion requirements [31]. It has been used in

a

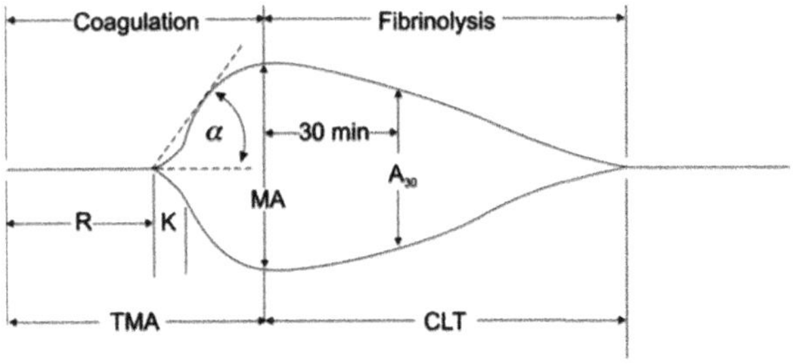

R	R time is the period of time of latency from the time that the blood was placed in the TEG® analyzer until the initial fibrin formation. This represents the enzymatic portion of coagulation.
K	K time is a measure of the speed to reach a certain level of clot strength. This represents clot kinetics.
α	α measures the rapidity of fibrin build-up and cross-linking (clot strengthening). This represents fibrinogen level.
MA	MA, or Maximum Amplitude, is a direct function of the maximum dynamic properties of fibrin and platelet bonding via GPIIb/IIIa and represents the ultimate strength of the fibrin clot. This represents platelet function/aggregation.
LY30	LY30 measures the rate of amplitude reduction 30 minutes after MA. This represents clot lysis.

b

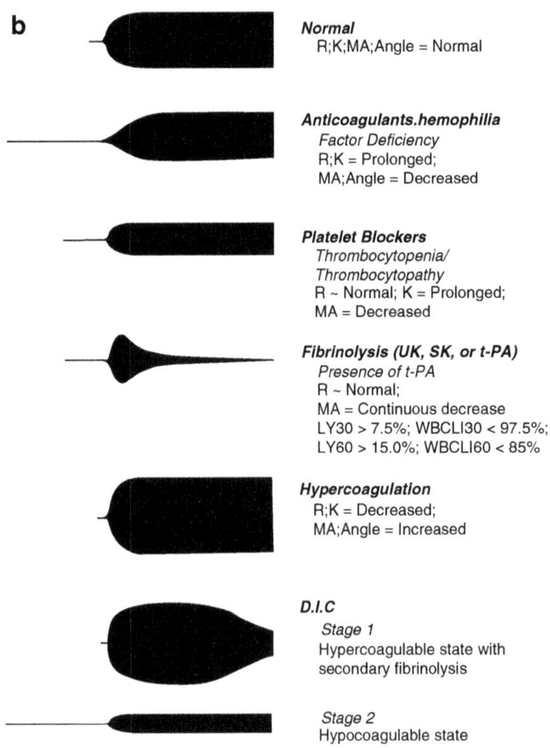

Fig. 5.10 (**a**) Thromboelastogram interpretation (TEG®5000 user manual). (**b**) Thromboelastogram qualitative analysis (TEG®5000 user manual)

various clinical settings, such as surgery and anesthesia, but rarely in neuro-interventional procedures [32]. Of note, TEG may be insensitive to samples from patients who have taken aspirin [33].

Hemodyne (Hemodyne Inc, Midlothian, VA) assesses platelet contractile forces (PCF) and clot rigidity. It is a simple test that detects the ability of platelets to interact with a fibrin network. PCF is decreased in thrombocytopenia, various acquired and genetic platelet abnormalities, and GP IIb/IIIa inhibitors. Overall, this is a nonspecific test in which low PCF values may predict bleeding risk, while higher values predict thrombotic tendencies [34].

Platelet Activation

Several tests have been developed to measure levels of platelet release products in plasma or blood to give an estimate of platelet activation in vivo. In particular, measurement of TXA2 may be useful in evaluating the efficacy of drugs inhibiting the COX pathway, such as aspirin. TXA2 is synthesized by platelets from arachidonic acid and is released on activation to amplify further platelet activation and recruit additional platelets to the site of injury. Although TXA2 has a very short half-life, its stable metabolites, thromboxane B2 (TXB2) and 11-dehydroxy-TXB2, can be measured in blood and urine via immunoassays or mass spectroscopy. Measurement of these metabolites may be altered by platelet activation during sampling.

References

1. Angiolillo DJ, Ueno M, Goto S. Basic principles of platelet biology and clinical implications. Circ J. 2010;74:597–607.
2. FitzGerald GA. Mechanisms of platelet activation: thromboxane A2 as an amplifying signal for other agonists. Am J Cardiol. 1991;68(7):11B–5.
3. Offerman S. Activation of platelet function through G protein-coupled receptors. Circ Res. 2006;99: 1293–304.
4. Duke WW. The relation of blood platelets to hemorrhagic disease. JAMA. 1910;55:1185.
5. Burns ER, Lawrence C. Bleeding time: a guide to its diagnostic and clinical utility. Arch Pathol Lab Med. 1989;113(11):1219–24.
6. Harrison P, Lordkipanidze M. Testing platelet function. Hematol Oncol Clin North Am. 2013;27(3): 411–41.
7. Lind SE. The bleeding time does not predict surgical bleeding time. Blood. 1991;77:2547–52.
8. Barber A, Green D, Galluzzo T, Ts'ao CH. The bleeding time as a preoperative screening test. Am J Med. 1985;78(5):761–4.
9. Gandhi CD, et al. Platelet function inhibitors and platelet function testing in neurointerventional procedures. J NeuroInterv Surg. 2014;6:567–77.
10. Harrison P, Horton A, Grant D, et al. Immunoplatelet counting: a proposed new reference procedure. Br J Haematol. 2000;108:228.
11. Bowles KM, Bloxham DM, Perry DJ, Baglin TP. Discrepancy between impedance and immunofluorescence platelet counting has implications for clinical decision making in patients with idiopathic thrombocytopenia purpura. Br J Haematol. 2006;134:320.
12. Born GV. Aggregation of blood platelets by adenosine diphosphate and its reversal. Nature. 1962;194:927–9.
13. Mascelli MA, Worley S, Veriabo NJ, et al. Rapid assessment of platelet function with a modified whole-blood aggregometer in percutaneous transluminal coronary angioplasty patients receiving anti-GP IIb/IIIa therapy. Circulation. 1997;96:3860.
14. Thompson NT, Scrutton MC, Wallis RB. Particle volume changes associated with light transmittance changes in the platelet aggregometer: dependence upon aggregating agent and effectiveness of stimulus. Thromb Res. 1986;41:615–26.
15. Nicholson NS, Panser-Knodle SG, Haas NF, et al. Assessment of platelet function assays. Am Heart J. 1998;135:S170–8.
16. Ozaki Y, Satoh K, Yatomi Y, et al. Detection of platelet aggregates with a particle counting method using light scattering. Anal Biochem. 1994;218:284.
17. Yamamoto T, Egawa Y, Shirasawa Y, et al. A laser light scattering in situ system for counting aggregates in blood platelet aggregation. Meas Sci Technol. 1995;6:174.
18. Breet NJ, van Werkum JW, Bouman HJ, et al. Comparison of platelet function tests in predicting clinical outcome in patients undergoing coronary stent implantation. JAMA. 2010;303(8):754–62.
19. Jakubowski JA, Li YG, Small DS, et al. A comparison of the VerifyNow P2Y12 point-of-care device and light transmission aggregometry to monitor platelet function with prasugrel and clopidogrel: an integrated analysis. J Cardiovasc Pharmacol. 2010;56:29–37.
20. EPIC Investigators. Use of a monoclonal antibody directed against the platelet glycoprotein IIb/IIIa receptor in high-risk coronary angioplasty. The EPIC investigation. N Engl J Med. 1994;330:956–61.
21. Fries D, Streif W. Point-of-care testing in critically ill patients. Semin Thromb Hemost. 2015;41:75–83.
22. Fressinaud E, Veyradier A, Sigaud M, et al. Therapeutic monitoring of von Willebrand disease: interest and limits of a platelet function analyser at high shear rates. Br J Haematol. 1999;106:777.

23. Favaloro EJ. Clinical utility of the PFA-100. Semin Thromb Hemost. 2008;34(8):709–33.
24. Fricke W, Kouides P, Kessler C, et al. A multicenter clinical evaluation of the Clot Signature Analyzer. J Thromb Haemost. 2004;2:763–8.
25. Gorog DA, Kovacs IB. Thrombotic status analyser. Measurement of platelet-rich thrombus formation and lysis in native blood. Thromb Haemost. 1995; 73:514.
26. Shenkman B, Inbal A, Tamarin I, et al. Diagnosis of thrombotic thrombocytopenic purpura based on modulation by patient plasma of normal platelet adhesion under flow condition. Br J Haematol. 2003;120:597.
27. Varon D, Dardik R, Shenkman B, et al. A new method for quantitative analysis of whole blood platelet interaction with extracellular matrix under flow conditions. Thromb Res. 1997;85(4):283–94.
28. Despotis GJ, Levine V, Filos KS, et al. Evaluation of a new point-of-care test that measures PAF-mediated acceleration of coagulation in cardiac surgical patients. Anesthesiology. 1996;85:1311.
29. Coiffic A, Cazes E, Janvier G, et al. Inhibition of platelet aggregation by abciximab but not by aspirin can be detected by a new point-of-care test, the hemostatus. Thromb Res. 1999;95:83.
30. Shore Lesserson L, Manspeizer HE, DePerio M, et al. Thromboelastography-guided transfusion algorithm reduces transfusions in complex cardiac surgery. Anesth Analg. 1999;88:312–9.
31. Afshari A, Wikkelso A, Brok J, et al. Thrombelastography (TEG) or thromboelastometry (ROTEM) to monitor haemotherapy versus usual care in patients with massive transfusion. Cochrane Database Syst Rev. 2011;3, CD007871.
32. Lombard FW, Welsby IJ, Alexander MJ. TEG detects inadequate response. Neurocrit Care. 2006;4:32–4. doi:10.1385/NCC:4:1:032.
33. Blais N, Pharand C, Lordkipanidzé M, et al. Response to aspirin in healthy individuals. Cross-comparison of light transmission aggregometry, VerifyNow system, platelet count drop, thromboelastography (TEG) and urinary 11-dehydrothromboxane B(2). Thromb Haemost. 2009;102:404.
34. Greilich PE, Carr ME, Zekert SL, Dent RM. Quantitative assessment of platelet function and clot structure in patients with severe coronary artery disease. Am J Med Sci. 1994;307:15.

Role of Antiplatelet Therapy in Neurosurgery: Efficacy and Safety Profiles

6

Nicholas Bowen and Shaker A. Mousa

Review of Aspirin and Clopidogrel

It is vital to understand the pharmacokinetic profile of antiplatelet agents and the reason why patients take the agents. Knowing the reason for antiplatelet therapy helps to determine the risks of its discontinuation. A patient using antiplatelet therapy for primary or secondary prevention of vascular events will have a lower risk of vascular events than a patient who is using antiplatelet therapy to prevent stent thrombosis. Depending on how long it has been since stent placement, the risk of stent thrombosis may outweigh the risk of increased bleeding. Knowing the half-life of the drug and its metabolite(s) and the time required for platelet homeostasis to return after antiplatelet discontinuation is important. This information determines how far in advance to discontinue a drug prior to surgery. If there is still delayed platelet inhibition or pharmacologically active drug in a patient, they could still be at increased risk of bleeding despite having stopped the medication. Other studies have been dedicated solely to the pharmacokinetics of aspirin and clopidogrel and are widely available, and thus the intent of this chapter is to cover the important details that relate to the current surgery recommendations.

N. Bowen, PharmD
S.A. Mousa, PhD, MBA, FACC, FACB (✉)
The Pharmaceutical Research Institute, Albany College of Pharmacy and Health Sciences, Rensselaer, NY 12144, USA
e-mail: shaker.mousa@acphs.edu

Aspirin

The antiplatelet effect of aspirin results from the irreversible acetylation of an important serine moiety of cyclooxygenase (COX-1) on the platelet. This acetylation impairs the COX-1 mediated synthesis of thromboxane A_2, which is responsible for platelet aggregation and vasoconstriction [1]. Figure 6.1 depicts the mechanism of action of antiplatelet agents [2, 3]. Despite aspirin having a short terminal half-life of 0.4 h before being metabolized to salicylate, platelets are rapidly rendered unable to regenerate COX-1 and subsequently thromboxane A_2 [4, 5]. Although salicylate has a longer half-life than aspirin (2.1 h), it does not possess any inhibitory effects on platelet COX-1 [5, 6]. No antidote is available for aspirin because it binds irreversibly. Fresh platelets that have not been exposed to aspirin must be created to have functioning COX-1 and thromboxane A_2 activity. Although a platelet's life span is 7–10 days, some authors have claimed it may take 12–14 days for normal levels of platelet COX-1 and thromboxane A_2 to return [7, 8]. The mechanism proposed for the extended delay in normalization was that the freshly produced platelets were created from

C.M. Loftus (ed.), *Anticoagulation and Hemostasis in Neurosurgery*,
DOI 10.1007/978-3-319-27327-3_6

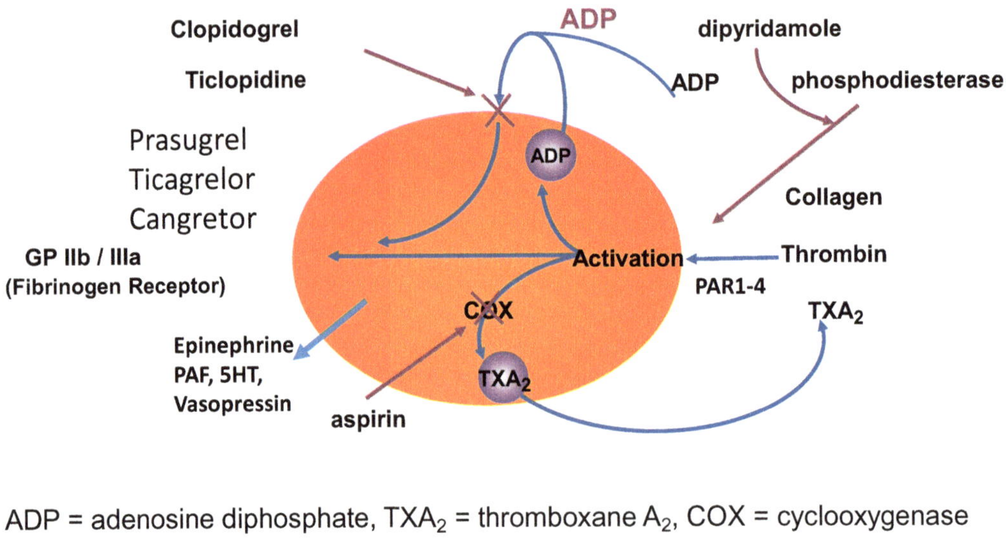

Fig. 6.1 Mechanism of action of antiplatelet agents

megakaryocytes with impaired COX-1 activity from prior aspirin exposure [7]. However, platelet aggregation recovers fully in 50 % of patients by day 3 and in 80 % of patients by day 4 [9]. Complete platelet function is achieved after approximately 7 days [8]. Recovery may have some variability between patients due to the dose ingested, bone marrow turnover, and the potential size of the platelet pool, determined by platelet count and patient size [10].

Clopidogrel

Clopidogrel is an oral, $P2Y_{12}$ receptor inhibitor. By irreversibly binding to the $P2Y_{12}$ receptor and modifying the adenosine diphosphate (ADP) receptor site, ADP is unable to bind, which prevents induction of platelet aggregation [11, 12]. Clopidogrel is a prodrug and requires hepatic activation to produce pharmacological activity. The antiplatelet efficacy is variable due to genetic variations in genes that are responsible for absorption and bio-activation of clopidogrel [13]. Maximum platelet aggregation inhibition of 40–60 % is achieved in 3–5 days [1]. Loading doses are often given to achieve therapeutic levels more rapidly [14]. Maximum platelet inhibition can be achieved within 6 h of a 300 mg loading dose [15]. Platelet inhibition can be seen within 2 h of ingestion [11]. Clopidogrel is concerning in surgery because some studies have reported carbon 14-labeled clopidogrel to have a half-life of >300 h at steady state [16]. However, the half-life of clopidogrel is roughly 6 h, and the active metabolite has a half-life of about 30 min [17]. Despite the concerning half-life of >300 h, normal platelet function returns after 7 days of discontinuation [18]. Similar to aspirin, there is no antidote for clopidogrel, which also binds irreversibly. A new pool of platelets must be created to replenish the platelets that have been irreversibly inhibited by clopidogrel. The week-long inhibition of platelet function can be problematic in patients who experience trauma or intracranial hemorrhage (ICH) because increased bleeding could potentially occur. Replenishing the platelet pool with uninhibited platelets via platelet transfusions may be the only way to reduce excessive bleeding in emergency situations such as trauma or ICH.

Utility of Aspirin and Clopidogrel

Aspirin is used in both primary and secondary prevention of atherothrombotic vascular events, myocardial infarction (MI), stroke, and vascular death. However, the utility of aspirin in primary prevention has been questioned [19]. Clopidogrel is often used in conjunction with aspirin in patients at high risk for ischemic events [20]. Clopidogrel may also be used for patients with allergies or intolerances to aspirin. Aspirin and clopidogrel are also used for dual antiplatelet therapy (DAPT) after stent placement. The differing mechanisms of platelet inhibition provide synergy in helping to prevent stent thrombosis. The challenge in prescribing these medications lies in balancing their risks and benefits.

The vascular protection provided by antiplatelet therapy was clearly demonstrated in a 2002 meta-analysis of 287 studies in patients ($n = 135{,}000$) at high risk for occlusive vascular events [21]. Antiplatelet therapy reduced serious vascular events by 22 %, nonfatal MIs by 34 %, nonfatal stroke by 28 %, and vascular mortality by 15 %. Aspirin was the most commonly investigated drug in the meta-analysis. The authors concluded that aspirin in daily doses of 75–150 mg appeared to be as effective as larger doses of aspirin for long-term treatment. In addition, clopidogrel could be used as an effective alternative for patients who were unable to take aspirin.

Despite vascular protection benefits, antiplatelet therapy comes with risks. The increased risk of bleeding is worrisome with these agents, especially in the setting of neurosurgery where proper hemostasis is essential. One of the primary difficulties in determining the bleeding risk associated with low dose aspirin is the variable definition of "low dose" aspirin therapy. It has been defined as 75–162 mg daily in the CHARISMA trial [22], 50–325 mg daily by Berger et al. [23], 75–325 mg daily by Mills et al. [24], 75–150 mg daily by Rodríguez et al. [25], 75–100 mg daily by the American College of Chest Physicians [26], and 75 mg daily in the SALT trial [27]. Thus, great attention to detail must be used when assessing the risk-reducing benefits and bleeding risks associated with low dose aspirin.

A meta-analysis by Serebruany et al. [28] included 51 randomized, controlled trials of 338,191 patients and divided antiplatelet therapy into 6 groups based on drug and dose. The data showed there was no difference in Thrombolysis in Myocardial Infarction (TIMI) major bleeds between the aspirin <100 mg daily group (1.7 %, 95 % CI [1.4–1.9 %]) and the aspirin 100–325 mg daily group (1.7 %, 95 % CI [1.5–1.85 %]). There was an increase in TIMI major bleeds in the aspirin >325 mg daily group (2.5 %, 95 % CI [1.7–3.3 %]) vs. the aspirin 100–325 mg daily group (1.7 %, 95 % CI [1.5–1.85 %]), but no P value was calculated. When looking at total bleeds (both major and minor), aspirin <100 mg daily was the safest option (3.6 %, 95 % CI [3.3–3.9 %]). Aspirin 100–325 mg daily and aspirin >325 mg were much more problematic in regard to total bleeds (9.1 %, 95 % CI [8.7–9.4 %] and 9.9 %, 95 % CI [8.4–11.4 %], respectively). It appears there is no difference in major bleeding between aspirin <100 mg daily and aspirin 100–325 mg daily, while doses >325 mg daily may lead to increased bleeding. For all bleeds, aspirin <100 mg daily was the safest while 100–325 mg daily and >325 mg daily were similar for total bleeds. For neurosurgery patients who need to be on aspirin, less than 100 mg daily is likely the safest option.

The rates of bleeding for clopidogrel use were less clear in the Serebruany et al. meta-analysis. Major bleeds were recorded in patients taking thienopyridines—a major bleeding rate of 2.1 % (95 % CI [1.9–2.3 %]). For total bleeds, the rate of bleeding was 8.5 % (95 % CI [8.1–8.8 %]) [28]. No P values were reported between aspirin and clopidogrel. However, given the increase in both major and total bleeds, it appears reasonable to use aspirin over clopidogrel whenever possible especially when one antiplatelet agent must be used for prevention of stent thrombosis during surgery.

Perioperative Use of Antiplatelet Agents

There are two primary concerns with antiplatelet therapy in the perioperative setting: continued use of antiplatelet agents during surgery could lead to increased bleeding during surgery and discontinuation of antiplatelet agents could result in the occurrence of vascular complications. A review by Korte et al. [29] reported that several studies showed an increase of bleeding and transfusion of blood products with the perioperative use of aspirin. However, there is a lack of studies that have investigated the use of aspirin in neurosurgery. A meta-analysis by Burger et al. [30] reported that aspirin at relatively higher doses possibly increased the risk of bleeding-related fatalities, and relatively "low-dose aspirin neither increases the level of the severity of bleeding complications nor the perioperative mortality because of bleeding complications." Palmer and colleagues reported that aspirin was not associated with any bleeding fatalities [31]. But they reported that the combination of such agents with certain pathologies may lead to an increased risk of postoperative hematomas. It is unclear if age, reason for first surgery, or other patient characteristics contributed to postoperative hematomas. Also, anticoagulants were not excluded, and it is unclear how many patients may have been on both anticoagulants and aspirin.

Suddenly discontinuing antiplatelet therapy can result in a rebound effect. There is a temporary period of increased thromboxane A_2 production and decreased fibrinolysis, which leads to increased prothrombotic activity [32–34]. A prospective study reported that patients who had recently discontinued aspirin, primarily for elective surgery, were responsible for 5.4 % of all patients admitted for acute coronary syndrome (ACS) [35]. The average time for ACS onset after aspirin withdrawal was 12 days. Recent aspirin withdrawers (patients who discontinued aspirin within 3 weeks prior to ACS) had significantly higher rates of death or myocardial infarction (21.9 % vs. 12.4 %, $P=0.04$) and bleeding complication (13.7 % vs. 5.9 %, $P=0.03$) than patients who discontinued aspirin earlier than 3 weeks prior to ACS. Retrospective studies have also seen increases in number of cardiovascular events ranging from 2.3 to 6.1 %. The timing from aspirin withdrawal and incidence of cardiovascular events was on average 8.5 days for ACS, 14.3 days for stroke, and 25.8 days for peripheral vascular events [36–38].

A meta-analysis of 50,279 patients taking aspirin for secondary prevention reported a threefold increase (OR = 3.14) in major cardiovascular events in aspirin withdrawers compared to those who remained on aspirin therapy [39]. The risk was even greater in patients with coronary stents (OR = 89.78). The average time from aspirin discontinuation to a thrombotic cardiovascular event was 10.7 days. The authors concluded that aspirin withdrawal in patients with ischemic heart disease or other apparent cardiovascular disease was associated with obvious, prognostically adverse consequences. They recommended only discontinuing aspirin therapy if the risk of bleeding far surpassed the risk of atherothrombotic consequences.

Clearly, there are risks associated with both the continued use of antiplatelet agents during surgery and the discontinuation of antiplatelets prior to surgery. Although it is likely that aspirin and other antiplatelet agents may lead to increased bleeding in neurosurgery, the real risk has not been determined. The high risk and consequences associated with excessive bleeding in a closed system have led researchers to rely on the results of continued aspirin use in other surgical studies. Guidelines for antiplatelet use in neurosurgery are also scarce. The guidelines for the perioperative use of antiplatelet agents typically come from The American College of Chest Physicians (CHEST), The American College of Cardiology (ACC), The American Heart Association (AHA), and The American Stroke Association (ASA), although they do not specifically address neurosurgery. The guidelines are clearer for patients who are on antiplatelet therapy and have planned surgery than for patients on antiplatelet therapy who require immediate surgery due to trauma or spontaneous ICH.

Patients who require antiplatelet therapy for prevention of stent thrombosis pose a challenging dilemma because the risk of stent thrombosis may outweigh the risk of bleeding even during neurosurgery. The type of stent used is also important. Bare metal stents are fully endothelialized in 4–6 weeks, however, drug-eluting stents require up to a year. The highest risk of thrombosis occurs during the endothelialization, and the risk is further increased when antiplatelet therapy is abruptly discontinued [40]. The 2014 ACC/AHA guidelines are very specific to patients with a previous percutaneous coronary intervention (PCI) and stent placement because they include both timing to surgery and antiplatelet use [41]. For timing of elective non-cardiac surgery in patients with previous PCI, the ACC and AHA made the following recommendations [41]:

Class I

1. "Elective non-cardiac surgery should be delayed 14 days after balloon angioplasty (*Level of Evidence:* C) and 30 days after bare metal stent (BMS) implantation. (*Level of Evidence:* B)"
2. "Elective non-cardiac surgery should be optimally delayed 365 days after drug-eluting stent (DES) implantation. (*Level of Evidence:* B)"

Class IIa

1. "In patients in whom non-cardiac surgery is required, a consensus decision among treating clinicians as to the relative risks of surgery and discontinuation or continuation of antiplatelet therapy can be useful. (*Level of Evidence*: C)"

Class IIb

1. "Elective non-cardiac surgery after DES implantation may be considered after 180 days if the risk of further delay is greater than the expected risks of ischemia and stent thrombosis. (*Level of Evidence*: B)"

Class III: HARM

1. "Elective non-cardiac surgery should not be performed within 30 days after BMS implantation or within 12 months after DES implantation in patients in whom dual antiplatelet therapy (DAPT) will need to be discontinued perioperatively. (*Level of Evidence*: B)"
2. "Elective non-cardiac surgery should not be performed within 14 days of balloon angioplasty in patients in whom aspirin will need to be discontinued perioperatively. (*Level of Evidence*: C)"

In addition to timing, the agent used can also influence the risk of bleeding. As stated before, clopidogrel may be associated with higher rates of bleeding and reversal of platelet inhibition occurs at a slower rate than with aspirin [9, 18, 28]. It is not surprising that the guidelines developed by the ACC and the AHA favor aspirin over clopidogrel. For the antiplatelet agent used in the perioperative setting, they made the following recommendations [41].

Class I

1. "In patients undergoing urgent non-cardiac surgery during the first 4–6 weeks after BMS or DES implantation, DAPT should be continued unless the relative risk of bleeding outweighs the benefit of the prevention of stent thrombosis. (Level of Evidence: C)"
2. "In patients who have received coronary stents and must undergo surgical procedures that mandate the discontinuation of $P2Y_{12}$ platelet receptor-inhibitor therapy, it is recommended that aspirin be continued if possible and the $P2y_{12}$ platelet receptor be restarted as soon as possible after surgery. (Level of Evidence: C)"
3. "Management of the perioperative antiplatelet therapy should be determined by a consensus of the surgeon, anesthesiologist, cardiologist, and patients, who should weigh the relative risk of bleeding with that of stent thrombosis. (Level of Evidence: C)"

Class IIb

1. "In patients undergoing nonemergency/nonurgent non-cardiac surgery who have not had previous coronary stenting, it may be reasonable to continue aspirin when the risk of potential increased cardiac events outweigh the risk of increased bleeding. (Level of Evidence: B)"

Class III: No Benefit

1. "Initiation or continuation of aspirin is not beneficial in patients undergoing elective non-carotid surgery who have not had previous coronary stenting (Level of Evidence: B), unless the risk of ischemic events outweighs the risk of surgical bleeding. (Level of Evidence: C)"

These recommendations could apply for patients taking aspirin for primary and secondary prevention of cardiovascular events because their recommendations rely on the risk vs. benefit of antiplatelet therapy. In neurosurgery, it is unlikely that the risk of cardiac events will outweigh the risk of bleeding, especially in patients without stents. In the 2012 CHEST supplement to The Antithrombotic Therapy and Prevention of Thrombosis Evidence-Based Clinical Practice Guidelines [26], a review of primary stoke prevention with aspirin, there was no significant reduction in number of strokes including nonfatal ischemic and hemorrhagic strokes in low, moderate, or high cardiovascular risk patients. The CHEST guidelines were similar to the ACC/AHA guidelines, however, they specifically mentioned secondary prevention: "For patients with established CAD including patients after the first year post-ACS and/or with prior CABG surgery: We recommend long-term single antiplatelet therapy with aspirin 75–100 mg daily or clopidogrel 75 mg daily over no antiplatelet therapy (Grade 1A). We suggest single over dual antiplatelet therapy with aspirin plus clopidogrel (Grade 2B)" [26].

Once again, risk vs. benefit applies to these recommendations. *In the setting of neurosurgery, discontinuation is likely the right decision nearly every time*. The risk of increased bleeding is more dangerous than the risk of a cardiovascular event while on the short discontinuation from antiplatelet therapy during surgery. The patients who experienced increased vascular events had discontinued aspirin and had remained off therapy. Patients who must take a short antiplatelet therapy hiatus for surgery may not see an increase in vascular events because resuming therapy may counteract the time of increased prothrombotic activity. The average time to vascular events after discontinuing antiplatelet therapy ranged from 8.5 to 25.8 days [35–39]. Patients would likely discontinue antiplatelet therapy for only 5–7 days, depending on the agent, prior to surgery and resume therapy shortly after surgery. Initiation of antiplatelet therapy would likely occur before the average time of increased vascular events. Quickly reinitiating antiplatelet therapy after surgery may prevent the occurrence of these vascular events.

As the guidelines recommend, timing of elective surgeries in patients with stents is important. In patients at high risk for surgical bleeding, $P2Y_{12}$ platelet receptor inhibitors should be discontinued, however, aspirin should be continued throughout surgery. The $P2Y_{12}$ platelet receptor inhibitor should be resumed as soon as possible after surgery. The management of the patient's antiplatelet therapy should be carefully discussed between the cardiologist, neurosurgeon, anesthesiologist, patient, and pharmacist. Pharmacists can provide a wealth of knowledge about mechanism of action, half-life, time form discontinuation to platelet normalization, and possible alternative options in the perioperative setting. Aspirin is the drug of choice when the patient must remain on one antiplatelet agent during surgery. Any antiplatelet medications discontinued prior to surgery should immediately be restarted once the patient is out of surgery and stabilized.

Does Antiplatelet Therapy Increase the Risk of Hematoma Expansion?

Thrombocytopenia and coagulopathy are common after traumatic brain injury and the occurrence of these abnormalities increases as severity of injury increases [42]. Potentially exacerbating hematoma expansion is the use of antiplatelet agents prior to head injury. The limited number of platelets remaining in the thrombocytopenic patient could potentially be irreversibly inactivated by aspirin or clopidogrel, leading to a further inability to prevent excessive bleeding.

The primary concern with hematoma expansion is its direct link to increased morbidity and mortality [42–47]. Some studies have associated anticoagulants, specifically warfarin, with increased hematoma expansion and mortality [43–45, 47, 48–50, 51]. It is reasonable to question if antiplatelet therapy would also have a similar association. Unfortunately, the data is less clear. The 2010 AHA and ASA guidelines developed for patients suffering ICH recommended warfarin reversal in INR-elevated patients [52]. They also recommended replacement therapy for severe coagulation factor deficiency patients. However, no recommendations regarding the reversal of antiplatelet therapy were provided because of limited and conflicting studies. When closely inspected, there is no surprise why there are no guidelines written based on the studies that have investigated the effect of antiplatelet therapy on hematoma expansion. There were large variations between studies as far as the definition of hematoma expansion, the inclusion window from symptom onset to hospital admission, and time from symptom onset until first computed tomography (CT) scan. Several studies contained significant flaws in data recording, lack of patient demographics, and poor study design. In the defense of some of these studies, the researchers were assessing other factors or agents besides antiplatelets on hematoma expansion and decided to include an analysis of their patients on antiplatelet therapy. Another common issue was that several studies failed to exclude patients who were on prior anticoagulants. Failing to exclude these from the study contaminates the results because anticoagulants are known to contribute to hematoma expansion and increase mortality. It would have been prudent to exclude warfarin from the studies because warfarin is well known to increase bleeding. Exclusion is particularly important in the studies that are directly investigating the effect of antiplatelet agents on hematoma expansion. Table 6.1 is a summary of some of the most substantial and relevant studies on the impact of antiplatelet therapy on hematoma expansion.

Flibotte and colleagues [53] were primarily assessing the risk of hematoma expansion and mortality in patients on warfarin, and determined that 40 % of the study population was on antiplatelets (more than were on warfarin). Although this study supports that antiplatelet therapy does not increase hematoma expansion, its limitations were a small sample size, contamination of results with data from patients on warfarin, and a lack of patient demographics. It was also unclear how many patients on antiplatelet therapy were also on warfarin.

Saloheimo and colleagues [54] did not report the exact time to first CT scan after symptom onset in their study. The first CT imaging was done in 73 % (32/44) of aspirin users and 70 % (97/138) of non-aspirin or warfarin users on day one of symptom onset. However, large variations can occur between groups because hematoma expansion occurs early and rapidly. Thus it is prudent to include time to first CT scan because most expansion occurs within 6 h of symptom onset. Although aspirin users had the smallest median volume of ICH (16 mL) compared with non-aspirin and warfarin users (20 mL), there was no significant difference in median volume between nonusers and aspirin users. The study did not find an association between aspirin and hematoma enlargement. However, the exclusion of numerous deaths and emergent surgeries in a small population may have accounted for lack of significance because these patients did not have a second CT. Only 56.5 % (78/138) of nonusers of aspirin or warfarin and 47.7 % (21/44) of aspirin users received a second CT scan. Age and comorbid conditions may also have impacted the results of the study because aspirin users were older than non-aspirin or warfarin users.

Toyoda and colleagues [55] recorded both the agent and dose of the antiplatelet for the three agents used at various doses and combinations. Of the 57 patients on antiplatelet therapy, 33 were included in calculating the influence of antiplatelet therapy on hematoma enlargement. Patients who were excluded from the analysis had died ($n=4$) or required surgery ($n=20$); the study may have been underpowered. A greater percentage of the patients in the antiplatelet group were over 70 years of age, had suffered more symptomatic ischemic strokes, and had higher rates of diabetes mellitus and heart disease than those patients not on antiplatelet agents.

Table 6.1 Studies on the role of antiplatelet therapy (APT) on hematoma expansion

Study	Population	APT agents + daily dose (mg)[a] + no. of patients (n)	ACT excluded? If not, no. of patients on ACT	Results
Flibotte 2004	183 patients <72 h of symptom onset prior to hospital admission and CT scan evidence of non-traumatic ICH	None specified	No; study designed to determine risk of hematoma expansion in W patients	APT not associated with increased initial hematoma volume, APT use 34.8 mL ± 40.5 mL vs. non-APT use 35.4 mL ± 38.7 mL, $P = 0.92$ APT not associated with hematoma expansion OR 0.42, 95 % CI [0.12–1.46]
Saloheimo 2005	44 ASA patients CT evidence of ICH or death record confirming ICH Control group = 138 patients not on ASA or W with CT evidence of ICH or death record confirming ICH	ASA median dose 250 (range 50–500)	No W users had their own group ($n = 26$)	No difference in hematoma expansion between non-ASA users (8 % [6/78]) and ASA users (19 % [4/21], no *P* value provided Significant increase in mean enlargement of hematomas by percentage in ASA users (12.8 % ± 22.6) vs. non-ASA users (4.8 % ± 16.1), $P = 0.006$
Toyoda 2005	57 patients on APT with non-traumatic ICH hospitalized within 24 h of stroke onset Control group = 194 patients not on APT with non-traumatic ICH hospitalized within 24 h of stroke onset	ASA 81 ($n = 15$) ASA 100 ($n = 16$) ASA 162 ($n = 1$) ASA 200 ($n = 1$) T 100 ($n = 2$) T 200 ($n = 9$) T 300 ($n = 1$) Cilostazol 100 ($n = 3$) ASA 100 + T 100 ($n = 2$) ASA 81 + T 200 ($n = 5$) ASA 100 + cilostazol 100 ($n = 1$) T 200 + cilostazol 200 ($n = 1$)	Yes	Hematoma enlargement >40 % within 2 hospital days was greater in patients on APT (27 % [9/33]) vs. patients not on APT therapy (8 % [12/147]), $P < 0.005$ On multivariate analysis, APT was associated with hematoma enlargement OR 7.67, 95 % CI [1.62–36.4], $P = < 0.01$ Multivariate analysis of the 31 patients on ASA 81–100 mg and the 194 patients not on APT showed that ASA was an independent predictor of hematoma enlargement, OR 5.81, 95 % CI [1.01–33.3], no *P* value provided
Sorimachi 2007	8 patients hematoma enlargement ≥20 % 180 patients no hematoma enlargement ≥20 %	Hematoma enlargement group ASA 80 or 100 ($n = 5$, 1 also on W) No hematoma enlargement no ASA dose specified, ($n = 14$)	No Hematoma enlargement group ($n = 1$ on W alone, $n = 1$ on ASA + W) No hematoma enlargement group ($n = 14$)	Hematoma expansion ≥20 %, observed in 26.3 % (5/19) of patients on ASA therapy

(continued)

Table 6.1 (continued)

Study	Population	APT agents + daily dose (mg)[a] + no. of patients (n)	ACT excluded? If not, no. of patients on ACT	Results
Toyoda 2008	180 patients on APT hospitalized within 24 h of non-traumatic ICH Control group=738 patients not on APT or ACT hospitalized within 24 h of non-traumatic ICH	ASA 81 (*n*=62) ASA 100 (*n*=41) ASA other doses (*n*=5) T 100 (*n*=9) T 200 (*n*=29) T 300 (*n*=3) Cilostazol 100 (*n*=3) Cilostazol 200 (*n*=3) Various other single agents (*n*=6) DAPT (mainly ASA 81 and T 100) (*n*=19)	No W users were in a separate study group	APT associated with increase in hematoma expansion, OR adjusted for age and sex: 1.71, 95 % CI [1.04–2.81], *P*=0.036 APT associated with increase in hematoma expansion, multivariate adjusted odds ratio: 1.92, 95 % CI [1.10–3.34], *P*=0.022 Multivariate analysis showed APT did not increase the risk of large hematomas ASA alone associated with increase in hematoma expansion, OR adjusted for age and sex: 1.80, 95 % CI [1.02–3.17], *P*=0.044 ASA alone associated with increase in hematoma expansion, multivariate adjusted OR: 1.99, 95 % CI [1.05–3.79], *P*=0.035
Moussouttas 2009	17 patients on APT with a spontaneous supratentorial ICH diagnosed within 6 h of onset and a follow-up CT ~48 h later Control group=53 patients not on APT with a spontaneous supratentorial ICH diagnosed within 6 h of symptom onset and a follow-up CT ~48 h later	ASA (*n*=15) C (*n*=2) No doses specified	Yes	Antiplatelet therapy not a predictor of ICH expansion >25 %, >33 % or >50 %, *P*=0.81, 0.93, 0.64, respectively No difference in initial CT scan volume (mL) between APT patients (13.8±11.4) vs. non-APT patients (19.2±15.4), *P*=0.25 No difference in second CT scan volume (mL) between APT patients (21.5±24.6) vs. non-APT patients (24.6 ±25.1), *P*=0.50 No difference in hematoma expansion (mL) between APT users (7.7±22.7) vs. non-APT users (5.5±14.3), *P*=0.94 No difference in hematoma expansion (%) between APT users (110.4±363.4) vs. non-APT users (20.8±47.9), *P*=1.0.
Sansing 2009	70 patients on APT with CT diagnosis of ICH within 6 h of symptom onset Control group=212 patients not on APT with CT diagnosis of ICH within 6 h of symptom onset	ASA (*n*=56) C (*n*=5) D (*n*=1) ASA + C (*n*=3) ASA + D (*n*=2) Triflusal (*n*=2) Indobufen (*n*=1) No doses specified	Yes	The relative risk with any hematoma expansion in APT patients was 0.85, UCI=1.03, *P*=0.16 No difference in initial ICH volume in patients on APT (median [IQR]: 13.1 [7.9–27.3]) vs. patients not on APT (median [IQR]: 15.7 [7.9–31.4]), *P*=0.037 No difference in percentage of patients with ICH growth >33 % in APT patients (24.2 %) vs. non-APT patients (26.2 %), *P*=0.75 No difference in percentage of patients with any ICH growth in APT patients (59.1 %) vs. non-APT patients (67.3 %), *P*=0.18

(continued)

Table 6.1 (continued)

Study	Population	APT agents + daily dose (mg)[a] + no. of patients (n)	ACT excluded? If not, no. of patients on ACT	Results
Yildiz 2011	52 patients on APT with CT diagnosis of ICH within 12 h of symptom onset and a follow up CT 72 h later Control group = 101 patients not on APT with diagnosis of ICH and a CT within 12 h of symptoms and a follow-up CT 72 h later	ASA (n=49) C (n=1) ASA + C (n=2) No doses specified	Yes	APT patients had hematoma expansion 42.9 % (15/35) vs. non-APT patients 17.5 % (10/57), P<0.01 More APT patients had hematoma expansion (42.9 % [15/35]) vs. non-APT patients (17.5 % [10/57]), P<0.01 APT patients had more increase between baseline and follow-up hematoma volume (3.6 mL [median IQR: 0.3–14.3]) vs. non-APT patients (0.0 mL [median IQR: 0.0–5.7]), P<0.01
Fabbri 2013	201 patients with mild, moderate or severe head trauma that worsened on follow-up head CTs Control group = 1357 patients with mild, moderate, or severe head trauma with stable or improved follow-up head CTs	Study group = 106 on APT Control group = 431 on APT ASA = 439 (usual dose 100 mg daily) T (n=69) C (n=28) No doses specified for T and C	No	APT patients at increased risk of worsening CT vs. those not treated, RR 2.09, 95 % CI [1.63–2.71] In mild head trauma, APT increased risk of worsening CT in patients with ≤2 lesions vs. no APT, RR 1.86, 95 % CI (1.06–3.30), P=0.032 In mild head trauma, APT increased risk of worsening CT in patients with ≥3 lesions vs. no APT, RR 3.34, 95 % CI (1.74–6.40), P=0.003 In moderate-severe head trauma, APT increased risk of worsening CT in patients with ≤2 lesions vs. no APT, RR 1.72, 95 % CI (1.21–2.45), P=0.002 In moderate-severe head trauma, APT increased risk of worsening CT in patients with ≥3 lesions vs. no APT, 33 %, [13/39] vs. 22.7 % [15/66], no RR or P calculated Neurosurgical intervention was required more often in APT patients (21.2 %) vs. non-APT patients (11.2 %), RR 1.90, 95 % CI (1.35–2.66), P<0.001

[a]Daily dose

ACT anticoagulant therapy, *APT* antiplatelet therapy, *ASA* aspirin, *C* clopidogrel, *CT* computed tomography, *D* dipyridamole, *DAPT* dual antiplatelet therapy, *ICH* intracerebral hemorrhage, *IQR*, interquartile range *OR* odds ratio, *T* ticlopidine, *UCI* upper limit of confidence interval, *W* warfarin

Despite using a smaller increase in percentage (≥20 %) to define increase in hematoma expansion compared to other studies, Sorimachi and colleagues [56] found eight patients who experienced hematoma expansion. They found that hematoma expansion occurred in 26.3 % of the patients on antiplatelet agents prior to the ICH, which might be due to warfarin.

An excellent 2008 study by Toyoda and colleagues [57] investigated the role of antiplatelet therapy on hematoma expansion. They included a very specific definition of hematoma expansion and included the specific dose of each agent used. There were detailed patient demographics and a multivariant adjustment based on risk factors and comorbidities. The authors prevented contamination of the data with warfarin by creating separate categories for antiplatelet agents, warfarin, and for patients on both antiplatelet agents and warfarin. The authors also recorded time from symptom onset to first CT scan, in which there was no difference between the control group and the antiplatelet group. One of the best aspects of the study was that the antiplatelet groups were differentiated into three groups: aspirin alone, antiplatelet agent other than aspirin, and dual antiplatelet agents. Multivariate-adjusted analysis was done on these groups to provide the best analysis on this highly controversial topic. The study limitations were reported as the study being retrospective and that hematoma expansion was not assessed in every patient because some patients died or received surgery before a second CT scan. This likely reduced the reported number of patients experiencing hematoma expansion. Despite these limitations, this study was one of the most carefully designed and well reported studies to date in analyzing the effect of antiplatelet therapy on hematoma expansion. One possible disadvantage is that the study population may be homogenous because the study was conducted in Japan.

Moussouttas and colleagues [58] recorded time to first CT scan, time between initial and second CT, as well as hematoma volumes and changes. Patient demographics were included, however, hypertension was the only comorbidity included. It is impossible to determine if any factors besides age and hypertension may have contributed to the results of the study. The main disadvantage of the study is that it was likely unpowered because the study consisted of 70 patients, of which only 17 were on antiplatelet therapy.

Data from the prospective, placebo arm of the Cerebral Hemorrhage and NXY-059 Treatment (CHANT) trial was analyzed by Sansing and colleagues [59]. This is one of the larger and more properly designed studies with attention to imaging timing, baseline demographics, and exclusion of anticoagulants. The authors differentiated the antiplatelet agents, however, no doses were recorded. This study was one of the few studies to conduct a power analysis. They reported an 80 % power to detect a 6.5 mL difference in hematoma expansion between study groups, using an alpha of 0.05 and a standard deviation of 16 mL. The majority of the studies reviewed up to this point lacked a power analysis. The authors concluded that aspirin, compared to the other antiplatelet agents, had comparable hemorrhage volumes and rates of hematoma expansion, although no analysis was shown. The population size was still not large enough to confidently make a generalized determination that antiplatelets do not contribute to hematoma expansion.

Yildiz and colleagues [60] provided excellent patient demographics, which included timing to first CT scan and an analysis of the agents used. However, no doses were recorded, even though 94 % of the antiplatelet patients were on aspirin monotherapy alone. Patients on aspirin had larger admission hematoma volumes, which would have required larger growth to qualify as expansions. The definition of expansion in this study was growth >12.5 mL or >33 % from baseline ICH volumes. Antiplatelet agents were determined to cause hematoma expansion, however, a large portion (33 %) of patients did not have a second CT scan. It is difficult to make a strong conclusion regarding the remaining patients because small changes have much more dramatic changes in percentages and *P* values. The study was likely underpowered, and a large portion of patients not being included in analysis only further eroded the ability to detect differences between the groups. The lack of a substantial population in this study makes it difficult to make a determination if antiplatelet therapy contributes to hematoma expansion.

Fabbri and colleagues [61] had a substantially sized study, with a primary interest in determining the short-term and long-term outcomes in subjects with head injuries. Their study included data about worsening lesions, however, they did not define what constituted a hematoma expansion. Worsening was defined as a "change of at least one point in Marshall Category between initial and follow up CT scan performed during serial controls within 24 h and the need for neurosurgical intervention because of clinical and/or radiological deterioration during the observation period (first 7 days after diagnosis)." No patient demographics were included comparing patients on antiplatelet therapy and those not on antiplatelet therapy. It is unclear if there were any significant differences between patients on antiplatelet therapy who had favorable outcomes vs. those who had unfavorable outcomes because no demographics of these groups were disclosed. It is unclear if patients on antiplatelets were older and/or sustained more severe injuries. These factors could have influenced the results of the study. The only demographics provided compared patients with worsening or stable/improved conditions between initial and follow up CT. Of the 201 patients who had worsening outcomes, 106 were on antiplatelet therapy. Patients in the worsening category had significantly lower Glasgow Coma Scale (GCS) scores (65.2 %) than those in the stable/improved group (22.7 %, $P<0.001$). Patients in the worsening group also had significantly more basal skull fractures (13.9 %) than those in the stable/improved group (8.6 %, $P=0.019$). Throughout this paper there were some inconsistencies in numbers reported when referring to the same value.

Several factors can determine if a researcher will conclude if hematoma expansion occurred. These factors include the definition of hematoma expansion and time to first CT scan. Several of the studies had differing definitions of hematoma expansion, as listed in Table 6.2, thus it may be difficult to directly compare the studies' results. An exaggeration of hematoma expansion may exist if a significant number of small hematomas enlarged slightly but due to increasing >33 %, qualified as an expanded hematoma. Substantial hematoma expansions of this nature could misrepresent the true risk. Future studies investigating hematoma expansion should adopt a uniform definition that prevents over-representation of small hematoma expansions. A more specific definition should include two qualifiers such as an increase >33 % and >12.5 mL. This definition was used in two of the studies reviewed. A double qualifier definition would exclude small hematomas that expanded only slightly but still surpassed the 33 % benchmark.

Table 6.2 Different trials' definitions of hematoma expansion

Author, year	Definition of hematoma expansion
Fabbri 2013	No clear definition. Head CTs were retrospectively reviewed by a blinded, independent, expert neurologist. No percentage or volume requirements given.
Flibotte 2004	≥33 %
Moussouttas 2009	No specific definition. Directly compared APT patients' hematomas vs. non-APT patients' hematomas volume.
Saloheimo 2005	≥33 %
Sansing 2009	>33 %
Sorimachi 2007	≥20 %
Toyoda 2005	>40 %
Toyoda 2008	>33 % or >12.5 mL
Yildiz 2011	≥33 %

APT Antiplatelet therapy

Data regarding hematoma growth indicates that most growth occurs within 6 h of symptom onset [62]. Studies that had extended time between onset of symptoms and first CT scan may have missed the opportune time to accurately determine hematoma expansion. Table 6.3 lists the inclusion criteria window that the studies discussed above allowed from symptom onset to admission. The lack of consistency in timing of the first CT could be a potential reason for the unknown role of antiplatelet therapy on hematoma expansion. Only three studies required patients to be diagnosed with ICH by CT scan within 6 h of onset. Interestingly, none of these studies showed an increase in hematoma growth with antiplatelet therapy.

One major event that cannot be overlooked in the role of antiplatelets (or any drug) in hematoma expansion is that patients may not receive a

Table 6.3 Inclusion window from time of first symptom onset until admission

Study	Inclusion window from symptom onset to admission (h)
Fabbri 2013	24
Flibotte 2004	72
Moussouttas 2009	6
Saloheimo 2005	No time period (any patient with documented ICH included)
Sansing 2009	6
Sorimachi 2007	24
Toyoda 2005	24
Toyoda 2008	24
Yildiz 2011	12

ICH intracerebral hemorrhage

second CT scan due to their prognosis. If a patient presents with a substantial hematoma and the decision by the medical staff and family is to withdraw care or proceed with surgery, a second CT may not be performed. In cases of surgery or death, it is likely that hematoma expansion occurred because the patient required surgery to prevent further expansion or died from the severity of the expanding hemorrhage. The amount of data that goes unrecorded by this mechanism may prevent detection of hematoma expansion in certain patient populations. An analysis of patients with a second CT scan should be conducted as well as a separate analysis that assumes that patients who required surgery or died also qualified as having hematoma expansion. In these studies, it may be clearer to determine the true risk of hematoma expansion in patients on antiplatelet therapy prior to traumatic brain injury or ICH.

Clearly, larger, multicenter studies need to be performed to determine the actual risk of hematoma expansion with prior antiplatelet use. Too many studies have been unpowered and were unable to determine the true risk. If several large hospitals agreed to prospectively follow patients and combine their data, the true risk may finally be determined. In order for such a trial to work, there needs to be an established definition of hematoma expansion. A consensus should be established on how long the inclusion window should be from symptom onset to first CT scan. With windows that extend up to 24 h, the hematoma may have already experienced its primary growth before a CT could be obtained. As several studies have shown, the most expansion occurs in the first 6 h after symptom onset [62]; limiting the inclusion window to patients having a CT scan within 6 h of symptom onset may be best. To ensure a large population for the study, anticoagulants may not necessarily have to be excluded from the analysis if they have their own study group. Patients who are on both anticoagulants and antiplatelet therapy should also be their own study group and not grouped into either the anticoagulant or antiplatelet groups. Names and doses of each antiplatelet therapy should also be recorded to potentially determine the safest antiplatelet agent.

Do Platelet Transfusions Reduce Mortality in Patients with Spontaneous or Traumatic Intracranial Hemorrhage?

Patients with inhibited platelet function may experience excessive bleeding. Correcting for platelet inhibition may reduce hematoma expansion in trauma and ICH patients. As previously discussed, platelets are irreversibly inhibited by aspirin and clopidogrel for the life of the platelet. The only way to reverse platelet inhibition would be to create new platelets. However, in a trauma situation, patients do not have a week to replenish platelets. Quick replenishment with new platelets appears to be a reasonable option to reverse the platelet inhibition. However, platelet transfusions are not a procedure to be taken lightly because they are associated with inherent risk. These risks prevent platelet transfusions from being performed in every patient who has been on antiplatelet therapy prior to an ICH or who has suffered severe trauma.

One of the most feared complications of platelet transfusions is transfusion-related acute lung injury (TRALI). Globally, TRALI is the primary mechanism for transfusion-related morbidity and mortality [63]. In the FDA's fatality summary report investigating blood collection and transfusions, TRALI was responsible for 47 % of all transfusion-related fatalities disclosed to the Center for Biologics Evaluation and Research (CBER) [64]. The incidence of TRALI is frequently reported as 1 in every 5000 recipients of blood products, although several recent studies have proposed that the true incidence may be closer to 1 in every 1000 recipients [65, 66]. Although the definition of TRALI has changed several times, it is characterized by acute onset of severe dyspnea, tachypnea, fever, new or worsening hypoxemia, occasional hypotension, cyanosis, and bilateral infiltrates on frontal chest radiographs that occur within 6 h of transfused blood products [63].

Due to the inherent risks associated with platelet transfusions, it is important to establish the usefulness of such a procedure. Currently, there are no guidelines recommending a platelet transfusion to a patient suffering an ICH who had previously been on antiplatelet therapy. Platelet transfusions are regarded as investigational and their usefulness is unknown in patients on antiplatelet therapy prior to an ICH [52]. One of the reasons for the lack of recommendations is the conflicting results from studies that have investigated the role of platelet transfusions in patients taking antiplatelet therapy prior to an ICH or head trauma. Additionally, many of the studies were plagued by poor design and lacked substantial study populations. Table 6.4 summarizes the results from the most substantial, relevant, and commonly referenced studies on the impact of platelet transfusion reducing mortality in patients on antiplatelet therapy prior to an ICH or head trauma.

Ohm and colleagues [67] designed a study to investigate the role of antiplatelet agents in mortality in the elderly, and the paper contained some information on platelet transfusions. Demographics were not given for patients on antiplatelet therapy who received a platelet transfusion vs. those on antiplatelet therapy who did not receive a platelet transfusion or for the antiplatelet therapy patients who received a platelet transfusion and the control patients. Patients on antiplatelet therapy had significantly more comorbid conditions. It is not known if the patients on antiplatelet therapy who received the platelet transfusions were older, had more comorbid conditions, or sustained more severe injuries vs. the control patients who received platelet transfusions. Without a comparison between groups it is hard to determine the actual relationship between platelet transfusions and mortality in this study.

Ivascu and colleagues [68] clearly differentiated which antiplatelet agents the study population was taking. However there were no demographics given for the patients on antiplatelet therapy who received or did not receive a platelet transfusion, or between the antiplatelet therapy patients who received a platelet transfusion and the control patients who received a platelet transfusion. It is hard to establish if there were any factors that may have contributed to increased mortality such as age, GCS scores, and injury severity score. Given the small number of patients who received platelet transfusions ($n=40$) in this study and the uncertainty of how many of these patients were on antiplatelet therapy, it is impossible to make any general recommendations on platelet transfusions based on this study.

In the study by Fortuna and colleagues [69] platelet transfusions were determined on a case-by-case basis. Platelet transfusion patients were significantly older (73 ± 2 years vs. 69 ± 1, $P=0.02$), were injured more severely (injury severity scale (ISS) 28 ± 1 vs. 24 ± 1, $P=0.001$) and had a lower GCS (11 ± 1 vs. 13 ± 0.2, $P=0.007$). Although this study was somewhat larger than the previous studies, the information is contaminated by anticoagulant data and lacks a strong platelet transfusion analysis. These reasons make it difficult to confidently make any recommendation about platelet transfusions and mortality based on this study.

Extensive demographics were provided by Creutzfeldt and colleagues [70] about patients in their study as to receiving antiplatelet therapy or not and whether receiving a platelet transfusion or not. Antiplatelet therapy patients had significantly more comorbid conditions in comparison to the

Table 6.4 The role of platelet transfusions (PT) on mortality in patients on antiplatelet therapy (APT)

Study	Class of ICH	No. patients on APT, in control group	No. of patients transfused	ACT excluded? If not, no. of patients on ACT	Results
Ohm 2005	TR	APT (*n* = 90) ASA (*n* = 50), C (*n* = 12), ASA + C (*n* = 20) Control (*n* = 89)	APT (*n* = 24) Control (*n* = 5)	No W + ASA (*n* = 6) W + C (*n* = 2) W + ASA + C (*n* = 2) 6/10 W + APT patients had normal INRs No patients in control group on ACT	Increased mortality in PT group (47.6 %, 10/21) vs. the non-PT group (25 %, 2/8), no *P* value calculated
Ivascu 2008	TR	ASA (*n* = 61) C (*n* = 17) ASA + C (*n* = 31) Control (*n* = 42)	*n* = 40, unclear how many patients from each ACT group were transfused	Unclear, no exclusion criteria listed and INR was recorded	No difference in mortality between PT patients and non-PT patients, 28 % [11/40] vs. 13 % [9/69], respectively, *P* = 0.064
Fortuna 2008	TR	APT (*n* = 126) ASA (*n* = 91), C (*n* = 17), ASA + C (*n* = 18) Control (*n* = 250)	66/166 CAW	No W (*n* = 29) W + ASA (*n* = 10) H (*n* = 1)	Increased mortality in patients on CAW who received PT (30 %) vs. those on CAW who did not receive PT (16 %), *P* = 0.01 Multivariate analysis suggested that mortality was impacted by age (OR 1.07, 95 % CI [1.03–1.10]) and ISS (OR 1.04, 95 % CI [1.01–1.08]) but not CAW use (OR 0.56, 95 % CI [0.28–1.14]) or PT, P not calculated
Creutzfeldt 2009	SP	All (*n* = 368) APT (*n* = 121) ASA (*n* = 105) ASA + C (*n* = 11) ASA + D (*n* = 2)	53/121 APT	No, only patients with INR <1.5 excluded	No difference in mortality in APT patients who received PT (26 %, 14/53) vs. APT patients who did not receive PT (38 %, 26/68), *P* = 0.17 PT likely associated with hospital death (OR 1.25, 95 % CI 0.28–5.54) and APT likely associated with hospital death (OR 2.44, 95 % CI 1.07–5.56) when adjusted for prognostic and propensity score Unadjusted data showed APT likely associated with a favorable outcome (OR 2.01, 95 % CI 0.97–4.17) and unlikely to result in hospital death (OR 0.58, 95 % CI 0.27–1.27) Unadjusted data showed APT likely associated with favorable outcomes (OR 1.20, 85 % CI 0.78–1.86) and APT unlikely to be associated with hospital death (OR 2.44, 95 % CI 1.07–5.56).

(continued)

Table 6.4 (continued)

Study	Class of ICH	No. patients on APT, in control group	No. of patients transfused	ACT excluded? If not, no. of patients on ACT	Results
Downey 2009	TR	All (*n*=328)	*n*=166: ASA (*n*=92), ASA + C (*n*=74) No PT (*n*=162): ASA (*n*=139), ASA + C (*n*=23)	No PT: W (*n*=147) non-PT: W (*n*=130)	No difference in mortality between PT (17.5 % [29/166]) and non-PT (16.7 % [27/162], *P*=0.85)
Bachelani 2011	TR	All (*n*=84) ASA (*n*=36) No ASA (*n*=48)	45 with an initial ART of <550	Yes	No difference in mortality between PT 11 % (4/36) vs. those non-PT 6.4 % (3/48), *P*=0.442 Trend toward increased mortality in non-responders to PT, *P*=0.09
Washington 2011	TR	All (*n*=108) on APT APT: ASA, C, or both	44	Yes	No difference in mortality rates between PT (5 %, 2/44) vs. non-PT (0 %, 0/64)
Suzuki 2014	SP	All (*n*=432) APT (*n*=66) ASA (*n*=50), ASA + C (*n*=12), C (*n*=2), T (*n*=2) non-APT (*n*=366)	APT=6/66 non-APT=10/366	No	Increased mortality at 7 days in APT patients who did not receive PT (50 %, 30/60) vs. APT patients who received PT (0 %, 0/6), *P*=0.03 Increased mortality at 90 days in APT patients who did not receive PT (77.5 %, 31/60) vs. APT patients who received PT (0 %, 0/6), *P* not calculated

ACT anticoagulant therapy, *APT* antiplatelet therapy, *ART* The Aspirin Response Test (ART;VerifyNow), *ASA* aspirin, *C* clopidogrel, *CAW* clopidogrel, aspirin and warfarin, *D* dipyridamole, *H* heparin, *ICH* intracranial hemorrhage, *MTBI* mild traumatic brain injury, *PT* Platelet transfusion, *SP* spontaneous, *T* ticlopidine, *TR* traumatic, *W* warfarin

control group and higher GCS score than the control patients. There were no significant differences between patients on antiplatelet therapy who received platelet transfusions and patients on antiplatelet therapy who did not receive platelet transfusions. However, there were significantly more women in the platelet transfusion group. Knowing that the groups were similar makes determining the benefit of platelet transfusions easier. Platelet transfusions were associated with likely favorable outcomes in every category (unadjusted, adjusted for prognostic score, adjusted for propensity score, and adjusted for both prognostic and propensity score). Platelet transfusions were likely associated with hospital death when adjusted for prognostic score and prognostic and propensity score combined, while hospital death was unlikely when the data was unadjusted and adjusted for propensity. The unadjusted data suggested that platelet transfusions were beneficial because of the unlikelihood of hospital death according to their odds ratio (Table 6.4), yet the authors did not report a benefit from platelet transfusions. All the patients in the platelet transfusion group who died, died after life support was withdrawn. However, six patients in the non-platelet transfusion group died from causes other than the removal of life support.

Downey et al. [71] provide demographics between the transfused and non-transfused patients that showed that patients in the platelet transfusion group were significantly older (77 ± 10.4 years) than non-platelet transfusion patients (73.0 ± 10.8 years, $P<0.001$). There were significantly more patients on warfarin in the platelet transfusion group (147 [89 %]) than patients in the non-platelet transfusion group (130 [80 %]). Warfarin may have affected the results of the study because mortality rates of patients on warfarin were higher (27.5 % [42/277]) than those not on warfarin (15.2 % [14/51]). The higher percentage of patients on warfarin should have put the platelet-transfused group at a disadvantage, however mortality rates were similar. The authors stated that there was no standardization of timing of platelet transfusion. Platelets took an average of 34 min to arrive once ordered, and more time was required to perform laboratory tests for abnormal platelet function. Transfusions performed earlier, possibly upon admission to the hospital, may have limited hemorrhage expansion and may have prevented mortality. The utility of this study is that it included a large number of patients and included many who were on warfarin, but this latter fact makes it difficult to confidently make a decision regarding platelet transfusions.

Excellent patient demographics were provided by Bachelani et al. [72]. Patients with platelet inhibition were significantly older (81 years, interquartile range (IQR) [74-86]) compared to patients without platelet inhibition (76 years, IQR [59-85]; $P=0.010$). All other factors were similar between groups including comorbid conditions, injury severity, and admission GCS. There was no significant difference in mortality between transfused and non-transfused patients. Because all factors besides age were similar, this is one of the few studies in which transfused patients were not worse off than non-transfused patients. However, the small size of the study made it difficult to find significant changes between groups. The authors conducted some additional analysis of platelet transfusions. Repeat Aspirin Response Tests (ARTs) were conducted after each platelet transfusion. In patients who received a platelet transfusion, 29 of 45 had a correction of their platelet inhibition, as evidenced by an ART of ≥550 aspirin response units. Of the 16 non-responders to the first platelet transfusion, nine were transfused again. Of the nine patients, six had reversal of their platelet inhibition. An additional patient was able to reverse platelet inhibition after a third transfusion. The remaining two patients were unable to correct their platelet inhibition with >3 transfusions. A trend toward increased mortality in patients who were non-responders to platelet transfusions was observed. Patients who did respond to platelet transfusion were given larger quantities/volumes (median, 6 [IQR 5–10] vs. 8 [IQR 6–10]; $P=0.13$). This likely represented a dose–response relationship for platelet transfusions. The authors reported an average increase of 70 ± 50 aspirin response units per 6-pack of platelets. The data showed that not every patient will respond to a single platelet transfusion.

The benefit of platelet transfusions in mild traumatic brain injury was investigated by Washington and colleagues [73]. The attending neurosurgeon made the decision to transfuse because there was no protocol for the initiation of transfusion. It appeared that platelet transfusions were reserved for worse-off or declining patients. The demographics showed that the patients who received platelet transfusions were more likely to be on clopidogrel (52 % [23/44] vs. 20 % [13/64]; $P=0.0005$), have a Marshall class VI hemorrhage (32 % [14/44] vs. 11 % [7/64]; $P=0.043$), and have larger ICH volumes (20.6 mL ± 26.5 vs. 8.2 mL ± 13.7; $P=0.02$) than patients who did not receive a platelet transfusion. Interestingly, there was no difference in any of the other outcome results (neurological decline, surgical intervention, cardiac event, respiratory event, Glasgow outcomes, or hematoma expansion) between groups. Patients who received platelet transfusions did experience more medical decline (14 % [6/44]) than those who did not receive a platelet transfusion (3 % [2/6]), however, this did not reach statistical significance ($P=0.06$). The medical decline may have been related to the fact that the patients who received platelet transfusions were in worse medical condition. There were no deaths in the non-transfused group and two deaths in the platelet transfusion group; both deaths occurred after platelet transfusions, one from a myocardial infarction and the other from a congestive heart failure exacerbation. It is unclear if these were directly related to platelet transfusions because the authors did not elaborate on the deaths.

Detailed demographics were also given in the study by Suzuki and colleagues [74]. They provided several excellent multivariate analyses investigating the role of antiplatelet therapy on mortality, as well as platelet transfusions on mortality. However, the study only included data on platelet transfusions in six patients on previous antiplatelet therapy prior to ICH. It would be impossible to discover any meaningful, significant differences between groups with such a small population.

A Dutch study, the Platelet Transfusion Intracerebral Hemorrhage (PATCH) trial [75], was designed to investigate the role of platelet transfusion in improving outcomes in patients previously on antiplatelet therapy who have a spontaneous ICH. This trial would be one of the largest studies to date, planned to have a sample size of 95 patients in the study group. Study patients would receive a platelet transfusion within 6 h of onset of intracerebral hemorrhage and within 1.5 h of CT scan, and 95 patients in the control group would receive the standard of care. Patients would be excluded if they are on vitamin K antagonists, if surgery was planned within 24 h after admission, or if death was imminent. These important exclusion criteria eliminate the influence of warfarin on results and try to ensure data outcomes for as many patients as possible. Many prior studies lacked substantial populations because patients who received surgery or died were not included in result outcomes. No information regarding the study results has been published yet.

It is clear that more extensive studies with larger populations need to be conducted. With some conflicting results from the studies reviewed here and small sample sizes in some cases, it is obvious why the AHA and the ASA consider platelet transfusions in patients with a history of antiplatelet use to be investigational and their role unclear [52]. One of the primary reasons why their benefit is unknown is that most platelet transfusion studies do not compare similar groups. Frequently, platelet transfusion patients had worse injuries or were in poorer medical condition than the patients who did not receive platelet transfusion. These patients were more likely to die, which could skew the results toward platelet transfusions not being beneficial in reducing mortality. When the decision to transfuse is left to the neurosurgeon, they may want to wait to transfuse patients who are in poorer health, declining, or more severely injured because platelet transfusions come with inherent risks. The concern with administering a platelet transfusion to a patient who is not critically ill or declining is the possibility of having the patient suffer complications from the transfusion. These complications could result in increased morbidity or death. A protocol similar to the one in the Bachelani study [72], in which the patient's condition did not affect the decision to transfuse, may be a good approach. Using a more objective test to determine when to initiate a platelet transfusion would help to reduce the tendency to only treat patients who are more likely to die. Using an aspirin response test in prior aspirin users may help determine which patients are initial responders and which require additional transfusions. The knowledge that all patients may not initially respond to the first transfusion is an important key to help reduce mortality. Similar testing for clopidogrel can also be done using the flow cytometric vasodilator-stimulated phosphoprotein phosphorylation (VASP)-assay and the VerifyNow $P2Y_{12}$ assay. Better designed trials should investigate the true role of platelet transfusions in reducing mortality. This is an important area of research that needs to be addressed because of the many patients on antiplatelet therapy and the high rate of mortality associated with ICH.

Review of Novel Antiplatelet Agents

Several novel antiplatelet agents have been developed that have improved pharmacokinetic properties and potential clinical benefits over the traditional antiplatelet agents like aspirin and clopidogrel. Some of these new antiplatelet agents are reversible, have shorter half-lives, and have more consistent inhibition than clopidogrel. These characteristics may provide a safer option for patients who require antiplatelet therapy during neurosurgery. However, these medications have not been tested in neurosurgery and bleeding risks must be evaluated based on non-neurosurgery studies.

Prasugrel

Prasugrel is an oral, third generation theinopyridine that selectively and irreversibly inhibits the $P2Y_{12}$ receptor [76]. Prasugrel, like clopidogrel, is a prodrug, but it is more potent than clopidogrel. In a study of a single oral dosing of prasugrel, there was a tenfold increase in the anti-aggregatory ability of prasugrel compared to clopidogrel [77]. Prasugrel has a faster onset and a greater and more consistent platelet inhibition compared with clopidogrel at the approved dose and as compared to clopidogrel.

Several trials have compared prasugrel and clopidogrel for bleeding risk and cardiovascular outcomes. In the TRILOGY-ACS trial ($n=9326$), fewer cardiovascular deaths, myocardial infarctions, or strokes were in the prasugrel arm than in patients who took clopidogrel based on angiographic analysis [78]. Prasugrel did not significantly increase the risk of Global Use of Strategies to Open Occluded Arteries (GUSTO) severe or life-threatening bleeds or TIMI major bleeds [79].

In another large study ($n=13{,}608$), prasugrel was compared to clopidogrel for death and bleeding risk for patients with moderate-to-high risk for acute coronary syndrome with a scheduled percutaneous coronary intervention. Prasugrel significantly reduced the number of nonfatal MIs (7.3 % vs. 9.5 %, $P<0.001$), urgent target-vessel revascularizations (2.5 % vs. 3.7 %, $P<0.001$), and stent thrombosis (1.1 % vs. 2.4 %, $P<0.001$) compared with clopidogrel. However, prasugrel was associated with more non-CABG-related TIMI major bleeding (2.4 % vs. 1.8 %, $P=0.03$), life-threatening bleeds (1.4 % vs. 0.9 %, $P=0.01$), fatal bleeding (0.4 % vs. 0.1 %, $P=0.002$), and CABG-related TIMI major bleeding (13.4 % vs. 3.2 %, $P<0.001$) [80].

Given the increased risk of bleeding and only minor improvements in protective effects, prasugrel is likely not a practical choice for neurosurgery.

Ticagrelor

Ticagrelor is an orally active adenosine triphosphate analog that reversibly binds the $P2Y_{12}$ receptor. Interestingly, ticagrelor is not a prodrug and does not need metabolic activation to effectively inhibit the $P2Y_{12}$ receptor, but approximately 1/3 of an administered ticagrelor dose undergoes hepatic conversion into an active metabolite that is essentially equipotent to the parent compound [81–83]. When ticagrelor binds to the $P2Y_{12}$ receptor, it almost completely inhibits platelet aggregation induced by adenosine diphosphate [81, 84]. A quicker and more extensive inhibition of platelet inhibition is achieved with ticagrelor compared with clopidogrel [81, 85]. However, there are similar concerns in the perioperative setting for ticagrelor as for prasugrel. First, the half-life of ticagrelor is 7 h (and 9 h for the active metabolite), which is similar to clopidogrel [86]. Second, the greater extent of platelet inhibition may also lead to increased bleeding. One large study investigated the role of cardiovascular events and bleeding risks in patients admitted to the hospital with acute coronary syndrome. In the ticagrelor PLATO study ($n=18{,}624$), ticagrelor reduced death vs. clopidogrel from vascular causes, MI, or stroke (9.8 % vs. 11.7 %, $P<0.001$) and occurrence of definite stent thrombosis (1.3 % vs. 1.9 %, $P=0.009$) [87]. There was no significant difference in major bleeding between ticagrelor vs. clopidogrel by study criteria (11.6 % vs. 11.2 %, $P=0.43$) or TIMI criteria (7.9 % vs. 7.7 %, $P=0.57$), or life-threatening or fatal bleeding (5.8 % vs. 5.8 %, $P=0.70$). There was a small increase in intracranial bleeding in the ticagrelor group compared to the clopidogrel group but it was not statistically significant. Patients who did have an intracranial bleed were more likely to have a fatal bleed while on ticagrelor vs. on clopidogrel (0.1 % vs. 0.001 %, $P=0.02$). The increased risk of intracranial bleeding and fatality associated with intracranial bleeds is a major concern with ticagrelor. Ticagrelor also appears not to be a possible alternative to clopidogrel for patients requiring neurosurgery.

Cangrelor

Cangrelor is an intravenous, short-acting, potent, reversible, competitive inhibitor of the $P2Y_{12}$ receptor. One of the most desirable characteristics of cangrelor is its short half-life of 3 min [76]. Platelet homeostasis can occur within 60 min of cangrelor discontinuation [88]. A shorter duration of platelet inhibition should allow for more manageable episodes of bleeding and hopefully fewer bleeding fatalities. Cangrelor can achieve steady state in 30 min and inhibits platelet aggregation more than clopidogrel [85, 88]. Despite these advantages, two cangrelor studies (CHAMPION PLATFORM [89] and CHAMPION PHOENIX [90]) were terminated early because cangrelor failed to achieve efficacy. In the CHAMPION PHOENIX study ($n = 11{,}145$), cangrelor use led to fewer primary endpoints: death from any cause, MI, ischemia-driven revascularization, or stent thrombosis vs. clopidogrel (4.7 vs. 5.9 %, $P = 0.005$). There was no difference in GUSTO-defined severe or life threatening bleeding for cangrelor vs. clopidogrel (0.2 % vs. 0.1 %, $P = 0.44$) or TIMI-defined major bleeding (0.1 % vs. 0.1 %, $P > 0.999$). However, there was an increase in GUSTO-defined severe or moderate bleeding in the cangrelor group vs. the clopidogrel group but without statistical significance. Given the lack of efficacy and the lack of reduction of bleeding risk associated with cangrelor, it also may not be the best alternative option to use in neurosurgery unless future studies can show a clear benefit.

Other novel agents are still in development and lack any substantial patient population studies. The data for prasugrel, ticagrelor, and cangrelor as replacement agents for the typical antiplatelet agents, aspirin and clopidogrel, is weak at best right now. The best option now may be to rely on aspirin and clopidogrel because they have the most data and have been used the longest. Knowing more about the bleeding threat that exists with aspirin or clopidogrel may be better than the unknown bleeding risks associated with the novel agents, especially in the setting of neurosurgery.

Conclusion

There are still many questions left unanswered by this review chapter, because there is little data regarding the use of antiplatelets in neurosurgery. Better designed studies in the future may help to discover the role of antiplatelet therapy in hematoma expansion as well as the benefit of platelet transfusions in patients with a prior history of antiplatelet therapy who experience an ICH or traumatic head injury. Although there is a lack of neurosurgical guidelines regarding the use of antiplatelet therapy, The American College of Chest Physicians, The American Heart Association, and The American Stroke Association provide the best guidance on antiplatelet therapy in the perioperative setting. In neurosurgery, discontinuation of all antiplatelet therapy agents is likely the best option unless the patient has recently had a stent placed. In these situations, discontinuation of all agents except aspirin appears to be the best recommendation at this time. More studies must be performed to determine the true benefit of the novel antiplatelet agents prasugrel, ticagrelor, and cangrelor. Although some of the novel agents may not be inferior, they may be associated with higher bleeding risks. Until more data is available, it appears that aspirin is the antiplatelet agent of choice when antiplatelet therapy must be continued during neurosurgery because aspirin has been extensively studied and the risks are well known. Using aspirin at doses <100 mg per day may help reduce the risk of bleeding in patients who require antiplatelet therapy during neurosurgery.

References

1. Harder S, Klinkhardt U, Alvarez JM. Avoidance of bleeding during surgery in patients receiving anticoagulant and/or antiplatelet therapy: pharmacokinetic and pharmacodynamic considerations. Clin Pharmacokinet. 2004;43(14):963–81. doi:10.2165/00003088-200443140-00002.

2. Hall R, Mazer CD. Antiplatelet drugs: a review of their pharmacology and management in the perioperative period. Anesth Analg. 2011;112(2):292–318. doi:10.1213/ANE.0b013e318203f38d.
3. Patrono C, Coller B, FitzGerald GA, Hirsh J, Roth G. Platelet-active drugs: the relationships among dose, effectiveness, and side effects: the Seventh ACCP Conference on Antithrombotic and Thrombolytic Therapy. Chest. 2004;126(3 Suppl):234S–64. doi:10.1378/chest.126.3_suppl.234S.
4. Patrono C. Aspirin as an antiplatelet drug. N Engl J Med. 1994;330(18):1287–94. doi:10.1056/NEJM199405053301808.
5. Schroder H, Schror K. Clinical pharmacology of acetylsalicylic acid. Z Kardiol. 1992;81 Suppl 4:171–5.
6. Cryer B, Feldman M. Cyclooxygenase-1 and cyclooxygenase-2 selectivity of widely used nonsteroidal anti-inflammatory drugs. Am J Med. 1998;104(5):413–21. doi: 10.1016/S0002-9343(98)00091-6
7. Feldman M, Shewmake K, Cryer B. Time course inhibition of gastric and platelet COX activity by acetylsalicylic acid in humans. Am J Physiol Gastrointest Liver Physiol. 2000;279(5):G1113–20.
8. Patrono C, Baigent C, Hirsh J, Roth G, American College of Chest P. Antiplatelet drugs: American College of Chest Physicians Evidence-Based Clinical Practice Guidelines (8th Edition). Chest. 2008;133(6 Suppl):199S–233. doi:10.1378/chest.08-0672.
9. Jimenez AH, Stubbs ME, Tofler GH, Winther K, Williams GH, Muller JE. Rapidity and duration of platelet suppression by enteric-coated aspirin in healthy young men. Am J Cardiol. 1992;69(3):258–62. doi:10.1016/0002-9149(92)91316-V
10. Achneck HE, Sileshi B, Parikh A, Milano CA, Welsby IJ, Lawson JH. Pathophysiology of bleeding and clotting in the cardiac surgery patient: from vascular endothelium to circulatory assist device surface. Circulation. 2010;122(20):2068–77. doi:10.1161/CIRCULATIONAHA.110.936773.
11. Patel PA, Augoustides JG. Progress in platelet medicine: focus on stent thrombosis and drug resistance. J Cardiothorac Vasc Anesth. 2010;24(4):722–7. doi:10.1053/j.jvca.2010.04.017.
12. Savi P, Pereillo JM, Uzabiaga MF, Combalbert J, Picard C, Maffrand JP, Pascal M, Herbert JM. Identification and biological activity of the active metabolite of clopidogrel. Thromb Haemost. 2000;84(5):891–6.
13. Jaitner J, Morath T, Byrne RA, Braun S, Gebhard D, Bernlochner I, Schulz S, Mehilli J, Schomig A, Koch W, Kastrati A, Sibbing D. No association of ABCB1 C3435T genotype with clopidogrel response or risk of stent thrombosis in patients undergoing coronary stenting. Circ Cardiovasc Interv. 2012;5(1):82–8. doi:10.1161/CIRCINTERVENTIONS.111.965400. S81-82.
14. Patel PA, Lane B, Augoustides JG. Progress in platelet blockers: the target is the P2Y12 receptor. J Cardiothorac Vasc Anesth. 2013;27(3):620–4. doi:10.1053/j.jvca.2013.01.008.
15. Maree AO, Fitzgerald DJ. Variable platelet response to aspirin and clopidogrel in atherothrombotic disease. Circulation. 2007;115(16):2196–207. doi:10.1161/CIRCULATIONAHA.106.675991.
16. Lins R, Broekhuysen J, Necciari J, Deroubaix X. Pharmacokinetic profile of 14C-labeled clopidogrel. Semin Thromb Hemost. 1999;25 Suppl 2:29–33.
17. Highlights of prescribing information, Plavix (clopidogrel bisulfate) tablets. http://www.accessdata.fda.gov/drugsatfda_docs/label/2013/020839s058lbl.pdf (2013). Accessed 1 April 2015.
18. Weber AA, Braun M, Hohlfeld T, Schwippert B, Tschope D, Schror K. Recovery of platelet function after discontinuation of clopidogrel treatment in healthy volunteers. Br J Clin Pharmacol. 2001;52(3):333–6. doi:10.1046/j.0306-5251.2001.01453.x.
19. Patrono C. Low-dose aspirin in primary prevention: cardioprotection, chemoprevention, both, or neither? Eur Heart J. 2013;34(44):3403–11. doi:10.1093/eurheartj/eht058.
20. Lordkipanidze M, Diodati JG, Pharand C. Possibility of a rebound phenomenon following antiplatelet therapy withdrawal: A look at the clinical and pharmacological evidence. Pharmacol Ther. 2009;123(2):178–86. doi:10.1016/j.pharmthera.2009.03.019.
21. Antithrombotic Trialists' Collaboration. Collaborative meta-analysis of randomised trials of antiplatelet therapy for prevention of death, myocardial infarction, and stroke in high risk patients. BMJ. 2002;324(7329):71–86.
22. CHARISMA Investigators. Clopidogrel and aspirin versus aspirin alone for the prevention of atherothrombotic events. N Engl J Med. 2006;354(16):1706–17. doi:10.1056/Nejmoa060989.
23. Berger JS, Brown DL, Becker RC. Low-dose aspirin in patients with stable cardiovascular disease: A meta-analysis. Am J Med. 2008;121(1):43–9. doi:10.1016/j.amjmed.2007.10.002.
24. Mills EJ, Wu P, Alberton M, Kanters S, Lanas A, Lester R. Low-dose aspirin and cancer mortality: A Meta-analysis of Randomized Trials. Am J Med. 2012;125(6):560–7. doi:10.1016/j.amjmed.2012.01.017.
25. Rodriguez LAG, Cea-Soriano L, Martin-Merino E, Johansson S. Discontinuation of low dose aspirin and risk of myocardial infarction: case-control study in UK primary care. Brit Med J. 2011;343:d4094. doi:10.1136/Bmj.D4094.
26. Vandvik PO. Primary and secondary prevention of cardiovascular disease: antithrombotic therapy and prevention of thrombosis, 9th ed: American College of Chest Physicians Evidence-Based Clinical Practice Guidelines. Chest. 2012;141(2 suppl):e637S–68. doi:10.1378/chest.11-2306.
27. The SALT Collaborative Group. Swedish Aspirin Low-Dose Trial (SALT) of 75 mg aspirin as secondary prophylaxis after cerebrovascular ischaemic events. Lancet. 1991;338(8779):1345–9.

28. Serebruany VL, Malinin AI, Eisert RM, Sane DC. Risk of bleeding complications with antiplatelet agents: meta-analysis of 338,191 patients enrolled in 50 randomized controlled trials. Am J Hematol. 2004;75(1):40–7. doi:10.1002/ajh.10451.
29. Korte W, Cattaneo M, Chassot PG, Eichinger S, von Heymann C, Hofmann N, Rickli H, Spannagl M, Ziegler B, Verheugt F, Huber K. Peri-operative management of antiplatelet therapy in patients with coronary artery disease: joint position paper by members of the working group on Perioperative Haemostasis of the Society on Thrombosis and Haemostasis Research (GTH), the working group on Perioperative Coagulation of the Austrian Society for Anesthesiology, Resuscitation and Intensive Care (OGARI) and the Working Group Thrombosis of the European Society for Cardiology (ESC). Thromb Haemost. 2011;105(5):743–9. doi:10.1160/TH10-04-0217.
30. Burger W, Chemnitius JM, Kneissl GD, Rucker G. Low-dose aspirin for secondary cardiovascular prevention - cardiovascular risks after its perioperative withdrawal versus bleeding risks with its continuation - review and meta-analysis. J Intern Med. 2005;257(5):399–414. doi:10.1111/j.1365-2796.2005.01477.x.
31. Palmer JD, Sparrow OC, Iannotti F. Postoperative hematoma: a 5-year survey and identification of avoidable risk factors. Neurosurgery. 1994;35(6):1061–4. discussion 1064-1065.
32. Beving H, Zhao C, Albage A, Ivert T. Abnormally high platelet activity after discontinuation of acetylsalicylic acid treatment. Blood Coagul Fibrinolysis. 1996;7(1):80–4.
33. Fatah K, Beving H, Albage A, Ivert T, Blomback M. Acetylsalicylic acid may protect the patient by increasing fibrin gel porosity. Is withdrawing of treatment harmful to the patient? Eur Heart J. 1996;17(9):1362–6.
34. Vial JH, McLeod LJ, Roberts MS. Rebound elevation in urinary thromboxane B2 and 6-keto-PGF1 alpha excretion after aspirin withdrawal. Adv Prostaglandin Thromboxane Leukot Res. 1991;21A:157–60.
35. Collet JP, Montalescot G, Blanchet B, Tanguy ML, Golmard JL, Choussat R, Beygui F, Payot L, Vignolles N, Metzger JP, Thomas D. Impact of prior use or recent withdrawal of oral antiplatelet agents on acute coronary syndromes. Circulation. 2004;110(16):2361–7. doi:10.1161/01.CIR.0000145171.89690.B4.
36. Albaladejo P, Geeraerts T, Francis F, Castier Y, Leseche G, Marty J. Aspirin withdrawal and acute lower limb ischemia. Anesth Analg. 2004;99(2):440–3. doi:10.1213/01.ANE.0000131965.61686.BD.
37. Collet JP, Himbet F, Steg PG. Myocardial infarction after aspirin cessation in stable coronary artery disease patients. Int J Cardiol. 2000;76(2-3):257–8. doi:10.1016/S0167-5273(00)00399-5.
38. Ferrari E, Benhamou M, Cerboni P, Marcel B. Coronary syndromes following aspirin withdrawal: a special risk for late stent thrombosis. J Am Coll Cardiol. 2005;45(3):456–9. doi:10.1016/j.jacc.2004.11.041.
39. Biondi-Zoccai GG, Lotrionte M, Agostoni P, Abbate A, Fusaro M, Burzotta F, Testa L, Sheiban I, Sangiorgi G. A systematic review and meta-analysis on the hazards of discontinuing or not adhering to aspirin among 50,279 patients at risk for coronary artery disease. Eur Heart J. 2006;27(22):2667–74. doi:10.1093/eurheartj/ehl334.
40. Di Minno MN, Prisco D, Ruocco AL, Mastronardi P, Massa S, Di Minno G. Perioperative handling of patients on antiplatelet therapy with need for surgery. Intern Emerg Med. 2009;4(4):279–88. doi:10.1007/s11739-009-0265-0.
41. Fleisher LA, Fleischmann KE, Auerbach AD, Barnason SA, Beckman JA, Bozkurt B, Davila-Roman VG, Gerhard-Herman MD, Holly TA, Kane GC, Marine JE, Nelson MT, Spencer CC, Thompson A, Ting HH, Uretsky BF, Wijeysundera DN, American College of C, American Heart A. 2014 ACC/AHA guideline on perioperative cardiovascular evaluation and management of patients undergoing noncardiac surgery: a report of the American College of Cardiology/American Heart Association Task Force on practice guidelines. J Am Coll Cardiol. 2014;64(22):e77–137. doi:10.1016/j.jacc.2014.07.944.
42. Brott T, Broderick J, Kothari R, Barsan W, Tomsick T, Sauerbeck L, Spilker J, Duldner J, Khoury J. Early hemorrhage growth in patients with intracerebral hemorrhage. Stroke. 1997;28(1):1–5. doi:10.1161/01.STR.28.1.1.
43. Cucchiara B, Messe S, Sansing L, Kasner S, Lyden P, Investigators C. Hematoma growth in oral anticoagulant related intracerebral hemorrhage. Stroke. 2008;39(11):2993–6. doi:10.1161/STROKEAHA.108.520668.
44. Davis SM, Broderick J, Hennerici M, Brun NC, Diringer MN, Mayer SA, Begtrup K, Steiner T, Recombinant Activated Factor VIIIHTI. Hematoma growth is a determinant of mortality and poor outcome after intracerebral hemorrhage. Neurology. 2006;66(8):1175–81. doi:10.1212/01.wnl.0000208408.98482.99.
45. Flaherty ML, Tao H, Haverbusch M, Sekar P, Kleindorfer D, Kissela B, Khatri P, Stettler B, Adeoye O, Moomaw CJ, Broderick JP, Woo D. Warfarin use leads to larger intracerebral hematomas. Neurology. 2008;71(14):1084–9. doi:10.1212/01.wnl.0000326895.58992.27.
46. Leira R, Davalos A, Silva Y, Gil-Peralta A, Tejada J, Garcia M, Castillo J, Stroke Project CDGotSNS. Early neurologic deterioration in intracerebral hemorrhage: predictors and associated factors. Neurology. 2004;63(3):461–7. doi:10.1212/01.WNL.0000133204.81153.AC.
47. Zubkov AY, Mandrekar JN, Claassen DO, Manno EM, Wijdicks EF, Rabinstein AA. Predictors of outcome in warfarin-related intracerebral hemorrhage. Arch Neurol. 2008;65(10):1320–5. doi:10.1001/archneur.65.10.1320.
48. Bonville DJ, Ata A, Jahraus CB, Arnold-Lloyd T, Salem L, Rosati C, Stain SC. Impact of preinjury warfarin and antiplatelet agents on outcomes of trauma patients. Surgery. 2011;150(4):861–8. doi:10.1016/j.surg.2011.07.070.

49. Franko J, Kish KJ, O'Connell BG, Subramanian S, Yuschak JV. Advanced age and preinjury warfarin anticoagulation increase the risk of mortality after head trauma. J Trauma. 2006;61(1):107–10. doi:10.1097/01.ta.0000224220.89528.fc.
50. Mina AA, Knipfer JF, Park DY, Bair HA, Howells GA, Bendick PJ. Intracranial complications of preinjury anticoagulation in trauma patients with head injury. J Trauma. 2002;53(4):668–72. doi:10.1097/01.TA.0000025291.29067.E9.
51. Pieracci FM, Eachempati SR, Shou J, Hydo LJ, Barie PS. Use of long-term anticoagulation is associated with traumatic intracranial hemorrhage and subsequent mortality in elderly patients hospitalized after falls: analysis of the New York State Administrative Database. J Trauma. 2007;63(3):519–24. doi:10.1097/TA.0b013e31812e519b.
52. Morgenstern LB, Hemphill 3rd JC, Anderson C, Becker K, Broderick JP, Connolly Jr ES, Greenberg SM, Huang JN, MacDonald RL, Messe SR, Mitchell PH, Selim M, Tamargo RJ, American Heart Association Stroke C, Council on Cardiovascular N. Guidelines for the management of spontaneous intracerebral hemorrhage: a guideline for healthcare professionals from the American Heart Association/American Stroke Association. Stroke. 2010;41(9):2108–29. doi:10.1161/STR.0b013e3181ec611b.
53. Flibotte JJ, Hagan N, O'Donnell J, Greenberg SM, Rosand J. Warfarin, hematoma expansion, and outcome of intracerebral hemorrhage. Neurology. 2004;63(6):1059–64. doi:10.1212/01.WNL.0000138428.40673.83.
54. Saloheimo P, Ahonen M, Juvela S, Pyhtinen J, Savolainen ER, Hillbom M. Regular aspirin-use preceding the onset of primary intracerebral hemorrhage is an independent predictor for death. Stroke. 2006;37(1):129–33. doi:10.1161/01.STR.0000196991.03618.31.
55. Toyoda K, Okada Y, Minematsu K, Kamouchi M, Fujimoto S, Ibayashi S, Inoue T. Antiplatelet therapy contributes to acute deterioration of intracerebral hemorrhage. Neurology. 2005;65(7):1000–4. doi:10.1212/01.wnl.0000179178.37713.69.
56. Sorimachi T, Fujii Y, Morita K, Tanaka R. Predictors of hematoma enlargement in patients with intracerebral hemorrhage treated with rapid administration of antifibrinolytic agents and strict blood pressure control. J Neurosurg. 2007;106(2):250–4. doi:10.3171/jns.2007.106.2.250.
57. Toyoda K, Yasaka M, Nagata K, Nagao T, Gotoh J, Sakamoto T, Uchiyama S, Minematsu K, Bleeding with Antithrombotic Therapy Study G. Antithrombotic therapy influences location, enlargement, and mortality from intracerebral hemorrhage. The Bleeding with Antithrombotic Therapy (BAT) Retrospective Study. Cerebrovasc Dis. 2009;27(2):151–9. doi:10.1159/000177924.
58. Moussouttas M, Malhotra R, Fernandez L, Maltenfort M, Holowecki M, Delgado J, Lawson N, Badjatia N. Role of antiplatelet agents in hematoma expansion during the acute period of intracerebral hemorrhage. Neurocrit Care. 2010;12(1):24–9. doi:10.1007/s12028-009-9290-0.
59. Sansing LH, Messe SR, Cucchiara BL, Cohen SN, Lyden PD, Kasner SE, Investigators C. Prior antiplatelet use does not affect hemorrhage growth or outcome after ICH. Neurology. 2009;72(16):1397–402. doi:10.1212/01.wnl.0000342709.31341.88.
60. Yildiz OK, Arsava EM, Akpinar E, Topcuoglu MA. Previous antiplatelet use is associated with hematoma expansion in patients with spontaneous intracerebral hemorrhage. J Stroke Cerebrovasc Dis. 2012;21(8):760–6. doi:10.1016/j.jstrokecerebrovasdis.2011.04.003.
61. Fabbri A, Servadei F, Marchesini G, Bronzoni C, Montesi D, Arietta L, Societa Italiana di Medicina d'Emergenza Urgenza Study G. Antiplatelet therapy and the outcome of subjects with intracranial injury: the Italian SIMEU study. Crit Care. 2013;17(2):R53. doi:10.1186/cc12575.
62. Mayer SA. Ultra-early hemostatic therapy for intracerebral hemorrhage. Stroke. 2003;34(1):224–9. doi:10.1161/01.STR.0000046458.67968.E4.
63. Benson AB, Moss M, Silliman CC. Transfusion-related acute lung injury (TRALI): a clinical review with emphasis on the critically ill. Br J Haematol. 2009;147(4):431–43. doi:10.1111/j.1365-2141.2009.07840.x.
64. Sridhar G, Menis M, Selvam N, Holness LG, Anderson SA, Wallace AE, Clark P, Daniel GW, Ball R, Izurieta HS. Transfusion-Related Acute Lung Injury (TRALI) Occurrence, Risk Factors, and Outcome: A Nested Case-Control Study. Int J Hematol. 2013;9(1).
65. Finlay HE, Cassorla L, Feiner J, Toy P. Designing and testing a computer-based screening system for transfusion-related acute lung injury. Am J Clin Pathol. 2005;124(4):601–9. doi:10.1309/1XKQKFF83CBU4D6H.
66. Popovsky MA. Transfusion-Related Acute Lung Injury: Incidence, Pathogenesis and the role of multicomponent apheresis in Its prevention. Transfus Med Hemother. 2008;35(2):76–9. doi:10.1159/000117811.
67. Ohm C, Mina A, Howells G, Bair H, Bendick P. Effects of antiplatelet agents on outcomes for elderly patients with traumatic intracranial hemorrhage. J Trauma. 2005;58(3):518–22.
68. Ivascu FA, Howells GA, Junn FS, Bair HA, Bendick PJ, Janczyk RJ. Predictors of mortality in trauma patients with intracranial hemorrhage on preinjury aspirin or clopidogrel. J Trauma. 2008;65(4):785–8. doi:10.1097/TA.0b013e3181848caa.
69. Fortuna GR, Mueller EW, James LE, Shutter LA, Butler KL. The impact of preinjury antiplatelet and anticoagulant pharmacotherapy on outcomes in elderly patients with hemorrhagic brain injury. Surgery. 2008;144(4):598–603. doi:10.1016/j.surg.2008.06.009. discussion 603-595.
70. Creutzfeldt CJ, Weinstein JR, Longstreth Jr WT, Becker KJ, McPharlin TO, Tirschwell DL. Prior antiplatelet therapy, platelet infusion therapy, and outcome after intracerebral hemorrhage. J Stroke

Cerebrovasc Dis. 2009;18(3):221–8. doi:10.1016/j.jstrokecerebrovasdis.2008.10.007.
71. Downey DM, Monson B, Butler KL, Fortuna Jr GR, Saxe JM, Dolan JP, Markert RJ, McCarthy MC. Does platelet administration affect mortality in elderly head-injured patients taking antiplatelet medications? Am Surg. 2009;75(11):1100–3.
72. Bachelani AM, Bautz JT, Sperry JL, Corcos A, Zenati M, Billiar TR, Peitzman AB, Marshall GT. Assessment of platelet transfusion for reversal of aspirin after traumatic brain injury. Surgery. 2011;150(4):836–43. doi:10.1016/j.surg.2011.07.059.
73. Washington CW, Schuerer DJ, Grubb Jr RL. Platelet transfusion: an unnecessary risk for mild traumatic brain injury patients on antiplatelet therapy. J Trauma. 2011;71(2):358–63. doi:10.1097/TA.0b013e318220ad7e.
74. Suzuki Y, Kitahara T, Soma K, Konno S, Sato K, Suzuki S, Oka H, Yamada M, Fujii K, Kitahara Y, Yamamoto Y, Otsuka T, Sugiura Y, Kanoh Y, Tamai Y, Ohto H. Impact of platelet transfusion on survival of patients with intracerebral hemorrhage after administration of anti-platelet agents at a tertiary emergency center. PLoS One. 2014;9(5), e97328. doi:10.1371/journal.pone.0097328.
75. de Gans K, de Haan RJ, Majoie CB, Koopman MM, Brand A, Dijkgraaf MG, Vermeulen M, Roos YB, Investigators P. PATCH: platelet transfusion in cerebral haemorrhage: study protocol for a multicentre, randomised, controlled trial. BMC Neurol. 2010;10:19. doi:10.1186/1471-2377-10-19.
76. Siller-Matula JM, Krumphuber J, Jilma B. Pharmacokinetic, pharmacodynamic and clinical profile of novel antiplatelet drugs targeting vascular diseases. Br J Pharmacol. 2010;159(3):502–17. doi:10.1111/j.1476-5381.2009.00555.x.
77. Sugidachi A, Asai F, Ogawa T, Inoue T, Koike H. The in vivo pharmacological profile of CS-747, a novel antiplatelet agent with platelet ADP receptor antagonist properties. Br J Pharmacol. 2000;129(7):1439–46. doi:10.1038/sj.bjp.0703237.
78. Wiviott SD, White HD, Ohman EM, Fox KA, Armstrong PW, Prabhakaran D, Hafley G, Lokhnygina Y, Boden WE, Hamm C, Clemmensen P, Nicolau JC, Menozzi A, Ruzyllo W, Widimsky P, Oto A, Leiva-Pons J, Pavlides G, Winters KJ, Roe MT, Bhatt DL. Prasugrel versus clopidogrel for patients with unstable angina or non-ST-segment elevation myocardial infarction with or without angiography: a secondary, prespecified analysis of the TRILOGY ACS trial. Lancet. 2013;382(9892):605–13. doi:10.1016/S0140-6736(13)61451-8.
79. Roe MT, Armstrong PW, Fox KA, White HD, Prabhakaran D, Goodman SG, Cornel JH, Bhatt DL, Clemmensen P, Martinez F, Ardissino D, Nicolau JC, Boden WE, Gurbel PA, Ruzyllo W, Dalby AJ, McGuire DK, Leiva-Pons JL, Parkhomenko A, Gottlieb S, Topacio GO, Hamm C, Pavlides G, Goudev AR, Oto A, Tseng CD, Merkely B, Gasparovic V, Corbalan R, Cinteza M, McLendon RC, Winters KJ, Brown EB, Lokhnygina Y, Aylward PE, Huber K, Hochman JS, Ohman EM, Investigators TA. Prasugrel versus clopidogrel for acute coronary syndromes without revascularization. N Engl J Med. 2012;367(14):1297–309. doi:10.1056/NEJMoa1205512.
80. Wiviott SD, Braunwald E, McCabe CH, Montalescot G, Ruzyllo W, Gottlieb S, Neumann FJ, Ardissino D, De Servi S, Murphy SA, Riesmeyer J, Weerakkody G, Gibson CM, Antman EM, Investigators T-T. Prasugrel versus clopidogrel in patients with acute coronary syndromes. N Engl J Med. 2007;357(20):2001–15. doi:10.1056/NEJMoa0706482.
81. Husted S, Emanuelsson H, Heptinstall S, Sandset PM, Wickens M, Peters G. Pharmacodynamics, pharmacokinetics, and safety of the oral reversible P2Y12 antagonist AZD6140 with aspirin in patients with atherosclerosis: a double-blind comparison to clopidogrel with aspirin. Eur Heart J. 2006;27(9):1038–47. doi:10.1093/eurheartj/ehi754.
82. James S, Akerblom A, Cannon CP, Emanuelsson H, Husted S, Katus H, Skene A, Steg PG, Storey RF, Harrington R, Becker R, Wallentin L. Comparison of ticagrelor, the first reversible oral P2Y(12) receptor antagonist, with clopidogrel in patients with acute coronary syndromes: Rationale, design, and baseline characteristics of the PLATelet inhibition and patient Outcomes (PLATO) trial. Am Heart J. 2009;157(4):599–605. doi:10.1016/j.ahj.2009.01.003.
83. Teng R, Butler K. Pharmacokinetics, pharmacodynamics, tolerability and safety of single ascending doses of ticagrelor, a reversibly binding oral P2Y(12) receptor antagonist, in healthy subjects. Eur J Clin Pharmacol. 2010;66(5):487–96. doi:10.1007/s00228-009-0778-5.
84. van Giezen JJ, Nilsson L, Berntsson P, Wissing BM, Giordanetto F, Tomlinson W, Greasley PJ. Ticagrelor binds to human P2Y(12) independently from ADP but antagonizes ADP-induced receptor signaling and platelet aggregation. J Thromb Haemost. 2009;7(9):1556–65. doi:10.1111/j.1538-7836.2009.03527.x.
85. Storey RF, Melissa Thornton S, Lawrance R, Husted S, Wickens M, Emanuelsson H, Cannon CP, Heptinstall S, Armstrong M. Ticagrelor yields consistent dose-dependent inhibition of ADP-induced platelet aggregation in patients with atherosclerotic disease regardless of genotypic variations in P2RY12, P2RY1, and ITGB3. Platelets. 2009;20(5):341–8. doi:10.1080/09537100903075324.
86. Chrvala C, Caspi A. Pharmacy and Therapeutics: Product Profiler: Brilinta™ (ticagrelor) Tablets. P&T Product Profiler 37 (4). http://www.ncbi.nlm.nih.gov/pmc/articles/PMC3353491/pdf/ptj3704s2.pdf (2012). Accessed 1 March 2015.
87. Wallentin L, Becker RC, Budaj A, Cannon CP, Emanuelsson H, Held C, Horrow J, Husted S, James S, Katus H, Mahaffey KW, Scirica BM, Skene A, Steg PG, Storey RF, Harrington RA, Investigators P, Freij A, Thorsen M. Ticagrelor versus clopidogrel in patients with acute coronary syndromes. N Engl J Med. 2009;361(11):1045–57. doi:10.1056/NEJMoa0904327.

88. Ferreiro JL, Ueno M, Angiolillo DJ. Cangrelor: a review on its mechanism of action and clinical development. Expert Rev Cardiovasc Ther. 2009;7(10):1195–201. doi:10.1586/erc.09.101.
89. Bhatt DL, Lincoff AM, Gibson CM, Stone GW, McNulty S, Montalescot G, Kleiman NS, Goodman SG, White HD, Mahaffey KW, Pollack Jr CV, Manoukian SV, Widimsky P, Chew DP, Cura F, Manukov I, Tousek F, Jafar MZ, Arneja J, Skerjanec S, Harrington RA, Investigators CP. Intravenous platelet blockade with cangrelor during PCI. N Engl J Med. 2009;361(24):2330–41. doi:10.1056/NEJMoa0908629.
90. Bhatt DL, Stone GW, Mahaffey KW, Gibson CM, Steg PG, Hamm CW, Price MJ, Leonardi S, Gallup D, Bramucci E, Radke PW, Widimsky P, Tousek F, Tauth J, Spriggs D, McLaurin BT, Angiolillo DJ, Genereux P, Liu T, Prats J, Todd M, Skerjanec S, White HD, Harrington RA, Investigators CP. Effect of platelet inhibition with cangrelor during PCI on ischemic events. N Engl J Med. 2013;368(14):1303–13. doi:10.1056/NEJMoa1300815.

Part 2

Coagulation Issues Across All Patient Spectrums

Congenital Coagulation Disorders 7

Danielle Sterrenberg and Sucha Nand

The congenital coagulation disorders encompass a wide variety of inherited diseases that can affect all aspects of coagulation including the disruption of both primary and secondary hemostasis. Most of these disorders are quite rare but some, such as von Willebrand disease, can be seen rather frequently. Given the disruption of the coagulation pathways, they all have in common an enhanced predilection for hemorrhagic episodes both spontaneous and as a result of hemostatic challenges like trauma or surgical procedures. As such, it is important to identify affected patients in order to prevent excessive bleeding in the perioperative period. Figure 7.1 is a summary of coagulation defects and their impact on either primary hemostasis, or formation of the platelet plug, and secondary hemostasis, i.e., generation of thrombin and clot stabilization. Inherited collagen vascular disorders are not discussed in this review. We review the inherited disorders of secondary hemostasis first as these disorders are encountered much more frequently in clinical practice and then move on to discuss disorders of primary hemostasis.

D. Sterrenberg, M.D. • S. Nand, M.D. (✉)
Loyola University Medical Center,
Maywood, IL, USA
e-mail: dsterrenberg@lumc.edu; snand@lumc.edu

Inherited Disorders of Secondary Hemostasis

Von Willebrand Disease

Von Willebrand disease (VWD) is the most common inherited disorder of coagulation affecting nearly 1 % of the general population [1]. Some epidemiologic studies suggest that 1:100 people have some form of VWD but only about 1:1000 are symptomatic [2, 3]. There are several forms of VWD, the most common of which are inherited in an autosomal dominant fashion and affect male and females nearly equally (Table 7.1).

Von Willebrand Factor

The von Willebrand factor (VWF) gene is located on the short arm of chromosome 12 at 12p13.3 and it encodes for the pro-coagulant adhesive protein, VWF. VWF is produced and stored as an ultralarge multimeric protein in endothelial cells and is also produced in megakaryocytes and stored in alpha granules of platelets. Endothelial cells release VWF constitutively into plasma whereas platelets release VWF into circulation only after their activation [4]. In the event of sheer stress, this ultralarge VWF binds collagen in exposed subendothelium and platelets forming a bridge. This exposes the A1 domain, a binding site for the cleavage protein, ADAMTS13. ADAMTS13 cleaves the ultralarge VWF into

C.M. Loftus (ed.), *Anticoagulation and Hemostasis in Neurosurgery*,
DOI 10.1007/978-3-319-27327-3_7

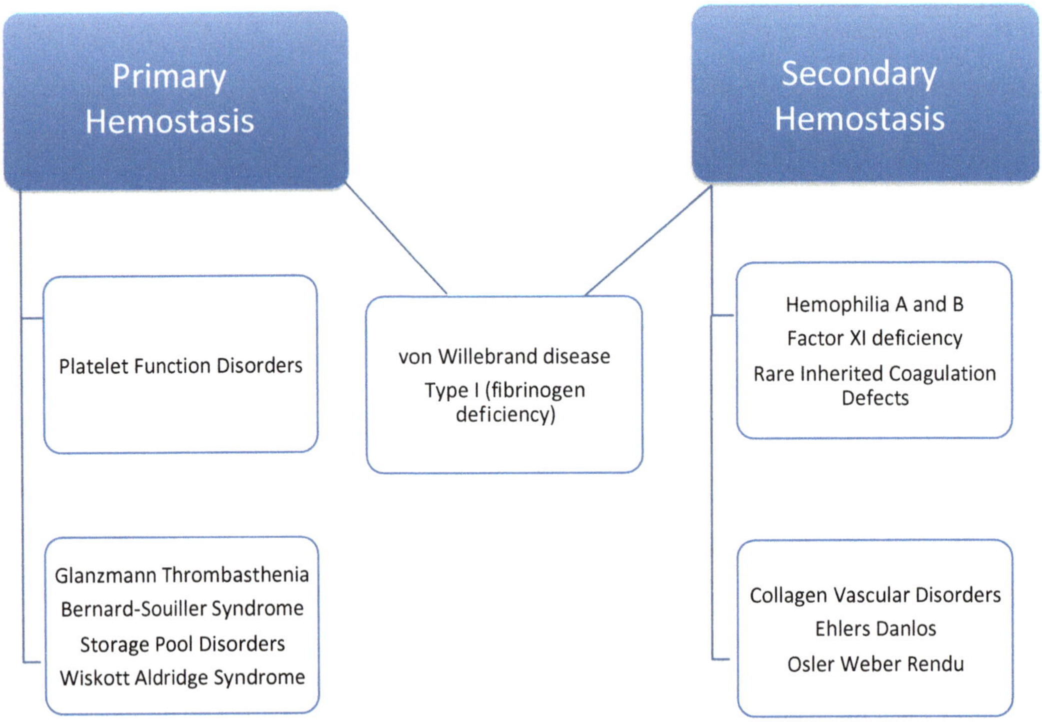

Fig. 7.1 Causes of congenital coagulation disorders and their effect on primary hemostasis, secondary hemostasis, or both

Table 7.1 Laboratory diagnosis of VWD [71]

Diagnosis	*VWF:RCo (IU/dL)	*VWF:Ag (IU/dL)	*Factor VIII	*Ratio of VWF:RCo to VWF:Ag	**RIPA	**VWF multimers
Type 1	↓ <30	↓ <30	↓ or normal	>0.6	Normal	Normal
Type 2A	↓ <30	↓ <30–200	↓ or normal	<0.6	↓	↓HMW multimers
Type 2B	↓ <30	↓ <30–200	↓ or normal	Usually <0.6	↑	↓HMW multimers
Type 2M	↓ <30	↓ <30–200	↓ or normal	<0.6	↓	Normal
Type 2N	↓ or normal; 30–200	↓ or normal; 30–200	↓↓	>0.6	Normal	Normal
Type 3	↓↓ <3	↓↓<3	↓↓↓ (<10 IU/dL)	NA	Absent	NA
Normal	50–200	50–200	100 IU/dL	>0.6	Normal	Normal

smaller multimers of various molecular weights, preventing the formation of platelet thrombi and enhancing the function of VWF [5].

Von Willebrand factor (VWF) is essential to both primary and secondary hemostasis. It is a bridging molecule with binding sites for factor VIII, platelet glycoprotein Ib, exposed collagen on the vessel wall, and platelet glycoprotein IIb/IIIa that allow for it to function at multiple steps in the hemostatic process [6]. VWF has 2 main roles in primary hemostasis; it mediates platelet adhesion to the sub endothelial surface through the GP1b/IX/V receptor and, in coordination with fibrinogen, allows for platelet aggregation via the GPIIb/IIIa receptor. Its role in secondary hemostasis is as a plasma stabilizer for the fragile factor VIII, carrying factor VIII and thereby preventing its proteolytic degradation in plasma by activated protein C and delivering it to sites of vascular injury [7].

Diagnosis and Classification

There are 3 main types of VWD characterized by a quantitative defect in the VWF, either partial loss of VWF as in Type I or full loss of the protein as is seen in Type 3, or by qualitative defects in the function of VWF as is seen in Type 2 VWD.

Initial laboratory evaluation for patients suspected of having VWD includes a complete blood count (CBC), which is usually normal but in certain variants of VWD can reveal a concurrent thrombocytopenia. Coagulation studies show an abnormal bleeding time, a normal prothrombin time (PT) and, depending on the variant of VWD, a normal or prolonged activated partial thromboplastin time (aPTT). Laboratory studies that are specific to VWD include the von Willebrand factor antigen (VWF:Ag) which measures circulating von Willebrand factor, von Willebrand Ristocetin cofactor assay (VWF:RCo) which measures the functional ability of VWF by mimicking the physiologic interaction between VWF and Gp1b on the platelet surface, and the factor VIII concentration (FVIII:C). The ratio of VWF:Ag to VWF:RCo can help to identify the subtype of VWD. For instance, in patients with quantitative defects in VWF, the ratio will be near 1 with the dysfunction of VWF related to the degree of deficiency of the protein. However, in the case of qualitative defects, the ratio will be <0.6 as the circulating antigen levels are near normal but their function is impaired. Once the patient is confirmed to have VWD with tests listed above, it is important to classify which type of VWD they have as the treatment, bleeding risk, and prognosis may vary. The two tests utilized most often in classifying VWD are ristocetin-induced platelet aggregation (RIPA), used to identify Type 2B in particular, and the VWF multimer analysis, used to distinguish Type 2A from Type 2M.

Type I VWD

Type I VWD is the most common subtype representing around 75–80 % of all cases. It is a quantitative defect in VWF leading to reduced, but not absent, levels in plasma. It is inherited in an autosomal dominant (AD) fashion, but has varying degrees of expression and penetrance making characterization of the responsible mutations and mechanisms of disease as well as diagnosis difficult. Furthermore, varying VWF levels throughout the aging process and throughout blood groups have made this even more challenging. For instance, VWF levels are known to increase with age and during times of stress or inflammation or pregnancy and to be higher in those individuals with AB blood types than in those with type O blood [8, 9]. However, recent studies have shown that the decreased VWF level seen in Type I VWD is likely due, in some instances, to enhanced clearance of VWF out of circulation or to intracellular retention of VWF [10]. Because the VWF function remains intact in Type I VWD, the use of desmopressin (DDAVP) may be useful.

Type 2 VWD

This subtype comprises a group of abnormalities in VWF that is further subdivided into four variants (2A, 2B, 2M, and 2N) all of which are characterized by qualitative deficits in VWF and collectively account for ~10–20 % of VWD. Essentially, the production and release of VWF is normal, but the protein itself is dysfunctional due to a variety of inherited mutations.

Type 2A: Most frequent form of Type 2 VWD, comprising 20–25 % of VWD. It is caused by genetic mutations that impair the multimerization of VWF or enhance its sensitivity to ADAMTS13 cleavage causing loss of high molecular weight (HMW) and intermediate molecular weight (IMW) multimers and decreased activity of the binding domains for GPIB on the surface of platelets. The key laboratory findings are both a reduced VWF:Ag and VWF:RCo level but with a disproportionate decrease in the functional component such that their ratio is <0.6, in addition to a VWF multimer profile exhibiting a loss of IMW and HMW multimers.

Type 2B: Gain of function mutations in the Gp1Ba binding domain, inherited in an Autosomal Dominant fashion, enable the VWF to bind platelets more avidly leading to enhanced clearance of HMW multimers and platelets. The hemostatic findings are identical to that seen in Type 2A, however, ristocetin induced platelet aggregation (RIPA) would show enhanced aggregation to low dose ristocetin, distinguishing Type 2A from 2B. In addition, Type 2B can be associated with thrombocytopenia. DDAVP is contraindicated in this subtype due to the risk of exacerbating thrombocytopenia.

Type 2M: Caused by loss of function mutations in the platelet or collagen binding domains that impair VWF dependent platelet adhesion. As with all Type 2 mutations, the ratio of VWF:Ag to VWF:RCo is <0.6 but VWF multimers remain normally distributed.

Type 2N (Normandy): This variant involves mutations inherited in an autosomal recessive (AR) fashion that interfere with the functional ability of VWF to bind and carry FVIII leading to enhanced proteolytic degradation of FVIII and a clinical syndrome that is similar to mild hemophilia A. Distinguishing hemophilia A from VWD Type 2N can be challenging as the VWF:Ag and VWF:RCo can be reduced or normal and factor VIII will be reduced. VWF multimers are usually normal as well. Distinction may require assays of factor VIII–VWF binding [11].

Type 3

This type is the most rare form of VWD, affecting only 1 in 1 million people and is the most severe [10]. It is caused by mutations, inherited as an autosomal recessive trait, that result in near total absence of VWF. This results in extremely low VWF:Ag and VWF:RCo as well as very low factor VIII levels that are in the range of those with severe hemophilia A. The clinical presentation of patients with Type 3 is different from all other forms of VWD as patients usually experience sever bleeding episodes with spontaneous hemorrhage into synovial space and musculature similar to that seen in severe hemophilia A. Given these patients have virtually no VWF, they do not respond to DDAVP.

Clinical Presentation

Patients with von Willebrand disease experience mucocutaneous bleeding, epistaxis, menorrhagia as well as prolonged and at times severe bleeding after surgery or trauma. One of the most common sources of hemorrhage in VWD patients is menorrhagia, with 20 % of women with menorrhagia having VWD [12]. Life threatening central nervous system (CNS) and gastrointestinal (GI) bleeding is rare but can occur in patients with Type 3 VWD or less frequently in type 2 VWD.

Treatment

There are 3 main therapeutic strategies for managing VWD. The first strategy involves enhancing the release of VWF from endogenous compartments into plasma through the use of DDAVP. The second strategy is to replace endogenous VWF with exogenous, virally inactivated plasma concentrates of VWF and factor VIII, and the third strategy is to enhance hemostatic control utilizing agents that are extraneous to the VWF/FVIII complex.

DDAVP is the treatment of choice for VWD. It is a synthetic derivative of vasopressin that facilitates the release of VWF from endothelial compartments via V2 receptors thereby increasing VWF levels in circulation [13]. It also raises FVIII levels, although this mechanism is not as well understood. All patients with VWD, except those with Type 2B, should undergo a DDAVP infusion test near the time of diagnosis to see if they respond to DDAVP as this treatment can be given to correct acute bleeding episodes or given prophylactically prior to necessary surgeries. Even though patients with Type 3 VWD usually do not respond to DDAVP, an infusion study should still be performed, as there are small subsets of patients who will respond to therapy [14].

Combination VWF and factor VIII concentrates are indicated in Type 2B VWD and in patients who are actively bleeding, for the prevention of excessive or delayed bleeding from trauma or surgical procedures with high risk of hemorrhage, and those patients who fail to respond to DDAVP. Humate-P is a VWF/factor VIII concentrate that is most commonly used in this setting as it has been the most studied. Its ratio of VWF/RCo to factor VIII is very similar to that seen in normal plasma and has been shown to have efficacy in restoring normal hemostasis. A new agent, BAX111, is a recombinant human VWF that has been shown to be efficacious in controlling bleeding in patients with VWD in phase I and Phase III trials [15]. It is currently awaiting FDA approval.

Other agents can be used to halt or prevent bleeding events in patients with VWD. For instance, oral contraceptives or intrauterine devices can be given to prevent menstrual blood loss while fibrin clot stabilizers such as epsilon aminocaproic acid (EACA or Amicar) or tranexamic acid (Cyklokapron) are often used to arrest minor mucosal bleeding or menorrhagia both in combination with DDAVP or factor replacement or as sole agents [16]. Both are available in oral, intravenous, and topical formulations and exert their effect by binding plasminogen and preventing its activation to plasmin, thereby preventing fibrinolysis [17]. They are contraindicated in patients with hematuria given the risk of clot formation in the renal collecting system leading to obstructive uropathy.

Perioperative Management of VWD

Preoperative evaluation of a patient with VWD should include a detailed history of previous bleeding episodes and surgical outcomes to fully assess the bleeding risk of the planned surgery or procedure. If the patient has not previously had a desmopressin infusion test performed, it should be done prior to surgery. Response patterns to DDAVP remain uniform throughout life, so if a patient has had a prior documented response to DDAVP, then this does not need to be repeated prior to surgery. Laboratory evaluations should include a CBC, PT, PTT, and factor VIII level as well as a VWF:Ag level and VWF:RCo assay. Clinical data suggest that the FVIII level is the best predictor of soft tissue, surgical, and delayed bleeding in VWD patients while the VWF:RCo is the component responsible for mucosal bleeding [16].

The ability to use DDAVP perioperatively to prevent bleeding depends on a variety of factors. Patient responsiveness is a main factor, but the extent of hemostatic challenge provided during the operation and the time needed to heal must be considered. In general, major surgery requires hemostasis for 7–14 days while minor surgeries only require hemostasis for 1–5 days. Common major and minor surgical procedures are listed in Table 7.1. If more than 3 days of hemostasis is necessary, then DDAVP is not the only agent needed to provide coverage given its propensity for tachyphylaxis after 3–4 doses. As such, factor replacement is necessary in these patients. Patients who are at very high risk of intraoperative bleeding due to the nature of the surgery should be covered by factor replacement as well. If the procedure is of mild hemorrhagic risk, such as a dental procedure, and the patient has been shown to have a response to DDAVP infusion, then the patient can be treated with DDAVP prior to surgery and then repeated every 8–24 h as needed for ~3 doses. However, factor VIII level and VWF:RCo should be checked after every administration because of the occurrence of tachyphylaxis. Usually for mild procedures, DDAVP is administered in conjunction with antifibrinolytics such as Amicar or tranexamic acid. The antifibrinolytics are usually continued for 5–7 days after mild procedures.

Humate P and Alphanate are two commercially available VWF factor replacements that are approved for the prophylactic prevention of bleeding in the surgical patient. However, Humate P is the most widely used and most studied in both the setting of reversing acute bleeding and in the prophylactic management of surgical patients. Several studies have shown that it achieves excellent to good hemostasis in 91–100 % of surgical procedures [18, 19]. Humate P is usually given once daily with the exact dose based on the risk of intraoperative bleeding. For instance, during major surgical procedures Humate P is given once daily and dosed to raise the factor VIII and VWF:RCo levels to 80–100 IU/dL the day of surgery and then maintained >50 IU/dL for 7–14 days after surgery. For minor procedures, FVIII and VWF:RCo target levels are >50 IU/dL on the day of surgery and then continued for a target level of >30 IU/dl for 1–5 days after surgery. For dental extractions or minimally invasive procedures, patients should receive a one-time dose of Humate P to raise their FVIII or VWF:RCo to >50 IU/dL [20].

Patients with VWD, despite their coagulopathy, can still develop thromboembolic disease. In fact, several studies have shown cases of deep venous thrombosis (DVT) or pulmonary embolism (PE) after factor VIII and VWF replacement in VWD patients undergoing surgery [21]. A review of the patients who developed these venous thromboembolic events (VTE) shows that several of them had very high FVIII levels and additional risks for VTE such as advanced age, estrogen use, and recent surgical procedures. Thus, care should be taken to not overcorrect the factor VIII level by checking both a FVIII in addition to VWF:RCo during factor replacement and to consider anticoagulant prophylaxis in surgical patients especially in those with other risk factors for VTE development [22].

Hemophilia

Hemophilia is a group of disorders resulting from genetic mutations in either factor VIII (hemophilia A) or factor IX (hemophilia B). Both genes are located on the long arm of the X chromosome at Xq28 and Xq27 respectively and thus are inherited in an X-linked fashion [23]. Most affected men display symptoms while carrier females are usually asymptomatic. With the use of molecular genetics, a wide spectrum of mutations in the factor VIII and factor IX genes have been identified and known to contribute to the respective clinical syndrome. In fact, according to an online database, www.factorviii-db.org, there are currently (as of February 2015) 2,015 unique mutations identified as causing hemophilia A. By far the most common mutations identified are intron 22 inversions that affects more than 45 % of severe hemophilia A patients. Hemophilia B has a similar online database at www.factorix.org that has identified 1095 unique variants of F9 mutations. Almost 70 % of patients with hemophilia B have causative missense mutations and inversions are in general not seen [24].

Hemophilia A is more prevalent, affecting around 1:5000 males with approximately 13,000 new cases identified per year. Hemophilia B affects approximately 1:30,000 males with around 3600 new cases of hemophilia B in the USA per year [25, 26].

Hemophilia A

Hemophilia A is an X-linked recessive (XLR) genetic deficiency of the functional plasma clotting factor, factor VIII (FVIII) resulting from mutations in the FVIII gene located on the long arm of the X chromosome. This results in low to absent factor VIII levels and a disruption in the intrinsic pathway of the coagulation cascade causing a lack of thrombin or fibrin generation and thus inability to stabilize the platelet plug formed during primary hemostasis resulting in excessive, often delayed, hemorrhage both in response to trauma or arising spontaneously. Over 70 % of cases are inherited in an XLR pattern, but around 30 % of cases arise as spontaneous mutations in the FVIII gene. Given its X linked pattern of inheritance it is a disease seen almost exclusively in males. However, mild hemophilia A and, very rarely, even a severe hemophilia phenotype are known to occur in heterozygous females due to various degrees of chromosomal X inactivation [27]. Given this and the fact that female carriers, while asymptomatic, can also have reduced factor VIII levels, monitoring of factor VIII levels should be considered in female patients with a family history of hemophilia or evidence of exaggerated hemorrhage in response to trauma or spontaneous hemorrhage.

The clinical severity, or risk of bleeding, in patients with hemophilia A can be predicted by the coagulation factor activity level present in plasma. Table 7.2 shows the clinical classification of patients with hemophilia A. In general, factor levels (<1 IU/dL) are considered severe with patients presenting, oftentimes in infancy, with episodes of spontaneous hemorrhage most commonly into their joints or muscles. Less severe phenotypes are associated with some

Table 7.2 Suggested duration of VWF replacement for different surgical procedures [72]

Major surgery (7–14 days)	Minor surgery (1–5 days)	Other procedures, if uncomplicated, single VWF treatment
Cardiothoracic	Biopsy: breast, cervical	Cardiac catheterization
Cesarean Section	Complicated dental extractions	Cataract surgery
Craniotomy	Gingival surgery	Endoscopy (without biopsy)
Hysterectomy	Central line placement	Liver biopsy
Open cholecystectomy	Laparoscopic procedures	Lacerations
Prostatectomy		Simple dental extractions

residual factor VIII levels and are characterized by excessive bleeding at sites of trauma. In general, factor VIII levels >30 % to that of normal are enough to prevent spontaneous hemorrhage and to maintain a normal hemostatic system. An epidemiologic survey conducted in the 1990s identified about 43 % of hemophiliacs as severe [28].

Both hemophilia A and B have identical inheritance patterns and clinical presentation but have different factor deficiencies. However, there are some studies suggesting a higher bleeding risk in patients with hemophilia A for the same level of factor activity [29]. Also, with hemophilia A the factor levels generally remain constant throughout a patients' life but with hemophilia B there can be some increase in FIX levels after puberty such that a patient with a moderate form of hemophilia may become more mild due to a small but clinically significant rise in FIX levels in response to androgen production during adolescence. Prior to modern factor replacement, the median overall survival for patients with severe hemophilia, A or B, was 11.3 years. However, more recent estimates in patients treated with factor replacement and after appropriate viral eradication of blood products was possible in them show an average survival of 63 years for males with severe phenotype and 73 years for males with mild to moderate hemophilia [30]. These numbers approach that seen with the normal population. As a consequence, more and more patients are developing additional medical comorbidities and are requiring surgical procedures for a number of common aging maladies such as heart disease and cancer.

FVIII Protein and the Pathophysiology of Hemophilia A

FVIII circulates in plasma as an inactive precursor that is in a complex with von Willebrand factor. It has no intrinsic enzymatic activity but rather functions as a cofactor for FIX in the activation of FX to its active form, FXa [31]. It is a highly unstable protein and requires the covalent binding of von Willebrand factor to prevent its proteolytic degradation in plasma. This instability of FVIII in plasma is why, in some forms of von Willebrand disease, FVIII levels can be low [32]. Factor VIII and factor IX deficiency results in the same coagulation derangement: namely, the inability to generate thrombin and fibrin to secure the primary platelet plug formed during primary hemostasis.

Hemophilia B

The clinical presentation of hemophilia B is nearly identical to that of hemophilia A. In addition, Both the FVIII and the FIX genes are located on the X chromosome in close proximity to one another. Also as seen in hemophilia A, 70 % of mutations are inherited in an XLR pattern but 30 % of mutations arise de novo.

FIX circulates in plasma as a serine protease zymogen that requires FVIII as a cofactor for its functional activity. Together with FVIII, a complex is formed that cleaves FX into its active form, FXa. However, unlike FVIII, FIX is dependent on posttranslational vitamin K-dependent processing by gamma carboxylase for full functional activity. Clinical severity and management of hemophilia B is also dependent on the amount of factor IX functional activity retained [33].

Clinical Manifestations of Hemophilia A and B

Bleeding is the hallmark of hemophilia. However, clinical presentation and prognosis in hemophilia varies significantly based on the residual factor levels. Patients with severe disease are often afflicted by recurrent non-traumatic bleeds. Birth represents the first hemostatic challenge in the life of a hemophiliac and is when some patients present with symptoms. Common sites of bleeding during the first month of life for patients with hemophilia include post-circumcision bleeds (~48 %), followed by intracranial hemorrhage (ICH) seen in 19 % of cases [34]. Multiple studies have shown that the rate of ICH in hemophilia, regardless of disease severity, is around 1–4 % with a 20 % mortality rate [34, 35]. After the neonatal period, patients tend to develop hemorrhage at alternative sites.

Hemarthrosis is the most common site of spontaneous hemorrhage. While any joint can be affected, this is seen most commonly in the knee, elbow and ankles usually starting after affected individuals begin to crawl or walk. Hemarthrosis results in chronic synovitis which can lead a patient to develop hemophilic arthropathy, which severely affects joint integrity and in cases of recurrent bleeds, can lead to a deformed and essentially dysfunctional joint [36].

Intramuscular hematomas are the second most common site of hemorrhage in hemophiliacs. The hematoma can be large and in severe cases, depending on the location, can be associated with compartment syndrome, major blood loss in the setting of iliopsoas hematomas, and local muscle or tendon damage [37].

Other common forms of hemorrhage include mucocutaneous, gastrointestinal and genitourinary. Intracranial hemorrhage is one of the most worrisome sequelae of hemophilia and remains a risk throughout the patients' life. In a case–control trial of hemophilia patients, high inhibitor titers, severe hemophilia, and a prior history of ICH were all associated with higher rates of ICH [38].

Diagnosis

Approximately 50–70 % of newborns with hemophilia have a positive family history and in these patients the diagnosis is usually made around the time of birth by checking factor VIII or factor IX levels on cord blood. In the remaining patients the disease is diagnosed when symptoms begin to manifest, which is usually very early in infancy for severe patients and later in childhood or in adulthood for mild cases. Workup consists of a detailed family history, a detailed bleeding history and surgical history, as well as appropriate laboratory testing. A CBC is necessary in the evaluation of a potential patient and is usually normal but can have an associated microcytic anemia depending on the amount of prior blood loss. The PT is normal but aPTT is prolonged. If performed, the bleeding time is usually normal. A mixing study will correct the aPTT to within normal range, but in patients with an inhibitor, the correction may be partial. Factor VIII or factor IX levels are reduced or absent in hemophilia A or B respectively. Because VWD, which is the most common congenital coagulation disorder, can also present with reduced factor VIII levels, it is important to rule this out via appropriate laboratory assessment prior to a formal diagnosis of hemophilia A.

Treatment

Replacement of the deficient factor with either plasma derived or recombinant factor VIII or factor IX concentrate is the hallmark of hemophilia therapy. Decisions regarding when to treat, what dose to use, and how often to administer depend on the severity of disease and whether or not there is active hemorrhage occurring or the patient is undergoing a surgical procedure.

The treatment of hemophilia is based on the clinical severity of the syndrome. Individuals with severe deficiency, require regular prophylactic administration of either plasma derived or recombinant factor VIII or factor IX to prevent spontaneous hemorrhage and consequent joint damage that occurs with synovial bleeds.

Multiple studies have been performed showing that in severe cases, prophylactic administration of factor replacement reduces the annual bleeding rates and subsequent joint damage seen in hemophilia patients versus on-demand replacement strategies [39]. Patients with mild to moderate forms can utilize on demand scheduling of factor replacement or alternative agents to reduce the bleeding risk. In cases of prophylactic administration or minor mucosal bleeding, raising factor VIII level to 30 % (~0.3 IU/dL) is usually sufficient for normal hemostasis.

Active Hemorrhage

During acute life threatening hemorrhage or major surgical procedures a normal factor VIII or factor IX level should be maintained at all times [40]. The half-life of both plasma derived and recombinant factor VIII is 8–12 h necessitating twice daily administration in the setting of active hemorrhage or major surgery, whereas the half-life of factor IX in serum is around 20 h allowing for daily dosing [41, 42]. The dose of concentrate to be administered is calculated based on the subtype of hemophilia, the baseline factor levels, and the target factor level. For mild/moderate bleeding, the target range for factor levels is around 0.3 IU/dL (30 % normal), however for acute severe hemorrhage, the goal is 1 IU/dL or near 100 % normal range [43]. Factor concentrates can be administered in bolus or continuous dosing, with some studies recommending a continuous infusion in cases of life threatening hemorrhage in order to prevent the peaks and troughs seen with bolus dosing.

Desmopressin (DDAVP)

Desmopressin, or DDAVP, can be used to treat patients with mild or moderate factor VIII deficiency in which a prior rise of their factor VIII levels in response to therapy has been demonstrated. DDAVP is a derivative of antidiuretic hormone and has been shown to increase plasma levels of factor VIII and von Willebrand factor through increasing the release of this complex from endothelial cells. It can therefore be used in cases of mild mucosal bleeding or perioperatively surrounding mild procedures, such as dental extractions, thereby decreasing or eliminating the use of homologous factor replacement in select patients [44]. Despite marked variability between patients, DDAVP can be seen to increase factor VIII levels three to fivefold that of baseline in patients with mild hemophilia A or von Willebrand disease and this increase is often enough to terminate mild bleeding episodes and provide adequate coverage for low risk surgical procedures. Patients with severe factor VIII deficiency or hemophilia B do not respond to DDAVP and this agent should not be considered.

The fibrin clot stabilizers Amicar and tranexamic acid are seldom utilized in hemophilia. However, they can be considered for mild mucosal or uterine bleeding or after dental extractions again in an effort to enhance local control of minor bleeding without the use of blood products. As mentioned earlier, they are contraindicated in patients with hematuria.

Inhibitors

Now that blood products used for replacement in hemophilia utilize adequate viral eradication strategies, the transmission of HIV and hepatitis that once plagued the hemophilia world and led to significant morbidity and mortality is essentially a concern of the past. However, the main concern now with the use of factor replacement is the development of inhibitors. These inhibitors are allo-antibodies to factor VIII and factor IX that decrease levels of endogenous factors and also neutralize the administration of exogenous factors during replacement strategies thus increasing a patient's risk of bleeding both spontaneously and in response to trauma and making the correction of their coagulopathy more difficult. In hemophilia A, about 30 % of patients with severe disease will develop inhibitors that can bind to factor VIII [45]. They are typically IgG4 and can render factor replacement completely ineffective. For reasons not completely known, they occur more frequently in patients with severe disease and are more common in African Americans, young patients undergoing replacement for the first time, patients getting factor replacement in preparation for surgery, and in those with certain genetic mutations responsible for hemophilia [46–48]. They occur less frequently in hemophilia B, usually in about 3 % of affected patients [45]. Not only do inhibitors increase a patient's bleeding risk but they also make the prophylaxis and treatment of hemophilia much more challenging.

The severity of inhibitors is based on the activity of the antibodies, which is measured in antibody titers. Patients with low-titer inhibitors, i.e., <5 BU/ml (Bethesda units), often have transient antibodies that can subside without therapy and can be treated with higher doses of factor VIII or factor IX alone. However, high-titer inhibitors (>5 BU/ml) often will not respond to increasing doses of factor replacement and require alternative forms of therapy. As in the patient without inhibitors, one can consider DDAVP, Amicar, and tranexamic acid to control or decrease the risk of bleeding. However, in patients with severe acute bleeding or at high risk of spontaneous hemorrhage, bypass agents are used.

Factor VIII Inhibitor Bypassing Agents (FEIBA)

FEIBA is an activated prothrombin complex concentrate (aPCC) containing all the vitamin K dependent coagulation factors (FII, FVII, FIX, and FX) and factor VIII in both zymogen and active forms. The mechanism of action is complex, but is thought to involve thrombin activation via prothrombin and factor X [49]. It has a half-life of 6–12 h and thus doses are usually repeated every 6–12 h depending of bleeding severity and clinical response.

Recombinant Factor VIIa (rVIIa)

rVIIa, also known as Novoseven, is a recombinant factor VIIa that facilitates hemostasis by activating FXa directly on platelet surfaces, thus bypassing the factor VIII complex entirely. It has a short half-life of 2.3 h and thus must be administered frequently in the setting of active major hemorrhage [50].

Immune Tolerance Induction Therapy (ITI)

The long-term treatment of inhibitor development in hemophilia is aimed at eliminating the causative antibodies. ITI is the most studied and efficacious therapy, eradicating inhibitors in about 70 % of patients. However, it takes 9–12 months of treatment to obtain this result. Therefore, bypassing agents are often required in patients prior to or during ITI or in the event of relapse. Immune tolerance is achieved using frequent and prolonged high doses of FVIII either with or without concurrent immunosuppressive therapy [51].

Perioperative Treatment of Hemophilia

The risk of bleeding is high for patients with hemophilia who require surgery and all appropriate preoperative measures should be taken. A detailed surgical and family history of all surgical patients should be recorded prior to their procedure and if a potential female hemophilia carrier is identified, then she would require a more in depth hematologic assessment, as her FVIII levels can be variably reduced, predisposing her to excessive perioperative hemorrhage and potentially requiring treatment prior to surgery. In anticipation of any elective surgical procedure, a multidisciplinary perioperative plan should be arranged. Care should to be taken to ensure that adequate factor replacement is available to administer to patients before, during, and after the procedure. A detailed presurgical workup should be performed a few weeks prior to surgery (in the case of elective procedures) and should include a repeat CBC, PT, aPTT, and factor levels. Laboratory assessment for the development of inhibitors should also be performed. Adequate preoperative testing can take more than a week to obtain results and should be planned accordingly.

Dosing of clotting factors varies on the type of surgery performed. For major surgery, FVIII and FIX levels should be around 100 % of normal. This can be accomplished with perioperative and postoperative administration of factor concentrate provided the patient has not developed any inhibitors. Treatment should begin prior to surgery and be continued for at least 10–14 days postoperatively and in some cases several weeks after major surgery depending on the ongoing bleeding risk. For moderate risk procedures, such as dental extractions, factor levels can be maintained around 50 % normal value and do not need to be continued weeks after the procedure. Factor replacement can be can be delivered in a bolus fashion (usually every 12 h for FVIII replacement and daily for FIX replacement) or as a continuous infusion. As in the setting of severe acute hemorrhage, some studies recommend continuous infusion perioperatively surrounding major surgical procedures with high bleeding risk.

In the event the hemophilic patient has developed either factor VIII or factor IX inhibitors, the perioperative management is more complicated. However, several treatment options are available, and the choice of treatment depends upon the severity of expected bleeding. It should be noted that patients with inhibitors have a higher risk of bleeding.

Novoseven (recombinant factor VII or rFVIIa) has been utilized in the perioperative management of hemophiliacs who have acquired inhibitors. Prothrombin factor concentrates (FEIBA, Autoplex) are also routinely used in this setting. However, the monitoring of their efficacy is more difficult, as one cannot rely upon the usual increase in factor levels. As such, the monitoring of their efficacy occurs largely by their ability to lower the aPTT level and clinically by the amount of hemostasis achieved in the patient.

Other agents such Amicar or tranexamic acid can be given after minor procedures such as dental extractions to decrease the risk of bleeding but their use and benefit in major neurologic procedures is minimal, if any. However, they should not be used in conjunction with bypassing agents as this could increase the patients' risk of thromboembolic phenomenon.

Factor XI Deficiency

Factor XI (FXI) deficiency, sometimes referred to as hemophilia C, is a rare autosomal recessive inherited coagulation disorder caused by a mutation in the F11 gene on the short arm of Chromosome 4. It affects about 1 in 100,000 people. However, it is much more prevalent in Ashkenazi and Iraqi Jewish populations, with one in eight Ashkenazi Jews being heterozygous for the F11 gene mutation and one in 190 having a homozygous deficiency [52].

Unlike hemophilia A and B, patients with FXI deficiencies usually do not develop spontaneous hemorrhage but rather have excessive bleeding due to surgery or trauma. Also unlike hemophilia, the plasma level of FXI does not correlate with bleeding risk of the patient. For example, homozygous patients with FXI levels <20 IU/dL can either have adequate hemostasis after trauma or surgery or experience significant bleeding risks. Heterozygotes with a partial deficiency and relatively high levels of FXI, around 60–70 IU/dL can also experience significant bleeding complications [53, 54]. As such, a detailed family history and prior bleeding history is of utmost importance because the phenotype of the patient and their family is the best way to truly assess bleeding risk as one cannot currently predict risk based on factor levels or other laboratory tests.

Diagnosis

As most FXI deficient patients are asymptomatic, the diagnosis of FXI deficiency is usually not made until late childhood or adulthood, generally after excessive bleeding is noted after surgery or during a preoperative workup of a prolonged aPTT. Similar to hemophilia A and B, initial workup of suspected individuals should include a detailed history and laboratory examination. CBC will usually be normal as will a prothrombin time but the aPTT will likely be prolonged. A workup for more common causes of excessive hemorrhage such as von Willebrand disease or hemophilia should be undertaken and ruled out. In certain patient populations such as Ashkenazi Jews, checking for factor XI deficiency should be considered prior to a workup for hemophilia or VWD given its higher frequency in this patient population. The diagnosis is confirmed after demonstration of low plasma factor XI levels. Of note, infants normally have low factor XI levels that then rise to normal levels after 6 months of age with no additional age related variations thereafter and patients with synthetic liver dysfunction will have lower factor XI levels as the liver is the primary site of FXI production [55].

Treatment

There is some anecdotal evidence that DDAVP can be helpful at inducing hemostasis in mild cases of bleeding with FXI deficiency due to an increase in FVIII levels and vWF levels following its administration and may be considered in mild cases of FXI deficiency [56]. However, its use is controversial. In general, the treatment includes either factor replacement or the use of antifibrinolytic agents.

Fresh Frozen Plasma (FFP), which contains all factors of the soluble coagulation system, was the initial treatment of choice for FXI deficiency and remains so in areas, such as the USA, where FXI concentrates (FXIC) are unavailable. Since the early 1990s, FXIC has overtaken FFP in centers where it is available, like the UK, as it has a longer half-life of around 45 h, infuses only factor XI and not additional pro-coagulant agents, and can be given in a much lower volume thereby reducing the risk of volume overload and other complications seen with FFP. For prophylactic treatment of major surgical procedures with high bleeding risk or in the treatment of severe acute bleeding, FXI concentrate, if available is the treatment of choice and is usually given every other day and continued for 10–14 days after major surgery and for 1 week postoperatively after minor procedures. In the USA, FFP given perioperatively for the same duration is the standard. There are a few risks that are unique to factor replacement for FXI deficiency. That is, with both FFP and FXI concentrates there is a risk of severe anaphylaxis in patients with IgA deficiency, a risk of inhibitor formation, and a risk of severe volume overload with the high volume of FFP needed to correct the deficiency. With FXIC, there is a well-documented risk of thrombosis that must be considered. Given the risks associated with factor repletion, studies are underway to develop laboratory measures that would adequately quantify bleeding risk in FXI deficiency in order to identify patients in whom factor replacement can be avoided. A thrombin generation test (TGT) has shown promise in some studies, but further validation is necessary [57]. At present, the standard approach is to give prophylactic therapy for all major surgical patients with either FFP or FXI depending on availability, assessing each patient for IgA levels, inhibitor formation, and comorbidities that may enhance their risk of volume overload with FFP prior to surgery in order to optimize factor replacement. Furthermore, given the risk of thrombotic events with both FFP and especially with FIXC, factor repletion aim for target levels around 60–70 IU/dL and, if given in a prophylactic setting, should have prophylactic anticoagulation administered simultaneously if safe.

As is the case with most inherited defects of coagulation, antifibrinolytic agents, given in either an oral or topical or intravenous route, can be used to stop or prevent minor cases of bleeding. However, their use in conjunction with FXI replacement should be avoided due to the risk of thrombotic events [58].

Factor XI Inhibitors

The development of FXI inhibitors after plasma infusion is rare, but can occur as frequently as 33 % in specific gene mutations within FXI deficiency [59]. In general, these inhibitors can be bypassed with rFVIIa [60].

Rare Inherited Coagulation Disorders

The Rare Inherited Coagulation disorders (RICD) comprise only 2–5 % of all inherited disorders of coagulation and include deficiencies of factor I (afibrinogenemia, hypofigrinogemia, dysfibrinogenemia), factor II (prothrombin), factor V, combined deficiency of factor V and factor VIII, factor VII deficiency, factor X deficiency, FXIII deficiency and combined deficiency of vitamin K dependent factors. Inheritance patterns, epidemiology, and treatment of these various deficiencies is listed in Table 7.3. These deficiencies are a clinically heterogeneous group of disorders that arise from autosomal recessive inheritance of DNA mutations in genes encoding the corresponding coagulation factors leading to decreased levels of the protein or, more rarely, dysfunction of the involved protein. The exceptions to this are in the combined FV and FVIII deficiency in which there is a mutation in a protein regulating intracellular transport of the two factors [61] and in the deficiency of vitamin K dependent Factors

(VKDFD) whereby a defect in genes encoding enzymes involved in the vitamin K dependent posttranslational modification of proteins lead to a deficiency of FII, VII, IX, and X (as well as procoagulant factors protein C and S) and systemic issues related to deranged vitamin K metabolism [62]. Bleeding is more common in homozygotes with RICD but heterozygotes can also have an increased propensity for bleeding after episodes of hemostatic stress.

The hallmark of RICD is excessive hemorrhage, the exception to this being FXII deficiency that is not associated with an increased bleeding risk and thus will not be discussed in this chapter. The clinical presentation of the RICD is variable with patients being diagnosed anywhere from infancy to late adulthood. In general, their bleeding risk is less than that seen with hemophilia A and B, but some of these syndromes are associated with serious bleeding complications and in the case of FXIII deficiency with relatively high rates of spontaneous intracranial hemorrhage (34 % in severe patients) [63].

In all forms of RICD, patients can develop menorrhagia, mucocutaneous bleeding and epistaxis and excessive bleeding following surgical procedures. In severe forms of the deficiencies, spontaneous hemorrhage into synovial spaces or muscles can occur as well. With some syndromes there is a clear correlation with factor level and bleeding risk but in others this linear correlation is less clear. Heterozygotes of these disorders can exhibit excessive bleeding but usually only after significant hemostatic challenge. The diagnosis usually is made by characteristic abnormalities in laboratory analysis of coagulation in addition to corresponding factor deficiencies.

Treatment

Treatment should be individualized to the patient and their specific deficiency but common themes exist. Acute bleeding is managed by replacement of the deficient factor via either recombinant forms or plasma concentrates, if such factors are available, or pooled plasma combination of factors listed below.

Table 7.3 The severity of bleeding manifestations in hemophilia A and B is correlated to residual clotting factor level

Severity	Clotting factor level % activity (IU/mL)	Bleeding episodes
Severe	1 % (<0.01)	Spontaneous bleeding, usually into joints or muscles. Prophylactic infusions of factor replacement is required.
Moderate	1–5 % (0.01–0.05)	Occasional spontaneous bleeding and severe bleeding with trauma or surgery. Prophylactic infusion of factor replacement is usually required.
Mild	4–40 % (0.05–0.40)	Severe bleeding with major trauma or surgery. Prophylaxis is not generally required.

Fresh Frozen Plasma

FFP is beneficial for several disorders as it contains all the factors of the coagulations system.

Prothrombin Complex Concentrates.

Prothrombin complexes are a combination of FII, VII, IX, and X and protein C and S prepared from fresh frozen human plasma.

Cryoprecipitated antihemophilic factor (cryoprecipitate).

Cryo is a frozen plasma product rich in fibrinogen and also containing factors VIII, VWF, and FXIII and is used most frequently in the treatment of factor I or fibrinogen deficiency.

As with other coagulation disorders, the antifibrinolytic agents can be useful in the setting of an acute bleeding episode, as well as to prevent perioperative hemorrhage alone in the setting of minor deficiencies and minor procedures or in combination with factor replacement. However, care should be given when using it with full dose rVII as this can potentiate thrombotic events. Treatment strategies for all RICD are listed in Table 7.3.

Inhibitors

Inhibitors can develop in RICD but at a lower frequency than that seen in hemophilia and is on the order of <5 %. This is usually managed with rVIIa similar to inhibitor development with hemophilia A, B, or C.

Inherited Disorders of Primary Hemostasis

Role of Platelets in Clot Formation

Platelets are the main actors in primary hemostasis. They are small enucleate cells that are released from the megakaryocyte and circulate inactive in plasma with an average life span of 10 days. However, after vessel wall damage, subendothelial components such as collagen and VWF are exposed and bind to and activate platelets. Exposed collagen binds the GPVI receptor and VWF binds to platelets via the GPIb/IX/V receptor anchoring them into place and recruiting other platelets to the site. Once there, the platelets are then activated by a variety of platelet agonists such as ADP and thromboxane that, through G protein receptor activation, cause a change in the platelet cytoskeleton that leads to alteration in the shape of platelets allowing them to spread and release the contents stored in their alpha and delta intracellular granules. This results in release of thromboxane A2 (TXA2) and production of a procoagulant surface whereby secondary hemostasis can be conducted, and activation of GPIIb/IIIa receptors resulting in platelet aggregation and the subsequent formation of a platelet plug limiting blood flow to the site of vascular damage [64].

Inherited Disorders of Platelets (IDP)

Genetic mutations causing alterations in any one of the steps involved in primary hemostasis can result in IDP. IDP are rare and very heterogeneous group of disorders, the true incidence of which is unknown [65]. They mostly result in mild to moderate mucocutaneous bleeding as well as an exaggerated hemorrhagic response following surgical procedures. Given the risk of enhanced perioperative bleeding, a detailed workup for IDP should be conducted in the patient with normal coagulation screening tests and a history of unexplained or exaggerated bleeding [66]. Please see Figs. 7.2 and 7.3 for a list of platelet disorders and where they affect platelet function. Our discussion will be limited to the most commonly occurring and most severe inherited disorder.

Glanzmann's Thrombasthenia (GT)

GT is the most severe of the IDP, and according to some reports, affects around 33 % of IDP patients. GT is a severe bleeding disorder with affected individuals presenting early in life with excessive bruising and bleeding in response to trauma but also with spontaneous hemorrhage including intracranial hemorrhage [67]. It is an autosomal recessive disorder that is caused by qualitative or quantitative defects in the GpIIb/IIIa (fibrinogen) receptors on the platelet surface [68]. This prevents platelets from aggregating and thus from forming a hemostatic plug.

Bernard Soulier Syndrome (BSS)

BSS can at times be a severe bleeding disorder. It is an autosomal recessive congenital bleeding disorder caused by quantitative or qualitative defects in the GPIb-IX-V VWF (VWF) receptor impairing normal adhesion of platelets to sites of vascular damage . It is characterized by thrombocytopenia and large platelets and a prolonged bleeding time. Like GT, the bleeding diathesis can be severe at times.

Storage Pool Disorders (SBP)

The storage pool disorders, listed in Table 7.4 and shown in Fig. 7.3, are a heterogeneous group of diseases characterized by deregulated platelet aggregation from various genetic mutations

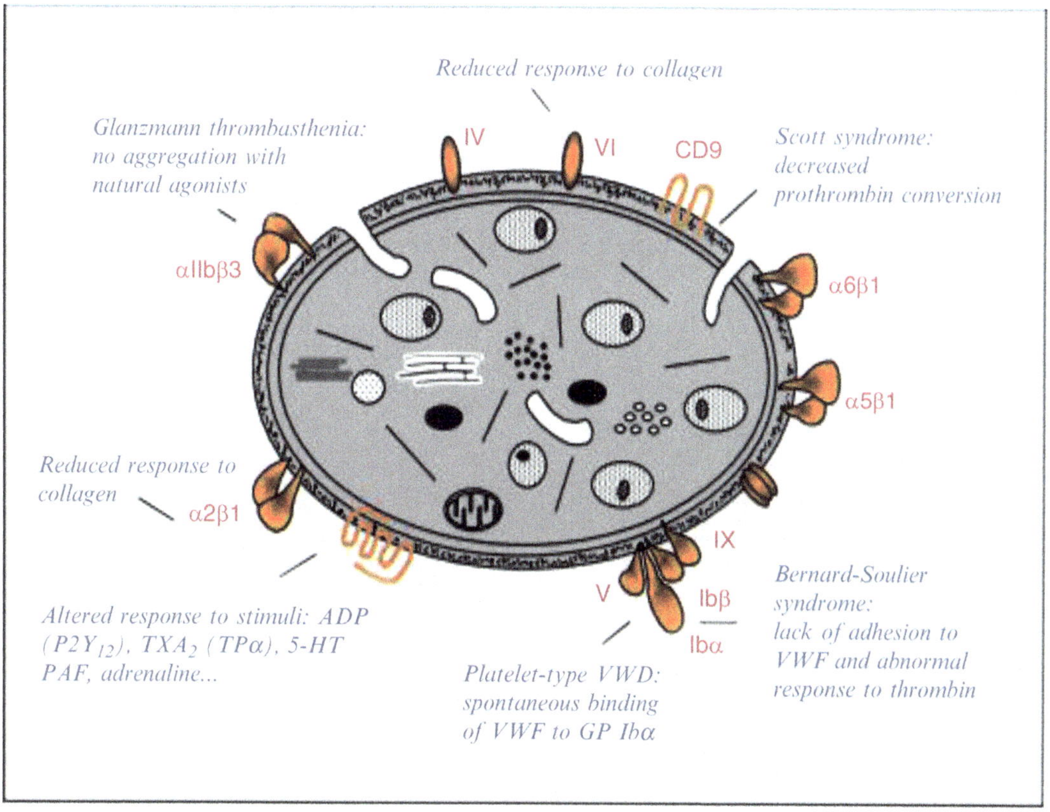

Fig. 7.2 Disorders that principally affect surface components of platelets [75]. Reprinted from Nurden and Nurden et al. *Congenital Disorders with Associated Platelet Dysfunction*

ultimately causing disordered release of platelet granular contents. The mutations involved in these disorders can extend beyond the megakaryocytic lineage causing a constellation of systemic findings that can include severe immunodeficiency, albinism and neurologic deficits [69].

Clinical Presentation

Patients can present in infancy or into early adulthood with a bleeding diathesis caused by IDP. Usually the bleeding manifestations of affected individuals include unexplained bruising, epistaxis, menorrhagia, mucocutaneous bleeding, and excessive bleeding following surgical procedures such as dental extractions or after traumatic events. Certain IPD can cause a severe bleeding diathesis that manifest as spontaneous mucocutaneous, gastrointestinal, genitourinary, or intracranial hemorrhage. Most of the defects are inherited in an autosomal recessive fashion, but there are rare X-linked and autosomal dominant.

Diagnosis

The diagnosis of IPD can be challenging. In general patients in whom there is concern for an IDP should undergo simultaneously workup for acquired disorders that could lead to platelet dysfunction or medications that could interfere with the function of platelets. A detailed drug history is important as many common over-the-counter medications can interfere with platelet function, most notable being NSAIDS. However, occasional herbal supplements can interfere with

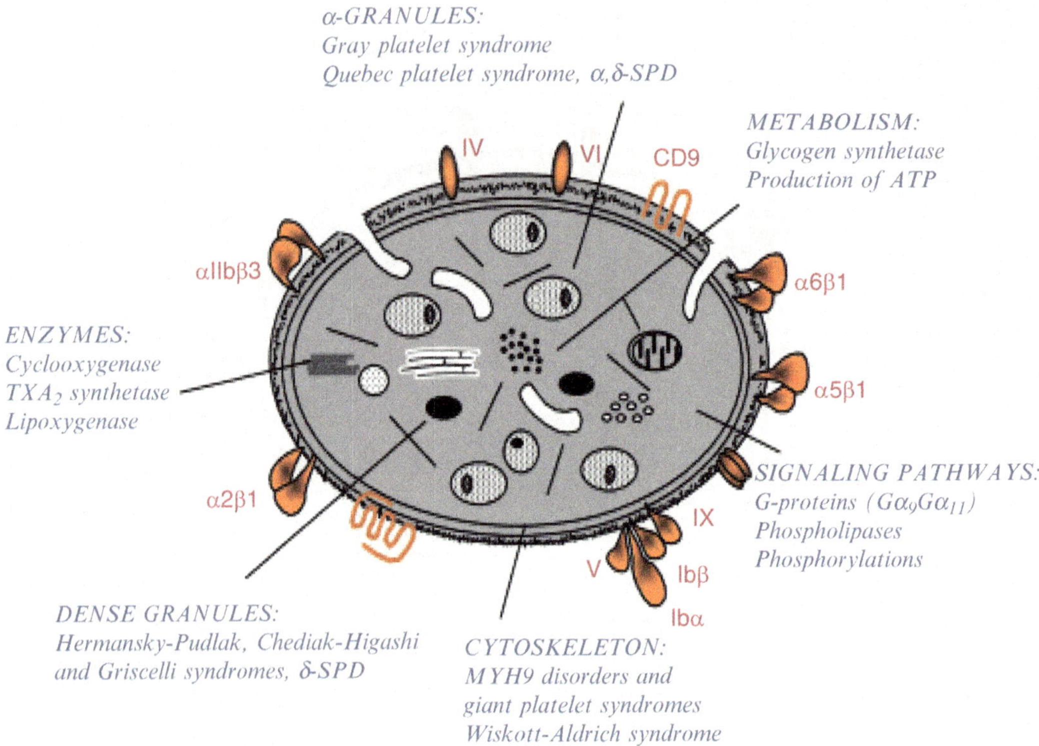

Fig. 7.3 Disorders affecting intracellular organelles or cytosolic portions of proteins of platelets [75]. Reprinted from Nurden and Nurden et al. *Congenital Disorders with Associated Platelet Dysfunction*

platelet function too. Patients should also undergo screening for more common causes of coagulopathy such as VWD or hemophilia. In practicality this often occurs alongside the workup for a platelet function disorder [70].

Laboratory examination should include a CBC with peripheral blood smear examination under the microscope looking primarily at the size and morphology of the platelets as well as any concurrent cellular changes in the leukocytes or red blood cells. All patients should have coagulation studies performed including a PT and aPTT, which are usually normal and a workup of VWD including a VWF:Ag and VWF:RCo. If a bleeding time is sent it can be normal, minimally prolonged, or severely prolonged depending on the disorder and its severity. The Platelet Function Analyzer-100 is a screening test measuring platelet adhesion to a variety of surfaces and is abnormal in most IPD, especially in Glanzmann Thrombasthenia or Bernard-Soulier where the closure time can be especially prolonged. However, there have been false negatives recorded with PFA-100 especially with the various SPD and as such a normal PFA-100 should not stop a workup for IDP. Platelet aggregations studies are generally the next step in the diagnosis of a possible IDP. They measure the ability of platelets to aggregate in response to typical agonists to aggregation, ADP, adrenaline, collagen, arachidonic acid, ristocetin, and thromboxane. Response curves are then generated for each agonist and compared to a reference range. However, this test can be inaccurate in the setting of NSAID use or thrombocytopenia. Once again a normal platelet aggregation study does not necessarily rule out a diagnosis of IDP, and if this remains a clinical concern patients should undergo specialized

Table 7.4 Prevalence, inheritance patterns, bleeding risk, and treatment of RICD [5, 8, 63, 73, 74]

Factor deficiency	Prevalence	Inheritance	Lab findings	Correlation of factor levels to bleeding risk	Spontaneous bleeding	ICH, % of patients	Other associations	Treatment
Factor I Afibrinogenemia Hypofibrinogenemia dysfibrinogenemia	1:1,000,000	AR AR AD	↑PT ↑PTT ↑TT ↑reptilase test	Strong	Yes	Yes, 5 %	Thrombosis, pregnancy loss	FIC cryo
Factor II prothrombin	1:2,000,000	AR	↑PT ↑ aPTT	Unknown	Yes	Yes, 7 %		PCC, FFP
Factor V	1:1,000,000	AR	↑PT ↑ aPTT	Weak	Yes	Yes, 8 %	thrombosis	FFP
Factor V + factor VIII	1:2,000,000	AR	↑PT ↑ aPTT	Strong	No	No		FFP
Factor VII	1:500,000	AR	↑PT nl aPTT	Weak	Yes	Yes, 20 %	Thrombosis	rVIIa
Factor X	1:1,000,000	AR	↑PT ↑ aPTT	Strong	Yes	Yes, 13 %	Pregnancy loss	PCC
Factor XIII	1:2,000,000	AR	nl PT nl aPTT	Strong	Yes	Yes, 34 %	Pregnancy loss, impaired wound healing	rXIII FXIIIC FFP
VKDFD		AR	↑PT ↑ aPTT	Unknown	Yes	Yes	Skeletal abnormalities	Vitamin K FFP PCC rVIIa

additional testing such as measurement of ATP/ADP content release via a platelet nucleotide/ATP release, platelet flow cytometry to measure platelet activation or surface glycoproteins, or dense granule release or phospholipid expression (GPIB/IX/V and GPIIb/IIIa), or molecular analysis can be considered [70]. These tests are only performed at a small number of specialized centers.

Treatment

Despite the clinical heterogeneity seen with IDPs their treatment is largely the same and involves the administration of donor platelets in order to achieve an adequate number of active platelets for normal hemostasis. Severe IDP such as Glanzmann Thrombasthenia or Bernard Soulier Syndrome may need prophylactic administration of platelets to prevent spontaneous hemorrhage.

The main concern with the use of platelets with these disorders is that patients may, and often will, become alloimmunized and thus refractory to platelet transfusions. Alloimmunity is the development of antibodies against either HLA Antigen mismatch on the surface of donor platelets or the development of antibodies against the GpIIb/IIIa or GPIb/V/IX receptors on donor platelets that are lacking on platelets of patients with GT or BSS, respectively. Once the patient becomes alloimmunized they are refractory to subsequent platelet transfusions. For patients who are alloimmunized due to an HLA mismatch, they can be given HLA matched single donor platelets if available. In all patients with a platelet function disorder, they should have leukocyte reduced platelet transfusions in order to try and prevent this from occurring. In addition, platelet transfusions should be performed only if necessary. Unfortunately for GT and BSS, these patients often require prophylactic administration of platelets in order to prevent spontaneous hemorrhage.

In milder phenotypes of IDP, patients can take antifibrinolytics or DDAVP perioperatively surrounding mild procedures or dental extractions or acutely in the setting of mild bleeding episodes in order to prevent platelet transfusions. However, in the setting of major surgical procedures and acute severe hemorrhage, platelet transfusions are required but can be given in addition to Amicar, tranexamic acid, or DDAVP. For patients

Table 7.5 Classification of inherited disorders of platelet function [69]

1. Disorders of Adhesion: Defects in platelet–vessel wall interaction
(a) von Willebrand disease
(b) Bernard–Soulier syndrome (deficiency or defect in GPIb)
2. Disorders of aggregation: Defects in platelet–platelet interaction
(a) Congenital afibrinogenemia (deficiency or dysfunctional plasma fibrinogen)
(b) Glanzmann's thrombasthenia (deficiency or defect in GPIIb-IIIa)
3. Disorders of platelet secretion and abnormalities of granules
(a) Storage pool deficiency
• α-granule disorders
– Gray platelet syndrome
– Quebec platelet disorder
• Dense granule disorders
– Hemansky–Pudlak syndrome
– Chediak–Higashi syndrome
– Idiopathic dense granule disease
4. Disorders of platelet secretion and signal transduction
(a) Receptor defects: Defects in platelet–agonist interaction with thromboxane a2, collagen, ADP, epinephrine
(b) Defects in G-protein activation
• Gαq deficiency
• Gαs abnormalities
• Gαi1 deficiency
(c) Defects in phosphatidylinositol metabolism: Phospholipase C-2 deficiency
(d) Defects in calcium mobilization
(e) Defects in protein phosphorylation (pleckstrin) PKD-y deficiency
(f) Abnormalities in arachidonic acid pathways and thromboxane A2 synthesis impaired liberation of arachidonic acid
• Cyclooxygenase deficiency
• Thromboxane synthase deficiency
5. Defects in cytoskeletal regulation
(a) Wiskott–Aldrich
6. Disorders of platelet–coagulant protein interaction (membrane phospholipid defects)
(a) Scott Syndrome
7. Miscellaneous

Table 7.6 Inherited thrombocytopenia: genetic mutations and associated phenotype [75]. Reprinted from Nurden and Nurden et al. *Congenital Disorders with Associated Platelet Dysfunction*

Syndrome	Affected gene chromosomal location	Inheritance	Associated phenotype
MYH9-related diseases: May–Hegglin anomaly, Fechtner, Epstein, and Sebastian syndromes	*MYH9* 22q12–13	AD	Various combinations of leukocyte inclusions, deafness, nephritis, cataracts. Large platelets
Mediterranean macrothrombocytopenia	*GPIBA*, possibly others 17p 13	AD	Large platelets
Bernard–Soulier syndrome	*GPIBA*, *GPIBB*, *GF9* 17p 13, 22q11, and 3q21	AR	Giant platelets, platelet adhesion defect, abnormal aggregation of thrombin
Platelet-type VWD	GPIBA 17p 13	AD	Enlarged platelets. Defective adhesion due DO spontaneous binding of VWF to GPIbα and cleavage of VWF multimers
Familial platelet disorder/acute myelogenous leukemia	*RUNXI (CBFA2, AMLI)* 21q22	AD	Myelodysplasia, propensity for leukemia. Platelet dysfunction
Chromosome 10/THC2	*FLJ14813* 10p 11–12	AD	None
Paris-Trousseau/Jacobsen syndromes	Hemizygous deletion including *FL11* 11q23	AD	Cardiac and facial defects, mental retardation Enlarged platelets and large granules
Gray platelet Syndrome	Unknown	Mostly recessive	Myelofibrosis, Enlarged platelets with no α-granules, platelet dysfunction
Congenital amegakaryocytic thrombocytopenia (CAMT)	*c-MPL* 1p34	AR	Severe thrombocytopenia at birth. Progressive aplasia
Thrombocytopenia and absent radii (TAR)	Large deletion 1q21.1	AR	Shortened/absent radii bilaterally
Amegakaryocytic thrombocytopenia with radio-ulnar synostosis	*HOXA11* 7pl5–14	AD	Fused radius, incomplete range of motion
Wiskott–Aldrich syndrome	WAS Xp 11.23-p11.22	X-linked	Immunodeficiency, eczema, lymphoma, small platelets. Defective platelet and lymphocyte function
X-linked thrombocytopenia (XLT)	*WAS*	X-linked	Small platelets, no immune problems
GATA-1-related thrombocytopenia with dyserythropoiesis	*GATAI* Xp11.23	X-linked	Dyserythropoiesis ± anemia, β-thalassemia in some patients (XLTT). Platelet dysfunction, large platelets

AD autosomal dominant, *AR* autosomal recessive

AP autosomal recessive inheritance, *AD* autosomal dominant inheritance. The DiGeorge velocardiofacial syndrome is occasionally familial but largely de novo in origin and is not included in the Table Type 2BVWD is accompanied by a familial thrombocytopenia is some families that have developed allo-immunity, there have been studies reporting adequate hemostasis after rVIIa (Novoseven), particularly in patients with GT (Tables 7.5 and 7.6).

References

1. Rodeghiero F, Castaman G, Dini E. Epidemiological investigation of the prevalence of von Willebrand's disease. Blood. 1987;69:454–9.
2. Werner EJ, Broxson EH, Tucker EL, Giroux DS, Shults J, Abshire TC. Prevalence of von Willebrand disease in children: a multiethnic study. J Pediatr. 1993;123:893–8.
3. Bowman M, Hopman W, Rapson D, Lilicrap D, Silva M, James P. Brief Report: A Prospective Evaluation of the Prevalence of Symptomatic von Willebrand Disease (VWD) in a Pediatric Primary Care Population. Pediatr Blood Cancer. 2010;55:171–3. doi:10.1002/pbc.
4. Goodeve AC. The genetic basis of von Willebrand disease. Blood Rev. 2010;24:123–34. doi:10.1016/j.blre.2010.03.003.
5. Zhang X, Halvorsen K, Zhang C-Z, Wong WP, Springer TA. Mechanoenzymatic cleavage of the ultralarge vascular protein von Willebrand factor. Science. 2009;324:1330–4. doi:10.1126/science.1170905.
6. James PD, Lillicrap D. The molecular characterization of von Willebrand disease: Good in parts. Br J Haematol. 2013;161:166–76. doi:10.1111/bjh.12249.
7. Koppelman SJ, van Hoeij M, Vink T, et al. Requirements of von Willebrand factor to protect factor VIII from inactivation by activated protein C. Blood. 1996;87:2292–300.
8. Conlan MG, Folsom AR, Finch A, et al. Associations of factor VIII and von Willebrand factor with age, race, sex, and risk factors for atherosclerosis: The Atherosclerosis Risk in Communities (ARIC) Study. Thromb Haemost. 1993;70:380–5.
9. Jenkins PV. O'Donnell JS. ABO blood group determines plasma von Willebrand factor levels: A biologic function after all? Transfusion. 2006;46:1836–44. doi:10.1111/j.1537-2995.2006.00975.x.
10. Sadler JE, Budde U, Eikenboom JCJ, et al. Update on the pathophysiology and classification of von Willebrand disease: a report of the Subcommittee on von Willebrand Factor. J Thromb Haemost. 2006;4:2103–14. doi:10.1111/j.1538-7836.2006.02146.x.
11. von Lillicrap D. Willebrand disease: advances in pathogenetic understanding, diagnosis, and therapy. Blood. 2013;122:3735–40. doi:10.1182/blood-2013-06-498303.
12. Ragni MV, Bontempo FA, Cortese HA. Von Willebrand disease and bleeding in women. Haemophilia. 1999; 5:313–7. doi:10.1046/j.1365-2516.1999.00342.x.
13. Kaufmann JE, Vischer UM. Cellular mechanisms of the hemostatic effects of desmopressin (DDAVP). J Thromb Haemost. 2003;1:682–9. doi:10.1046/j.1538-7836.2003.00190.x.
14. Castaman G, Lattuada A, Mannucci PM, Rodeghiero F. Factor VIII:C Increases after Desmopressin in a Subgroup of Patients with Autosomal Recessive Severe von Willebrand Disease. Br J Haematol. 1995;89(1):147–51.
15. Mannucci PM, Kempton C, Millar C, et al. Pharmacokinetics and safety of a novel recombinant human von Willebrand factor manufactured with a plasma-free method: A prospective clinical trial. Blood. 2013; 122:648–57. doi:10.1182/blood-2013-01-479527.
16. Rodeghiero F, Castaman G, Tosetto A. How I treat von Willebrand disease. Blood. 2009;114:1158–65. doi:10.1182/blood-2009-01-153296.
17. Verstraete M. Clinical application of inhibitors of fibrinolysis. Drugs. 1985;29:236–61. doi:10.2165/00003495-198529030-00003.
18. Thompson AR, Gill JC, Ewenstein BM, Mueller-Velten G, Schwartz BA. Successful Treatment for Patients with von Willebrand Disease Undergoing Urgent Surgery Using Factor VIII/VWF Concentrate (Humate-P). Haemophilia. 2004;10(1):42–51.
19. Federici AB, Castaman G, Franchini M, et al. Clinical use of Haemate P in inherited von Willebrand's disease: a cohort study on 100 Italian patients. Haematologica. 2007;92:944–51. http://www.ncbi.nlm.nih.gov/pubmed/17606445.
20. Franchini M. Surgical prophylaxis in von Willebrand's disease: A difficult balance to manage. Blood Transfus. 2008;6 Suppl 2:s33–8. doi:10.2450/2008.0035-08.
21. Makris M, Colvin B, Gupta V, Shields ML, Smith MP. Venous thrombosis following the use of intermediate purity FVIII concentrate to treat patients with von Willebrand's disease. Thromb Haemost. 2002;88:387–8. doi:10.1267/THRO88020987.
22. Mannucci PM. Treatment of von Willebrand's disease. N Engl J Med. 2004;351:683–94. doi:10.1056/NEJMra040403.
23. Mannucci PM. Back to the future: A recent history of haemophilia treatment. Haemophilia. 2008;14:10–8. doi:10.1111/j.1365-2516.2008.01708.x.
24. Giangrande PLF. The molecular basis of hemophilia. In: Molecular Hematology: Third Edition; 2010:219–232. doi:10.1002/9781444318531.ch18.
25. Stonebraker JS, Bolton-Maggs PHB, Michael Soucie J, Walker I, Brooker M. A study of variations in the reported haemophilia A prevalence around the world. Haemophilia. 2010;16:20–32. doi:10.1111/j.1365-2516.2009.02127.x.
26. Kasper CK, Lin JC. Prevalence of sporadic and familial haemophilia. Haemophilia. 2007;13:90–2. doi:10.1111/j.1365-2516.2006.01397.x.
27. Di Michele DM, Gibb C, Lefkowitz JM, Ni Q, Gerber LM, Ganguly A. Severe and moderate haemophilia A and B in US females. Haemophilia. 2014;20(2):e136–43. doi:10.1111/hae.12364.

28. Soucie JM, Evatt B, Jackson D. Occurrence of hemophilia in the United States. The Hemophilia Surveillance System Project Investigators. Am J Hematol. 1998;59:288–94. doi:10.1002/(SICI)1096-8652(199812)59:4<288::AID-AJH4>3.0.CO;2-I [pii].
29. Mannucci PM, Franchini M. Is haemophilia B less severe than haemophilia A? Haemophilia. 2013;19:499–502. doi:10.1111/hae.12133.
30. Plug I, Van Der Bom JG, Peters M, et al. Mortality and causes of death in patients with hemophilia, 1992-2001: a prospective cohort study. J Thromb Haemost. 2006;4:510–6. doi:10.1111/j.1538-7836.2006.01808.x.
31. Bowen DJ. Haemophilia A, and haemophilia B: molecular insights. Mol Pathol. 2002;55:127–44. doi:10.1136/mp.55.2.127.
32. Federici AB. The factor VIII/von Willebrand factor complex: basic and clinical issues. Haematologica. 2003;88:EREP02.
33. Lillicrap D. The molecular basis of haemophilia B. Haemophilia. 1998;4:350–7.
34. Kulkarni R, Presley R, Lusher J, et al. Complications of hemophilia in children in the first two years of life: A report from the centers for disease control (CDC) universal data collection (UDC) system. Haemophilia. 2012;18.
35. Richards M, Lavigne Lissalde G, Combescure C, et al. Neonatal bleeding in haemophilia: A European cohort study. Br J Haematol. 2012;156:374–82. doi:10.1111/j.1365-2141.2011.08967.x.
36. Valentino LA. Blood-induced joint disease: The pathophysiology of hemophilic arthropathy. J Thromb Haemost. 2010;8:1895–902. doi:10.1111/j.1538-7836.2010.03962.x.
37. Sørensen B, Benson GM, Bladen M, et al. Management of muscle haematomas in patients with severe haemophilia in an evidence-poor world. Haemophilia. 2012;18:598–606. doi:10.1111/j.1365-2516.2011.02720.x.
38. Witmer C, Presley R, Kulkarni R, Michael Soucie J, Manno CS, Raffini L. Associations between intracranial haemorrhage and prescribed prophylaxis in a large cohort of haemophilia patients in the United States. Br J Haematol. 2011;152:211–6. doi:10.1111/j.1365-2141.2010.08469.x.
39. Iorio A, Marchesini E, Marcucci M, Stobart K, Chan AK. Clotting factor concentrates given to prevent bleeding and bleeding-related complications in people with hemophilia A or B. Cochrane Database Syst Rev. 2011;9, CD003429. doi:10.1002/14651858.CD003429.pub3.
40. Josephson N. The hemophilias and their clinical management. ASH Educ Progr B. 2013;2013:261–7. doi:10.1182/asheducation-2013.1.261.
41. Collins PW, Björkman S, Fischer K, et al. Factor VIII requirement to maintain a target plasma level in the prophylactic treatment of severe hemophilia A: Influences of variance in pharmacokinetics and treatment regimens. J Thromb Haemost. 2010;8:269–75. doi:10.1111/j.1538-7836.2009.03703.x.
42. Barnes C. Importance of pharmacokinetics in the management of hemophilia. Pediatr Blood Cancer. 2013;60 Suppl 1:S27–9. doi:10.1002/pbc.24339.
43. Srivastava A, Brewer AK, Mauser-Bunschoten EP, et al. Guidelines for the management of hemophilia. Haemophilia. 2013;19(1):e1–47. doi:10.1111/j.1365-2516.2012.02909.x.
44. Mannucci PM. Desmopressin (DDAVP) in the treatment of bleeding disorders: the first 20 years. Blood. 1997;90:2515–21.
45. Brettler DB. Inhibitors in congenital haemophilia. Baillieres Clin Haematol. 1996;9:319–29. doi:10.1016/S0950-3536(96)80066-7.
46. Gouw SC, Van Den Berg HM, Oldenburg J, et al. F8 gene mutation type and inhibitor development in patients with severe hemophilia A: Systematic review and meta-analysis. Blood. 2012;119:2922–34. doi:10.1182/blood-2011-09-379453.
47. Astermark J, Oldenburg J, Escobar M, White GC, Berntorp E. The Malmö International Brother Study (MIBS). Genetic defects and inhibitor development in siblings with severe hemophilia A. Haematologica. 2005;90:924–30.
48. Astermark J, Berntorp E, White GC, Kroner BL. The Malmo International Brother Study (MIBS): further support for genetic predisposition to inhibitor development in hemophilia patients. Haemophilia. 2001;7:267–72.
49. Turecek PL, Váradi K, Gritsch H, Schwarz HP. FEIBA: mode of action. Haemophilia. 2004;10 Suppl 2:3–9. doi:10.1111/j.1365-2516.2004.00934.x.
50. Lindley CM, Sawyer WT, Macik BG, et al. Pharmacokinetics and Pharmacodynamics of Recombinant Factor VIIa. Clin Pharmacol Ther. 1994;55:638–48.
51. Kempton CL, White GC. How we treat a hemophilia A patient with a factor VIII inhibitor. Blood. 2009;113:11–7. doi:10.1182/blood-2008-06-160432.
52. Asakai R, Chung DW, Davie EW, Seligsohn U. Factor XI deficiency in Ashkenazi Jews in Israel. N Engl J Med. 1991;325:153–8. doi:10.1056/NEJM199107183250303.
53. Bolton-Maggs PHB, Patterson DA, Wensley RT, Tuddenham EGD. Definition of the bleeding tendency in factor XI-deficient kindreds: A clinical and laboratory study. Thromb Haemost. 1995;73:194–202.
54. Bolton-Maggs PH, Young Wan-Yin B, McCraw AH, Slack J, Kernoff PB. Inheritance and bleeding in factor XI deficiency. Br J Haematol. 1988;69:521–8.
55. Kadir RA, Lee CA, Sabin CA, Pollard D, Economides DL. Pregnancy in women with von Willebrand's disease or factor XI deficiency. Br J Obstet Gynaecol. 1998;105:314–21.
56. Castaman G, Tosetto A, Rodeghiero F. Reduced von Willebrand factor survival in von Willebrand disease: pathophysiologic and clinical relevance. J Thromb Haemost. 2009;7 Suppl 1:71–4. doi:10.1111/j.1538-7836.2009.03381.x.

57. Livnat T, Martinowitz U, Mansharov R, Ariella Z. Thrombin Generation Test Can Predict Bleeding Tendency In Patients With Severe Factor XI Deficiency. Blood. 2013;122:3600. http://bloodjournal.hematologylibrary.org/content/122/21/3600.abstract.
58. Bolton-Maggs PHB, Perry DJ, Chalmers EA, et al. The rare coagulation disorders - Review with guidelines for management from the United Kingdom Haemophilia Centre Doctors' Organisation. Haemophilia. 2004;10:593–628. doi:10.1111/j.1365-2516.2004.00944.x.
59. Salomon O, Zivelin A, Livnat T, et al. Prevalence, causes, and characterization of factor XI inhibitors in patients with inherited factor XI deficiency. Blood. 2003;101:4783–8. doi:10.1182/blood-2002-09-2794.
60. Livnat T, Tamarin I, Mor Y, et al. Recombinant activated factor VII and tranexamic acid are haemostatically effective during major surgery in factor XI-deficient patients with inhibitor antibodies. Thromb Haemost. 2009;102:487–92. doi:10.1160/TH09-03-0172.
61. Nichols WC, Seligsohn U, Zivelin A, et al. Mutations in the ER-Golgi intermediate compartment protein ERGIC-53 cause combined deficiency of coagulation factors V and VIII. Cell. 1998;93:61–70. doi:10.1016/S0092-8674(00)81146-0.
62. Napolitano M, Mariani G, Lapecorella M. Hereditary combined deficiency of the vitamin K-dependent clotting factors. Orphanet J Rare Dis. 2010;5:21. doi:10.1186/1750-1172-5-21.
63. Acharya SS, Coughlin A, Dimichele DM, et al. Rare bleeding disorder registry: Deficiencies of factors II, V, VII, X, XIII, fibrinogen and dysfibrinogenemias. J Thromb Haemost. 2004;2:248–56. doi:10.1111/j.1538-7836.2003.t01-1-00553.x.
64. Bolton-Maggs PHB, Chalmers EA, Collins PW, et al. A review of inherited platelet disorders with guidelines for their management on behalf of the UKHCDO. Br J Haematol. 2006;135:603–33. doi:10.1111/j.1365-2141.2006.06343.x.
65. Knöfler R, Streif W. Strategies in Clinical and Laboratory Diagnosis of Inherited Platelet Function Disorders in Children. Transfus Med Hemother. 2010;37:231–5. doi:10.1159/000320762.
66. Hayward CPM, Rao AK, Cattaneo M. Congenital platelet disorders: Overview of their mechanisms, diagnostic evaluation and treatment. Haemophilia. 2006;12:128–36. doi:10.1111/j.1365-2516.2006.01270.x.
67. Knöfler R, Olivieri M, Weickardt S, Eberl W, Streif W. First results of the THROMKID study: a quality project for the registration of children und adolescents with hereditary platelet function defects in Germany, Austria, and Switzerland. Hamostaseologie. 2007; 27:48–53. doi:07010048 [pii].
68. Salles II, Feys HB, Iserbyt BF, De Meyer SF, Vanhoorelbeke K, Deckmyn H. Inherited traits affecting platelet function. Blood Rev. 2008;22:155–72. doi:10.1016/j.blre.2007.11.002.
69. Handin RI. Inherited platelet disorders. Hematology Am Soc Hematol Educ Program. 2005:396–402. doi:10.1182/asheducation-2005.1.396.
70. Kirchmaier CM, Pillitteri D. Diagnosis and management of inherited platelet disorders. Transfus Med Hemother. 2010;37:237–46. doi:10.1159/000320257.
71. Yawn B, Nichols WL, Rick ME. Diagnosis and management of von Willebrand disease: guidelines for primary care. Am Fam Physician. 2009;80: 1261–8.
72. Nichols WL, Hultin MB, James AH, et al. von Willebrand disease (VWD): evidence-based diagnosis and management guidelines, the National Heart, Lung, and Blood Institute (NHLBI) Expert Panel report (USA). Haemophilia. 2008;14:171–232. doi:10.1111/j.1365-2516.2007.01643.x.
73. Escobar MA. Advances in the treatment of inherited coagulation disorders. Haemophilia. 2013;19:648–59. doi:10.1111/hae.12137.
74. Acharya SS, Dimichele DM. Rare inherited disorders of fibrinogen. Haemophilia. 2008;14:1151–8. doi:10.1111/j.1365-2516.2008.01831.x.
75. Nurden P, Nurden AT. Congenital disorders associated with platelet dysfunctions. Thromb Haemost. 2008;99:253–63. doi:10.1160/TH07-09-0568.

Acquired Coagulation Disorders

8

Kimberly Kruczek, Kathrine Cooper, Hanh Mai, and Sucha Nand

Introduction

Hemostasis is a complex, regulated sequence of interactions involving platelets, the blood vessel endothelium, and coagulation factors. Primary hemostasis involves platelet activation and culminates in the formation of the platelet plug. Secondary hemostasis follows with the activation of the coagulation cascade on the surface of platelets, leading to the formation of a stable fibrin clot. Under physiologic conditions, an equilibrium exists between the formation of a clot and its degradation. Fibrinolysis is a series of reactions that limit the extent of thrombosis. Our understanding of the normal coagulation cascade has changed substantially over the last two decades and is focused on thrombin generation, which is initiated by the activation of factor VII by tissue factor and is amplified at multiple steps (Fig. 8.1) [1]. However, in a conceptual sense, one can still divide the cascade into the intrinsic and extrinsic pathways as it helps interpret the commonly used tests – prothrombin time (PT) and activated partial thromboplastin time (aPTT) (Fig. 8.2). The initiation of the intrinsic pathway involves activation of factor XII by the serine protease prekallikrein, which leads to the subsequent activation of factors XI and IX. The extrinsic pathway is activated when tissue factor is exposed and activates factor VII at the site of endothelial damage. Both intrinsic and extrinsic pathways converge onto the common pathway with the activation of factor X and factor V, culminating in the generation of thrombin and subsequent fibrin formation.

Abnormal bleeding can occur when the normal equilibrium no longer exists and can result from disorders of the coagulation system, platelets, or blood vessels. Disorders of the coagulation system can be acquired or hereditary, the former resulting from nutritional deficiencies, systemic diseases, formation of factor inhibitors, and drugs [2]. This chapter will address the most common and clinically relevant acquired coagulation disorders including vitamin K deficiency, liver dysfunction, factor deficiencies, and inhibitors. We will conclude with a discussion of the antiphospholipid antibody (APLA) syndrome, which is primarily a prothrombotic state and rarely causes bleeding.

K. Kruczek, D.O. (✉) • K. Cooper, M.D.
H. Mai, D.O. • S. Nand, M.D.
Department of Hematology/Oncology,
Loyola University Medical Center, Maywood,
IL 60153, USA
e-mail: kkruczek@lumc.edu;
Kathrine.cooper@lumc.edu;
hmai@lumc.edu; snand@lumc.edu

C.M. Loftus (ed.), *Anticoagulation and Hemostasis in Neurosurgery*,
DOI 10.1007/978-3-319-27327-3_8

Fig. 8.1 Modern view of coagulation pathways. (**a**) Initiation phase in which a small amount of thrombin is generated. (**b**) Amplification phase in which thrombin generation is significantly increased (Furie B, et al. New Eng J Med 2008)

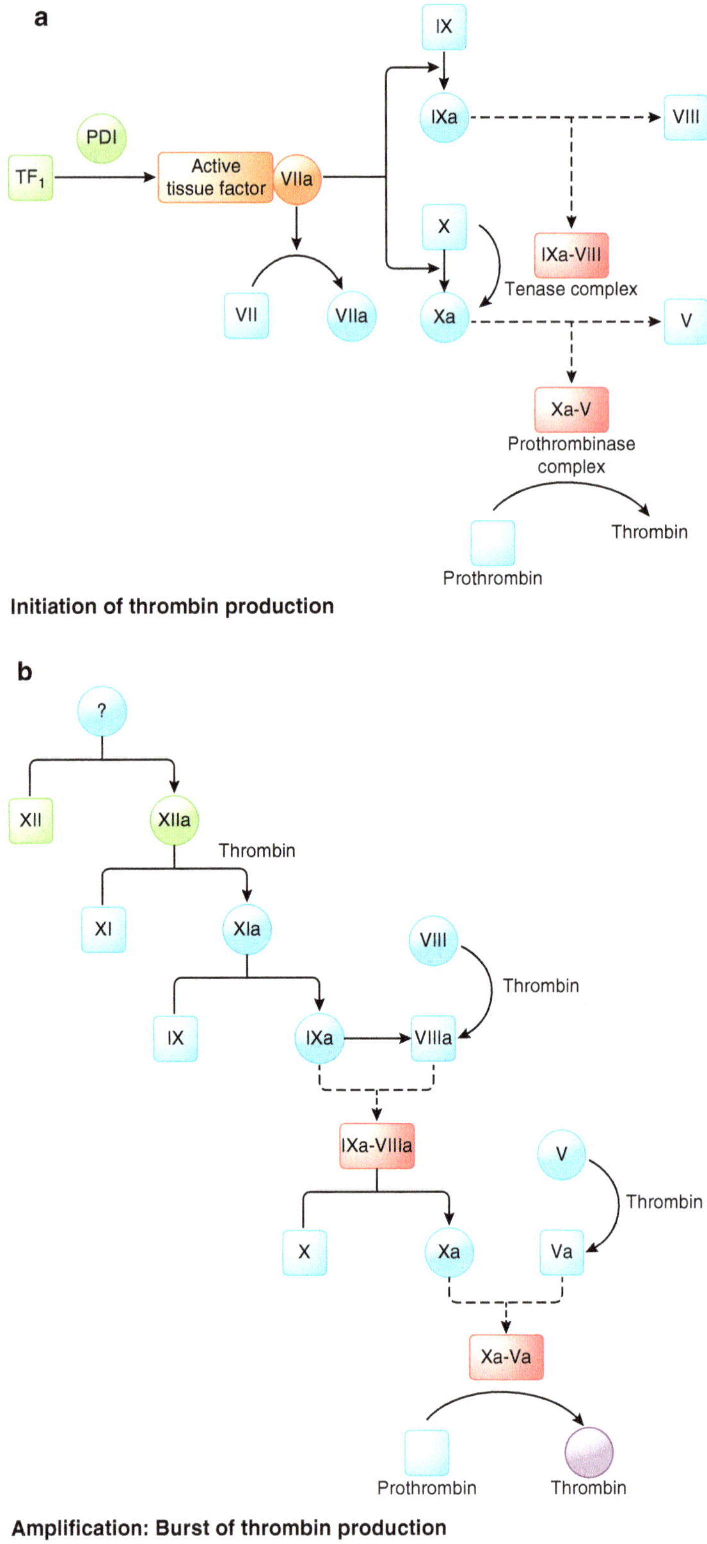

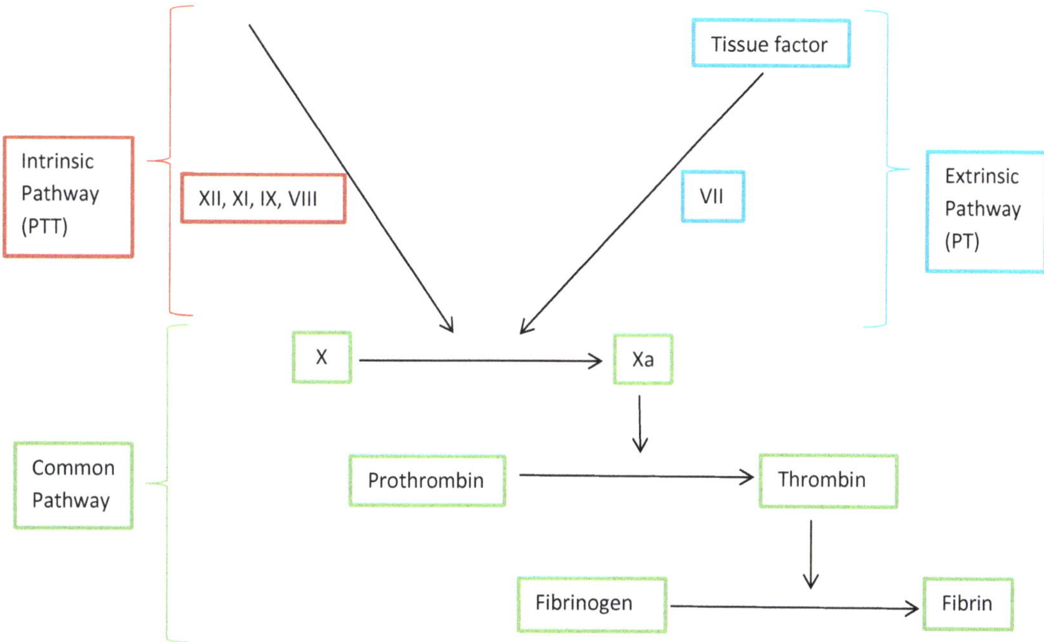

Fig. 8.2 Coagulation cascade

Vitamin K Disorders

Disorders of vitamin K can result from multiple etiologies including the use of vitamin K antagonists such as warfarin, inadequate dietary intake, malabsorption syndromes, or the chronic use of antibiotics. Vitamin K is a cofactor required for the activity of several key proteins containing carboxyglutamic acid residues important in the coagulation cascade. Hepatocytes contain carboxylase enzymes, which are necessary for the activation of coagulation factors II, VII, IX, and X. These residues facilitate the binding of coagulation factors to calcium ions on the negatively charged phospholipids [3]. Therefore, vitamin K deficiency can lead to decreased synthesis of these coagulation factors and render them ineffective, leading to coagulation abnormalities [4, 5].

The term "vitamin K" was first coined more than 50 years ago. Henrik Dam of Denmark reported the "anticlotting" factor that had the capability of reversing dietary-induced bleeding disorders in chicks. In fact, the name comes from the German/Danish word *koagulationsvitamin* (clotting vitamin) [5]. Doisy and colleagues first isolated vitamin K from alfalfa sprouts [4, 6]. There are multiple sources of vitamin K. Dietary vitamin K1 (i.e., phylloquinone or phytonadione), which is fat soluble, is mostly found in green leafy vegetables such as spinach and broccoli [7]. Its absorption requires intact pancreatobiliary function and fat absorptive mechanisms. Vitamin K2 is synthesized by microflora colonizing the GI tract, i.e., colon and terminal ileum [8]. Vitamin K, a lipophilic molecule, is protein-bound in the bloodstream and therefore requires proteolytic enzymes to liberate the active vitamin K component within the small intestines. Bile salts then solubilize vitamin K into micelles, which are absorbed into enterocytes, incorporated into chylomicrons, and then absorbed into the intestinal lymphatic system and portal circulation for transportation to the liver [9].

The normal physiologic requirement of vitamin K is 0.5 μg/kg/day [10]. Inadequate intake may deplete vitamin K stores in the body in as little as 7 days. Clinical signs and symptoms of vitamin K deficiency are characterized by easy bruising and mucosal bleeding. A prolonged PT that corrects with mixing study is a characteristic of vitamin K deficiency. When the deficiency is mild, only the PT is prolonged, but in severe cases, both the PT and aPTT may be affected. Repletion of vitamin K can be provided by oral, subcutaneous, and intravenous routes. Intravenous vitamin K carries a small risk of anaphylaxis. The PT begins to improve within 12 h and should completely normalize in 24–48 h.

Antibiotic Use and Malabsorption

Acquired vitamin K deficiency can occur secondary to the use of drugs such as antibiotics or in patients receiving total parenteral nutrition (TPN). Chronic antibiotic use can lead to alteration of the normal gut flora responsible for the synthesis of vitamin K2. In addition, antibiotics can directly affect the activation of vitamin K in the liver. Prolonged starvation or the fasting state can also decrease vitamin K levels. Since vitamin K is a fat-soluble vitamin, dysregulation in the fat absorption pathway can result in vitamin K deficiency. Disorders of bile or pancreatic enzyme secretion, including cystic fibrosis, primary biliary cirrhosis, primary sclerosing cholangitis, biliary atresia, familial intrahepatic cholestasis, and inherited disorders associated with cholestasis, as well as intestinal diseases such as celiac disease, inflammatory bowel disease, and short bowel syndrome, can result in vitamin K deficiency. Any prior history of intestinal resection, especially at the terminal ileum which is responsible for fat absorption, can result in vitamin K deficiency.

Liver Dysfunction

The liver produces most of the procoagulants, natural anticoagulants, and fibrinolytic proteins [11]. In fact, all coagulation factors are synthesized in the liver, except von Willebrand factor and factor VIII. Thus, liver dysfunction can lead to coagulation abnormalities secondary to decreased synthesis of coagulation factors, decreased clearance of activated factors, dysregulation of fibrinolysis, and production of abnormal fibrinogen [11]. Reduction of factor V distinguishes liver disease from vitamin K deficiency [10]. The degree of coagulopathy is proportional to the extent of liver parenchymal cell damage. For instance, mild to moderate liver dysfunction is associated with slightly prolonged PT, which is caused by a decrease in factor VII since it has the shortest circulating half-life. More advanced liver disease is characterized by additional factor deficiencies, including factors II, IX, and X, fibrinogen, and factor V. Factor VIII is often preserved in severe liver disease due to extrahepatic synthesis.

Acute liver injury is usually not associated with bleeding as loss of coagulation factors is compensated by a similar loss of anticoagulant proteins [12]. Even though disseminated intravascular coagulation (DIC) is seen in a small number of patients with acute hepatic necrosis and shock liver, it is not clear that hepatic injury is directly responsible for disseminated intravascular coagulopathy. Fulminant hepatic failure is characterized by activated fibrinolysis and impaired clot formation due to increasing levels of tissue plasminogen activator (t-PA) and urokinase plasminogen activator [11]. In patients with chronic liver failure, the clinical picture is frequently complicated by splenomegaly and thrombocytopenia. In both acute and chronic liver failure, patients have a risk of bleeding as well as thrombosis [13].

Vitamin K Antagonists

Vitamin K antagonists (VKAs) are often used on a long-term basis in patients with prosthetic heart valves, high-risk atrial fibrillation, venous thromboembolism, or others at high risk of thrombotic or embolic events including stroke. VKAs such as warfarin, which has a similar structure to vitamin K, block the synthesis of factors II, VII, IX, and X and anticoagulant proteins C, S, and Z (a cofactor for the inhibition of activated factor X). In particular, it interrupts the cycling of vitamin K between its oxidized and reduced state, thus preventing the gamma-carboxylation of glutamic acid residues on vitamin K-dependent proteins [11, 13]. Treatment with a VKA results in decreased synthesis and thus reduced activity of such proteins. After ingestion, warfarin is rapidly absorbed from the GI tract and reaches maximal concentration in the blood in approximately 90 min. It then accumulates in the liver where it is metabolized by P450 cytochromes CYP2C9, CYP1A2, and CYP3A4. Its half-life is roughly 36–42 h. It has a narrow therapeutic index and thus can be challenging to monitor. In addition, there are multiple food-drug and drug-drug interactions. Various patient factors affect the anticoagulant response, including age, body weight, dietary habits, gender, ethnicity, and genetic polymorphisms [3]. Its anticoagulant effect is monitored by the international normalized ratio (INR). The annual incidence of any warfarin-associated major bleeding is 0–16 %, whereas the annual incidence of warfarin-associated fatal bleed is 0–2.9 % [14]. A significantly elevated INR predicts a high risk of major bleeding. For example, Hylek et al. prospectively reported that the risk of bleeding doubles for each single point of increase in the INR above 3.0, with major bleeding occurring at a rate of 2.4–8 % per patient-year [15]. The most devastating bleeding complication is intracranial hemorrhage (ICH), which is estimated to occur at a rate of nearly 1 % per patient-year. ICH carries an estimated mortality rate of 60 %. Published guidelines to date on management of ICH are largely based on expert opinion rather than randomized clinical trials [8].

Management of VKA-Associated Coagulopathy

Treatment of VKA-associated bleeding depends on the degree of anticoagulation, clinical manifestations, and urgency at which reversal is required. Reversal agents include vitamin K, fresh frozen plasma (FFP), or prothrombin complex concentrate (PCC). Intravenous vitamin K carries a small risk of anaphylaxis, especially if formulations contain polyethoxylated castor oil, which is used to maintain vitamin K in solution [8]. The estimated risk of anaphylaxis according to one study is approximately 3 per 10,000. Several randomized controlled trials have demonstrated that low doses of oral vitamin K are effective in reducing an elevated INR in this setting. No studies have directly compared the efficacy of different doses of oral vitamin K to reverse VKA-associated coagulopathy.

In the case of a non-bleeding patient with a moderately elevated INR (less than 5), a potential management strategy includes withholding the VKA and allowing the INR to drift down. It is also reasonable to withhold the VKA and administer low-dose oral vitamin K. It is not recommended to administer FFP or coagulation factor concentrates in this setting. A number of studies have demonstrated that the incidence of 30-day major bleeding in patients with an INR greater than 9 was high (9.6 %) compared to only 1 % with INR over 5–6 [8]. If the INR is greater than 9 without associated bleeding, it is generally accepted to hold warfarin and give oral vitamin K at a dose of 2–5 mg, which can reduce the INR within 24–48 h. If the INR is between 5 and 9 and the patient is not bleeding, warfarin should be held and the administration of low-dose vitamin K is optional.

The urgency of anticoagulation reversal in the setting of VKA-associated bleeding complications depends on the severity, bleeding site, and degree of INR elevation. The VKA should be withheld and intravenous vitamin K and/or coagulation factor replacement administered in cases of VKA-associated major bleeding. With intact hepatic function, the INR generally starts to improve within 8–12 h of vitamin K administration and reaches the normal range within 24 h in most patients. The management of acute major life-threatening bleeding includes the administration of intravenous vitamin K, FFP, and PCC.

FFP is obtained from either whole blood donations or automated plasmapheresis techniques. It is widely available but provides only partial reversal of coagulopathy through replacement of factors II, VII, IX, and X. It contains all the natural pro- and anticoagulant factors at concentration of 1 U/ml. Thus, it is administered at a dose of 15 ml/kg, which usually requires infusion of volumes over 1 L. A lower dose of 5–8 ml/kg may be appropriate in cases of urgent reversal. There are advantages and disadvantages to its use [9, 14].

PCCs are pooled human plasma-derived products containing factors II, IX, and X with variable amounts of factor VII, proteins C and S, and antithrombin. It is supplied as a powder and diluent, which are reconstituted prior to administration. Products must be warmed to room temperature if previously refrigerated [3]. There are two types: a nonactivated and an activated form. Nonactivated PCCs can be classified as three factor (3F-PCC) or four factor (4F-PCC). The former contains factors II, IX, and X with a small amount of VII concentrate. The latter contains sufficient levels of all vitamin K-dependent factors. Thus, 3-F PCC and 4-F PCC differ by amount of FVII. In the United States, 4F-PCC (Kcentra) was approved in April 2013 for reversal of acquired coagulopathy due to vitamin K antagonists. However, this product has been used in Canada and Europe for many years [14]. PCC provides a rapid and effective method for replacing deficient clotting factors and correcting the INR. In a randomized clinical trial, 18 over-anticoagulated patients were randomized to receive PCC or intravenous vitamin K [16]. The authors concluded that patients who received PCC had a more rapid INR correction compared those treated with vitamin K. In another study comparing the use of PCC versus FFP, Makris et al. reported that complete correction of the INR occurred within 15 min in 28 out of 29 patients treated with PCC, compared to none of the 12 patients treated with FFP [17]. The optimal dose of PCC is not established. The dose of PCC can be adjusted based on weight, initial INR, and target INR. The effect of PCC lasts only 12–24 h. Thus, vitamin K should be coadministered with PCC as the INR may rebound due to the persistent effects of warfarin. PCC therapy is generally safe. A systematic review of 14 studies involving 460 patients demonstrated only 7 total thrombotic complications (3 strokes, 2 myocardial infarctions, 2 deep vein thromboses) after the use of PCC [8].

Fresh Frozen Plasma Versus Prothrombin Complex Concentrates

PCCs do not require ABO compatibility or thawing. The volume of PCC necessary for reversal is smaller than FFP since PCCs contain 25 times the concentration of vitamin K-dependent factors relative to an equal volume of plasma. At present, it is recommended that PCCs should be given for reversal of VKA-associated major bleeding based on the ability of PCCs to rapidly correct a supratherapeutic INR. However, it is unclear if rapid reversal of the INR translates to improved patient outcomes. A prospective, randomized controlled trial comparing the efficacy and safety of 4F-PCC to FFP demonstrated the following conclusions: 4F-PCC is non-inferior, achieves rapid reduction in INR (62.2 % vs. 9.6 %), requires a shorter infusion time, results in a lower incidence of fluid overload (5 % vs. 13.2 %), and has a similar safety profile [18]. Doses reported in the literature range from 8 to 50 U/kg. Risk of thrombotic complications and high cost are potential barriers to use of 4F-PCC by clinicians [9]. In contrast to the use of PCCs, FFP requires thawing for approximately 30 min at 30–37 °C and ABO typing prior to administration; in addition, it carries a small risk of transmissible infections and has the potential for causing volume overload [8, 9, 14]. Although more costly, PCC can normalize INR faster (15 min vs. 1–2 h), reduces the need for PRBC transfusions, requires a smaller infusion volume, and does not increase adverse events in comparison to FFP [3, 19]. In addition, PCCs undergo a viral inactivation process to reduce transmission of infective agents.

In cases of major or life-threatening bleeding associated with VKA use, intravenous vitamin K and coagulation factor replacement are recommended [8].

Recombinant Factor VIIa

Recombinant factor VIIa (rFVIIa) can reverse VKA-associated coagulopathy in patients with serious bleeding complications. It is currently approved for treatment of bleeding complications in patients with hemophilia who develop antibodies to factor VIII or IX. Its primary mechanisms of action include activation of tissue factor at the site of endothelial injury to activate factor X and the reversal of platelet defects. There are a paucity of data to support its clinical efficacy in patients with vitamin K deficiency or antagonism. The use of rFVIIa is associated with the development of arterial thrombosis. Since the therapeutic effect of rFVIIa lasts only about 12–24 h, vitamin K must be administered as well.

US and European guidelines, including the American College of Chest Physicians, recommend PCCs as primary treatment for anticoagulation reversal in life-threatening bleeding and increased INR, with rFVIIa as a possible alternative. The VKA should be discontinued and intravenous vitamin K should be concomitantly administered.

Perioperative Management of Patients Receiving Vitamin K Antagonists

The management of patients receiving a VKA who require surgical procedures can be challenging. There is an increased risk of thromboembolism when anticoagulation is interrupted for a surgical procedure. However, invasive surgeries are associated with inherent bleeding risk, which is magnified in patients who are on anticoagulation. Thus for each patient, a balance between reducing risk of thromboembolism and preventing excess bleeding must be reached at the time of surgery. One should take into account the estimated thromboembolic risk, the bleeding risk inherent to the procedure, the timing of VKA interruption, and whether or not bridging anticoagulation is indicated. Most published guidelines are based on expert opinion since data from randomized clinical trials in this setting are lacking [3, 18, 20–22].

For an elective procedure, the VKA should be discontinued about 6 days prior to planned surgery. PT/INR should be obtained 1 day prior to surgery. If procedure is planned after 24 h, vitamin K administration is reasonable. Subcutaneous vitamin K can be given if the INR remains greater than 1.5 despite receiving oral vitamin K. The INR should be in the normal range in patients undergoing procedures associated with a high bleeding risk, i.e., intracranial, spinal, or urologic surgeries, and/or any procedure requiring neuroaxial anesthesia. Discontinuation of the VKA for several days will result in subtherapeutic anticoagulation. Bridging with a subcutaneous or intravenous short-acting agent, i.e., low molecular weight heparin or unfractionated heparin for approximately 2–3 days prior to surgery in patients deemed at high or very high risk of thromboembolism, may be indicated. For urgent procedures requiring rapid INR normalization, additional reversal agents can be utilized. The appropriate reversal agent for VKA-induced coagulopathy depends on the degree of anticoagulation, urgency of the procedure, and bleeding risk. For semi-urgent reversal, which is often defined as within 1–2 days, the VKA should be withheld and vitamin K (either oral or IV) can be given. In contrast, when immediate reversal is desired (i.e., active major bleeding and/or emergent surgery), PCC or FFP along with vitamin K is recommended [3, 18, 20–22].

Acquired Factor Deficiencies and Inhibitors

Acquired Factor X Deficiency

Factor X is a vitamin K-dependent coagulation factor which may be deficient in a variety of clinical scenarios, including patients with liver disease or vitamin K deficiency. Acquired factor X deficiency has been described in patients with certain malignancies, such as spindle cell thymoma, renal or adrenal carcinoma, gastric carcinoma, and acute leukemia. *Mycoplasma pneumoniae* infection may cause a transient decrease in factor X levels [23]. Acquired factor X deficiency is well-described in patients with AL amyloidosis.

Factor X Deficiency in AL Amyloidosis

AL amyloidosis is a plasma cell disorder in which abnormal protein fibrils deposit in tissues, resulting in organ failure. AL refers to the amyloid light chain-derived subtype of amyloidosis, which occurs in 8 per million people per year [24]. It is more common in men and occurs most commonly in the sixth or seventh decade of life. In most patients, a monoclonal protein will be detected by serum or urine immunofixation and free light chain assays. Common sites of amyloid fibril deposition include the liver, heart, soft tissues, kidneys, and nerves. This entity is diagnosed by tissue biopsy of an involved organ or tissue with positivity by Congo red staining, showing apple-green birefringence under polarized light. Patients may present with fatigue, weight loss, macroglossia, neuropathy, heart failure symptoms, hepatomegaly, or nephrotic range proteinuria. AL amyloid may occur in isolation or in association with another B-cell disorder, such as multiple myeloma or non-Hodgkin lymphoma. Other common subtypes of amyloidosis include AA amyloidosis, which is associated with chronic inflammatory diseases, hereditary amyloidosis, and age-related "senile" systemic amyloidosis, the detailed discussion of which is outside the scope of this chapter.

Acquired deficiency of factor X is the most common coagulation factor deficiency seen in patients with AL amyloidosis [25]. However, less than 5 % of patients with AL amyloidosis present with factor X deficiency [26]. The mechanism involves increased clearance of factor X from circulation due to adherence to amyloid fibrils [27]. This is likely independent of proteinuria and liver dysfunction [25]. Bleeding in this scenario can be life-threatening and can present a therapeutic challenge. Factor X is rapidly removed from circulation in this disease, and therefore factor replacement with products such as fresh frozen plasma or prothrombin complex concentrates is often ineffective [28]. Patients with amyloidosis can also have bleeding due to other mechanisms, including fragile blood vessels, hyperfibrinolysis, platelet dysfunction, and other less common factor deficiencies (II, VII, IX, V) [25, 29, 30]. Severe bleeding is generally seen in patients with plasma factor X levels below 25 % of normal [25]. Moderate to severe bleeding can occur in patients with factor X levels 25–50 % of normal [25]. Patients with acquired factor X deficiency may have a prolonged PT or PTT, with a mixing study which corrects with the addition of normal plasma.

Extensive binding of factor X to amyloid fibrils can occur in the spleen. If the patient has significant splenic involvement by amyloidosis, splenectomy may improve the coagulopathy by removal of amyloid deposits [31]. RFVIIa has been used perioperatively for splenectomy or other surgical procedures to reduce bleeding risk [28, 32, 33]. However, the benefits of rFVIIa must be balanced with the risk of thrombosis. Ultimately, treatment of the underlying AL amyloidosis is necessary to reverse the coagulopathy. The preferred therapy is high-dose melphalan followed by autologous stem cell transplantation (ASCT). If not eligible for ASCT, patients may receive chemotherapy with agents such as bortezomib, melphalan, alkylating, or immunomodulatory agents.

Acquired Factor XIII Deficiency

Factor XIII is a tetramer which plays an important role in the formation of the fibrin clot. It consists of two active A subunits and two B subunits, which protect the A subunits in circulation. In addition to congenital factor XIII deficiency (see Chap. 7), a variety of medical conditions can result in an acquired deficiency of factor XIII, such as major surgery, sepsis, DIC, pulmonary embolism, malignancy, stroke, cirrhosis, or an autoimmune disorder. Severe factor XIII deficiency is defined as a factor XIII level less than 5 %, with moderate 5–10 %, and mild greater than 10 %. Patients with factor XIII deficiency will have a normal PT, PTT, and thrombin time; the test of choice to evaluate for this condition is a factor XIII activity assay. In general, patients with acquired factor XIII deficiency do not reach levels less than 30 % and therefore do not require replacement therapy. If necessary, factor XIII concentrate is the preferred treatment for this disorder, with fresh frozen plasma an alternative option. Patients with autoantibodies against factor XIII should be considered for plasma exchange and/or immunosuppressive medications [34].

Acquired von Willebrand Syndrome (Factor VIII Deficiency)

Von Willebrand disease (VWD) is an inherited bleeding disorder in which patients may experience mucosal or skin bleeding, as well as hemostatic dysfunction perioperatively. This condition occurs when there is dysfunctional or deficient von Willebrand factor (VWF), a plasma protein which facilitates the binding of platelets to each other and to sites of tissue injury. VWF also acts as a carrier for coagulation factor VIII. Therefore, the bleeding diathesis seen in patients with VWD occurs due to a reduction in factor VIII levels and impaired adhesion of platelets to sites of tissue injury. See Chap. 7 for a detailed discussion of the evaluation and management of patients with inherited von Willebrand disease.

Acquired von Willebrand syndrome (AVWS) occurs when there is a deficiency or defect in the function of von Willebrand factor as a consequence of another medical condition. This disorder is relatively rare and is usually associated with an underlying lymphoproliferative or myeloproliferative disorder. It can also be seen in patients with other malignancies, cardiovascular conditions, those with autoimmune diseases, or as a result of certain medications. Its prevalence may be increasing due to a greater use of left ventricular assist devices (LVADs). It is more common in elderly patients [35]. There are three mechanisms which lead to AVWS: destruction of VWF from shear stress, autoimmune destruction or inhibition of VWF, or increased binding of VWF to platelets or other surfaces [36]. Patients with this syndrome as a result of cardiac valvular disease or another vascular condition may have a decrease in VWF multimers due to destruction from shear stress. Patients may present with mucocutaneous bleeding and usually will not have a past or family history of bleeding. Diagnostic evaluation generally reveals a normal PT and a normal or prolonged PTT. Additional studies may show a decrease in factor VIII activity, VWF activity (ristocetin cofactor activity), and/or VWF antigen.

Treatment of AVWS is aimed at controlling acute bleeding, preventing perioperative bleeding, and treating the underlying disorder if possible. This can include desmopressin, which causes release of VWF stores into circulation, although not all patients will respond to this therapy. If possible, patients should have a therapeutic trial of desmopressin with measurement of plasma VWF activity and factor VIII levels prior to and at intervals following administration to ensure adequate response. The typical dose used is 0.3 μg/kg over 30 min once daily. Patients should be monitored for the common adverse effects of hyponatremia and volume overload [35]. Tachyphylaxis can occur and therefore desmopressin should not be used more than once per day for up to 3 days. If patients do not respond to desmopressin or if response is unknown, VWF/factor VIII concentrates can be effective, although these products can have a short half-life, especially in patients with inhibitors to VWF [35]. Intravenous immunoglobulin (IVIG) is another therapy which may provide benefit if patients do not respond to desmopressin or VWF/factor VIII concentrates [37]. In patients with immune-mediated AVWS, plasma exchange, steroids, or immunosuppression may be effective. Successful use of rFVIIa has been reported in patients with AVWS, although benefits must be balanced with the risk of thrombosis. Treatment of the underlying malignancy or surgical correction of the cardiac defect if possible may eliminate the coagulopathy. In patients with thrombocytosis and AVWS, correction of the thrombocytosis will often correct the coagulopathy. Patients with hypothyroidism may develop AVWS, which is treated with thyroid hormone replacement [36].

Acquired Hemophilia A (Factor VIII Inhibitor)

Hemophilia A is the congenital deficiency of coagulation factor VIII, which is active in the intrinsic pathway of the coagulation cascade. The acquisition of an inhibitor to factor VIII, or acquired hemophilia A, can be idiopathic, or secondary to various medical conditions, including autoimmune disorders, malignancy, the postpartum period, infections, or certain medications [38]. It occurs more commonly in elderly patients. Factor VIII inhibitors are rare, with an incidence of 1–4 per million people per year [38]. This condition causes severe and often life-threatening bleeding, with a high mortality rate (8–22 %) [38]. In contrast to patients with congenital hemophilia A, who often experience hemarthrosis, patients with an acquired factor VIII inhibitor may present with mucosal or subcutaneous bleeding, hematuria, or GI bleeding. Evaluation reveals a prolonged PTT which does not correct with the addition of normal plasma by mixing study. Additional workup should include a factor VIII level and factor VIII inhibitor activity.

Treatment of a bleeding patient with a factor VIII inhibitor should include one of two strategies: raising the factor VIII level (generally only if a low titer factor VIII inhibitor is present, less than 5 Bethesda units (BU)) or bypassing factor VIII. Patients with a low titer inhibitor can be treated with human factor VIII concentrates, 20 IU/kg for each BU of inhibitor plus 40 IU/kg intravenously [38].

If the titer is greater than or equal to 5 BU, a bypassing agent should be used. RFVIIa is frequently used as a first-line agent, with a recommended dose of 90–120 μg/kg every 2–3 h, as the half-life is approximately 2.5 h [39, 40]. RFVIIa leads to the generation of thrombin. The benefit of this agent must be balanced against the risk of thrombosis, particularly in elderly patients. Activated prothrombin complex concentrate (aPCC) is an alternative bypassing agent, which provides the vitamin K-dependent clotting factors. The recommended dose range of aPCC is 50–100 IU/kg every 8–12 h [39, 40]. In order to eliminate the inhibitor, various immunosuppressive agents have been employed. Steroids alone or in combination with cyclophosphamide are frequently used for this indication. Intravenous immunoglobulin may also be effective when combined with immunosuppressive agents. Plasma exchange, immune tolerance protocols, cyclosporine, and rituximab have been used to eradicate factor VIII inhibitors as well. In patients with a minor bleeding episode, desmopressin can be considered. There is a high risk of infectious complications from immunosuppressive therapy. These therapies should be administered after consultation with a hematologist.

Antiphospholipid Antibody Syndrome

The antiphospholipid antibody syndrome (APS) is an acquired condition resulting in a prothrombotic state. APS can be a primary condition or can be associated with an underlying disorder such as a rheumatologic disease or malignancy. The syndrome requires the presence of both laboratory and clinical components for diagnosis, including an autoantibody in the plasma and either a venous or arterial thrombosis or recurrent obstetrical complications. In a surgical setting, it is important to identify a preexisting history of this syndrome as patients are prone to thrombosis and may require anticoagulant therapy. In some settings, preoperative workup may reveal a prolonged aPTT, which prompts further investigation with a mixing study and evaluation for circulating inhibitors. The APLAs implicated in this syndrome include anticardiolipin antibodies (aCL), anti-β_2-glycoprotein I antibodies (aβ_2GPI), and the lupus anticoagulant (LA). Perioperative management of patients with known APS includes holding warfarin prior to planned intervention and reversing warfarin if urgent surgery is required. Prophylactic doses of anticoagulation should be started as soon as possible postoperatively, and therapeutic anticoagulation should be reinitiated as soon as safe from a surgical standpoint. Here we will review the pathophysiology, laboratory diagnosis, clinical presentation, and treatment of APS. We will also include a brief discussion of catastrophic APS (CAPS).

Pathophysiology

APS is an autoimmune process associated with circulating autoantibodies to phospholipid protein complexes. Although these antibodies were first detected in patients with systemic lupus erythematosus (SLE), the disorder is not limited to those with SLE. Subtypes of the antiphospholipid antibodies include aCL, aβ_2GPI, and LA. Positivity for all three of these tests is associated with the highest risk for thrombosis and pregnancy loss. There are a number of proposed mechanisms for how the presence of these antibodies results in an increased risk of thrombosis, including the effects of antibodies on platelets, endothelial cells, monocytes, and trophoblasts and interference with complement activation. Cell signaling pathways such as the phosphatidyl-inositol 3-kinase (PI3K)/AKT pathway may also be involved in pathogenesis [41].

Antiphospholipid antibodies can be detected in a variety of clinical settings including healthy individuals, in the presence of autoimmune or rheumatologic diseases, with infections, medication related, or in the presence of malignancy. The most frequent rheumatologic condition associated with APS is SLE, and approximately 31 % of patients with SLE will have a LA. Although LA is the most prevalent antibody in the setting of SLE, aCL or aβ_2GPI antibody may also be identified. Bacterial, viral, and parasitic infections can be associated with APLA. Such infections include HIV, mononucleosis, rubella, hepatitis, syphilis, Lyme disease, tuberculosis, malaria, and toxoplasmosis, among others. Common medications associated with the development of APLA include procainamide, phenothiazines, phenytoin, hydralazine, quinidine, quinine, ethosuximide, alpha interferon, amoxicillin, chlorothiazide, oral contraceptives, and propranolol. Associations with malignancies including solid tumors, Hodgkin and non-Hodgkin lymphoma, leukemias, and myeloproliferative disorders have been reported [42].

Diagnosis

Diagnosis of APS requires the presence of clinical and laboratory findings. Diagnostic workup may be pursued in the setting of (1) more than one otherwise unexplained thrombosis or thromboembolic events, (2) more than one pregnancy-related complications, or (3) otherwise unexplained prolongation of the aPTT or thrombocytopenia. The following laboratory studies should be obtained: IgG and IgM aCL antibodies, IgG and IgM aβ_2GPI antibodies, and LA testing. The aCL and aβ_2GP I antibodies are evaluated by enzyme-linked immunosorbent assay (ELISA). The LA is evaluated with an initial dilute Russell viper venom time (dRVVT), and if positive, a confirmatory test should follow. If any of the initial laboratory tests are positive, they need to be repeated and confirmed a second time, 12 weeks later.

The Sapporo criteria, now referred to as the revised Sapporo criteria or the Sydney criteria, are used to make a diagnosis of definite APS. According to these criteria, definite APS can be considered if at least one of the following clinical and one of the following laboratory criteria are present. The clinical criteria include (1) vascular thrombosis or (2) pregnancy morbidity. Specifically the vascular thrombosis must be a venous, arterial, or small vessel thrombosis with unequivocal imaging or histologic evidence. This does not include the presence of superficial thrombosis. Pregnancy-related morbidity is defined as unexplained fetal death at ≥10 weeks gestation of a normal fetus or one or more premature births before 34 weeks because of eclampsia, preeclampsia, or placental insufficiency or three or more early (<10 weeks) pregnancy losses unexplained by other etiologies.

The laboratory findings that are required for the diagnosis of APS include the presence of one or more of the following: (1) IgG and/or IgM anticardiolipin antibodies in moderate or high titer (>40 GPL or MPL units or greater than the 99th percentile for the laboratory testing), (2) antibodies to beta2-glycoprotein I of IgG or IgM isotype at a titer greater than the 99th percentile for the testing laboratory when tested according to recommended procedures, or (3) lupus anticoagulant activity detected according to published guidelines [43]. As previously stated, if any of the above tests are positive, the finding must be confirmed a second time, 12 weeks later, to rule out a false-positive result. False-positive tests can be observed in the setting of oral anticoagulants, older patients, or only mildly positive lupus anticoagulant results. False-negative results also occur and are usually related to laboratory processing. Checking for APLA at the time of acute thrombosis is not recommended as they can decrease temporarily or may be transiently positive.

Clinical Presentation

Clinical presentation of APS includes manifestations of venous or arterial thrombosis and/or pregnancy complications or loss. On physical exam, findings may include livedo reticularis, digital ischemia, asymmetric lower extremity edema from a deep venous thrombosis (DVT), or neurologic findings from stroke. Additional clinical manifestations may include thrombocytopenia, coronary artery disease, valvular heart disease, pulmonary hypertension, peripheral arterial disease, retinal disease, adrenal failure, and gastrointestinal manifestations. Venous thrombosis is more common than arterial thrombosis and the calf veins are the most common sites of DVT [44]. APS should be considered in young patients with history of stroke and no other risk factors for cerebrovascular disease or recurrent thrombotic events in the absence of other risk factors.

Additional hematologic manifestations may include thrombocytopenia, thrombotic microangiopathy, or bleeding. Thrombocytopenia is the most commonly seen hematologic manifestation and the usual platelet count ranges from 50,000 to 140,000/μl [45]. Thrombocytopenia does not preclude the development of thrombosis and should not preclude the use of anticoagulant therapy if the platelet count remains above 50,000.

Treatment

Once a diagnosis of APS has been reached and confirmed, timely treatment should be initiated. Treatment may include the use of anticoagulants such as heparin or warfarin and possibly antiplatelet agents such as aspirin. In the setting of an acute thrombosis associated with APS, the thrombosis should be treated in the same manner as thrombosis independent of APS. Heparin or low molecular weight heparin is frequently initiated with the simultaneous initiation of warfarin. The heparin product should be continued until the INR has been in the target therapeutic range for 48–72 h. Unfractionated heparin may be preferred in the setting of hemorrhagic complications as it can be rapidly reversed. The use of unfractionated heparin requires additional consideration when the aPTT is elevated at baseline. In this setting, the aPTT may not be a reliable measure of heparin levels and instead monitoring with anti-factor Xa levels may be more appropriate.

There must be consideration for long-term, possibly lifelong anticoagulation in the setting of unprovoked, spontaneous thromboembolism in the context of APS. There are no prospective data to support higher intensity anticoagulation therapy with an INR goal of 3.0–4.0 in APS. Clinical trials have demonstrated that there is no reduction in the rate of recurrent thrombosis with a higher INR goal as compared to a standard INR goal of 2.0–3.0 [46]. There are also no prospective data to support the use of direct factor Xa inhibitors or direct thrombin inhibitors in APS and thus these agents are not recommended.

In patients with a prolonged PT/INR at baseline, it may be necessary to confirm a therapeutic level of anticoagulation by monitoring factor II activity level or measuring chromogenic factor X assay. Whole blood point of care testing may be unreliable in the setting of APLA and therefore it should be correlated with a plasma INR from a peripheral blood draw prior to accepting point of care testing as an accurate measurement. Patients should be counseled regarding the potential medication and dietary interactions while on warfarin therapy. Home self-monitoring INR is a potential option in a carefully selected patient population.

The antiplatelet agents studied for therapeutic use in APS include aspirin and clopidogrel. There are some studies to suggest aspirin at a dose of 81 mg/day may decrease the risk of thrombosis in patients with APS; however, the routine use of aspirin should be driven primarily by the cardiovascular risk factors of the patient [47]. There are no data from randomized studies to support the routine use of clopidogrel in treatment of APS and this is not recommended [48]. There have been studies investigating the use of prophylactic aspirin in patients with positive APLA, but no history of thrombosis. However, these trials have failed to document a benefit from the addition of daily aspirin [49].

Catastrophic Antiphospholipid Antibody Syndrome

The catastrophic antiphospholipid antibody syndrome (CAPS) is a potentially life-threatening condition involving widespread thrombosis despite appropriate anticoagulation that results in multiorgan failure. Mortality rates have been reported as high as 30 % in some studies [50]. Criteria for the diagnosis of this syndrome include (1) evidence of involvement of three or more organs, systems, and/or tissues; (2) development of manifestations simultaneously or within 1 week of each other; (3) confirmation by histopathology of small vessel occlusion in at least one organ tissue; and (4) laboratory confirmation of the presence of APLAs. The diagnosis of definite CAPS requires the presence of all four criteria. If less than all four criteria are present, the diagnosis of probable CAPS may be reached [51]. Treatment of CAPS is focused on treating the thrombotic events and also the underlying cytokine storm that ensues. Patients with CAPS may benefit from combined treatment with anticoagulants, glucocorticoids, plasma exchange, and/or intravenous immune globulin (IVIG). Rituximab has been studied in the setting of resistant CAPS and may provide some benefit [52].

A preexisting history of APS in the neurosurgical patient is important to identify, as careful attention to perioperative anticoagulation is required. The goal of treatment should be to safely resume anticoagulation as soon as safe from a surgical perspective as these patients are at high risk of thrombosis. At times, a new diagnosis of APS may be identified by a neurosurgical service with an appropriate level of suspicion based on clinical and laboratory findings. Consultation with a hematologist is appropriate in the setting of APS.

References

1. Furie B, Furie B. Mechanisms of thrombus formation. NEJM. 2008;359:938–49.
2. Cashen AF. *The Washington manual subspecialty consult series: Hematology and oncology subspecialty consult.* 2nd ed. Philadelphia: Lippincott Williams & Wilkin; 2008. p. 49–57, 74–75.
3. Levy JH. Peri-operative hemostatic management of patients treated with vitamin K antagonists. Anesthesiology. 2008;109:918.
4. Dam H. The anti-hemorrhagic vitamin of the chick: occurrence and chemical nature. Nature. 1935;135:652.
5. Vermeer C, Schurgers LJ. A comprehensive review of vitamin K and vitamin K antagonists. Hematol Oncol Clin North Am. 2000;14:339.
6. Shearer MJ, Vitamin K. Lancet. 1995;345:229.
7. Sconce E, Avery P, Wynne H, Kamali F. Vitamin K supplementation can improve stability of anticoagulation for patients with unexplained variability in response to warfarin. Blood. 2007;109(6):2419–23.
8. Dentali F, Crowther MA. Management of excessive anticoagulant effect due to vitamin K antagonists. Hematology Am Soc Hematol Educ Program. 2008;2008(1):266–70. ASH Education Book.
9. Yates SG, Sarode R, et al. New strategies for effective treatment of vitamin K antagonist-associated bleeding. J Thromb Haemost. 2015;13 Suppl 1:S180–6.
10. Spaet TH. Clinical implications of acquired blood coagulation abnormalities. Blood. 1964;23(6):839–42.
11. Hambleton J, Leung LL, Levi M. Coagulation: consultative hemostasis. Hematology Am Soc Hematol Educ Program. 2002;2002:335–52.
12. Bernal W, Wendon J. Acute liver failure. N Eng J Med. 2013;369:2525–34.
13. Tripodi A, Mannucci M. The coagulopathy of chronic liver disease. N Eng J Med. 2011;365:147–56.
14. Le Roux P, Pollack Jr CV, Milan M, Schaefer A. Race against the clock: overcoming challenges in the management of anticoagulant-associated intracerebral hemorrhage. J Neurosurg. 2014;121(Suppl):1–20.
15. Fitzmaurice DA, Blann AD, Lip GYH. Bleeding risks of antithrombotic therapy. BMJ. 2002;325:828.
16. Taberner DA, Thomson JM, Poller L. Comparison of Prothrombin complex concentrate and vitamin K1 in oral anticoagulant reversal. BMJ. 1976;2:83.
17. Makris M, et al. Emergency oral anticoagulant reversal: the relative efficacy of infusions of Fresh Frozen Plasma and clotting factor concentrate on correction of the coagulopathy. Thromb Haemost. 1997;77:477–80.
18. Sarode R. Efficacy and safety of a 4F PCC in patients on VKA presenting with major bleeding: a randomized, plasma controlled, phase IIIb study. Circulation. 2013;128:1234.
19. Parry-Jones AR, Di Napoli M, Goldstein JN, Schreuder FH, et al. Reversal strategies for vitamin K antagonists in acute intracerebral hemorrhage. Ann Neurol. 2015;78(1):54–62.
20. Douketis JD. Peri-operative management of anti-thrombotic therapy: anti-thrombotic therapy and prevention of thrombosis, 9th ed: ACCP evidenced-based clinical practice guidelines. Chest. 2012;141, e326S.
21. Kearon C. Management of anticoagulation before and after elective surgery. N Engl J Med. 1997;336:1506.
22. Larson BJ. A feasibility study of continuing dose-reduced Warfarin for invasive procedures in patients with high thromboembolic risk. Chest. 2005;127:922.
23. Uprichard J, Perry DJ. Factor X deficiency. Blood Rev. 2002;16:97–110.
24. Kyle RA, et al. Incidence and natural history of primary systemic amyloidosis in Olmsted County, Minnesota, 1950 through 1989. Blood. 1992;79(7):1817–22.
25. Choufani EB, et al. Acquired factor X deficiency in patients with amyloid light-chain amyloidosis: incidence, bleeding manifestations, and response to high-dose chemotherapy. Blood. 2001;15:97(6).

26. Ericson S, et al. Fatal bleeding due to acquired factor IX and X deficiency: a rare complication of primary amyloidosis; case report and review of the literature. Clin Lymphoma Myeloma Leuk. 2014;14(3):e81–6.
27. Furie B, et al. Mechanism of factor X deficiency in systemic amyloidosis. NEJM. 1981;2:304(14).
28. Boggio L, Green D. Recombinant human factor VIIa in the management of amyloid-associated factor X deficiency. Br J Hematol. 2001;112:1074–5.
29. Gamba G, et al. Clotting alterations in primary systemic amyloidosis. Haematologica. 2000;85.
30. Mumford AD, et al. Bleeding symptoms and coagulation abnormalities in 337 patients with AL-amyloidosis. Br J Hematol. 2000;110.
31. Greipp PR, et al. Factor X deficiency in primary amyloidosis – resolution after splenectomy. NEJM. 1979;301:1050–1.
32. Takabe K, et al. Successful perioperative management of factor X deficiency associated with primary amyloidosis. J Gastrointest Surg. 2004;8(3):358–62.
33. Ma JF, et al. Refractory hematuria from amyloidosis successfully treated by splenectomy. Urology. 2006;67(5):1085e13–5.
34. Tahlan A, Factor AJ, XIII. Congenital deficiency factor XIII, acquired deficiency, factor XIII a-subunit, and factor XIII B-subunit. Arch Pathol Lab Med. 2014;138(2):278–81.
35. Tiede A, et al. How I treat the acquired von Willebrand syndrome. Blood. 2011;23:117(25).
36. Nichols WL, et al. Von Willebrand disease (VWD): evidence-based diagnosis and management guidelines, the national heart, lung and blood institute (NHLBI) expert panel report (USA). Hemophilia. 2008;14:171–232.
37. Federici AB, et al. Acquired von Willebrand syndrome: data from an international registry. Thromb Haemost. 2000;84:345–9.
38. Franchini M, Giuseppe L. How I treat acquired factor VIII inhibitors. Blood. 2008;112(2):250–5.
39. Franchini M, Mannucci PM. Inhibitors of propagation of coagulation (factors VIII, IX and XI): a review of current therapeutic practice. Br J Clin Pharmacol. 2011;74(4):553–62.
40. Hay CRM, et al. The diagnosis and management of factor VIII and IX inhibitors: a guideline from the United Kingdom haemophilia centre doctors organisation. Br J Haematol. 2006;133:591–605.
41. Canaud G, Biemaime F, Tabarin F, et al. Inhibition of the mTORC pathway in the antiphospholipid syndrome. N Engl J Med. 2014;371:303.
42. Cervera R, Asherson RA. Clinical and epidemiological aspects in the antiphospholipid syndrome. Immunobiology. 2003;207:5.
43. Giannakopoulos B, Passam F, Ioannou Y, Krilis SA. How we diagnose the antiphospholipid syndrome. Blood. 2009;113:985.
44. Gromnica-Ihle E, Schossler W. Antiphospholipid syndrome. Int Arch Allergy Immunol. 2000;123:67.
45. Cervera R, Piette JC, Font J, et al. Antiphospholipid syndrome: clinical and immunologic manifestations and patterns of disease expression in a cohort of 1,000 patients. Arthritis Rheum. 2002;46:1019.
46. Crowther MA, Ginsberg JS, Julian J, et al. A comparison of two intensities of warfarin for the prevention of recurrent thrombosis in patients with the antiphospholipid antibody syndrome. N Engl J Med. 2003; 349:1133.
47. Barbhaiya M, Erkan D. Primary thrombosis prophylaxis in antiphospholipid antibody-positive patients: where do we stand? Curr Rheumatol Rep. 2011; 13:59.
48. Bick RL. Antiphospholipid thrombosis syndromes. Hematol Oncol Clin North Am. 2003;17:115.
49. Erkan D, Harrison MJ, Levy R, et al. Aspirin for primary thrombosis prevention in the antiphospholipid syndrome: a randomized, double-blind, placebo-controlled trial in asymptomatic antiphospholipid antibody-positive individuals. Arthritis Rheum. 2007; 56:2382.
50. Bucciarelli S, Espinosa G, Cervera R, et al. Mortality in the catastrophic antiphospholipid syndrome: causes of death and prognostic factors in a series of 250 patients. Arthritis Rheum. 2006;54:2568.
51. Ashercon RA, Cervera R, de Groot PG, et al. Lupus. 2003;12:530.
52. Berman H, Rodriguez-Pinto I, Cervera R, et al. Rituximab use in the catastrophic antiphospholipid syndrome: descriptive analysis of the CAPS registry patients receiving rituximab. Autoimmun Rev. 2013; 12:108.

9 Regulation and Dysregulation of Fibrinolysis

Omer Iqbal, Paul O'Malley, and Nil Guler

Introduction

Claude Bernard (1813–1878), a French physiologist, first coined the term *milieu intérieur* (the environment within), now known as homeostasis. Hemostasis is one such homeostatic process. Hemostasis could be defined as a state of physiologic homeostasis resulting from a dynamic equilibrium between coagulation and fibrinolysis. The endothelium, a single layer of cells, which line the intimal surface of the entire cardiovascular system (estimated to be 1000–5000 square meters), is by far the largest endocrine, paracrine, and autocrine gland ever known to man and plays a central role in maintaining blood fluidity. The coordinated interplay of primary hemostasis (platelet-vessel wall interactions), secondary hemostasis (fibrin formation), and fibrinolysis ensures arrest of blood flow at sites of injury and restoration of vascular patency during wound healing by local activation of plasminogen to plasmin. This finely tuned balance enables healing of a vascular lesion without compromising the stability of the clot and to contain the fibrinolytic activity to the injured area. This can be achieved by the intricate fine balance between coagulation, fibrinolysis, and proteolytic and inhibitory proteins [1].

O. Iqbal, M.D., F.A.C.C., F.E.S.C. (✉)
Department of Pathology, Loyola University Health System, 2160 South 1st Avenue, Maywood, IL 60153, USA

Department of Ophthalmology, Loyola University Health System, 2160 South 1st Avenue, Maywood, IL 60153, USA
e-mail: oiqbal@luc.edu

P. O'Malley, M.S.P., M.B.A. • N. Guler, M.D.
Department of Pathology, Loyola University Health System, 2160 South 1st Avenue, Maywood, IL 60153, USA
e-mail: pomalley1@luc.edu; nilvecay@yahoo.com

Regulation of Fibrinolysis

The fibrinolytic system is an important endothelium-dependent mechanism for limiting fibrin accumulation [2]. Plasmin plays a central role in fibrinolysis and is formed from plasma zymogen, plasminogen, by the action of plasminogen activators derived from the endothelium. The endogenous plasminogen activators are, namely, tissue-type plasminogen activator (tPA) and urokinase-type plasminogen activator (uPA) which themselves exist in zymogenic forms, tPA as single-chain tPA and uPA as prourokinase [3]. The tPA is fibrin selective since its catalytic activity is enhanced significantly following binding to fibrin. Specific cell surface membrane receptors also allow plasminogen activation by tPA and uPA and thereby promote dissolution of fibrin clot from the microenvironment of the endothelial cell, macrophages, or platelet surface [3].

C.M. Loftus (ed.), *Anticoagulation and Hemostasis in Neurosurgery*,
DOI 10.1007/978-3-319-27327-3_9

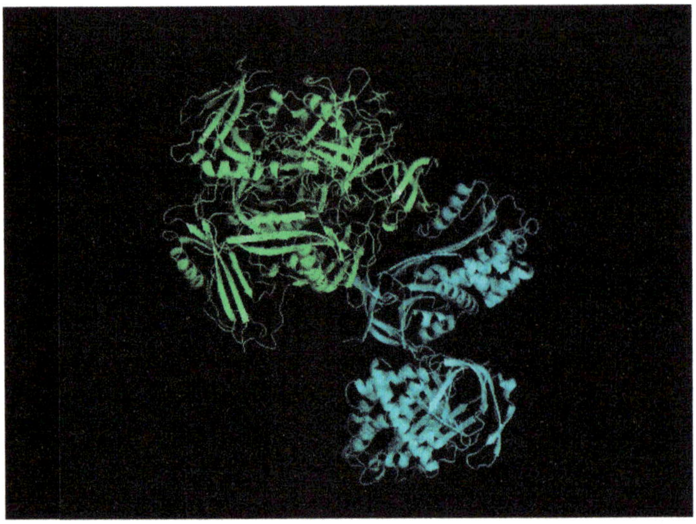

Fig. 9.1 Plasmin shown in *green* is regulated via plasminogen activator inhibitor-1 (PAI-1) in *blue*

Once plasmin is formed it degrades the fibrin and forms fibrin degradation products (FDPs) and by virtue of their competition with fibrin monomer for fibrin binding sites and with fibrinogen for platelet surface glycoprotein IIb/IIIa (GPIIb/IIIa) binding sites, they have anticoagulant properties [3]. Plasmin besides lysing the fibrinogen is also known to split prothrombin, thereby triggering thrombin generation and causing a procoagulant effect. Plasminogen activation is regulated by α2-antiplasmin, and plasmin activity is regulated by plasminogen activator inhibitors (PAI-1 and PAI-II) by forming one-to-one stoichiometric complexes with the active enzymes (see Fig. 9.1) [3]. Another non-plasmin fibrinolytic pathway described involves binding of fibrin to the pluripotent macrophage integrin Mac-1 (DC11b/CD18), and then the fibrinogen-Mac-1 complex is then internalized in the macrophage, and then the fibrin is degraded by the action of cathepsin D into FDPs [4]. This macrophage-mediated, non-plasmin fibrinolytic pathway takes place during the process of recanalization of the vessel [3].

The proteases involved in fibrinolysis include plasmin and tissue-type plasminogen activator (tPA) and urinary-type plasminogen activator (uPA) or urokinase which like the serine proteases exist as zymogens. The plasmin cleaves the α-chain of fibrinogen to release the αC Fragments, thereby producing Fragment X of about 260 kDa, and upon further plasmin action produces Fragment Y and Fragments D and E. However, through enzymatic actions of thrombin and FXIIIa, cross-linked fibrin is formed which upon action by plasmin forms D-dimer and E complex. The human plasminogen is the zymogenic form of plasmin. It is a single-chain glycoprotein of 92 kDa. All plasminogen activators cleave the Arg561-Val562 bond in plasminogen. There are several variants of plasminogen which could result from glycosylation and genetic polymorphism besides limited proteolysis and activation processes. The physiologic plasminogen activators include tPA and uPA. Another activation system, the contact plasminogen activator pathway, is dependent on the FXII, prekallikrein, and high molecular weight kininogen. There are some plasminogen activators from bacteria and vampire bat such as staphylokinase and vampire bat plasminogen activator.

Tissue-type plasminogen activator: It is a serine protease of 68 kDa, which, having secreted by the endothelial cells, exerts its effects in the vessels. Besides the circulating amount of approximately 5 μg/L (70 pM), the rest complexes with its primary inhibitor plasminogen activator inhibitor (PAI-1). The tPA cleaves the Arg561-Val562 bond in plasminogen but is ineffective activator of plasminogen in the absence of fibrin. Mutations engineered in tPA alter its characteristics which may make tPA resistant to the action of PAI-1 or make more effective agents such as new mutant tenecteplase (TNK-tPA).

Urinary-type plasminogen activator: Although found in the urine at 40–80 μg/L, it is synthesized by cells with a fibroblast-like morphology and also epithelial cells, monocytes, and macrophages. It activates plasminogen by cleaving Arg561-Val562 bond, but does not require fibrin. While tPA functions in the vasculature, uPA has a role in degradation of extracellular matrix and cell migration which may have effects on wound healing, inflammation, and embryogenesis and invasion of tumor cells and metastases. However, this does not discount its role in fibrin degradation.

Contact pathway system: The contact system comprising of FXII, prekallikrein, FXI, and high molecular weight kininogen. The negatively charged surfaces such as kaolin, ellagic acid, sulfatides, and dextran sulfate activate FXII to FXIIa and prekallikrein to kallikrein. Factor XIIa further activates the FXI to FXIa, triggering the coagulation cascade. The contact factor, FXII, although a clotting factor, is structurally similar to tPA, uPA, and plasminogen and causes fibrinolysis at least by three mechanisms such as (1) direct activation of plasminogen by FXIIa, (2) generation of kallikrein by FXII-dependent and FXII-independent pathways triggering activation of scuPA, and (3) indirect stimulation of fibrinolysis caused by kallikrein cleavage of high molecular weight kininogen, generating bradykinin, which is a potent stimulator of tPA release from the endothelial cells. In plasma, the presence of fourfold higher concentration of FXII than tPA and uPA is suggestive of its important role in activation of plasminogen as effective as urokinase. The contact pathway regulates fibrinolysis by these mechanisms.

Other Plasminogen Activators

Streptokinase: Streptokinase is not an enzyme but an extracellular protein produced by streptococci and is capable of activating the human fibrinolytic system, by forming a 1:1 stoichiometric complex with plasminogen. The activated streptokinase-plasminogen complex binds with another molecule of plasminogen and cleaves it at Arg541-Val562 that forms plasmin. The activated streptokinase-plasminogen complex retains its ability to bind to the fibrin and is protected by inhibitory effects of α2-antiplasmin. Streptokinase causes systemic conversion of plasminogen to plasmin and depletion of circulating fibrinogen, plasminogen, and FV and FVIII. Streptokinase is antigenic.

Staphylokinase is also not an enzyme but a protein produced by *Staphylococcus aureus*, which forms a stoichiometric complex with plasminogen. Staphylokinase is fibrin-dependent and hence in the absence of fibrin does not activate plasminogen. Trace amount of plasmin on the surface of fibrin cleaves ten residues from the amino terminus of staphylokinase, allowing staphylokinase to bind with plasminogen and interacting with fibrin-bound plasminogen forming free plasmin. The free plasmin converts the staphylokinase-plasminogen complex to staphylokinase-plasmin complex which is not vulnerable to inactivation by α2-antiplasmin. Staphylokinase is antigenic.

Vampire bat plasminogen activator: Four plasminogen activators in the salivary glands of vampire bat (*Desmodus rotundus*) were identified, namely, DSPAα1 and DSPAα2 and DSPAβ and DSPAγ. DSPA unlike other plasminogen activators is very fibrin specific and the activity of DSPAα1 is in fact 105,000-fold higher in the presence of fibrin than in its absence. Enhanced fibrin specificity and long clearance time are some of its important properties.

Inhibitors of the fibrinolytic system: While plasminogen activator inhibitor-1 is the main inhibitor of tPA and uPA, α2-antiplasmin inhibits plasmin. **PAI-1 and α2-antiplasmin are members of the serpin family which includes antithrombin and heparin cofactor II**.

Plasminogen activator inhibitor-1 (PAI-1): There are several sources of production of PAI-1, such as platelets, megakaryocytes, endothelial cells, hepatocytes, and adipocytes; however, the source of resting plasma PAI-1 is not known. The source of increased PAI-1 levels as an acute phase response is hepatocytes. Half of the circulating PAI-1 is known to come from the platelets and its large amounts accumulate in the thrombi. While PAI-1 inhibits tPA and uPA, it does not inhibit scuPA which is largely inactive. Once bound to uPAR on the surface of monocytes, the activity of scuPA is profoundly increased. The receptor-bound scuPA initiates proteolytic activity. The conversion of receptor-bound scuPA to uPA and the vulnerability of uPA to the inhibitory effects of PAI-1 are considered to be ways of regulating fibrinolysis. PAI-1 deficiency is quite rare and leads to bleeding.

PAI-1 inhibitors: Inhibition of PAI-1, which is a major inhibitor of tPA and uPA, results in increased endogenous fibrinolytic activity. PAI-1 synthesis is decreased in vitro by lipid lowering drugs such as niacin and fibrates [5, 6]. Similarly, peptides that block PAI-1 activities are also identified which prevent insertion of the reactive center loop upon cleavage by the target protease [7] or by converting PAI-1 into a latent conformation [8]. Development of small molecule PAI-1 inhibitors, some of which may have antithrombotic properties in vivo, may be quite interesting [9].

α2-antiplasmin: It is a fast-acting inhibitor of plasmin. The circulating concentration of α2-antiplasmin is 70 mg/L. It is synthesized in the liver and obviously is decreased in patients with hepatic insufficiency. It exists in several forms in the plasma and its inhibitory capability resides in the core of the protein. **α2-antiplasmin causes interference in the interaction of plasminogen, plasmin, tPA, and fibrin**. Plasminogen and tPA may interact directly with fibrin, by acting as a cofactor in plasminogen activation resulting in fibrin degradation due to action of plasmin. α2-antiplasmin can bind with plasminogen and prevent binding of plasminogen to fibrin. α2-antiplasmin can also cross-link to fibrin preventing plasmin binding to fibrin and by binding to plasmin prevents plasmin's action, thereby inhibiting fibrin degradation. Deficiency of α2-antiplasmin results in delayed bleeding and normal initial hemostasis characteristic of fibrinolytic defects.

TAFI: As the name implies, thrombin activatable fibrinolytic inhibitor is a fibrinolytic inhibitor, activated by thrombin generated by the coagulation cascade. As an intermediate between coagulation and fibrinolysis, it cross-regulates coagulation and fibrinolysis. TAFI is a procarboxypeptidase U (pro-CPU) and is a zymogen of the active enzyme TAFIa, a plasma carboxypeptidase B (pCPB). The generation of C-terminal lysyl residues serves as an important feedback mechanism and enables the plasminogen to bind to fibrin in enhancing fibrinolysis. TAFIa removes these C-terminal lysyl residues, thereby regulating the fibrinolytic process. Thus TAFI is activated by thrombin-thrombomodulin complex and by plasmin in a reaction that is enhanced by glycosaminoglycans (see Fig. 9.2). TAFI is produced in the liver and circulates in the blood at approximately 75 nM concentration, and only a small proportion is necessary for activation to have complete function. Due to polymorphisms in TAFI gene, there could be wide ranges of its concentration in healthy population and does not necessarily correlate with disease. There is no known endogenous inhibitor of TAFIa. As an acute phase reactant, the TAFI levels are increased in inflammation. Elevated levels of TAFI and PAI-1 and associated hypofibrinolysis may pose a risk for venous thrombosis. Deficiency of TAFI in mice has shown to increase the risk of cerebral thrombosis and ischemic stroke in mice. Hemophilic patients show defective activation of TAFI that leads to increased fibrinolysis and increased bleeding. Most of the clot is formed after the formation of a clot by the intrinsic pathway activation of FXI by thrombin. Clots formed in vitro in the presence of FIX deficient plasma lysed prematurely and could be reversed by the addition of FIX and thrombomodulin to the plasma. Normal fibrinolysis could be achieved, if TAFI, thrombomodulin, and FVIII are added to the plasma from hemophilic patient. Administration of Factor XIa antibodies and inhibition of TAFI in rabbit models is reported to have shown twofold increased endogenous fibrinolysis.

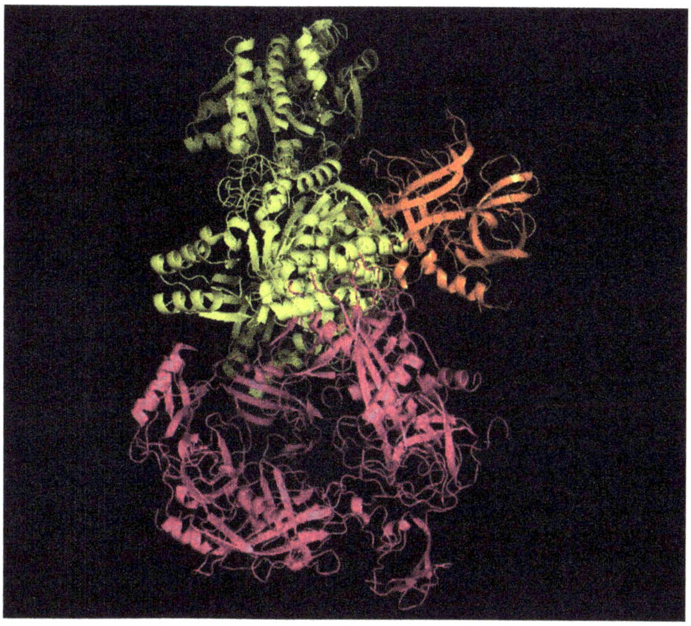

Fig. 9.2 TAFI seen in *yellow* is activated by the thrombin-thrombomodulin complex in addition with plasmin seen in *pink*. This reaction is also enhanced by glycosaminoglycans. The *orange* protein seen above is thrombin

TAFI cross-regulates coagulation and fibrinolysis. Hemophilia A is caused by the deficiency of FVIIIa and the bleeding, as a result of defective clot formation. The defective role of TAFI in hemophilia plays a role in less protection of the clot. It is interesting to note the degree of bleeding in hemophilic patients due to defective clot formation or defective clot protection as a result of defective TAFI activation. It is also interesting to know as to how much does activation of TAFI contribute to the increased risk of venous thrombosis associated with high levels of coagulation factors II, VIII, IX, and XI.

Interactive role of thrombin-thrombomodulin complex, TFPI, protein C, APC, TAFI, and fibrinolytic pathways in severe sepsis: Tissue factor-induced thrombin generation is downregulated by TFPI and the functional protein C pathway [10]. Thrombin-TM complex links coagulation with the fibrinolysis by TAFI [11, 12]. In a severe septic state, increased thrombin and reduced APC inhibition of thrombin generation, leading to increased thrombin levels, promote TAFI activity, thereby inhibiting fibrinolysis. When the TM levels are increased, TAFI activity is promoted and there is more fibrinolytic deficit.

Protein C also combines with PAI-1 to prevent inhibition of fibrinolysis. In sepsis there is reduced protein C/APC activity. This formed the basis of administering protein C to patients with meningococcal septicemia where changes in TM and EPCR result in purpura fulminans [13–15]. Maruyama demonstrated in rodent and primate models of TF-induced DIC that recombinant soluble TM may prevent DIC even when the AT levels are low [16, 17].

Other Inhibitors

PAI-2: PAI-2 is a urokinase inhibitor in placenta. Monocytes being the important source of PAI-2, it gets into the clot and causes fibrin stability by cross-linking with fibrin. PAI-2 is known to inhibit two-chain tPA. By its intracellular presence, it is led to believe that, besides inhibition of plasminogen activator, it may have protective effects on the cells from cytopathic effects of alpha virus infection.

Alpha2-macroglobulin: It is a glycoprotein circulating in the blood in the amounts of 2.5 g/L. It inhibits several proteases including plasmin but initiates its activity when the activity

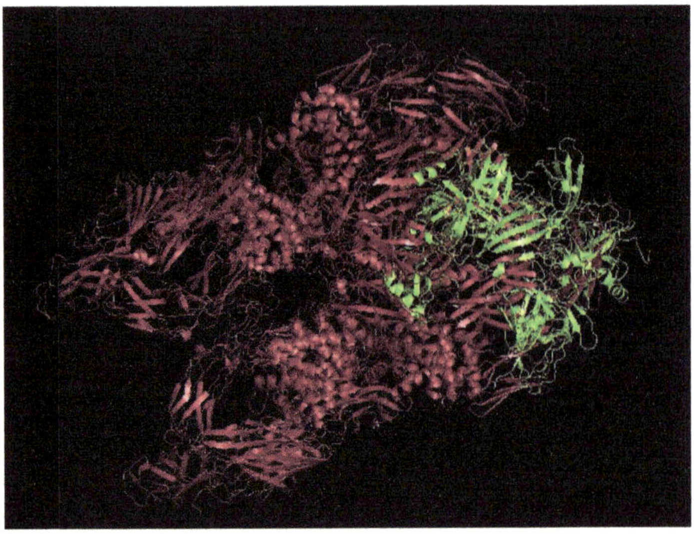

Fig. 9.3 Alpha2-macroglobulin seen in *red* interacting with plasmin in *yellow*. Alpha2-macroglobulin inhibits several proteases, including plasmin when the activity of α2-antiplasmin is diminished. In addition it can form complexes with tPA and uPA

of α2-antiplasmin is worn off. It forms complexes with tPA and uPA (see Fig. 9.3).

C1-inhibitor: It is a highly glycosylated serpin, circulating in the blood at a concentration of 1.7 μM. Besides inhibiting the activated complements of Cl, namely, Clr and Cls, it also inhibits the FXIIa, FXIa, plasma kallikrein, plasmin, tPA, and uPA. Although the precise function of C1-inhibitor is not known, it may regulate fibrinolysis by virtue of its inhibition of contact proteases and the conversion of scuPA to uPA.

Lipoprotein (a): Circulating in the blood at 50–1000 mg/L, lipoprotein (a) binds to fibrin, extracellular matrix, platelets, and cells. It competes with plasminogen and tPA for binding sites on fibrin, thereby exerting an antifibrinolytic effect.

Histidine-rich glycoprotein: Histidine-rich glycoproteins are synthesized in the liver and are taken up by the platelets and megakaryocytes and released upon thrombin activation. HRG may combine with plasminogen and circulate as a complex, thereby decreasing the plasminogen available for fibrin. Although rare, congenital heterozygous HRG deficiency may lead to thrombotic complications.

Balance of plasminogen activation and regulation of fibrinolysis: Conversion of plasminogen to active plasmin only takes place on the fibrin and cell surfaces; otherwise, the plasmin activity may cause generalized fibrinolysis, proteolysis, and degradation of clotting factors FV, FVIII, vWF, and platelet glycoproteins. Once fibrin is formed, the plasminogen is activated to plasmin which acts on the fibrin converting it into very early FDP and FDP. The very early FDP converts the plasminogen to plasmin in the presence of fibrin. However, the thrombin-thrombomodulin complex converts TAFI into TAFIa which removes the formed CT lysines from the FDP, which does not allow it to activate plasminogen to plasmin.

Dysregulation of Fibrinolysis

In disseminated intravascular coagulation (DIC), both the processes of coagulation and fibrinolysis are dysregulated. The activation of coagulation is evident in DIC, by the presence of intravascular thrombi, manifested by increased levels of activated coagulation factors, tissue factor (TF), D-dimer, and decreased fibrinogen [18, 19]. The lipopolysaccharide can initiate clotting by triggering the contact activation of the intrinsic pathway of clotting process and TF activating the extrinsic pathway of coagulation activation, leading to the generation of thrombin. Thrombin once formed can combine with thrombomodulin to activate the protein C to activated protein C. Thrombin will also directly activate the TAFI to TAFIa which can result in fibrinolytic deficit (see Fig. 9.2). In severe sepsis, activation of the coagulation system can activate the endothelial cells, resulting in the potentiation of the pro-inflammatory responses and the production of cytokines such as TNF-α and IL-1. Anticoagulants in the form of antithrombin, TFPI, APC, anti-Xa inhibitors, anti-IIa inhibitors, TM, TAFI inhibitors, etc. control the activation of the coagulation. The dysregulated fibrinolytic process, manifested by an increased level of plasminogen activator inhibitor-1, can be targeted for therapeutic intervention and by supplementing the decreased endogenous anticoagulant agents such as APC, AT, and TFPI in sepsis [17]. Activation of coagulation and dysregulated fibrinolytic process can lead to intravascular deposition of soluble fibrin, platelet, and leukocyte activation, leading to multiple organ failure in severe sepsis. Leukocytes are found in high numbers in venous thrombi. The leukocytes and activated platelets can form rosettes mediated by P-selectin expression on the activated platelets [20, 21]. Prevention of this interaction between inflammatory cells and platelets resulted in inhibition of both arterial and venous thrombi in animal models [22, 23]. Activation of the endothelium due to thrombin results in increased leukocyte adhesion due to P- and E-selectin expression [20, 24]. Thrombin is an agonist for the formation of platelet-activating factor (PAF), and the adherent neutrophils on the endothelium are vulnerable to the action of PAF, resulting in the release of proteases and oxidants which might increase damage to the endothelium [25]. Furthermore, the factor VIIa-TF complex and FXa are known to activate cells through protease-activated receptors, thereby generating cellular responses similar to those initiated by thrombin activation of protease receptor 1 [25]. Procalcitonin is reported to be as a marker of systemic inflammatory response and as a potential biomarker of sepsis [26, 27]. A recent randomized, double-blind, placebo-controlled phase 2b study to evaluate the safety and efficacy of recombinant human soluble thrombomodulin (ART-123), in patients with sepsis and DIC, reported that there was an increase in procalcitonin, PAI-1, C5a, IL-6, IL-10, and myeloperoxidase (MPO) and a decrease in protein C [28]. Furthermore, the levels of procalcitonin, PAI-1, IL-6, and IL-10 were reported to be much higher than that of both overt and nonovert and normal controls, and the protein C antigen and functional levels were decreased in a larger extent in the overt group [28].

Diabetes mellitus is known to cause increased cardiovascular morbidity and mortality. Hyperglycemia stimulating the coagulation process and hyperinsulinemia impairing fibrinolysis in healthy humans has been reported earlier [29]. A recent study, in which whether elevated antigen levels of tPA, PAI-1, and tPA/PAI-complex, or von Willebrand factor (vWF) precede the diagnosis of type II diabetes, was evaluated and concluded that elevated levels of fibrinolytic variables in fact precede the manifestation of type II diabetes after adjusting for metabolic and cardiovascular risk factors and can be detected several years before the changes in glucose tolerance occur [30]. Association of obesity with chronic inflammation [31] and activation of endothelial cells that produce vWF by inflammatory markers [32] have been reported earlier. Similarly, CRP causing upregulation of PAI-1 gene expression in human aortic endothelial cells has also been shown [33]. Obesity-induced development of diabetes manifested by resident macrophages in the adipose tissue producing cytokines such as transforming growth factor (TGF)-β and TNF-α causing increase in PAI-1 is reported [34, 35]. The upregulation of PAI-1 early in the development of type II diabetes may be as a result of metabolic syndrome [30].

The important implication of the intricacies of regulation and dysregulation of fibrinolysis is in the cautious use of fibrinolytic drugs especially in neurosurgical patients. There has been a paradigm shift in the management of patients with acute ischemic stroke very recently. While the results of studies, such as the International Management of Stroke (IMS III) [36], Mechanical Retrieval and Recanalization of Stroke Clots Using Embolectomy (MR RESCUE) [37], and SYNTHESIS Expansion [38], presented and published 2 years ago provided evidence that mechanical thrombectomy was ineffective in treating acute stroke secondary to emergent large vessel occlusion (ELVO), there has been a dramatic significant paradigm shift. The current evidence based on large studies such as the Multicenter Randomized Clinical trial of Endovascular treatment for Acute ischemic stroke in the Netherlands (MR CLEAN) [39], the Endovascular treatment for Small Core and Anterior circulation Proximal occlusion with Emphasis on minimizing CT to recanalization times (ESCAPE) [40], the Extending the Time for Thrombolysis in Emergency Neurological Deficits-Intra-Arterial (EXTEND-IA) [41], and the Solitaire FR With the Intention For Thrombectomy as Primary Endovascular Treatment for Acute Ischemic Stroke (SWIFT PRIME) [42] provides evidence on the contrary that thrombectomy is profoundly beneficial in patients with ELVO. Thus, based on the results of these new trials, the focus in the management of patients with acute ischemic stroke will shift from intravenous thrombolysis to thrombectomy. While currently 24 % of patients with stroke are transferred to inpatient rehabilitation services and 31 % transferred to skilled nursing facilities and of those returning home directly, 32 % use home healthcare services [43]. The projected total direct medical stroke-related costs between 2012 and 2030 are expected to triple from 71.6 billion to 184.1 billion [44] with 70 % of the first year poststroke costs due to inpatient hospital costs [45]. Due to decreased length of stay for patients undergoing thrombectomy, the overall costs are anticipated to significantly decrease [46].

References

1. Mutch NJ, Booth NA. Plasminogen activation and regulation of fibrinolysis. In: Marder VJ, Aird WC, Bennett JS, Schulman S, White II GC, editors. Hemostasis and thrombosis. 6th ed. Philadelphia, PA: Walters Kluwer/Lippincott Williams & Wilkins; 2013.
2. Collen D, Lijnen HR. Basic and clinical aspects of fibrinolysis and thrombosis. Blood. 1991;78: 3114–24.
3. Loscalzo J, Schafer AI. Overview of hemostasis and fibrinolysis. In: Sasahara AA, Loscalzo J, editors. New therapeutic agents in thrombosis and thrombolysis. 2nd ed. New York: Marcel Decker Inc.; 2003.
4. Simon DI, Ezratty AM, Francis SA, et al. Fibrin(ogen) is internalized and degraded by activated human monocytoid cells via Mac-1 (DC11b/DC18): a nonplasmin fibrinolytic pathway. Blood. 1993;82: 2414–22.
5. Brown SL, Sobel BE. Attenuation of the synthesis of plasminogen activator inhibitor type 1 by niacin: a potential link between lipid lowering and fibrinolysis. Circulation. 1995;92:767–72.
6. Fuji S, Sawa H, Sobel BE. Inhibition of endothelial cell expression of plasminogen activator inhibitor type-1 by gemfibrozil. Thromb Haemost. 1993;70: 642–7.
7. Kvassman J, Lawrence D, Shore J. The acid stabilization of plasminogen activator inhibitor-1 depends on the protonation of a single group that affects loop insertion into b-sheet A. J Biol Chem. 1995;270: 27942–7.
8. Eitzman DT, Fay WP, Lawrence DA, et al. Peptide-mediated inactivation of recombinant and platelet plasminogen activator inhibitor-1 in vitro. J Clin Invest. 1995;95:2416–20.
9. Frederich PM, Levi M, Biemond B, et al. Novel low molecular weight inhibitor of PAI-1 (XR5118) promotes endogenous fibrinolysis and reduces post-thrombolysis thrombus growth in rabbits. Circulation. 1997;96:916–21.
10. Iba T, Yagi Y, Kidoworo A, et al. Increased plasma levels of soluble thrombomodulin in patients with serpin and organ failure. Jpn J Surg. 1995;25:585–90.
11. Lopez-Aguirre Y, Paramo JA. Endothelial cell and homeostatic activation in relation to cytokines in patients with sepsis. Thromb Res. 1999;94:95–101.
12. Drake TA, Cheng J, Chang A, et al. Expression of tissue factor, thrombomodulin and E-selectin in baboons with lethal E. coli sepsis. Am J Pathol. 1993;142: 1458–70.
13. Laszik Z, Carson CW, Nadasdy T, et al. Lack of suppressed renal thrombomodulin expression in a septic rat model with glomerular thrombotic microangiopathy. Lab Invest. 1994;70:862–7.
14. Rivard GE, David M, Farrell C, et al. Treatment of purpura fulminans in meningococcemia with protein C concentrate. J Pediatr. 1995;126:646–52.
15. Smith OP, White B. Infectious purpura fulminans. Diagnosis and treatment. Br J Haematol. 1999;104: 202–7.
16. Maruyama I. Recombinant thrombomodulin and activated protein C in the treatment of disseminated intravascular coagulation. Thromb Haemost. 1999; 104:202–7.
17. Iqbal O, Messmore H, Fareed J, et al. Antithrombotic agents in the treatment of severe sepsis. Expert Opin Emerg Drugs. 2002;7(1):111–39.

18. Camerota A, Creasey A, Patla V, Larkin V, Fink M. Delayed treatment with recombinant human tissue factor pathway inhibitor improves survival in rabbits with Gram-negative peritonitis. J Infect Dis. 1988; 177:668–76.
19. Park T, Creasey A, Wright S. Tissue factor pathway inhibitor blocks cellular effects of endotoxin by binding to endotoxin and interfering with transfer to CD14. Blood. 1997;89:4268–74.
20. Schaub RG, Simmons CA, Koets MH, Romano PJ, Stewart GJ. Early events in the formation of a venous thrombus following local trauma and stasis. Lab Invest. 1984;51:218–24.
21. Yang J, Furie BC, Furie B. The biology of P-selectin glycoprotein ligand-1: its role as a selectin counter receptor in leukocyte endothelial and leukocyte platelet interaction. Thromb Haemost. 1999;81:1–7.
22. Palabrica T, Lobb R, Furie BC, et al. Leukocyte accumulation promoting fibrin deposition is mediated in vivo by P-selectin on adherent platelets. Nature. 1992;359:848–51.
23. Wakefield TW, Strieter RM, Schaub R, et al. Venous thrombosis prophylaxis by inflammatory inhibition without anticoagulant therapy. J Vasc Surg. 2000;31: 309–24.
24. Coughlin SR. Thrombin receptor function and cardiovascular disease. Trends Cardiovasc Med. 1994;4: 77–83.
25. Lorante DE, Patel KD, McIntire TM, McEver RP, Prescott SM, Zimmerman GA. Co-expression of GMP-140 and PAF by endothelium stimulated by histamine or thrombin: a juxtacrine system for adhesion and activation of neutrophils. J Cell Biol. 1991; 115:223–34.
26. Reinhart K, Karzai W, Meisner M. Procalcitonin as a marker of the systemic inflammatory response in infection. Intensive Care Med. 2000;26(9):1193–200.
27. Erickson Y, Samia N, Bedell B, Friedman K, Atkinson B, Raife T. Elevated procalcitonin and C-reactive protein as potential biomarkers of sepsis in a subpopulation of thrombotic microangiopathy patients. J Clin Apher. 2009;24(4):150–4.
28. Hoppensteadt D, Tsuruta K, Hirman J, Kaul I, Osawa Y, Fareed J. Dysregulation and inflammatory hemostatic markers in sepsis and suspected disseminated intravascular coagulation. Clin Appl Thromb Hemost. 2015;21(2):120–7.
29. Stegenga MB, van der Crabben SN, Levi M, de Voss AF, Tanck MW, Sauerwein HP, van der Poll T. Hyperglycemia stimulates coagulation and hyperinsulinemia impairs fibrinolysis in healthy humans. Diabetes. 2006;55:1807–12.
30. Hernestal-Boman J, Norberg M, Jansson J-K, Eliasson M, Erickson JW, Lindahl B, Johansson L. Signs of dysregulated fibrinolysis precede the development of type 2 diabetes mellitus in a population-based study. Cardiovasc Diabetol. 2012;11:152. http://www.cardiab.com/content/11/1/52.
31. Wellen KE, Hotamisligil GS. Obesity-induced inflammatory changes in adipose tissue. J Clin Invest. 2003;112:1785–8.
32. Ker R, Stirling D, Ludlam CA. Interleukin-6 and haemostasis. Br J Haematol. 2001;115:3012.
33. Devraj S, Xu DY, Jialal I. C-reactive protein increases plasminogen activator inhibitor-1 expression and activity in human aortic endothelial cells: implications for the metabolic syndrome and atherothrombosis. Circulation. 2003;107:398–404.
34. Cigonoli M, Tonoli M, Borgato L, Frigotto L, et al. Expression of plasminogen activator inhibitor-1 in human adipose tissue: a role of TNF-α? Atherosclerosis. 1999;143:81–90.
35. Alessi MC, Bastelica D, Morange P, et al. Plasminogen activator inhibitor-1, transforming growth factor-beta1, and BMI are closely associated in human adipose tissue during morbid obesity. Diabetes. 2000;49:1374–80.
36. Broderick JP, Palesch YY, Demchuk AM, et al. Endovascular therapy after intravenous t-PA versus t-PA alone for stroke. N Engl J Med. 2013;368:893–903.
37. Kidwell CS, Jahan R, Gombein J, et al. A trial of imaging selection and endovascular treatment for ischemic stroke. N Engl J Med. 2013;368:914–23.
38. Ciccone A, Valvassori L, Nichellati M, et al. Endovascular treatment for acute ischemic stroke. N Engl J Med. 2013;368:904–13.
39. Berkhemer OA, Fransen PS, Beumer D, et al. A randomized trial of intraarterial treatment for acute ischemic stroke. N Engl J Med. 2015;372:11–20.
40. Goyal M, Demchuk AM, Menon BK, et al. Randomized assessment of rapid endovascular treatment of ischemic stroke—for the ESCAPE Trial Investigators. N Engl J Med. 2015;372:1019–30.
41. Campbell BCV, Mitchell PJ, Kleinig TJ, et al. for the EXTEND-IA Investigators. Endovascular therapy for ischemic stroke with perfusion-imaging selection. N Engl J Med 2015;372:1009–1018.
42. Saver J. SWIFT PRIME Results. Paper presented at International Stroke Conference Annual Meeting; 2015 Feb 11; Nashville, TN, USA.
43. Buntin MB, Garten AD, Paddock S, et al. How much is postacute care use affected by its availability? Health Serv Res. 2005;40:413–34.
44. Ovblagele B, Goldstein LB, Higashida RT, et al.; on behalf of the American Heart Association Advocacy Coordinating Committee and Stroke Council. Forecasting the future of stroke in United States: a policy statement from the American Heart Association and American Stroke Association. Stroke 2013;44:2361–75.
45. Taylor TN, Davis PH, Tomer JC, et al. Lifetime cost of stroke in the United States. Stroke. 1996;27: 1459–66.
46. Fiorella DJ, Fargen KM, Mocco J, et al. Thrombectomy for acute ischemic stroke: an evidence-based treatment. J NeuroInterv Surg. 2015. doi:10.1136/neurintsurg-2015-011707.

Risks Associated with Administration of Allogeneic Blood Components

10

Phillip J. DeChristopher

Background

In the United States annually, at a direct cost of at least $4 billion, more than 9 million allogeneic volunteer blood donors provide around 20.9 million qualified and tested blood components to over 5 million patients, for the treatment of a wide variety of clinical conditions including, but not limited to, acute blood loss, other chronic or acquired anemias and cytopenias, and protein clotting factor deficiencies [1]. By regulatory authority, the US Food and Drug Administration (FDA) mandates establishment of the processes necessary to assure the safety, purity, potency, and effectiveness of blood components. It accomplishes this using multiple overlapping layers of safety which include donor screening and selection, donor deferral lists, disease testing of donated blood, storage, transportation, quarantining, and correction of manufacturing deficiencies of blood components to protect both donors and recipients [2].

Over the past 40 years, as a result of remarkable successes of these combined precautions and safeguards, the US blood supply is considered among the safest in the world, due chiefly to the reduction in infectious disease risks [3]. Current tests required by the US FDA for all blood donated for transfusions are noted in Table 10.1. Over 25 years ago, because blood transfusions remain high volume, high cost, high risk, and problem prone, blood transfusions were characterized as "*unavoidably unsafe*" [4]. These attributes and risks remain so because, despite how "safe" the blood resource is made, two fundamental difficulties with transfusing blood remain: There are the inherent and *irreducible* risks of transfusing allogeneic tissue transplants derived from other human beings (blood components are sterile parenteral drugs and "biologics"); and these therapies are delivered by complex series of processes carried out by imperfect humans who are error-prone (see Fig. 10.1). Blood transfusions are the only tissues casually transplanted with the stroke of a pen or click of a computer mouse.

This chapter focuses on the acute adverse effects of transfusion which are usually manifest within hours of administration, as well as important concerns which impact both the informed consenting process and the actual decisions to transfuse. Risks associated with blood transfusion include the residual infectious disease risks, transfusion decision-making, blood administration errors, and noninfectious complications, some of which may be delayed. The latter problems remain the most common ones and are determined chiefly on the fact that blood donors

P.J. DeChristopher, M.D., Ph.D. (✉)
Department of Pathology, Loyola University Health System, 2160 South First Avenue, Bldg. 103, Room 0306D, Maywood, IL 60153, USA
e-mail: pdechristopher@lumc.edu

C.M. Loftus (ed.), *Anticoagulation and Hemostasis in Neurosurgery*,
DOI 10.1007/978-3-319-27327-3_10

Table 10.1 Tests required by the US FDA for all blood components

Collected for transfusion
• ABO group and Rh type
• Antibody screening and identification of clinically significant rbc alloantibodies
• Multiple serologic tests (FDA-cleared, usually EIA methods) for
– Syphilis (serologic RPR or VDRL)
– Hepatitis B & C (HBsAg, anti-HBc, anti-HCV)
– Retroviruses (anti-HIV-1/2, anti-HTLV-I/II)
– Anti-*trypanosoma cruzi* (Chagas' disease)
– Anti-*Babesia* (NAT format assays also available), pilot testing under an FDA IND, in FY 2016
• Nucleic acid testing, using genomic amplification methods
– HIV-1
– HCV
– WNV

EIA enzyme immunoassay, *FDA* US Food and Drug Administration, Hepatitis B and C viruses, HBV and HCV, respectively. *HBc* hepatitis B core, *HBsAg* hepatitis B surface antigen, *HCV* hepatitis C virus, *HTLV* human T-cell lymphotropic virus, *rbc* red blood cell, *IND* investigational new (drug) device, *WNV* West Nile virus

and recipients are genetically, phenotypically, and immunologically nonidentical (comprehensive reviews of all adverse effects of blood transfusion are available [3, 5–8]).

Actionable Intelligence [9]

Like decisions to transfuse blood, the decisions to "sound" a "transfusion reaction" assessment are clinical and are best made with bedside patient evaluation. Standards of care require stereotypical protocols to be established and followed by both transfusionists and the laboratory when acute adverse effects of transfusion are reported. These are noted in Table 10.2.

Whereas the vast majority of blood transfusions are well tolerated and uneventful, a significant fraction of transfusion episodes are associated with serious adverse effects. Because it is well recognized that immediate transfusion reactions in patients receiving any blood component are both underrecognized and underreported, transfusionists are frequently caught off-guard and unprepared. The most important acute transfusion reactions, which remain actionable, very commonly involve changes in vital signs, which require clinical recognition, judgement, and speedy management. For example, in the setting of transfusion, a fever [defined at a temperature ≥38 °C or a rise of ≥1 °C (1.8 °F) from pretransfusion value] includes the differential of bacterial contamination of the unit, a febrile nonhemolytic reaction (FNHTR), immune (such as ABO)-incompatibility, and even transfusion-related acute lung injury (TRALI). Because the etiology of febrile reactions cannot be distinguished at the bedside, it is always prudent to stop the transfusion and evaluate what else is happening to the patient. In bacterial septic reactions, the fevers might be associated with any of the following: rigors, tachycardia, hypotension, shock, dyspnea, nausea/vomiting. However, acute fevers associated with respiratory signs and symptoms include the differentials of TRALI, TACO (transfusion-associated circulatory overload) (Tables 10.3 and 10.4), and severe anaphylaxis, each of which must be managed individually and appropriately. Comparative clinical features of TRALI and TACO are noted in Table 10.6.

Albeit representing only a microcosm of what actually occurs in medical practice, metrics used to quantify serious adverse effects of transfusion include *reported* transfusion fatalities. "Serious Hazards of Transfusion" (SHOT) is a professionally led, nationalized hemovigilance system in the United Kingdom (UK) which has been collecting, analyzing information on and monitoring the adverse effects and reactions of transfusion recipients in the UK [17]. SHOT is a very robust program, in effect since 1996, that annually includes >99 % of all healthcare institutions involved in transfusing blood. From over 3000 reports in 2014, two deaths were definitely related to transfusion (one case of acute hemolysis; one case of TACO) and three deaths were attributed to delays in transfusion. The risk of transfusion-related death for this period was 5.6 per million components issued (~1:17,900). The risk of

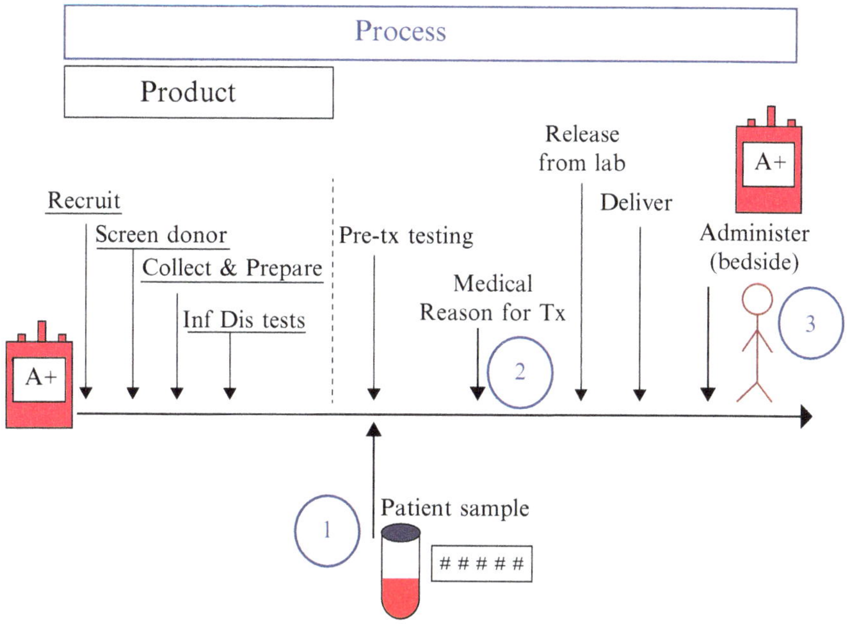

Fig. 10.1 Safe transfusions require the safe manufacturing of blood components and the safe delivery of blood via complex processes that are error-prone. (*1*) represents specimen acquisition, identification, labeling, and acceptability; (*2*) represents the clinical decision(s), which may or may not be evidence-based, to transfuse blood; (*3*) represents all the errors that can be made during blood administration, such as component-patient identification processes, imperfect/inappropriate storage conditions, drug adulteration by admixture with incompatible drugs or IV fluids, infection control considerations, etc.

Table 10.2 Immediate responses to acute adverse effects to blood transfusion

• **Stop (interrupt) the transfusion** • **The transfusionist performs evaluative functions at the bedside, related to**	
The patient • Repeat documented clerical identification check • Keep the IV line open with 0.9 % saline • If hemolysis is suspected/cannot be ruled out or other life-threatening events are inferred, discontinue and disconnect the component from the patient • Administer supportive care	**The blood component** • Repeat documented clerical check • Report the event to the blood bank/transfusion service, per existing protocol • Obtain posttransfusion blood specimen and send to the transfusion service • Send the blood bag, administration set, and any attached IV fluid bag with the patient's specimen
Laboratory functions are designed to rule out acute hemolysis	
• **Clerical check**: Examine and compare the patient's specimen, blood container labeling, and other records, as appropriate • Perform a visual check for hemolysis in the posttransfusion specimen, compared to the pretransfusion specimen • Perform a posttransfusion direct antiglobulin test (DAT) • Perform repeat ABO/Rh testing on the patient • (Additional studies are performed per policies and procedures, as indicated, clinically correlated to the event)	

major morbidity (febrile, serious allergic, and TACO), which contributed to death, occurred in 63.5 per million components issued (~1:1600). Importantly, the 2014 SHOT data also logs what are known as "*near misses*" (occurrences that would have caused harm had they not been detected) and "wrong blood in tube" (WBIT) errors, i.e., patient identification or tube labeling error, uncomfortably accounting for 44 % of the reports analyzed. The imbedded messages of these latter episodes are that they are certainly preventable.

Table 10.3 Acute adverse effects of transfusion: classification and frequency of occurrence [1, 3, 5–8]

Adverse effect	Estimated "reported" frequency per unit or comment (most *reactions* are considered underreported)
Immune mediated	
Fever without hemolysis (FNHTR) • Differential diagnosis includes acute hemolysis, bacterial contamination of components, and TRALI	• May or may not be associated with chills/rigors • Associated with WBC alloimmunization in recipients and BRMs which accumulate in stored components • Prevalence varies with recipient populations – 1–3:1000, all hospitalized patients – 1–3 %, hematology/oncology patients – 0.19 % in pediatric patients [10]
Simple cutaneous type 1 hypersensitivity reactions ("allergic") • Confined to cutaneous manifestations	• Manifest as pruritus and urticaria, typically nonprogressive • Mediators largely unknown, plasmatic protein in nature • 1:1500 transfusion episodes • 0.27 % in pediatric patients [10] • 1–3 % in heavily transfused populations
TRALI (noncardiogenic pulmonary edema), clinical criteria: (a) Acute lung injury • Hypoxemia • $PaO_2/FiO_2 < 300$ or $SpO_2 < 90\,\%$ on RA • Bilateral infiltrates on CXR • No evidence of left atrial hypertension • During 6 h of transfusion (b) No pre-existing acute lung injury (c) Occurs within 6 h of transfusion (most cases within 1–2 h)	• Onset includes fever, chills, dyspnea, cyanosis, hypotension, new-onset bilateral pulmonary edema • True incidence unknown, but is not the same in all populations of patients [11] • 1:1200–1:190,000 • Associated with donor antibodies against HLA, Class I and Class II, and neutrophil (HNA) antigens • (Less commonly) associated with bioactive lipopolysaccharides or cytokines • TRALI is the leading reported cause of transfusion-related mortality in the USA, the UK, and France [12] • **TACO** (see Table 10.6), bacterial contamination and acute hemolysis are in the differential
Acute hypotensive transfusion reaction	• Associated with storage-lesion bradykinin accumulation • Closely associated with use of ACE medication • 1:18, 500 (0.005 %) in all recipients • 0.29 % in pediatric patients [10]
Acute hemolysis, *nonfatal* (e.g., ABO incompatibility)	• 1:6000–1:33, 000 • Commonly associated with WBIT which occurs as often as 1:1986 [13]
Severe allergic reactions including anaphylaxis	• 1:20, 000–50, 000 • Associated with plasmatic factors that are rarely identified
Acute hemolysis, *fatal* (e.g., ABO and other RBC incompatibilities)	• Mortality, 1:2.7 million per unit (SHOT data)
Non-immune-mediated adverse effects	
TACO [14] (hydrostatic pulmonary edema)	• No single diagnostic findings or accepted diagnostic criteria • B/L pulmonary infiltrates on CXR; clinically evident left atrial hypertension • Dyspnea, orthopnea, hypoxemia, cyanosis, tachycardia, increased BP; elevated BNP • Incidence varies widely: passive reporting systems, 1:5561 RBC transfusions; fatality rate 1–3 % • 1:68–1:1566 in plasma recipients • 1:356 transfused ICU patients • Mortality rate of 1–3 % • Risk factors: – Extremes of age (60 % ≥ 70 years old) – Positive fluid balance/low body weight – Left ventricular dysfunction – Acute myocardial infarction • Differential includes TRALI and anaphylaxis

(continued)

Table 10.3 (continued)

Adverse effect	Estimated "reported" frequency per unit or comment (most *reactions* are considered underreported)
Bacterial sepsis	• Clinical sepsis in 1:100,000 platelet transfusions • Platelets harboring relevant bacteria, ~1:3000 • Per patient risk of bacterial sepsis, ~1:1000 • RBC, 1:1,000,000 (most commonly due to GN)

ACE angiotensin-converting enzyme antihypertensive medications, *BNP* brain natriuretic peptide, *BRM* biologic response modifiers (e.g., proinflammatory cytokines such as IL-1, IL-6, IL-8, and TNF-α), *CXR* chest x-ray, *FNHTR* febrile nonhemolytic transfusion reaction, *GN* gram-negative bacteria, *HLA* human leukocyte antigens, *HNA* human neutrophil antigens, *RA* room air, *RBC* red blood cell, *SHOT* serious hazards of transfusion (United Kingdom), *TACO* transfusion-associated circulatory overload, *TRALI* transfusion-related acute lung injury, *WBIT* wrong blood in tube

Table 10.4 Comparison of some features of TRALI and TACO [15]

Features	TRALI	TACO
Diagnostic criteria		• **No universally agreed-upon definition**
Clinical features 1. Body temperature 2. Blood pressure 3. Respiratory symptoms 4. Neck veins 5. Auscultation 6. Chest radiograph 7. PA occlusion pressure 8. Fluid balance 9. Peripheral WBC 10. BNP 11. Response to diuretic	1. Fever can be present 2. Hypotension 3. Acute onset of dyspnea 4. Unchanged 5. Pulmonary rales 6. Diffuse bilateral infiltrates 7. ≤18 mmHg 8. Positive, even, negative 9. Transient leukopenia 10. <200 pg/mL 11. Minimal	1. Unchanged 2. Hypertension 3. Acute dyspnea 4. Can be distended 5. Rales, S3 may be present 6. Diffuse bilateral infiltrates 7. ≥18 mmHg 8. Positive 9. Unchanged 10. >1200 pg/mL 11. Significant
Onset from start of transfusion	• Within 6 h of transfusion • No exiting ALI prior to transfusion	Within or during several hours of transfusion
Mitigation strategies [16]	"*All-male*" Plasma or Apheresis Platelets donated by males, nulligravida females, or HLA-antibody-tested and seronegative females	
Risk factors		
Treatment	Reverse the progressive hypoxemia with supplemental O_2 or ventilator support	Diuresis is helpful

ALI acute lung injury, *BNP* brain natriuretic peptide, *Hg* mercury, *HLA* human leukocyte antigen, *pg* picogram, *WBC* white blood cells

The US FDA annually compiles data on reported transfusion fatalities [18]. Although the absolute numbers of deaths appear small, in combined FDA reports from FYs 2010 through 2014, TRALI caused the highest number of reported fatalities (41 %), followed by TACO (22 %), hemolytic transfusion reactions (21 % of the total); hemolytic transfusion reactions (total 21 %, due to non-ABO [14 %] and ABO [7 %] incompatibilities. Microbial infections and anaphylactic reactions accounted for 8 % and 6 % of reported fatalities, respectively. In the USA over the past several years, the Centers for Disease Control and Prevention (CDC)/National Healthcare Safety Network has organized a national system slated to be harmonized internationally with other programs such as SHOT [19]. When US hemovigilance becomes an extant and robust exercise, the hope of such programs is that opportunities for improvement will be identified and there will be means to monitor the effects of the implementation of recommendations. In the USA, this program remains a work in progress.

Currently, bacteria represent the most common transfusion-transmitted infectious disease (TTID, Tables 10.5 and 10.6). It is clearly recognized that the historical processes of layering on more and more reactive, pathogen-specific test developments are not sufficient to protect transfusion recipients. Therefore, the latest innovations to address the current and ongoing threats of microorganisms contaminating blood have been what are known as pathogen reduction systems (PRS). Pathogen-reduced pooled plasma (Octaplas™), manufactured by Octapharma using solvent/detergent treatment, was FDA approved in January 2013. Such plasma products have been safely and effectively used for a number of years, approved by the European Union (Table 10.7). In December 2014, the Cerus Corporation obtained FDA approval for pathogen inactivation technology (the INTERCEPT® process using a photosensitizing chemical and UVA light irradiation) for the manufacture of pathogen-reduced plasma and platelet concentrates. All PRS technologies which have been decades in development offer hope to contain TTIDs, but their implementation remains problematic. Although FDA approved, these technologies are not yet "mandated," are costly, and their reimbursement is far from settled. Also, in the USA, there is no position that use of PRS will somehow make currently required testing (Table 10.1) automatically unnecessary. As noted in a recent editorial [26], "*…we now have the means to protect patients from existing and emerging blood-borne threats – all we need is the will.*"

Another important advance, related directly to safe transfusion that has gained considerable footing in medical practice, is Patient Blood Management (PBM) [25]. PBM is the multidisciplinary and multimodal approach of using evidence-based experience to optimize the care of patients who require transfusion. The goals of PBM programs are to optimize patient care by taking steps to reduce the probability of transfusions being necessary. The details of such programs are beyond the scope of this chapter, but they are predicated on the truism expressed 40 years ago by Dr. R. W. Beal [27]:

> Blood transfusion is like marriage: it should not be entered upon lightly, unadvisedly or wantonly, or more often than is absolutely necessary.

Table 10.5 Residual transfusion-transmitted (TT) infectious disease risks of some organisms in the United States and other comments [3, 5–8]

Infectious agent	Estimated risk per unit donated (or comment) [20]
Viruses	
HBV	1:843,000–1:1,208,000
HCV	1:1,149,000
HIV-1	1:1470, 000
HIV-2	• No TT cases reported in the USA • <10 positive ARC donors detected since 1992
HTLV-I/II	• Rare, last reported case in 1989 [21] • One TT HTLV-I in US Army soldier deployed in Afghanistan, 2010 [22]
WNV	• One 2012 case, reported in 2013, since NAT testing implemented [23]
Hepatitis A	• Fecal/oral transmission • TT, but exceedingly rare • Low incidence in the USA; lack of carrier state • (No FDA-cleared screening test for blood supply)

(continued)

Infectious agent	Estimated risk per unit donated (or comment) [20]
Hepatitis E [24]	• Fecal/oral transmission and zoonotic • TT, but exceedingly rare; none in the USA • (No FDA-cleared screening test for blood supply)
CMV	• 50–80 % by age 40 • ~1 % of seropositive donors transmit CMV • Selected seronegative populations protected using either seronegative donors or leukoreduction
Human parvovirus B-19	• Associated with aplastic anemia in patients with chronic congenital anemias • TT in blood components and plasma pools • (No FDA-cleared screening test or testing requirement for blood supply)
HHV-6	• High seroprevalence in the USA • (No FDA-cleared screening test for blood supply)
HHV-8 (also known as KSHV)	• Seroprevalence, general population 2–10 % • Seroprevalence, US blood donors, 2–4 % • (No FDA-cleared screening test for blood supply)
Bacteria	
GP or GN bacteria	• 1:2000–3000 platelet transfusions • Most neither interdicted or recognized • 1 in 2500 result in clinical sepsis • 1:20,000 for RBC
Borrelia burgdorferi (spirochete, transmitted by *Ixodes* ticks), Lyme disease	• Bacteria can live in donated blood for short periods • No TT Lyme disease yet reported in the USA
Treponema pallidum	No TT syphilis reported in the USA during the last 45 years
Parasitic infections	
Babesiosis, transmitted by *Babesia* species of ticks	• At least 160 TT cases reported in the USA, contributing to at least 28 associated deaths (1979–2009) • Intraerythrocytic parasite causing hemolytic anemia, severe morbidity including death • Screening test of the US blood supply by an FDA-approved assay for blood donors in pilot testing in FY2016 • Residual TT risk ~1:20,000 units transfused in *Babesia*-endemic areas
Trypanosoma cruzi, agent causing Chagas' disease	• Seroprevalence high in California and the southern tier of US states • *Triatominae* insect vectors now inhabit southern USA • US blood supply tested since December, 2011

ARC American Red Cross, *CMV* cytomegalovirus, *EIA* enzyme immunoassay, *FDA* food and drug administration, *HBc* hepatitis B core, *HCV* hepatitis C virus, *HHV* human herpes virus, *HTLV* human T-cell lymphotropic virus, *RBC* red blood cell, *KSHV* Kaposi sarcoma herpes virus, *NAT* nucleic acid testing, *RBC* red blood cells, *TT* transfusion-transmitted, *WNV* West Nile virus

Table 10.6 Emerging/re-emerging infectious disease risks to the US blood supply

Infectious agent	Commentary
Dengue virus	• Vectors, day-feeding mosquitos, *Aedes aegypti* and *albopictus* – Mosquito vectors also transmit WNV, Japanese encephalitis, and yellow fever – Last US epidemic in Louisiana, 1945 • Current locally acquired cases in Florida and Texas • No vaccine • No screening test for blood donors
Chikungunya virus	• Emerged in Caribbean, 2013 • Local transmission of 750 cases in Florida • No vaccine • No screening test for blood donors

Table 10.7 Available mitigation strategies that reduce the risks of allogeneic blood transfusion-related morbidity and mortality (including US FDA-licensed/approved devices, platforms, or systems)

Strategy or manufacturing technology	Demonstrated or potential patient benefit
Prestorage leukoreduction of cellular blood components (using selective depth filtration methods)	• Minimizes alloimmunization to WBC/HLA antigens • Potential impact on reducing incidence of platelet-transfusion refractoriness • Confirmed reduced incidence of mediastinitis in open heart surgeries • Lowers incidence of FNHTRs • Provides CMV-"safe" RBCs and platelets (equivalent in most circumstances to CMV-seronegative components)
Validated Hospital and Laboratory Information Systems (numerous commercial suppliers)	• Document dispositions of all units in inventory • Authenticate identity of intended recipients • Corroborate the identity of blood units and recipients • Proffer both CPOE and clinical decision-support tools, such as evidence-based practice guidelines • Stipulate selected attributes required for individual recipients (e.g., antigen-negative, irradiated, CMV-seronegative, etc.)
"*All-male*" Plasma or Apheresis Platelets donated by males, nulligravida, or HLA-tested and seronegative females	• Established TRALI mitigation for plasma • Strategies for TRALI mitigation in platelets less well studied and not universally implemented
• Verax PGD platform	• *Point-of-Issue* bacteriologic testing of platelets • Licensed to detect GP and GN bacteria • Licensed for all forms of US-licensed platelet components • Established improved, effective supplement to culture methods
Pathogen reduction technologies	
Plasma: • Octaplas™ (Octapharma) • Cerus Intercept® Blood System	• Octaplas is plasma pools treated with solvents and detergents • The Cerus system uses Psoralen and UVA light exposure; cross links DNA and RNA
Platelets: • Cerus Intercept® Blood System	• Psoralen and UVA light exposure; cross links DNA and RNA • FDA approved, December, 2014 • CE marked
Patient blood management [25]	• Institutionalized programs to optimize blood usage

CE (Conformité Européenne) denotes conformance with the requirements of the European Union, *CPOE* computerized provider order entry, *CMV* cytomegalovirus, *FDA* US Food and Drug Administration, *FNHTR* febrile nonhemolytic transfusion reactions, *GP* gram-positive, *GN* gram-negative, *HLA* human leukocyte antigen, *TRALI* transfusion-related acute lung injury, *WBC* white blood cell

References

1. Whitker B, Hinkins S. The 2011 national blood collection and utilization survey. Report (most recent published). http://www.bloodsurvey.org. Accessed 28 Aug 2015.
2. http://www.fda.gov/BiologicsBloodVaccines/BloodBloodProducts/default.htm. Accessed 28 Aug 2015.
3. Galel SA. Infectious disease screening (Chapter 8). In: Fung MK, Grossman BJ, Hillyer CD, Westhoff CM, editors. Technical manual. 18th ed. Bethesda, MD: AABB; 2014. p. 179–212.
4. Zuck TF. How should we test the tests? Transfusion. 1989;29(1):3–4.
5. Popovsky MA, editor. Transfusion reactions. 4th ed. Bethesda, MD: AABB Press; 2012.
6. Nester T, Jain S, Poisson J. Hemotherapy decisions and their outcomes (Chapter 20). In: Fung MK, Grossman BJ, Hillyer C, Westhoff CM, editors. Technical manual. 18th ed. Bethesda, MD: AABB Press; 2014.
7. Maynard K. Administration of blood components (Chapter 21). In: Fung MK, Grossman BJ, Hillyer C, Westhoff CM, editors. Technical manual. 18th ed. Bethesda, MD: AABB Press; 2014.
8. Mazzei CA, Popovsky MA, Kopko PM. Noninfectious complications of blood transfusion (Chapter 27). In: Fung MK, Grossman BJ, Hillyer C, Westhoff CM, editors. Technical manual. 18th ed. Bethesda, MD: AABB Press; 2014.
9. Sazama K, DeChristopher PJ, Dodd R, et al. Practice parameter for the recognition, management and prevention of adverse consequences of blood transfusion. Arch Pathol Lab Med. 2000;124(1):61–71.

10. Oakley FD, Woods M, Arnold S, Young PP. Transfusion reaction in pediatric compared with adult patients: a look at rate, reaction type and associated products. Transfusion. 2015;55:563–70.
11. Toy P, Gaji O, Bacchetti P, et al. Transfusion-related acute lung injury: incidence and risk factors. Blood. 2012;119(7):1757–67.
12. American Association of Blood Banks (AABB). TRALI risk mitigation for plasma and whole blood for allogeneic transfusion. Bulletin # 14-02, 20 Jan 2014.
13. Bolton-Maggs PHB, Wood EM, Wiersum-Osselton JC. Wrong blood in tube – potential for serious outcomes: can it be prevented? Br J Haematol. 2015;168:3–13.
14. Alam M, Lin Y, Lima A, et al. The prevention of transfusion-associated circulatory overload. Transfus Med Rev. 2013;27(2):105–12.
15. Skeate RC, Eastlund T. Distinguishing between transfusion related acute lung injury and transfusion associated circulatory overload. Curr Opin Hematol. 2007;14:682–7.
16. Dunbar NM. Current options for transfusion-related acute lung injury risk mitigation in platelet transfusions. Curr Opin Hematol. 2015;22(6):554–8.
17. Annual SHOT Report, 2014 Summary. [http://www.shotuk.org]. Accessed 20 Oct 2015.
18. Fatalities Reported to FDA Following Blood Collection and Transfusion. Annual Summary for Fiscal Year 2014. http://www.fda.gov/downloads/biologicsbloodvaccines/safetyavailability/reportaproblem/transfusiondonationfatalities/ucm459461.pdf. Accessed 02 Oct 2015.
19. Center for Disease Control and Prevention National Healthcare Safety Network, Biovigilance Component, Hemovigilance Module Surveillance Protocol, August 2014.
20. Stramer SL. Current risks of transfusion-transmitted agents (a review). Arch Pathol Lab Med. 2007; 131:702–7.
21. Kleinman S, Swanson P, Allain JP, et al. Transfusion transmission of human T-lymphotropic virus types I and II: serologic and polymerase chain results in recipients identified through look-back investigations. Transfusion. 1993;33(1):14–8.
22. Hakre S, Manak MM, Murray CK, et al. Transfusion-transmitted human T-lymphotropic virus Type I infection in a United States military emergency whole blood transfusion recipient in Afghanistan, 2010. Transfusion. 2013;53:2176–82.
23. Centers for Disease Control and Prevention (CDC). Fatal West Nile virus infection after probable transfusion-associated transmission – Colorado, 2012. MMWR Morb Mortal Wkly Rep. 2013;62(31):622–4.
24. Dalton HR, Hepatitis E. The "new kid on the block" or an old friend? Transfus Med Hemother. 2014;41:6–9.
25. An AABB White Paper. Building a better patient blood management program: identifying tools, solving problems and promoting patient safety. Bethesda, MD: AABB Press; 2015.
26. Snyder EL, Stramer SL, Benjamin RJ. The safety of the blood supply- time to raise the bar. N Engl J Med. 2015;372:1882–5.
27. Beal RW. The rational use of blood. Aust N Z J Surg. 1976;46(4):309–13.

Common Coagulation Disorders That May Arise Intraoperatively: Specifically DIC

11

Srikanth Nagalla and Geno Merli

Neurosurgical patients could have preexisting congenital or acquired systemic coagulation disorders that can complicate their intraoperative management. Further conditions like traumatic brain injury, major trauma, sepsis, and malignancy can cause coagulopathy complicating the course of the neurosurgical patient. Antithrombotic therapy for preexisting conditions adds to the complexity of the situation either exacerbating bleeding or by delaying the surgical procedure. Similarly there are disorders of coagulation that could occur in the postoperative period, one of which is the increased risk of thrombosis in the neurosurgical patients. All of the above-mentioned disorders have been dealt with in detail in other sections of this textbook. The most important coagulation disorder that may arise intraoperatively is disseminated intravascular coagulation (DIC).

S. Nagalla, M.B.B.S., M.S., F.A.C.P. (✉)
Department of Medicine/Hematology, Sidney Kimmel Medical College at Thomas Jefferson University, 1015 Chestnut Street, Suite 1321, Philadelphia, PA 19107, USA
e-mail: srikanth.nagalla@jefferson.edu

G. Merli, M.D.
Department of Surgery, Sidney Kimmel Medical College at Thomas Jefferson University, 111 S 11th Street, Gibbon Bldg., Ste. 6210, Philadelphia, PA 19107, USA
e-mail: Geno.merli@jefferson.edu

Disseminated Intravascular Coagulation

Introduction

The hemostatic response is tightly regulated so that there is effective control of bleeding at the site of local injury. The platelets, von Willebrand factor, coagulation factors, naturally occurring anticoagulants, fibrinolytic system, and endothelium work in a meticulous fashion to result in a controlled hemostatic response. Disseminated intravascular coagulation (DIC) is the result of a pathological overstimulation of the hemostatic pathway that could present as a simultaneous hemorrhagic and thrombotic process [1]. An individual patient can be either at the thrombotic or at the hemorrhagic end of the spectrum at any given point of time. DIC increases the mortality in trauma patients [2]. DIC is a highly heterogeneous condition with different phases and varying degrees of severity. In 2001 the International Society of Thrombosis and Hemostasis defined DIC as "an acquired syndrome characterized by the intravascular activation of coagulation without a specific localization and arising from different causes. It can originate from and cause damage to the microvasculature, which if sufficiently severe, can produce organ dysfunction [3]."

C.M. Loftus (ed.), *Anticoagulation and Hemostasis in Neurosurgery*,
DOI 10.1007/978-3-319-27327-3_11

Clinical Manifestations

The clinical presentation of DIC could be acute or chronic and the severity can range from mild to severe. DIC can be mild in some presentations that it may be identified only on laboratory testing without any overt clinical symptoms or signs. In the more severe and acute forms there is activation of the coagulation cascade resulting in the formation of micro- and macrovascular thrombosis followed by fibrinolysis of the microthrombi resulting in the increase of fibrin degradation products. Severe DIC can result in thrombosis in the vascular beds of almost all organ systems. There is evidence of microangiopathic hemolytic anemia due to fragmentation of red blood cells as they pass through the microvasculature laden with thrombi. Some of the clinical manifestations of these widespread microthrombi include acute renal failure, respiratory distress syndrome, dermal necrosis, and altered mental status.

The uncontrolled activation of the coagulation cascade also results in the consumption of the clotting factors and platelets. The above process combined with fibrinolysis can result in hemorrhagic manifestations in multiple organs. There can be widespread mucocutaneous bleeding, hematuria, bleeding from central and peripheral venous catheter sites, and intracerebral bleeding. Bleeding into the adrenal glands can result in adrenal cortical failure.

In summary the neurological manifestations in DIC can include thrombotic and hemorrhagic strokes, altered mental status, coma, and convulsions.

Pathophysiology of DIC

Tissue factor (TF) plays an important role in the initiation of DIC in neurosurgical procedures [4]. Brain tissue and tumors are rich in tissue factor and manipulation of the tissues during procedures can initiate DIC medicated by TF. Decreased levels of naturally occurring anticoagulants, like Antithrombin, Protein C, and Tissue factor pathway inhibitor, can exacerbate DIC [5]. Patients could have lower levels of these anticoagulants due to consumption in the clotting process. Plasmin is the key enzyme involved in fibrinolysis. As thrombin generated by the tissue factor initiated clotting process converts the fibrinogen to fibrin, plasmin breaks down the fibrin clot. The balance between the thrombin and plasmin levels determines the clinical phenotype of DIC which can range from extensive thrombosis to overt bleeding.

Laboratory Parameters in DIC

There is no single test or a set of tests that can accurately diagnose DIC. All laboratory testing should be combined with the clinical scenario to help with a diagnosis and management of DIC. Some of the tests that are routinely performed and readily available are prothrombin time (PT), activated partial thromboplastin time (aPTT), platelet count, fibrinogen, and d-dimer. D-dimer is a cross-linked fibrin degradation product. PT, aPTT, platelet count, and fibrinogen are usually low in moderate to severe DIC with an elevated d-dimer. There are numerous confounding variables in the interpretation of the above-mentioned tests. The coagulation parameters in a patient with liver disease may be similar to a patient in DIC. Factor VIII is synthesized in the endothelial cells whereas all the other factors are synthesized by the liver parenchyma. Getting Factor II, V, X, and VIII levels may help to distinguish coagulopathy of liver disease from DIC. Factor VIII is usually normal or high in early to mid stages of liver failure with the other factors being low. Since DIC is a process where all factors are consumed in the clotting process even Factor VIII is low. Fibrinogen is an acute phase reactant and the levels of the protein may be high in infections and inflammation. So it is important to follow serial levels to evaluate for a decrease in the fibrinogen level due to consumption rather than a one-time test looking for a below normal value. Similarly there are other conditions that can result in a high D-dimer level apart from DIC. Evaluation of the peripheral blood smear by a hematologist may demonstrate red cell fragments and decreased platelet count.

The schistocytes in DIC are not markedly elevated unlike other microangiopathic hemolytic anemias and schistocytes are not required for making a diagnosis of DIC.

Tests like thrombin-antithrombin complexes, soluble fibrin, and prothrombin fragment 1.2 are better than the standard tests discussed previously in the evaluation of DIC. Since these tests are not readily available in most hospitals, their use in the real-time management of DIC is limited.

Assays of global hemostasis are being used commonly during cardiac and hepatic surgeries. These points of care (POC) devices could give an overview of the entire coagulation system including the platelet-clot interaction and fibrinolysis. This is in stark contrast to the commonly performed tests that only evaluate a particular aspect of the clotting cascade. Further these POC devices can be used in the operating room helping with real-time management decisions. Devices like thromboelastogram (TEG), rotational thromboelastometry (ROTEM), and thrombin generation assay (TGA) could aid in the management of DIC during neurosurgical procedures [6]. Unlike the conventional tests these POC devices may help in the early diagnosis of DIC and also inform the surgeon if the patient is in the hypercoagulable phase or hyperfibrinolytic phase of DIC.

DIC Development During Neurosurgical Procedures

DIC can occur intraoperatively during resection of brain tumors or with excessive use of hemostatic products like prothrombin complex concentrates (PCCs) and recombinant factor VIIa (rVIIa).

Resection of Tumors

Neurosurgical procedures for brain tumors can be complicated by the development of DIC. DIC in this setting increases the mortality rate for the patient. Surgical resection of meningioma, oligodendroglioma, neuroblastoma, glioblastoma multiforme, and metastatic adenocarcinoma has been reported in the literature to be complicated by DIC [7]. Rarely DIC can develop after embolization of brain tumors [8].

DIC in the above-mentioned neurosurgical procedures was predominantly hemorrhagic in nature. DIC was caused by the intraoperative manipulation of the tumor. Apart from supportive transfusion therapy with platelets, plasma, and cryoprecipitate, resection of the tumor was important for control of DIC. Tissue factor released from the intraoperative manipulation of meningiomas could have contributed to DIC in this setting. Meningiomas associated with a hemorrhagic complication stained positive for tissue factor by immunohistochemistry compared to meningiomas without hemorrhagic complications [9].

DIC with the Use of Hemostatic Therapy

Neurosurgeons are in situations where complex surgical procedures are needed in patients with congenital or acquired clotting factor deficiencies with inhibitors and these surgeries are usually performed under the cover of inhibitor bypassing agents like prothrombin complex concentrates (PCCs) and recombinant factor VIIa (rVIIa). Similarly the above-mentioned hemostatic agents are used in patients who present with life-threatening intracranial hemorrhage due to supratherapeutic INR on warfarin or target-specific anticoagulants (Rivaroxaban, Apixaban, Edoxaban, and Dabigatran). These hemostatic agents in large doses can result in DIC. PCCs can either be non-activated (containing factor II, VII, IX, and X) or activated (aPCCs—containing factors IIa, VIIa, IXa, and Xa). The non-activated PCCs have a lower incidence of DIC than the aPCCs. It is very important to monitor the patient closely for any symptoms and signs of DIC and laboratory parameters of DIC while receiving systemic hemostatic treatments.

Treatment of DIC

The most important step in the management of DIC is to treat the underlying cause of DIC. The patient has to be supported aggressively with blood product replacement therapy and pharmacological agents depending on whether the patient has bleeding or thrombotic manifestations of DIC. The supportive management plays a crucial role when DIC develops during a neurosurgical procedure for a tumor. The patient will need replacement therapy if there is evidence of bleeding with abnormal DIC labs or if the patient requires a procedure. Cryoprecipitate is used as a replacement for low fibrinogen. Fresh frozen plasma is used for factor replacement if PT and PTT are prolonged despite correcting the fibrinogen. Unactivated prothrombin complex concentrates may be used in conjunction with small doses of FFP if there are volume overload issues. Platelet transfusions are recommended (goal platelet count of >100,000/μl) in a bleeding neurosurgical patient with DIC. When patient has excessive fibrinolysis the use of anti-fibrinolytic agents in the form of lysine analogues (EACA or tranexamic acid) can be considered. Rarely despite the use of the replacement therapy the DIC may be so severe that it is difficult to maintain the coagulation factor levels and fibrinogen at hemostatic levels. In this situation low-dose infusion of heparin at 500 units/h can be considered along with the appropriate factor replacement therapy.

In patients with the thrombotic spectrum of DIC, therapeutic heparin infusion is the recommended treatment of choice.

References

1. Levi M. Current understanding of disseminated intravascular coagulation. Br J Haematol. 2004;124(5): 567–76.
2. Saggar V, Mittal RS, Vyas MC. Hemostatic abnormalities in patients with closed head injuries and their role in predicting early mortality. J Neurotrauma. 2009;26(10):1665–8.
3. Taylor Jr FB, Toh CH, Hoots WK, et al. Towards definition, clinical and laboratory criteria, and a scoring system for disseminated intravascular coagulation. Thromb Haemost. 2001;86(5):1327–30.
4. Heesen M, Winking M, Kemkes-Matthes B, et al. What the neurosurgeon needs to know about the coagulation system. Surg Neurol. 1997;47(1):32–4.
5. Esmon CT. Regulation of blood coagulation. Biochim Biophys Acta. 2000;1477(1–2):349–60.
6. Beynon C, Unterberg AW, Sakowitz OW. Point of care coagulation testing in neurosurgery. J Clin Neurosci. 2015;22(2):252–7.
7. Brecknell JE, McLean CA, Hirano H, Malham GM. Disseminated intravascular coagulation complicating resection of a malignant meningioma. Br J Neurosurg. 2006;20(4):239–41.
8. Velez AM, Friedman WA. Disseminated intravascular coagulation during resection of a meningioma: case report. Neurosurgery. 2011;68(4):E1165–9. discussion E1169.
9. Niiro M, Ishimaru K, Hirano H, Yunoue S, Kuratsu J. Clinico-pathological study of meningiomas with haemorrhagic onset. Acta Neurochir (Wien). 2003; 145(9):767–72.

12 Evaluation and Management of Untoward Intraoperative Bleeding

Michael P. Wemhoff and W. Scott Jellish

Introduction

The evaluation of intraoperative blood loss in neurosurgical procedures requires diligent attention from the surgeon and anesthesiologist to coordinate appropriate assessment and subsequent management of any untoward bleeding. While the history of hemostasis in surgical procedures has yielded invaluable time-honored techniques of tamponade pressure, vessel ligation, or electrocautery, many delicate aspects of neurosurgical procedures require finer control with less mechanical disruption or force applied to neural tissue. Additionally, the often small, confined surgical corridors in which neurosurgical procedures are performed are susceptible to complete obscuration from even small quantities of hemorrhage. In the case of recalcitrant bleeding, where hemorrhage does not appear isolated, underlying etiologies must be sought out. Multiple modalities now exist in order to evaluate the patient's ability to clot blood, and point of care testing can isolate the problem to platelet dysfunction, coagulation cascade abnormality, or some other global phenomenon. This chapter will elucidate the current methods available to surgical and anesthesia teams to evaluate and address excessive intraoperative blood loss.

A Brief History of Hemostasis in Neurosurgery

One of the first hemostatic issues encountered by early twentieth-century neurosurgeons arose from highly vascularized scalp tissue which often would lead to unacceptable blood loss if left unaddressed. Heinrich Braun first described the use of scalp infiltration by vasoconstrictive agents along the incision line, which was found to greatly reduce blood loss [1]. After making incision, the application of pressure from various tourniquet devices was initially tried with limited success [2]. Hemostatic sutures along the base of the scalp flap and upward along the incision line were preferred by many surgeons and had to be removed 10 days after the operation. Other surgeons preferred vessel ligation before surgery, and Charles Frazier recommended exposure of the common carotid artery before cranial surgery to allow for its subsequent occlusion in case of excessive hemorrhage [3]. Frazier also wrote about the use of pressure applied from gauze and

M.P. Wemhoff, M.D. (✉)
Department of Neurological Surgery, Loyola University Medical Center,
2160 S. 1st Ave, Maywood, IL 60153, USA
e-mail: michaelwem@gmail.com

W.S. Jellish, M.D., Ph.D.
Department of Anesthesiology, Loyola University Medical Center, 2160 S. 1st Ave, Maywood, IL 60153, USA
e-mail: wjellis@lumc.edu

C.M. Loftus (ed.), *Anticoagulation and Hemostasis in Neurosurgery*,
DOI 10.1007/978-3-319-27327-3_12

hemostats along the edge of the incision margin, and while effective, the hemostats cluttered the operative exposure. With the introduction of steel clips to the United States from France in the 1930s, scalp hemostasis could be achieved without obstructing the operative field. Raney clips, which utilized a spring-like clamping action when applied, were subsequently developed within the decade and continue to have relevance in successful scalp hemostasis [4].

Once adequate scalp hemostasis was achieved, bleeding that occurred from edges of bone during creation of the craniotomy was difficult to control. In 1888, Sir Victor Horsley introduced a formulation of antiseptic beeswax which allowed the surgeon to spread the substance along bone edges to plug the diploe and stem bleeding [5]. This innovation rapidly gained notoriety and continues to be used in modified form today.

Intracranial bleeding was perhaps the most challenging problem for early neurosurgeons who relied on a number of innovative devices, but did not have elaborate chemical means of stemming hemorrhage. The application of general surgical methods of applying pressure or clamping and ligating vessels carried great morbidity in neurosurgical procedures. Thermal cautery, a known technique since ancient times, was first attempted in neurosurgical procedures by heating the tip of a needle and selectively burning bleeding tissues, though this was controversial within the neurosurgical community. Others used the application of gentle pressure from gauze with hot irrigation.

In the 1920s the landmark innovation of surgical electrocautery was developed by William Bovie and Harvey Cushing, who first used it in an operation in 1926 [6]. This method achieved hemostasis by heat induction (rather than conduction or radiation) and thus limited damage to surrounding tissues. Though the initial iteration of this technology was cumbersome, Cushing and others saw its vast potential, which ultimately paved the way for bipolar electrocautery in 1940.

Since these early days, improved knowledge of platelet function and the coagulation cascade as well as medications and monitoring that allow practitioners to detect and correct aberrances in hemodynamics have improved the evaluation and correction of untoward bleeding.

Chemical Hemostatic Agents

Some of the aforementioned historical methods of hemostasis remain the workhorses in neurosurgical operations where there are identifiable vessels that can be safely electrocauterized with bipolar, compressed by cottonoid patties, or clamped with a vascular clip. Adjuvant methods may be used along with these primary methods, including warm irrigation or the use of hemostatic chemical agents (Table 12.1). The proposed mechanism for the role of warm saline irrigation in hemostasis, derived from animal epistaxis models, is twofold: edema from the surrounding tissue induces mechanical compression of the oozing vessels, and vasodilation of the vessels decreases the intraluminal pressure, slowing blood flow and producing hemostasis [7].

With the continued advancement in technology based on biochemical knowledge of coagulation, chemical agents have taken on a large role in hemostasis. Among the first agents developed were absorbable gelatin sponges. Developed in 1945, they work by allowing local lattice formation, which provides a framework for clot formation. The porous surface of the sponge allows for absorption of up to 45 times its weight in whole blood. This increase in weight eventually tamponades the underlying bleeding tissue [8, 9]. Despite this ideal increase in size and weight for hemostasis, the consequence of gelatin sponges compressing neural tissue has also been reported, and this can result in severe neurologic compromise from damage to the underlying neural tissue [10, 11].

Microfibrillar collagens have been in use since the late 1960s and are a class of materials that promote platelet aggregation though they have no direct effect on the intrinsic components of the coagulation cascade [9]. These agents are very hydrophilic and are best handled with forceps, as they will strongly adhere to surgical gloves.

Table 12.1 A comparison of commonly used hemostatic agents

Agent	Mechanism of action	Uses	Risks and shortcomings
Warm saline irrigation	Twofold: mechanical compression from edema and decreased intraluminal pressure from vasodilation	Copious irrigation is applied to the field with sensitivity to neural tissue damage from overly brisk irrigation	Temperature must be carefully monitored to minimize risk to tissue
Gelatin sponge	Local lattice formation provides a framework for clot formation	Applied over bleeding surface, can act as a compress	Can absorb 45 times its weight in whole blood, may swell and compress neural tissue
Microfibrillar collagen	Promotes platelet aggregation	Applied as powder to irregular surface (e.g., cancellous bone) or sheet that can be packed as a compress	Effectiveness is reduced with thrombocytopenia or platelet dysfunction
Oxidized cellulose/oxidized regenerated cellulose	Acidic properties react with blood to precipitate an artificial coagulum, provide substrate for further intrinsic coagulation	Applied to bleeding surface as sheet or strips, can act as compress if packed	Acidic properties may denature other hemostatic agents (e.g., thrombin)
Microporous polysaccharide hemospheres	Polysaccharides absorb fluid to concentrate soluble components of coagulation	Sprayed directly onto bleeding surface	Dependent upon an intact coagulation cascade
Thrombin	Enzymatic catalysis of soluble fibrinogen to insoluble fibrin	May be used on its own or commonly as a medium for soaking other agents (e.g., gelatin sponges) to enhance their effectiveness	Decreased effectiveness in fibrinogen deficiency (e.g., disseminated intravascular coagulation)
Fibrin glue	Uses exogenous human fibrinogen and thrombin to form cross-linked fibrin clot	Sprayer combines the two substrates when sprayed onto bleeding surface	May be denatured by oxidized cellulose

Both a powder and sheet form are available, with powder form being ideal for irregular surfaces and cancellous bone bleeding, while the sheet form is packed in place to provide additional compressive hemostasis. It should be noted that given the dependence of the mechanism of this agent on platelet function, platelet dysfunction and severe thrombocytopenia will decrease its effectiveness [12].

Oxidized cellulose and oxidized regenerated cellulose function by nature of their acidic properties that react with blood to precipitate an artificial coagulum, acting as a substrate for further coagulation of the intrinsic soluble components of the coagulation cascade [13]. Initially, after discovery of the hemostatic properties of oxidized cellulose in the 1940s, it was thought to have a mechanical effect. It was not until subsequent studies demonstrated that the caustic nature of this substance contributed to a chemical mechanism whereby, upon encountering blood, the oxidized cellulose reacts to form the hematin-containing coagulum. Though manufactured by different chemical processes, these agents have similar hemostatic properties.

Microporous polysaccharide hemospheres are absorbable hemostatic agents that consist of particles manufactured from biologically inert plant polysaccharides derived from potato starches. The fluid components of the patient's blood are absorbed immediately, concentrating platelets and clotting factors and promoting the formation of a gel matrix of proteins and blood cells on the surface of the particles [14].

It is important to note that the commonality among these agents is the requirement of an intact clotting cascade and their relative inefficiency in patients with thrombocytopenia. One way to ameliorate this limitation is to soak the hemostatic agent in thrombin. This method, however, is not fool proof. Thrombin's mechanism of action is the enzymatic catalysis of soluble fibrinogen to insoluble fibrin; thus, any situation where fibrinogen is deficient (e.g., a patient with disseminated intravascular coagulation) is one in which thrombin (and other thrombin-based hemostatic agents) would have limited efficacy [15]. Otherwise, in situations where upstream deficiencies in the coagulation cascade exist, thrombin can induce clotting as long as fibrinogen is present. Though thrombin is manufactured as a powder which can be directly applied to the operative site, its most common use is in solution with sterile saline. This solution can be used to soak gelatin sponges which readily absorb the thrombin to enhance their effect on coagulation. Thrombin will not improve the hemostatic properties of all agents; in particular, it is denatured by the low pH of oxidized cellulose [16]. Also, manufactured thrombin (derived from bovine prothrombin being converted into thrombin by thromboplastin) has been shown to induce an antigenic response in patients. Cases of bovine-derived thrombin products entering the vascular system of patients demonstrated a development of bovine thrombin-associated factor V antibodies, which themselves can lead to life-threatening hemorrhage [17].

Fibrin glue utilizes a combination of human thrombin and fibrinogen. Upon delivery to the tissue, the two components of the solution generate a cross-linked fibrin clot, thus functioning to induce coagulation completely independent of the patient's intrinsic coagulation cascade [18]. Neurosurgeons may be more familiar with fibrin glue because of its notable ability to act as a sealant which has led to its widespread off-label use for the repair of durotomies [19].

Thrombin has also been combined with gelatin to produce a gelatin-thrombin matrix sealant. It is applied via syringe applicator and has a viscous gel-like property which allows for its use on irregular surfaces such as cancellous bone where it is particularly useful in inducing hemostasis. It can produce hemostasis from a tamponading effect as well as providing a framework for the formation of fibrin clot via catalysis from the thrombin component of the agent [20].

As with any foreign body, the smallest effective amount of a hemostatic agent should be used to reduce the risk of infection. It also bears repeating that the smallest amount of gelatin sponge should be used to decrease the possibility of the substance acting as an expansive lesion.

Nonchemical Means of Enhancing Hemostasis

Controlled hypotension is usually defined as reducing mean arterial blood pressure to 50–75 mmHg. Systolic blood pressure is usually reduced in the range of 80–90 mmHg [21]. Controlled hypotension can be produced with the use of inhalational agents; intravenous medications such as propofol; beta-blockers such as esmolol, propranolol, and/or labetalol; and calcium channel blockers such as nicardipine or diltiazem. Arterial and venous dilators such as nitroglycerin and sodium nitroprusside, hydralazine, and combinations of the above drugs may also be used to reduce blood pressure. The use of controlled hypotension during anesthesia must be based on clinical judgment. Contraindications to the use of controlled hypotension include cardiovascular disease with uncontrolled hypertension or severe coronary artery disease. Cerebral vascular disease and hepatic and renal failure are also contraindications to controlled hypotension (Table 12.2). Deliberate hypotension to control blood loss improves the surgeon's operative field and decreases the need for blood transfusion with a reduction in infection risk and fluid overload. The risk of mortality related to hypotension is a concern, but the incidence is infrequent. Most studies that have evaluated the use of deliberate hypotension have noted minimal complications with low morbidity. Morbidity with controlled hypotension usually focuses on the threat of reduced perfusion to the central organs. The most concerning has to do with cerebral hypoperfusion. If mean arterial pressure is maintained above central venous pressure and oncotic pressure is also maintained (30–40 mmHg), cerebral perfusion should be adequate in otherwise healthy individuals [22]. However, a built-in margin of safety places the lower limit for perfusion at 50 mmHg. This level of pressure is also the lowest pressure at which autoregulation of cerebral blood flow occurs. Other determinants of cerebral blood flow, carbon dioxide, and oxygen tension must also be taken into consideration. In normotensive patients, cerebral blood flow changes at 2 mL/100 g/mmHg CO_2 [23]. The slope of this relationship is modified by controlled hypotension. In patients with hypertension or cerebral vascular disease, this lower level should be adjusted upward (Fig. 12.1). In patients with cerebrovascular disease or hypertension, their margin of safety may require a higher lower limit of blood pressure. Several studies have evaluated the safety of controlled hypotension and found that morbidity and mortality was approximately 0.1 %, most often due to hypoperfusion of the cerebral vasculature [24]. In hypertensive patients, the autoregulating curve for cerebral perfusion is shifted to the right which means that the lower limit of normal perfusion is also increased. Another concern of induced hypotension is in relation to the heart and adequate oxygen supply to meet myocardial demand. The heart maximally extracts oxygen, and an increase in myocardial oxygen requirements necessitates an increase in coronary blood flow. Hypotension reduces the coronary vasodilatory reserve. If the patient has atherosclerotic coronary artery disease, systemic hypotension with this scenario will directly reduce myocardial perfusion, possibly leading to ischemia [25]. Depending on the drug used to induce controlled hypotension, agents such as nitroprusside, adenosine, and possibly isoflurane could produce coronary arterial vasodilation with the possibility of coronary steal [26]. Nitroglycerine, however, which produces epicardial vasodilation and unloads the heart, will reduce the potential for myocardial ischemia.

Table 12.2 Factors that could contraindicate the use of controlled hypotension

1. Pregnancy
2. Anemia
3. Cardiovascular disease
4. Coronary artery disease
5. Hepatic disease
6. Renal failure
7. Severe hypertension
8. Cerebral vascular insufficiency
9. Hypovolemia
10. Pulmonary disease with hypertension

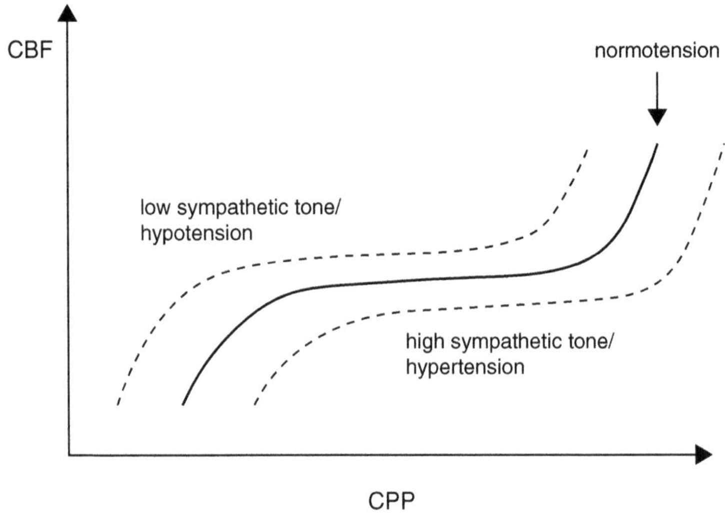

Fig. 12.1 Change in autoregulatory curve with hypertension and hypotension

With controlled hypotension, the MAP is reduced to 50–60 mmHg. At this pressure urine flow rate, endogenous creatinine clearance and osmolar clearance fall. Controlled hypotension leads to stimulation of the renin-angiotensin system in response to decreased renal perfusion. This also results in activation of the autonomic nervous system. Certain agents used to produce hypotension will activate catecholamines and the renin-angiotensin system. Sodium nitroprusside is one such agent, while drugs such as trimethaphan inhibit this response [27]. Isoflurane with labetalol also blocks this response, while drugs such as nitroglycerine and prostaglandin E increase renin activity [28]. Rebound hypertension has been known to occur after induced hypotension, especially if sodium nitroprusside is the agent used to reduce blood pressure. Most studies to date have shown that controlled hypotension maintained within autoregulatory limits is not detrimental to the liver.

The use of controlled hypotension, especially in the prone position during spine surgery with large blood loss, has been shown to be associated with visual loss from ischemic optic neuropathy [29]. An increase in intraocular pressure from large fluid administration producing dependent edema, coupled with diminished MAP, could produce lower perfusion pressure to the optic nerve head. The hypoxia that develops leads to destruction of axonal integrity with the free radicals formed during reperfusion further damaging the nerves. When applying deliberate hypotension, the anesthesiologist must keep in mind the physiology of hemorrhage and shock and continuously evaluate the patient for the development of metabolic acidosis from reduced perfusion.

If bleeding seems excessive for the neurological procedure performed and tumor cells or infected material is not anticipated to be in the blood, possible cell salvage and autotransfusion may be utilized to reduce transfusion requirements. The American Association of Blood Banks recommends the following indications for cell salvage: blood loss approaching 20 % or more of the patient's estimated blood volume. In addition, if a majority of the patients undergoing the procedure require one or more units of blood, the cost of blood salvaged from the surgical site is much less than the cost of allogenic blood.

Accurately predicting the probability of sizeable blood loss and the need for allogenic transfusion can be problematic. Implementation of cell salvage should initially start with a collecting system, a cardiotomy reservoir, a suction line, and anticoagulant to maintain the collected blood. In cases where large blood loss is almost certain, it is reasonable to set up all components

Table 12.3 Relative contraindications to blood salvage

1. Contaminants	
(a)	Stool
(b)	Amniotic fluid
(c)	Bone fragments
(d)	Bacteria
(e)	Fat emboli
(f)	Urine
(g)	Methylmethacrylate
2. Malignancy—tumor cells	
3. Sickle cell disease	
–	Patients with thalassemia
4. Carbon monoxide	
–	Catecholamines
5. Pharmacologic agents: clotting agents, irrigating fluids, Betadine, or topical antibiotics	

necessary to process blood. The patient's starting hematocrit, gender, age, and weight can influence the risk of receiving blood products [30]. There are certain contraindications for blood salvage that should be considered before a system is operationalized (Table 12.3). Many of the contraindications are theoretical, with little clinical evidence for support. Definite contraindications would include any process that involves red cell lysis. This would include blood that has been exposed to sterile water, alcohol, or hydrogen peroxide. Red cell hemolysis could result in renal failure, elevated serum lactate dehydrogenase, increased total bilirubin, and disseminated intravascular coagulation [31]. Blood collected from contaminated wounds, obstetrics, or malignancy, though contraindicated, can be considered safe in certain circumstances or under life-threatening conditions. Bacterial contamination of blood with bowel surgery, trauma, or in surgeries with an infected wound could reintroduce bacteria into the circulation if reinfused. Studies on blood contaminated with bacteria found that washing of blood cells was capable of reducing contamination from 5 to 23 % of the original bacterial load [32]. A 99 % reduction of the starting bacterial load still left a large bacterial contamination [33]. Studies have noted that bacterial contamination of blood from cell salvage during cardiac surgery approached 30 % [34]. In liver surgery, 9 % of cell-salvaged blood during these procedures had bacterial contamination [35]. In most surgical procedures, broad spectrum antibiotics are given. Studies have suggested that drugs such as these improve the safety of contaminated blood if readministered [36].

Cell salvage during cancer surgery is another issue of concern since immunomodulation occurs with allogenic transfusion, and this could affect tumor growth. There is considerable retrospective evidence to suggest that the outcome is worse for patients undergoing cancer surgery when they receive allogenic blood [37]. Administration of tumor-laden blood cells from cell salvage would also seem to be undesirable, yet during tumor surgery, hematogenous spread of cancer cells is common and does not correlate with outcome [38]. If using cell salvage during tumor surgery, the use of leukocyte depletion filters is advocated. These filters have been used to remove tumor cells during urologic cancer surgery, pulmonary surgery, and other tumor cell types [39, 40]. These studies concluded that leukocyte depletion filters were highly effective in removing tumor cell contamination.

Care must be taken during blood salvage as complications such as air embolus could occur if the collection bag is not de-aired prior to administration of the blood under pressure. If using leukocyte depletion filters, they should be changed after every 500 mL of blood administered. The bag should be pressurized to 300 mmHg to move blood through the filter. In some instances, blood salvaged during surgery will contain contaminants which could affect hemodynamics. Blood collected from neuroendocrine tumors, for example, could contain epinephrine or norepinephrine which could produce extreme hypertension or arrhythmia with reinfusion [41]. Other chemical contaminants from the surgical site could also be contained in salvaged blood. These contaminants could affect blood pressure, and administration of these blood products should be done slowly until the effect on hemodynamic variables is totally ascertained.

Pharmacologic Methods of Hemostasis

There are also pharmacologic methods to reduce abnormal bleeding during different neurosurgical procedures where unanticipated hemorrhage occurs (Table 12.4). Desmopressin (DDAVP) is a synthetic analogue of vasopressin. DDAVP causes an increase in the levels of factor VIII and stimulates the vascular endothelium to release large multimers of von Willebrand factor [42]. The drug also releases tissue plasminogen activator and prostacyclin from the vascular endothelium. DDAVP preserves plasma levels of factor VIII by protecting it from proteolytic enzymes and also stimulating its synthesis [43]. DDAVP has been used to reduce bleeding time and correct platelet dysfunction. The drug has been found to decrease blood loss and transfusion requirements with multiple surgeries. DDAVP may be most useful in patients with mild to moderate forms of hemophilia or von Willebrand disease who are undergoing surgery. In addition, patients with uremic platelet dysfunction and those with chronic liver disease may also have some benefit [44]. Some centers use thromboelastography to determine patients with platelet dysfunction and use this as a guide for DDAVP therapy.

Epsilon-aminocaproic acid and its analogue, tranexamic acid, are derivatives of the amino acid lysine. Both drugs inhibit the proteolytic activity of plasmin and the conversion of plasminogen to plasmin by plasminogen activation. Plasminogen is the precursor of plasmin, the main proteolytic enzyme of the fibrinolytic system. Plasmin cleaves fibrinogen by initially removing peptides from the A alpha chain and then from the B beta chains, leaving fragment X. This fragment undergoes asymmetric cleavage of all three chains, releasing fragment D and leaving fragment Y [45]. Plasmin has also been shown to decrease the activity of factors V, VIII, and IX and can also activate complements via the C1 esterase [46].

Table 12.4 Pharmacologic methods to reduce bleeding

1. Factor VIIa
2. Aprotinin
3. Epsilon-aminocaproic acid
4. Tranexamic acid
5. DDAVP (desmopressin)

Drugs that inhibit activation of plasminogen to plasmin and interfere with the lysis of fibrinogen and fibrin are noted to be antifibrinolytic agents. They are omega aminocarboxylic acids of lysine that bind to the kringles of plasminogen and plasmin which occupies the binding site for fibrinogen and fibrin, interfering with the fibrinolytic process [47]. These agents attach to lysine-binding sites on both plasminogen and plasmin to inhibit binding of lysine residues on fibrinogen and fibrin. Since plasminogen is now unable to bind to fibrin, it is unable to lyse it. All antifibrinolytic drips are water soluble and therefore are distributed through both intravascular and extravascular compartments. Tranexamic acid is six to ten times more potent than epsilon-aminocaproic acid (EACA) secondary to changes in molecular structure that mimics lysine. EACA loading doses should be around 75–150 mg/kg over 15–30 min followed by an infusion of 10–15 mg/kg/h. Tranexamic acid is administered with loading doses around 1 g (10–15 mg/kg) followed by an infusion of 1 mg/kg/h. Minimal side effects are reported with these drugs, the worst being hypotension from a rapid intravenous administration. There are few reports of either EACA or tranexamic-producing thrombosis [48].

Aprotinin is a serine protein inhibitor derived from bovine lung. Its broad spectrum of protease inhibition provides numerous avenues for decreasing bleeding. By inhibiting plasmin, aprotinin is able to inhibit fibrinolysis [49]. In addition, aprotinin inhibits kallikrein which helps to amplify and accelerate contact activation of factor XII. Inhibiting kallikrein also alters potential adverse effects of contact activation and protects platelets from activation. Kallikrein also is an activator of the fibrinolytic system and blocking its effects inhibits fibrinolysis. The precise mechanism of action of aprotinin in reducing blood loss and transfusion requirements is not clear. However, part of the mechanism of action is a better functioning platelet, possibly because of preservation of the glycoprotein 1b receptor which mediates adhesion of platelets [50]. The activity of aprotinin is expressed in kallikrein inactivator units where one inactivator unit is that quantity that inhibits one unit of kallikrein. Dosing is usually started at a 280 mg loading dose over 20 min followed by an infusion of 70 mg/h. Aprotinin has been utilized for its ability to decrease bleeding and transfusion requirements in cardiac and other surgical procedures. In these trials, aprotinin decreased bleeding without the risk of thromboembolic complications [51]. At present, aprotinin is off the market and unavailable for use in the United States secondary to studies that aprotinin use increased the risk of death after surgery. The studies noted that patients who received aprotinin had a much higher risk of heart complications after surgery including heart attack, stroke, and renal failure. Aprotinin is not accessible in the US market but still available in Europe and Asia.

There are several recombinant coagulation products used to manage bleeding. These include antihemophilic factor, factor IX concentrates, factor VIIa, and factor IX [46]. These agents, though specifically approved for patients with hematologic disorders, are also used to manage acute bleeding episodes in surgery. *The agent most often used is recombinant-activated factor VIIa that is approved to facilitate hemostasis in life-threatening refractory bleeding despite the use of hemostatic factors and platelets in patients with acquired hemostatic disorders in both cardiac and noncardiac surgeries* [52]. *Dosing of 30–45 mcg/kg has been reported to be effective in patients with uncontrolled surgical bleeding.*

Prothrombin complex concentrates can also be used to reverse coagulopathy from excessive or unexpected hemorrhage. This concentrate contains all of the vitamin K-dependent coagulation factors (II, VII, IX, X). In some patients with mild forms of hemophilia, IgG antibodies develop and inhibit factor VIII. The presence of these inhibitors can be reversed by prothrombin complex which has been used to successfully reverse abnormal bleeding. The use of this product has become somewhat restricted due to its excessive thrombogenic qualities.

Assessment and Workup of Intraoperative Hemostatic Perturbations

Bleeding is first assessed through clinical observation. One must assess the amount of blood loss and the presence or absence of clot formation in the field. The initial assessment would consist of a coagulation profile with blood sent for platelet count, fibrinogen level, prothrombin, and partial thromboplastin times which are important to get an initial impression of blood loss. Fibrin degradation product level and euglobulin lysis time may also be important to assess the bleeding. A minimum platelet count of 50,000 per μL is recommended to maintain coagulation. Counts up to 100,000 per μL may be needed to maintain clot formation during brisk bleeding. There is no level of blood loss or euvolemic hemodilution at which prophylactic platelet transfusions should be given. As blood is lost, there is a slow and often predictable level of hemodilution that occurs. The actual measured platelet count never fits what would be expected by hemodilution alone. There is no reason to transfuse platelets for any given amount of blood loss, especially if the platelet count was assessed to be normal prior to the bleed. One can expect at least one blood volume to be lost before the platelet count reaches a critical level [53].

Fibrinogen concentration can be assayed by either using thrombin as an activator in different dilutions of plasma or by immunoassay. *Fibrinogen concentrations of more than 100 mg/dL are sufficient to have normal clot function.* Following fibrinogen as an indicator of hemodilution is not necessarily accurate because fibrinogen is released from hepatic stores in response to stress. If one is transfusing packed red blood cells, it should be noted that these carry only small amounts of plasma and fibrinogen. As such, their levels in the circulation will consequently decrease as blood is administered.

Another test of whole blood clot formation which looks at overall protein function is the ACT (activated clotting time) [54]. This test uses either celite or kaolin to activate the intrinsic cascade. The ACT is not a predictor of abnormal

Fig. 12.2 (**a**) Variables and normal values measured by thromboelastography (**b**) TEG patterns of normal and disease states

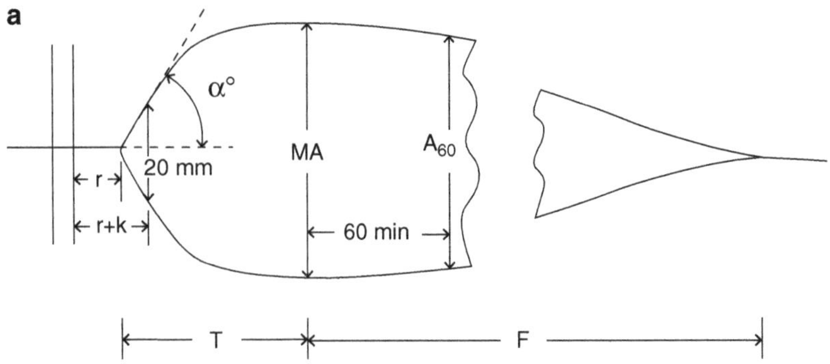

r	Reaction time	6–8 min
r + k	Coagulation time	10–12 min
α	Clot formation rate	>50°
MA	Maximum amplitude	50–70 mm
A_{60}	Amplitude at 60 min after MA	
A_{60}/MA* 100	Whole blood clot lysis index	>85%
F	Whole blood clot lysis time	>300 min

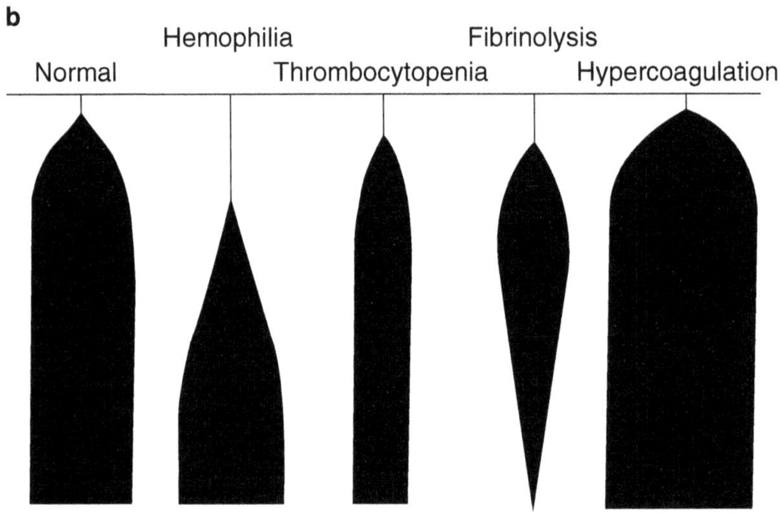

bleeding. Clearly, moderate prolongation of the ACT might suggest a risk of bleeding but normal ACT is meaningless because of the low sensitivity of the test. ACT gives a bioassay of heparin activity in whole blood. Comparisons of Hepcon-managed vs ACT-managed coagulation during cardiopulmonary bypass have shown some improvement with the Hepcon system for perioperative bleeding [55]. Usually these systems, though easily accessed for POC testing, are not well suited to direct therapy for product administration during abnormal bleeding or hemorrhage.

The TEG (thromboelastography) is a test of whole blood clot strength over time. It functions by maintaining a piston that does not touch the walls of a cup stable in an electromagnetic field. There is no connection between the cup and piston until whole blood is placed in the cup and coagulation begins. The TEG examines whole blood coagulation from the time of initiation through acceleration, control, and even lysis (Fig. 12.2). *The use of TEG in guiding coagulation therapy and in determining who would benefit from hemostatic therapy has been used to successfully guide desmopressin therapy to improve platelet function* [56]. *TEG is a good predictor for platelet function, for determination of trace amounts of heparin, and for assessing hypercoagulability.* A modification of TEG removes thrombin from the assay and studies the non-thrombin clot strengthened by the addition of ADP. Thromboelastography measures the clot's physical properties. The most important variables affecting clot strength are the fibrinogen concentration, platelet function, and platelet count. TEG has been successfully used to predict excessive bleeding and guide transfusion therapy during intraoperative bleeding.

Another means of assessing platelet dysfunction is by fluorescent flow cytometry. The measurement of specific serum markers of platelet activation such as beta-thromboglobulin and PF4 can be performed. However, the plasma collection techniques for these tests are cumbersome and the assays are often affected by other metabolic functions. Flow cytometry is ideal for dilution of low concentrations of specific protein within a large population of cells. These proteins may be either static portions of the platelet surface or dynamic products of platelet aggregation. Flow cytometry has helped in the diagnosis of disorders of platelet function. However, it is of questionable use during the management and diagnosis of intraoperative bleeding.

Abnormal or excessive bleeding during neurosurgical procedures could have devastating consequences. The use of hemostatic agents and alterations in hemodynamics may help to reduce this blood loss and allow the surgeon to identify and control the source of bleeding. If bleeding is excessive, blood salvage techniques may be utilized to reduce the amount of allogenic blood products received. Diagnostic techniques and point of care testing may also be utilized to help facilitate hemostasis and direct the administration of medication to help improve platelet function and reduce or inhibit thrombolysis. A coordinated effort with both the neurosurgeon and anesthesiologist actively involved will help to control and treat the blood loss and increase the chances of a successful outcome with minimized associated morbidity.

References

1. Braun H, Shields P. Local anesthesia: its scientific basis and practical use. Philadelphia: Lea & Febinger; 1914.
2. Cushing H. Technical methods of performing certain cranial operations. Surg Gynecol Obstet. 1908;6:227–46.
3. Frazier CH. Remarks upon the surgical aspects of operable tumors of the cerebrum. In: Mills CK, editor. Tumors of the cerebrum, their focal diagnosis, and surgical treatment. Philadelphia: Pennock; 1906.
4. Walker AE. A history of neurological surgery. New York: Hafner; 1967.
5. Horsley V. Antiseptic wax. Br Med J. 1892;1:1165.
6. Cushing H, Bovie WT. Electro-surgery as an aid to the removal of intracranial tumors. Surg Gynecol Obstet. 1928;47:752–84.
7. Stangerup SE, Thomsen HK. Histological changes in the nasal mucosa after hot-water irrigation. An animal experimental study. Rhinology. 1996;34:14–7.
8. Council on Pharmacy and Chemistry. Absorbable Gelatin sponge—new and nonofficial remedies. JAMA. 1947;135:921.
9. Gerald AG. Update on hemostasis: neurosurgery. Surgery. 2007;142:S55–60.
10. Herndon JH, Grillo HC, Risenborough EJ, et al. Compression of the brain and spinal cord following use of gelfoam. Arch Surg. 1972;104:107.
11. Friedman J, Whitecloud 3rd TS. Lumbar cauda equina syndrome associated with the use of gelfoam: case report. Spine. 2001;26:E485–7.
12. Abbot WM, Austen WG. The effectiveness and mechanism of collagen-induced topical hemostasis. Surgery. 1975;78:723–9.
13. Levy ML, Amar AP. The use of oxidized regenerated cellulose in neurosurgical procedures. Surg Technol Int. 1998;7:467–71.
14. Tschan CA, Nie M, Schwandt E, et al. Safety and efficacy of microporous polysaccharide hemospheres in neurosurgery. Neurosurgery. 2011;69(1 (Suppl Operative)):49–63.
15. Arand AG, Sawaya R. Intraoperative chemical hemostasis in neurosurgery. Neurosurgery. 1986;18:223–33.
16. Lew W, Weaver F. Clinical use of topical thrombin as a surgical hemostat. Biologics. 2008;2(4):593–9.
17. Streiff MB, Ness PM. Acquired FV inhibitors: a needless iatrogenic complication of bovine thrombin exposure. Transfusion. 2002;42:18–26.
18. Martinowitz U, Saltz R. Fibrin sealant. Curr Opin Hematol. 1996;3(5):395–402.
19. Shaffrey CI, Spotnitz WD, Shaffrey ME, et al. Neurosurgical applications of fibrin glue: augmentation of dural closure in 134 patients. Neurosurgery. 1990;26(2):207–10.
20. Oz MC, Rondinone JF, Shargill NS. FloSeal Matrix: new generation topical hemostatic sealant. J Card Surg. 2003;18:486–93.

21. Sollevi A. Hypotensive anesthesia and blood loss. Acta Anaesthesiol Scand Suppl. 1988;89:39–43.
22. Fahmy NM. Indications and contraindications for deliberate hypotension with a review of its cardiovascular effects. Int Anesthesiol Clin. 1979;17(1):175–87.
23. Shapiro HM. Physiology and pharmacologic regulation of cerebral blood flow. In: ASA refresher course in anesthesiology. Philadelphia, Pa: J.B. Lippincott; 1977. p. 161–78.
24. Pasch T, Huk W. Cerebral complications following induced hypotension. Eur J Anaesthesiol. 1986;3(4):299–312.
25. Hickey RF, Verrier ED, Baer RW, et al. A canine model of acute coronary artery stenosis: effects of deliberate hypotension. Anesthesiology. 1983;59(3):226–36.
26. Hartman JC, Kampine JP, Schmeling WT, et al. Steal-prone coronary circulation in chronically instrumented dogs: isoflurane versus adenosine. Anesthesiology. 1991;74(4):744–56.
27. Knight PR, Lane GA, Hensinger RN, et al. Catecholamine and renin-angiotensin response during hypotensive anesthesia induced by sodium nitroprusside or trimethaphan camsylate. Anesthesiology. 1983;59(3):248–53.
28. Fukayama H, Ito H, Shimada M, et al. Effects of hypotensive anesthesia on endocrine systems in oral surgery. Anesth Prog. 1989;36(4-5):175–7.
29. Dilger JA, Tetzlaff JE, Bell GR, et al. Ischaemic optic neuropathy after spinal fusion. Can J Anaesth. 1998;45(1):63–6.
30. Scott BH, Seifert FC, Glass PS, et al. Blood use in patients undergoing coronary artery bypass surgery: impact of cardiopulmonary bypass pump, hematocrit, gender, age and body weight. Anesth Analg. 2003;97:958–63.
31. Pierce LR, Gaines A, Varricchio F, et al. Hemolysis and renal failure associated with use of sterile water for injection to dilute 25% human albumin solution. Am J Health Syst Pharm. 1998;55:1057–70.
32. Boudreaux JP, Bornside GH, Cohn Jr I. Emergency autotransfusion: partial cleansing of bacteria-laden blood by cell washing. J Trauma. 1983;23:31–5.
33. Waters JH, Tuohy MJ, Hobson DF, et al. Bacterial reduction by cell salvage washing and leukocyte depletion filtration. Anesthesiology. 2003;99:652–5.
34. Bland LA, Villarino ME, Arduino MJ, et al. Bacteriologic and endotoxin analysis of salvaged blood used in autologous transfusions during cardiac operations. J Thorac Cardiovasc Surg. 1992;103:582–8.
35. Kang Y, Aggarwal S, Pasculle AW, et al. Bacteriologic study of autotransfusion during liver transplantation. Transplant Proc. 1989;21:35–8.
36. Smith RN, Yaw PB, Glover JL. Autotransfusion of contaminated Intraperitoneal blood: an experimental study. J Trauma. 1978;18:341–4.
37. Vamvakas EC. Perioperative blood transfusion and cancer recurrence: meta-analysis for explanation. Transfusion. 1995;35:760–8.
38. Fisher ER, Turnbull Jr RB. Cytologic demonstration and significance of tumor cells in the mesenteric venous blood in patients with colorectal carcinoma. Surg Gynecol Obstet. 1955;100:102–5.
39. Edelman MJ, Potter P, Mahaffey KG, et al. The potential for reintroduction of tumor cells during intraoperative blood salvage: reduction of risk with use of the RC-400 leukocyte depletion filter. Urology. 1996;47:179–81.
40. Perseghin P, Vigano M, Rocco G, et al. Effectiveness of leukocyte filters in reducing tumor cell contamination after intraoperative blood salvage in lung cancer patients. Vox Sang. 1997;72:221–4.
41. Smith DF, Mihm FG, Mefford I. Hypertension after intraoperative autotransfusion in bilateral adrenalectomy for pheochromocytoma. Anesthesiology. 1983;58:182–4.
42. Cash JD, Gader AMA, De Costa J. The release of plasminogen activator and factor VIII by LVP, AVP, DDAVP, AT III, and OT in man. Br J Haematol. 1984;30:363–4.
43. Cooney KA, Ginsburg D, Ruggeri ZM. von Willebrand disease. In: Loscalzo J, Schafer AL, editors. Thrombosis and hemorrhage. Boston, MA: Blackwell Scientific Publications; 1994. p. 657–82.
44. Mannucci PM, Remuzzi G, Pusineri F. Deamino-8-D-arginine vasopressin shortens the bleeding time in uremia. N Engl J Med. 1983;308:8–12.
45. Janssens M, Joris J, David JL, et al. High-dose aprotinin reduces blood loss in patients undergoing total hip replacement surgery. Anesthesiology. 1994;80:23–9.
46. Levi MM, Vink R, de Jonge E. Management of bleeding disorders by prohemostatic therapy. Int J Hematol. 2002;72 suppl 2:139–44.
47. Murkin JM, Lux J, Shannon NA, et al. Aprotinin significantly decreases bleeding and transfusion requirements in patients receiving aspirin and undergoing cardiac operations. J Thorac Cardiovasc Surg. 1994;107:554–61.
48. Tanaka K, Takao M, Yada I. Alterations in coagulation and fibrinolysis associated with cardiopulmonary bypass during open heart surgery. J Cardiothorac Anesth. 1989;3:181–8.
49. Davis R, Whittington R. Aprotinin: a review of its pharmacology and therapeutic efficacy in reducing blood loss associated with cardiac surgery. Drugs. 1995;49:954–83.
50. Rinder CS, Mathew JP, Ringer HM, et al. Modulation of platelet surface adhesion receptors during cardiopulmonary bypass. Anesthesiology. 1991;75:563–70.
51. Levy JH, Schwieger IM, Zaidan JR, et al. Evaluation of patients at risk for protamine reactions. J Thorac Cardiovasc Surg. 1989;98:200–4.
52. Stratmann G, Russell IA, Merrick SH. Use of recombinant factor VIIa as a rescue treatment for intractable

bleeding following repeat aortic arch repair. Ann Thorac Surg. 2003;76(6):2094–7.
53. Weiss EJ, Bray PF, Tayback M, et al. A polymorphism of a platelet glycoprotein receptor as an inherited risk factor for coronary thrombosis. N Engl J Med. 1996;334:1090–4.
54. Jobes DR, Schwartz AJ, Ellison N, et al. Monitoring heparin anti-coagulation and its neutralization. Ann Thorac Surg. 1981;31(2):161–6.
55. Gravlee GP, Rogers AT, Dudas LM, et al. Heparin management protocol for cardiopulmonary bypass influences postoperative heparin rebound but not bleeding. Anesthesiology. 1992;76(3):393–401.
56. Mongan PD, Hosking MP. The role of desmopressin acetate in patients undergoing coronary artery bypass surgery. A controlled clinical trial with thromboelestographic risk stratification. Anesthesiology. 1992;77(1):38–46.

Treatment of Disseminated Intravascular Coagulation (DIC)

13

Marcel Levi

Introduction

A variety of disorders, including (brain) trauma and injury but also infectious and inflammatory conditions or malignant disease, will lead to systemic activation of coagulation. In many cases, this activation of coagulation will not lead to clinical complications and will not even be detected by routine laboratory tests, but can only be measured with sensitive molecular markers for activation of coagulation factors and pathways [1, 2]. However, if activation of coagulation is sufficiently strong, the platelet count may decrease and global clotting times may become prolonged. In its most extreme form, systemic activation of coagulation is known as disseminated intravascular coagulation (DIC). DIC is characterized by the simultaneous occurrence of widespread (micro)vascular thrombosis, thereby compromising blood supply to various organs, which may contribute to organ failure [3, 4]. Because of ongoing activation of the coagulation system and other factors, such as impaired synthesis and increased degradation of coagulation proteins and protease inhibitors, consumption of clotting factors and platelets may occur, resulting in bleeding from various sites.

The diagnosis of DIC may be hampered by the nonspecific nature of many indicators of coagulation activation, although newly developed scoring algorithms based on readily available routine laboratory parameters show promising diagnostic accuracy [5]. Owing to the complexity of the clinical presentation, the variable and unpredictable course, and the multitude of therapies given to patients with DIC, properly conducted clinical trials are difficult to perform and even to devise. Management relies on limited evidence from clinical trials in combination with small studies employing surrogate outcome endpoints and experience from case series, as well as from an understanding of the underlying pathophysiologic mechanisms [6].

Epidemiology

Activation of coagulation in concert with trauma and associated inflammatory activation can result in microvascular thrombosis [7, 8]. In support of this concept, postmortem findings in patients with coagulation abnormalities and DIC include diffuse bleeding, hemorrhagic necrosis of tissues, microthrombi in small blood vessels and thrombi in mid-size and larger arteries and veins. Ischemia and necrosis was invariably the result of fibrin deposition in small and mid-size vessels.

M. Levi, M.D. (✉)
Department of Medicine, Academic Medical Center, University of Amsterdam, Meibergdreef 9, 1105 AZ Amsterdam, The Netherlands
e-mail: m.m.levi@amc.uva.nl

C.M. Loftus (ed.), *Anticoagulation and Hemostasis in Neurosurgery*,
DOI 10.1007/978-3-319-27327-3_13

Importantly, intravascular thrombi appear to be the driver of the organ dysfunction. Fibrin deposition in various organs also is a characteristic finding in animal models of DIC. Thus, experimental traumatic (brain) injury or bacteremia causes intravascular and extravascular fibrin deposition in the kidneys, lungs, liver, brain, and other organs [9]. Amelioration of the hemostatic defect by various interventions in these models reduces fibrin deposition, improves organ function and, in some cases, reduces mortality. Finally, results of clinical studies also support the concept that activation of coagulation is as important a determinant of clinical outcome. DIC has shown to be an independent predictor of organ failure and mortality [10]. In a consecutive series of patients with severe sepsis, 43 % of patients with DIC were compared with 27 % in those without DIC. In this study, the severity of the coagulopathy was also directly related to mortality [11].

In addition to microvascular thrombosis and organ dysfunction, coagulation abnormalities may have other harmful consequences. Thrombocytopenia in patients with trauma places them at increased risk of bleeding. Overall, critically ill patients with a platelet count of $<50\times10^9$/L have a four- to fivefold higher risk for bleeding as those with higher platelet counts [12]. Although the overall risk of intracerebral bleeding in patients in the ICU is less than 0.5 %, up to 88 % of patients with this complication have platelet counts less than 100×10^9/L. The use of anticoagulants in patients with thrombocytopenia further increases the risk of bleeding. Regardless of the cause, multivariate analyses indicate that thrombocytopenia is an independent predictor of ICU mortality and increases the risk of death by 1.9- to 4.2-fold. In particular, thrombocytopenia that persists more than 4 days after ICU admission, or 50 % or greater decrease in platelet count during the ICU stay, is associated with a four- to sixfold increase in mortality. In fact, the platelet count appears to be a stronger predictor for ICU mortality than composite scoring systems, such as the Acute Physiology and Chronic Evaluation (APACHE) II or Multiple Organ Dysfunction Score (MODS). Decreased levels of coagulation factors, as reflected by prolonged global coagulation times, also increase the risk of bleeding. Prolongation of the prothrombin time (PT) or activated partial thromboplastin time (aPTT) to over 1.5 times the control is associated with an increased risk of bleeding and mortality in critically ill patients.

Pathobiology

Traditionally, DIC was thought to be the result of activation of both the extrinsic and intrinsic pathways of coagulation. The classical concept was that the extrinsic pathway was initiated by a tissue-derived component, which activated factor VII, leading to the direct conversion of prothrombin to thrombin. This process would proceed as long as there was tissue damage from systemic infection, trauma, solutio placentae, or malignancy. In contrast, the intrinsic or contact pathway of coagulation was initiated by contact activation of factor XII which, together with its cofactors, kallikrein and kininogen, then activated factor XI with subsequent activation of factor IX. The initiators of contact activation were poorly understood until recently, but were thought to include collagen and artificial surfaces. In recent years, the molecular mechanisms of coagulation pathways have been defined (Fig. 13.1). This has provided new insight into the pathogenesis of DIC. In general, current thinking is that thrombin and fibrin generation in patients with DIC is largely driven via the extrinsic pathway; as the brain is a rich source of tissue factor in brain injury the role of tissue factor as initiator of coagulation activation is obvious. The role of the contact (kallikrein-factor XII) system in brain injury remains uncertain [9, 13].

Tissue Factor–Factor VII(a) Pathway

The extrinsic pathway is initiated by the tissue factor (TF)–factor VIIa complex. TF is a membrane-bound 4.5kD protein that is constitutively expressed

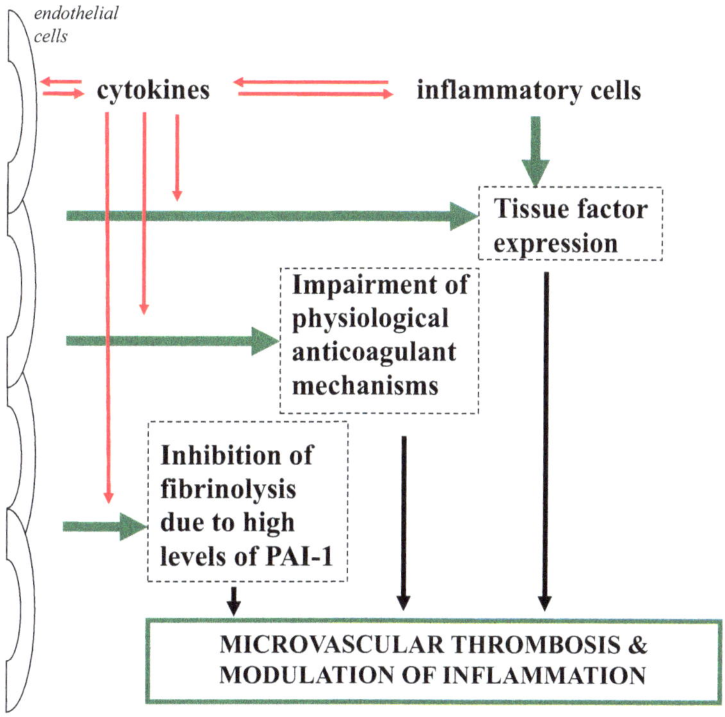

Fig. 13.1 Pathogenesis of disseminated intravascular coagulation. Pathways involved in the activation of coagulation in DIC. Both perturbed endothelial cells and activated mononuclear cells may produce proinflammatory cytokines that induce tissue factor expression, thereby initiating coagulation. In addition, downregulation of physiological anticoagulant mechanisms and inhibition of fibrinolysis promotes intravascular fibrin deposition. PAI-1: plasminogen activator inhibitor, type 1

on cells that are mostly in tissues not in direct contact with blood, such as the adventitial layer of larger blood vessels [12]. Subcutaneous tissue also contains substantial amounts of TF. When expressed on the cell surface, TF interacts with factor VII, either in its zymogen or activated form. The TF–factor VIIa complex catalyzes the activation of both factor IX and factor X. Factors IXa and Xa enhance the activation of factors X and prothrombin, respectively. In cells in contact with the blood circulation, TF is induced by the action of mediators such as cytokines, C reactive protein, and advanced glycosylation end products. Inducible TF is predominantly expressed by monocytes and macrophages. Monocyte TF expression is enhanced in the presence of platelets and granulocytes in a P-selectin dependent fashion. This may reflect NFkB activation that occurs when activated platelets bind to neutrophils or mononuclear cells. These cell–cell interactions also stimulate the production of IL-1b, IL-8, MCP-1, and TNFa. Under cell culture conditions, cytokines such as TNFa, and IL-1, can induce TF expression by vascular endothelial cells, but the in vivo relevance of this finding is uncertain. Studies in vivo suggest that IL-6 is the dominant mediator of TF expression by mononuclear cells.

With trauma, such as extensive surgery, brain injury, or burns, it is likely that constitutively expressed TF at the site of injury is the primary source of procoagulant material. Increased monocyte TF expression and procoagulant activity has been demonstrated in DIC associated with sepsis, cancer, or coronary disease. Tissue expression of TF appears to be localized to certain organs and vascular beds, but it is uncertain whether its expression is under genetic control in an organ-specific fashion.

Cytokines and Other Amplification Pathways

Activation of blood coagulation requires several cofactors. For development of DIC, the surfaces of cell remnants or intact cells, inflammatory mediators, and coagulation proteins are required. The stimulus for activation depends on the underlying disease and may range from bacterial cell compounds, such as endotoxin, TF on host or cancer cells, other cancer cell procoagulants, TF or fat or amniotic fluid emboli by unknown pathways. Each of these triggers interacts with other mediators: TF assembles on anionic phospholipid surfaces, which can be provided by activated platelets, leukocytes or by cancer cells, cytokines interact with receptors and induce signaling pathways that induce TF expression and other proinflammatory components via the NFκB complex.

The molecular mechanisms underlying endotoxin-induced activation of coagulation have been studied in primates and baboons. In endotoxin or *E. coli* models of sepsis, inhibition of the TF pathway abolishes the activation of coagulation, highlighting the importance of TF. IL-6 is an important mediator of procoagulant effects, whereas TNFa is involved in the fibrinolytic response to endotoxin. Inhibition of TF with TFPI reduces IL-6 levels in the baboon model, suggesting that there is extensive cross talk between coagulation and inflammatory mediators (see below). Monocytes that express TF bind factor VII(a), shed TF, or bind to the damaged vessel wall. After interacting with platelets, circulating monocytes may trigger DIC. Microvesicles may accelerate this process, and the complex interaction between cells, membrane fragments, soluble mediators, and proteins may trigger the DIC syndrome. The severity and duration of the consumptive process are mainly determined by the potency of the triggers and the capacity of inhibitory mechanisms.

Cross Talk Among Coagulation Proteases Results in Pro-inflammatory Effects

In addition to activating coagulation protein zymogens, coagulation proteases also interact with specific cell receptors and trigger signaling pathways that elicit pro-inflammatory mediators [8]. Factor Xa, thrombin and the factor VIIa–TF complex have such effects. Factor Xa injection into rats induces localized inflammation, probably as a result of its interaction with EPR-1 and not because of thrombin generation. Exposure of cultured endothelial cells to factor Xa stimulates the production of monocyte chemotactic protein 1 (MCP-1), and IL-6 and IL-8, and upregulates the expression of adhesion proteins that tether neutrophils to the cell surface. Further evidence for the cross talk between inflammation and coagulation comes from the observations that IL-6 and IL-8 elicit TF-dependent procoagulant activity in monocytes and IL-6 has been identified as the critical mediator of procoagulant activity either on its own or after endotoxin challenge in vivo. Therefore, cytokine production induced by factor Xa may be an important driver of coagulation in DIC.

In addition to its procoagulant functions, thrombin has a variety of non-coagulant effects. Thrombin induces the release of MCP-1 and IL-6 from fibroblasts, epithelial cells, and mononuclear cells in vitro. Thrombin also induces IL-6 and IL-8 production in endothelial cells. When generated in whole blood, IL-8 production, which has a procoagulant effect that is TF dependent. Cell activation by thrombin is likely mediated by protease activated receptor. The factor VIIa–TF complex also activates cells by binding PAR 2.

Direct evidence of the in vivo relevance of these phenomena comes from a study showing that recombinant factor VIIa infusion in volunteers induces an increase in plasma levels of IL-6 and IL-8. Although the concentrations of factor VIIa infused far exceed those found in patients with sepsis, it is possible that factor VIIa-induced cytokine production is of physiological importance. Thus, this information adds to the concept that several coagulation proteases induce pro-inflammatory mediators that augment procoagulant activity and amplify the consumptive process. Endogenous anticoagulant pathways are essential to regulate these proteases and prevent uncontrolled DIC.

Endogenous Anticoagulant Pathways in DIC

The development of DIC is counteracted by several mechanisms. First, coagulation inhibitors regulate the coagulation mechanism. Those inhibitors include antithrombin (AT), the protein C system, and tissue factor pathway inhibitor (TFPI) (Fig. 13.2) [8]. AT, which complexes and inhibits thrombin and factor Xa, is one of the

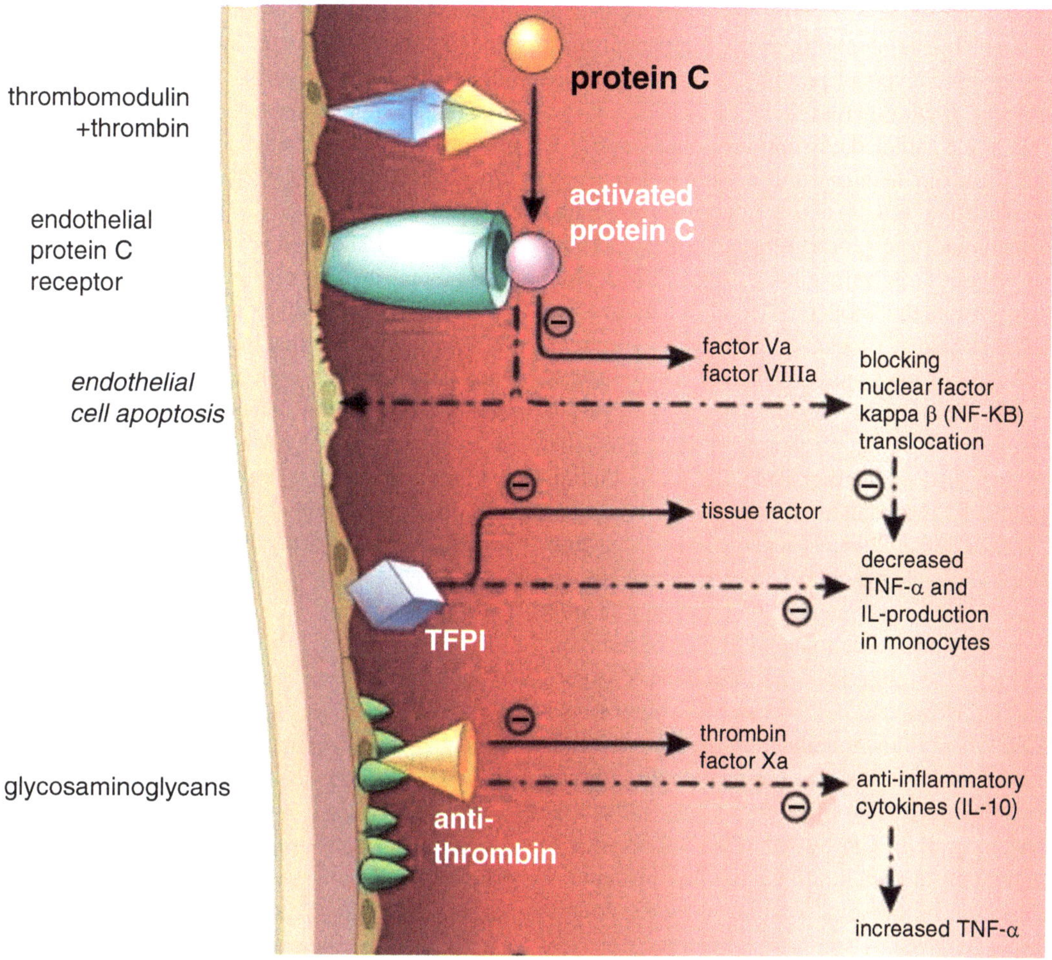

Fig. 13.2 Physiological anticoagulant mechanisms in DIC. Physiological anticoagulant mechanisms (activated protein C system, tissue factor pathway inhibitor (TFPI), and antithrombin) are not only involved in blocking thrombin generation and thrombin activity but also affect inflammatory pathways

most important inhibitors, and reduced AT levels are a characteristic of DIC. Reduction in AT levels reflects a combination of reduced protein synthesis as well as increased clearance through the formation of protease-AT complexes, and by degradation by neutrophil elastase. In addition, cytokines may impair proteoglycan synthesis in the vessel wall thereby reducing the availability of heparin sulfate for potentiation of AT activity.

Activated protein C and its cofactor protein S form a second line of defense. Thrombin binds to the endothelial cell membrane associated molecule thrombomodulin, and this complex converts protein C to its active form, activated protein C (APC) [14]. In addition, the thrombin–thrombomodulin complex accelerates the conversion of the thrombin activatable fibrinolytic inhibitor (TAFI). APC activates factors Va and VIIIa by proteolytic cleavage, thus slowing down the coagulation cascade. Endothelial cells, primarily of large blood vessels, express an endothelial protein C receptor (EPCR), which augments the activation of protein C at the cell surface. Activated protein C has anti-inflammatory effects on mononuclear cells and granulocytes, which may be distinct from its anticoagulant activity. Administration of APC prevented thrombin-induced thromboembolism in mice, mainly through its antithrombotic effect. In addition, several studies have demonstrated anti-inflammatory effects of APC.

In contrast, defects in the protein C mechanism enhance the vulnerability to DIC. In patient studies lowered levels of protein C and protein S are associated with increased mortality. Mice with a one allele targeted disruption of the protein C gene, causing heterozygous protein C deficiency, displayed a more severe DIC and associated inflammatory response. Blockade of the activity of protein C by infusion of C4 binding protein turns a sublethal model of *E. coli* in baboons into a lethal model. Blockade of EPCR by a neutralizing monoclonal antibody also increased mortality in the *E. coli* baboon model. Vice versa, infusion of PC in the same model, protected against DIC and dying. Thus, it appears that the protein C mechanism is of great importance in the host defense against sepsis and DIC. In situations associated with DIC and systemic inflammation, TNFa and interleukin-1 may significantly downregulate the cellular expression of thrombomodulin, as suggested by cell culture experiments. However, in vivo studies suggest that EPCR is not downregulated in sepsis, but upregulated and that this effect is mediated by thrombin. The formation of thrombin may induce the shedding of EPCR by the endothelium, due to activation of metalloproteinases by thrombin. It is presently unknown whether thrombomodulin is also cleaved by similar mechanisms.

A third inhibitory mechanism constitutes tissue factor pathway inhibitor (TFPI). This molecule, which exists in several pools (either endothelial cell associated or lipoprotein bound in plasma), inhibits the TF–factor VIIa complex by forming a quaternary complex in which factor Xa is the fourth component. Clinical studies in septic patients have not provided clues as to its importance, because in the majority of patients the levels of TFPI are not diminished as compared to normals. This may be explained by the lack of downregulatory effects of inflammatory mediators on cultured endothelial cells. The relevance of TFPI in DIC is illustrated by two lines of experimentation. First, the depletion of TFPI sensitized rabbits to DIC induced with tissue factor infusion. Second, TFPI infusion protected against the harmful effects of *E. coli* in primates. In this second study, TFPI not only blocked DIC but all baboons challenged with lethal amounts of *E. coli* showed a marked improvement in . vital functions and survived the experiment without apparent complications. An experimental study in volunteers confirmed the potential of TFPI to block the procoagulant pathway triggered by endotoxin.

In general, the presence of intact function and normal plasma levels of inhibitors appears to be important in the defense against DIC. It should be noted, however, that there are no strong indications that human with congenital deficiencies of inhibitors would suffer a greater chance of developing DIC, but this issue remains to be explored. In addition, the influence of inhibitors in modifying the interaction between coagulation and inflammation deserves further attention.

Fibrinolysis

In experimental models of DIC fibrinolysis is activated, demonstrated by an initial activation of plasminogen activation, followed by a marked impairment caused by the release in blood of plasminogen activator inhibitor, type 1 (PAI-1). The latter inhibitor strongly inhibits fibrinolysis causing a net procoagulant situation. The molecular basis is cytokine-mediated activation of vascular endothelial cells; TNFα and Il-1 decreased tPA and increased PAI-1 production. TNFa increased uPA production in endothelial cells. Endotoxin and TNFα stimulated PAI-1 production in liver, kidney, lung and adrenals of mice. The net procoagulant state is illustrated by a late rise in fibrin breakdown fragments after *E. coli* challenge of baboons. Experimental data also indicate that the fibrinolytic mechanism is active in clearing fibrin from organs and circulation. Endotoxin induced fibrin formation in kidneys and adrenals was most dependent on a decrease in urokinase type plasminogen activator (uPA). PAI-1 knockout mice challenged with endotoxin did not develop thrombi in the kidney in contrast to wild type animals. Endotoxin administration to mice with a functionally inactive thrombomodulin gene (TMProArg mutation) and defective protein C activator cofactor function caused fibrin plugs in the pulmonary circulation, while wild type animals did not develop macroscopic fibrin. This phenomenon proved to be temporary, with detectable thrombi at 4 h after endotoxin, and disappearance of clots at 24 h in animals sacrificed at that timepoint. These experiments demonstrate that fibrinolytic action is required to reduce the extent of intravascular fibrin formation.

Fibrinolytic activity is markedly regulated by PAI-1, the principal inhibitor of this system. Recent studies have shown that a functional mutation in the PAI-1 gene, the 4G/5G polymorphism, not only influenced the plasma levels of PAI-1, but was also linked to clinical outcome of meningococcal septicemia. Patients with the 4G/4G genotype had significantly higher PAI-1 concentrations in plasma and an increased risk of death. Further investigations demonstrated that the PAI-1 polymorphism did not influence the risk of contracting meningitis as such, but probably increased the likelihood of developing septic shock from meningococcal infection. These studies are the first evidence that genetically determined differences in the level of fibrinolysis influences the risk of developing complications of a gram-negative infection. In other clinical studies in cohorts of patients with DIC, high plasma levels of PAI-1 were one of the best predictors of mortality. These data suggest that DIC contributes to mortality in this situation, but as indicated earlier, the fact that PAI-1 is an acute phase protein, a higher plasma concentration may also be a marker of disease rather than a causal factor.

Clinical Manifestations

The clinical manifestation of DIC may vary dependent on the underlying disorder. The extreme end of the spectrum is acute, severe DIC, which often occurs in the setting of major trauma, brain injury, sepsis, obstetric calamities, and severe immunologic responses. Diffuse multiorgan bleeding, hemorrhagic necrosis, microthrombi in small blood vessels, and thrombi had unequivocal clinical and laboratory signs of DIC may not have confirming postmortem findings. Conversely, some patients in whom clinical and laboratory signs were not consistent with DIC had typical autopsy findings. This occasional lack of correlation among clinical, laboratory, and pathologic findings is partly due to extensive postmortem changes in the blood for example, excessive fibrinolysis, but remains unexplained in most instances. Organs most frequently involved by diffuse microthrombi are the lungs and kidneys, followed by the brain, heart, liver, spleen, adrenal glands, pancreas, and gut. Specific immunohistological techniques and ultrastructural analysis have revealed that most thrombi consist of fibrin monomers or polymers in combination with platelets. In addition, involvement of activated mononuclear cells and other signs of inflammatory activation are frequently present. In cases of long lasting DIC, organization and endothelialization of the microthrombi are often observed. Acute tubular necrosis is more frequent than renal cortical necrosis. Clinically, thrombotic occlusive events occur first, as the result of microthrombi of fibrin or platelets that obstruct the microcirculation of organs. These thrombi result from clots that form either in the circulation or in situ in arterioles, capillaries, or venules. Circulatory obstruction produces organ hypoperfusion and even ischemia, infarction, and necrosis. The process is disseminated throughout the microcirculation; therefore, all organs are potentially vulnerable.

In contrast to the acutely ill patient with complicated, severe DIC, other patients may have mild or protracted clinical manifestations of consumption or even subclinical disease manifest by only laboratory abnormalities [1]. The clinical picture of subacute to chronic DIC generally occurs in patients with malignancy, in particular with mucin-producing adenocarcinomas and APL. The latter usually is dominated by a hemorrhagic presentation, whereas venous thrombotic manifestations are more common in the former. In addition, patients with solid tumors may develop nonbacterial thrombotic endocarditis with systemic arterial embolization and infarction. Another cause of subacute to chronic DIC is the retained dead fetus syndrome. These patients

Table 13.1 Clinical conditions that are most frequently complicated by DIC

• Trauma/brain injury
• Sepsis/severe infection
• Malignancy
– Solid tumors
– Hematological malignancies
• Obstetrical conditions
– Amniotic fluid embolism
– Abruptio placentae
• Vascular abnormalities
– Kasabach–Merrit syndrome
– Other vascular malformations
– large aneurysms
• Severe allergic/toxic reactions
• Severe immunologic reactions (e.g., transfusion reaction)

have an extremely variable presentation from asymptomatic to mild or moderate skin and mucous membrane bleeding.

It is important to stress that DIC is not a disease in itself but is always secondary to an underlying disorder that causes the activation of coagulation. The underlying disorders most commonly known to be associated with DIC are listed in Table 13.1.

DIC in Neurosurgical Patients

In adults and children with head injuries, a high rate of mortality occurred when DIC was present. A laboratory DIC score has predictive value for prognosis in patients with head injuries, thereby supplementing the Glasgow coma score. Brain injury can be associated with DIC, most likely because the injury exposes the abundant TF of brain to blood. Specimens of contused brain, obtained during surgery in patients with head injury and of liver, lungs, kidneys, and pancreas obtained during autopsy, revealed microthrombi in arterioles and venules [15].

Trauma and Traumatic Brain Injury

Early trauma death is often due to coagulopathy and bleeding complications [16]. The time interval between trauma and medical intervention correlates with the development and magnitude of DIC. Experience during wars proved that fast evacuation and prompt medical care reduce the risk of DIC. Extensive exposure of TF to the blood circulation and hemorrhagic shock probably are the most immediate triggers of DIC in such instances, although direct proof of this mechanism is lacking [17, 18]. An alternative hypothesis is that cytokines play a pivotal role in the occurrence of DIC in trauma patients. In fact, the changes in cytokine levels are virtually identical in trauma patients and septic patients [19, 20]. The levels of TNF-α, IL-1β, PAI-1, circulating TF, plasma elastase derived from neutrophils, and soluble thrombomodulin all can be elevated in patients with signs of DIC, predicting MOD (ARDS included) and death [21, 22]. Careful monitoring of laboratory signs of DIC, reduced fibrinolytic activity, and perhaps low AT levels also are useful for predicting the outcome of such patients [23].

Laboratory Manifestations

Thrombocytopenia or a rapidly declining platelet count is an important diagnostic hallmark of DIC. However, only 35–44 % of critically ill patients develop thrombocytopenia (platelet count $<150\times10^9$/L). Consequently, the specificity of thrombocytopenia for the diagnosis of DIC is limited [12]. A platelet count of $<100\times10^9$/L is seen in 50–60 % of DIC patients, whereas 10–15 % of patients have a platelet count $<50\times10^9$/L. In surgical or trauma patients with DIC, over 80 % of patients have platelet counts less than 100×10^9/L. In traumatic brain injury an early occurring platelet dysfunction had been described as well [24].

Consumption of coagulation factors leads to low levels of coagulation factors in patients with DIC. In addition, impaired synthesis, for example due to impaired liver function or a vitamin K deficiency, and loss of coagulation proteins, due to massive bleeding, may play a role in DIC as well. Although the accuracy of the measurement of one-stage clotting assays in DIC has been contested (due to the presence of activated coagulation factors in plasma), the level of coagulation factors appears to correlate well with the severity of the DIC. The low level of coagulation factors is reflected by prolonged coagulation screening tests, such as the prothrombin time (PT) or the activated partial thromboplastin time (aPTT). A prolonged PT or aPTT occurs in 14–28 % of intensive care patients but is present in more than 95 % of patients with DIC.

Plasma levels of factor VIII are paradoxically increased in most patients with DIC, probably due to massive release of von Willebrand factor from the endothelium in combination with acute phase behavior of factor VIII. Recent studies have pointed to a relative insufficiency of the von Willebrand cleaving protease ADAMTS-13, thereby causing high concentrations of ultralarge von Willebrand multimers in plasma, which may facilitate platelet–vessel wall interaction and the subsequent development of thrombotic microangiopathy, which may contribute to organ dysfunction [25].

Measurement of fibrinogen has been widely advocated as a useful tool for the diagnosis of DIC but in fact is not very helpful to diagnose DIC in most cases [26]. Fibrinogen acts as an acute-phase reactant and despite ongoing consumption plasma levels can remain well within the normal range for a long period of time. In a consecutive series of patients the sensitivity of a low fibrinogen level for the diagnosis of DIC was only 28 % and hypofibrinogenemia was detected in very severe cases of DIC only.

Markers of Fibrin Generation and Degradation

Plasma levels of fibrin split products are frequently used for the diagnosis of DIC [27]. Fibrin split products are detectable in 42 % of a consecutive series of intensive care patients, in 80 % of trauma patients and in 99 % of patients with sepsis and DIC. Fibrin degradation products (FDP's) may be detected by specific ELISA's or by latex agglutination assays, allowing rapid and bed-side determination in emergency cases. None of the available assays for fibrin degradation products discriminates between degradation products of cross-linked fibrin and fibrinogen degradation, which may cause spuriously high results. The specificity of high levels of fibrin degradation products is therefore limited and many other conditions, such as trauma, recent surgery, inflammation or venous thromboembolism, are associated with elevated FDP's. Because FDPs are metabolized by the liver and secreted by the kidneys, FDP levels are influenced by liver and kidney function. Other tests are specifically aimed at the detection of neo-antigens on degraded cross-linked fibrin. One of such tests detects an epitope related to plasmin-degraded cross-linked γ-chain, resulting in fragment D-dimer. These tests better differentiate degradation of cross-linked fibrin from fibrinogen or fibrinogen degradation products. D-dimer levels are high in patients with DIC, but also poorly distinguish patients with DIC from patients with venous thromboembolism, recent surgery or inflammatory conditions. Theoretically, measurement of soluble fibrin or fibrin monomers in plasma could be helpful to diagnose intravascular fibrin formation in DIC. Indeed, initial clinical studies indicate that if the concentration of soluble fibrin has increased above a defined threshold, a diagnosis of DIC can be made. The only problem so far is that a reliable test is not available for quantitating soluble fibrin in plasma. Since soluble fibrin in plasma can only be generated intravascularly, this test will not be influenced by extravascular fibrin formation, which for example may occur during local inflammation or trauma.

Endogenous Coagulation Inhibitors

Antithrombin is the principal inhibitor of thrombin and may be readily exhausted during continuous thrombin generation. Patients with brain injury may present with low levels of antithrombin {Genet, 2013 6578 /id} {Nekludov, 2007 6581 /id}. Plasma levels of antithrombin have been shown to be potent predictors for survival in patients with DIC. During severe inflammatory responses, antithrombin levels are markedly decreased not only due to consumption but also due to impaired synthesis (as a result of a negative acute phase response) and degradation by elastase from activated neutrophils.

Plasma levels of physiological coagulation inhibitors, such as protein C or antithrombin may be useful indicators of ongoing coagulation activation [27]. Low levels of these coagulation inhibitors are found in 40–60 % of critically ill patients and in 90 % of DIC patients. Levels of protein C may indicate the severity of the DIC. In patients with meningococcal septicemia, very low plasma levels of protein C are observed and this may play a pivotal role in the occurrence of purpura fulminans in these patients. In fact, also the plasma level of protein C may be regarded as a strong predictor for the outcome in DIC patients. Observations in patients with severe gram-negative septicemia indeed confirmed the downregulation of thrombomodulin in vivo and impaired activation of protein C. Low levels of free protein S (the cofactor of activated protein C) may further compromise an adequate function of the protein C system.

Fibrinolytic Markers

Fibrinolytic activation in DIC may be monitored by measurement of plasma levels of plasminogen and α2-antiplasmin. Low levels may indicate consumption of these proteins. In brain injury a deficiency of antiplasmin was shown to play a crucial role {Reed, 2014 6582 /id}. Due to the relatively low plasma concentration of α2-antiplasmin, the determination of this protease inhibitor is a helpful test for judging the dynamics of fibrinolysis. Plasmin generation may be best judged by measurement of plasmin–α2-antiplasmin (PAP) complexes, which are indeed moderately elevated in patients with DIC. However, because the concentration of α2-antiplasmin is relatively low and therefore sensitive to relatively rapid exhaustion, this test may underestimate total fibrinolytic activity. At low concentrations of α2-antiplasmin, other protease inhibitors, such as antithrombin, α2-macroglobulin, α1-antitrypsin, and C1-inhibitor may act as plasmin inhibitor as well. The apparent insufficient fibrinolytic activity in patients with DIC is attributed to high levels of the inhibitor of plasminogen activation, plasminogen activator inhibitor type I (PAI-1). Indeed, plasma levels of PAI-1 are elevated in patients with DIC and various underlying conditions, and are strongly correlated with an unfavorable outcome. Of interest, studies have shown that a functional mutation in the PAI-1 gene, the 4G/5G polymorphism, not only influenced the plasma levels of PAI-1, but was also linked to clinical outcome of meningococcal septicaemia and associated DIC. Patients with the 4G/4G genotype had significantly higher PAI-1 concentrations in plasma and an increased risk of death.

Point of Care Tests

Thrombelastography (TEG) is a method that has been developed decades ago and provides an overall picture of ex vivo coagulation. Modern techniques, such as rotational thrombelastography (ROTEM) enable bedside performance of this test and has again become popular recently in acute care settings, including brain trauma [28] {Tauber, 2011 6579 /id}. The theoretical advantage of TEG over conventional coagulation assays is that is provides an idea of platelet function as well as fibrinolytic activity. Hypercoagulability and hypocoagulability as demonstrated with TEG was shown to correlate with clinically relevant morbidity and mortality in several studies, although its superiority over conventional tests has not unequivocally been established. Also, TEG seems to be overly sensitive to some interventions in the coagulation system, such as administration of fibrinogen, of which the therapeutic benefit remains to be established. There are no systematic studies on the diagnostic accuracy of TEG for the diagnosis of DIC, however, the test may be useful for assessing the global status of the coagulation system in critically ill patients.

Table 13.2 Diagnostic algorithm for the diagnosis of overt DIC[a]

1. Presence of an underlying disorder known to be associated with DIC	
(no = 0, yes = 2)	
2. Score global coagulation test results	
• Platelet count *(>100 = 0; <100 = 1; <50 = 2)*	
• Level of fibrin markers (e.g., D-dimer, fibrin degradation products)	
(no increase: 0; moderate increase: 2; strong increase: 3)[b]	
• Prolonged prothrombin time	
(<3 s. = 0; > 3 s. but < 6 s. = 1; > 6 s. = 2)	
• Fibrinogen level	
(>1.0 g/L = 0; < 1.0 g/L = 1)	
3. Calculate score	
4. If ≥ 5: compatible with overt DIC; repeat scoring daily	
If < 5: suggestive (not affirmative) for non-overt DIC; repeat next 1–2 days	

[a]According to the Scientific Standardization Committee of the International Society of Thrombosis and Haemostasis [5]

[b]Strong increase > 5× upper limit of normal; moderate increase is > upper limit of normal but <5× upper limit of normal

Diagnostic Algorithm for DIC

For the diagnosis of overt DIC a simple scoring system has been developed by the subcommittee on DIC of the International Society on Thrombosis and Hemostasis (ISTH) (Table 13.2) [5]. The score can be calculated based on routinely available laboratory tests, i.e., platelet count, prothrombin time, a fibrin-related marker (usually D-dimer), and fibrinogen. Tentatively, a score of 5 or more is compatible with DIC, whereas a score of less than 5 may be indicative but is *not* affirmative for non-overt DIC. For non-overt DIC more refined scoring systems have been developed, which are currently being evaluated. A recent study showed that the INR can be used (instead of PT prolongation), further facilitating international exchange and standardization. By using receiver-operating characteristics curves, an optimal cutoff for a quantitative D-dimer assay was determined, thereby optimizing sensitivity and the negative predictive value of the system. Prospective studies show that the sensitivity of the DIC score is 93 %, and the specificity is 98 %. Studies in series of patients with specific underlying disorders causing DIC (e.g., cancer patients or patients with obstetric complications) show similar results. The severity of DIC according to this scoring system is related to the mortality in patients with sepsis [11]. Linking prognostic determinants from critical care measurement scores such as Acute Physiology and Chronic Health Evaluation (APACHE-II) to DIC scores is an important means to assess prognosis in critically ill patients. Similar scoring systems have been developed and extensively evaluated in Japan. The major difference between the international and Japanese scoring systems seems a slightly higher sensitivity of the Japanese algorithm, although this may be due to different patient populations as Japanese series typically include relatively large numbers of patients with hematological malignancies.

Therapy

Adequate management of patients with DIC depends on vigorous treatment of the underlying disorder to alleviate or remove the inciting injurious cause. For sepsis-induced DIC, treatment includes aggressive use of intravenous organism-directed antibiotics and source control (e.g., by surgery or drainage). Other examples of vigorous treatment of underlying conditions are cancer surgery or chemotherapy, uterus evacuation in patients with abruptio placentae, resection of aortic aneurysm, and debridement of crushed tissue

Table 13.3 Mainstays of supportive treatment of DIC

Modality	Details	Expectations/rationale
Treating the underlying disorder	Dependent on the primary diagnosis	Inhibit or block the complicating pathologic mechanism of DIC in parallel with the response (if any) of the disorder
Antithrombotic agents	Prophylactic heparin to prevent venous thromboembolic complications (Low dose) therapeutic heparin in case of confirmed thromboembolism or if clinical picture is dominated by (micro) vascular thrombosis and associated organ failure	Risk of thromboembolism is increased in critically ill patients, trauma patients, or patients with cancer Prevent fibrin formation; tip the balance within the microcirculation toward anticoagulant mechanisms and physiologic fibrinolysis; allow reperfusion of the skin, kidneys, and brain
Transfusion	Infuse platelets, plasma and fibrinogen (cryoprecipitate) if there is overt bleeding or a high risk of bleeding	Bleeding should diminish and stop over the course of hours Platelet count, coagulation tests and fibrinogen should return toward normal
Anticoagulant Factor Concentrates	Recombinant human activated protein C may be effective in sepsis and DIC (24 μg/kg/h for 4 days)	Restore anticoagulation in microvascular environment and may have anti-inflammatory activity
Fibrinolytic inhibitors	Tranexamic acid (e.g., 500–1000 mg-q8–12 h or ε-aminocaproic acid 1000–2000 mg q8–12 h)	May be useful if there is (hyper) fibrinolysis Bleeding ceases, but there is a risk of microvascular thrombosis and renal failure

in case of trauma. In addition of intensive support of vital functions supportive treatment aimed at the coagulopathy may be helpful (Table 13.3) [6], as outlined in the following:

Platelet and Plasma Transfusion

Low levels of platelets and coagulation factors may increase the risk of bleeding. However, plasma or platelet substitution therapy should not be instituted on the basis of laboratory results alone; it is indicated only in patients with active bleeding and in those requiring an invasive procedure or who are at risk for bleeding complications [6]. The presumed efficacy of treatment with plasma, fibrinogen concentrate, cryoprecipitate, or platelets is not based on randomized controlled trials but appears to be rational therapy in bleeding patients or in patients at risk of bleeding who have a significant depletion of these hemostatic factors. The suggestion that administration of blood components might "add fuel to the fire" has never been proven in clinical or experimental studies.

Replacement therapy for thrombocytopenia should consist of 5–10 U platelet concentrate to raise the platelet count to $20–30 \times 10^9$/L and in cases in patients who need an invasive procedure, to 50×10^9/L.

One of the major challenges of infusion of fresh-frozen plasma in DIC and bleeding, which is necessary to correct the coagulation defect, is the propensity of the added volume to exacerbate capillary leak. This situation can increase the risk of inducing or worsening pulmonary edema and, by extension, can predispose to ARDS, and can induce ascites. Coagulation factor concentrates, such as prothrombin complex concentrate, may partially overcome this obstacle, but do not contain essential factors, such as factor V. Moreover, caution is advocated with the use of prothrombin complex concentrates in DIC, because it may worsen the coagulopathy due to traces of activated factors that are present in these concentrates. Specific deficiencies of coagulation factors, such as fibrinogen, may be corrected by administration of purified coagulation factor concentrates.

Cryoprecipitate (if available) can be used to rapidly raise the fibrinogen and von Willebrand/factor VIII levels, particularly when bleeding is part of the DIC and fibrinogen level is less than 1 g/L. Cryoprecipitate has at least four to five times the mass of fibrinogen per milliliter of infusate compared to fresh frozen plasma. Fresh frozen plasma contains fibrinogen in sufficient amounts for treatment of patients with mild to moderate hypofibrinogenemia.

Anticoagulant Treatment

Heparin therapy in patients with DIC remains controversial. Experimental studies have shown that heparin can at least partly inhibit the activation of coagulation in DIC. However, a beneficial effect of heparin on clinically important outcome events in patients with DIC has not been demonstrated in controlled clinical trials. Also, the safety of heparin treatment is debatable in DIC patients who are prone to bleeding. A large trial in patients with severe sepsis showed a slight, but nonsignificant benefit, of low dose heparin on 28-day mortality in patients with severe sepsis and no major safety concerns [29].

There is general consensus that administration of heparin is beneficial in some categories of DIC, such as metastatic carcinomas, purpura fulminans, and aortic aneurysm (prior to resection). Heparin also is indicated for treating thromboembolic complications in large vessels and before surgery in patients with chronic DIC. Heparin administration may be helpful in patients with acute DIC when intensive blood component replacement fails to improve excessive bleeding or when thrombosis threatens to cause irreversible tissue injury (e.g., acute cortical necrosis of the kidney or digital gangrene).

Heparin should be used cautiously in all these conditions. In patients with chronic DIC because of metastatic carcinoma or aortic aneurysm, continuous infusion of unfractionated heparin 500–750 U/h without a bolus injection has been advocated. If no response is obtained within 24 h, escalating dosages can be used. In hyperacute DIC cases, such as amniotic fluid embolism, septic abortion, and purpura fulminans, intravenous bolus injection of 5000–10,000 U heparin may be given simultaneously with replacement therapy with blood products. Some experts, however, would not administer a bolus dose of heparin even under these circumstances. Continuous infusion of 500–1000 U/h heparin may be necessary to maintain the benefit until the underlying disease responds to treatment. Apart from all these considerations, current guidelines dictate the universal use of prophylactic doses of heparin or low molecular weight heparin to prevent venous thromboembolic events in critically ill patients [6].

Theoretically, the most logical anticoagulant agent to use in DIC is directed against TF activity. Potential agents include recombinant TFPI, inactivated factor VIIa, and recombinant NAPc2, a potent and specific inhibitor of the ternary complex of TF/factor VIIa and factor Xa. Phase II trials of recombinant TFPI in patients with sepsis showed promising results but phase III trials in patients with severe sepsis or severe pneumonia and organ failure did not show an overall survival benefit in patients who were treated with TFPI [30].

Recombinant human soluble thrombomodulin binds to thrombin to form a complex that inactivates thrombin's coagulant activity and activates protein C, and thus, is a potential drug for the treatment of patients with DIC. In a phase III randomized double-blind clinical trial in patients with DIC, administration of the soluble thrombomodulin had a significantly better effect on bleeding manifestations and coagulation parameters than heparin. Currently ongoing trials with soluble thrombomodulin focus on DIC, organ failure and mortality rate.

Physiological Anticoagulant Factor Concentrates

Restoration of the levels of physiological anticoagulants in DIC may be a rational approach [31, 32]. Based on successful preclinical studies, the use of AT concentrates and heparin in patients with DIC has been examined mainly in randomized controlled trials that included patients with sepsis, septic shock, or both. All trials have shown some beneficial effect in terms of improvement of laboratory parameters, shortening of the duration of DIC, or even improvement in organ function. In several small clinical trials, use of very high doses of AT concentrate showed even a modest reduction in mortality, however, without being statistically significant. A large-scale, multicenter, randomized controlled trial also showed no significant reduction in mortality of patients with sepsis [33]. Interestingly, post hoc subgroup analyses of the latter study indicated some benefit in patients who did not receive concomitant heparin, but this observation needs validation. In a small randomized trial in patients with burns and DIC, AT administration decreased mortality, reduced multiple organ failure, and improved coagulation parameters compared to placebo-control patients.

Because a decreased function of the protein C system contributes to the pathogenesis of DIC, therapy by activated protein C (APC) was predicted to be beneficial [34]. Indeed, a dose-ranging controlled trial using continuous infusion of recombinant human APC disclosed that a dose of 24 μg/Kg per hour was optimal, judged by a decrease of D-dimer level in plasma. A subsequent phase III trial of APC concentrate in patients with sepsis was prematurely stopped because of efficacy in reducing mortality in these patients [35]. All cause mortality at 28 days after inclusion was 24.7 % in the APC group versus 30.8 % in the control group (a 19.4 % relative risk reduction). Amelioration of coagulation abnormalities and less organ failure were noted in patients who received the concentrate. Part of the success of therapy could be ascribed to the anti-inflammatory effect of APC. Interestingly, patients who manifested "overt DIC" (see DIAGNOSIS, above) benefited more from the therapy with APC than patients who did not have overt DIC [11]. The relative risk reduction in mortality of patients with both sepsis and DIC was 38 %, while patients with sepsis but no DIC only had a risk reduction of 18 %. This seems to underscore the importance of the coagulation derangement in the pathogenesis of sepsis and implies that the restoration of the protein C pathway in the microvasculature is essential for cure in patients with sepsis. However, meta-analyses of published literature conclude that the basis for treatment with APC, even in patients with a high disease severity, is not very strong or even insufficient. The series of negative trials in specific populations of patients with severe sepsis has added to the skepticism regarding the use of APC. On top of that, there is uncertainty regarding the bleeding risk of APC in patients with severe sepsis. In a phase 3 study conducted in patients with severe sepsis, the incidence of major bleeding (i.e., bleeding reported as a serious adverse event) during the infusion period was 2.4 % in the APC group as compared with 1.0 % in the control group ($P=0.02$). During the 28-day study period, the incidence of major bleeding was 3.5 % in the APC group and 2.0 % in the placebo group ($P=0.06$). Gastrointestinal bleeding was the most frequent bleeding complication in both groups. Most bleeding episodes were procedure related or occurred in patients with a severely deranged coagulation system (partial thromboplastin time [PTT] > 120 s or INR > 3.0), whereas spontaneous bleeding was rare. The bleeding rate in the clinical trials seems to be acceptable, but it may be that in the "real world" the risk of bleeding, including intracranial bleeding is higher. A recently completed placebo-controlled trial in patients with severe sepsis and septic shock was prematurely stopped due to the lack of any significant benefit of APC. *Subsequently, the manufacturer of APC has decided to withdraw the product from the market, which has resulted in a revision of current guidelines for treatment of DIC.*

Fibrinolytic Inhibitors

Most guidelines recommend against the use of antifibrinolytic agents, such as ε-aminocaproic acid or tranexamic acid, in patients with DIC. This is because these drugs block already suppressed endogenous fibrinolysis, and may further compromise tissue perfusion. In support of this concept, there are reports of severe thrombosis in DIC patients treated with these agents.

However, in patients with DIC accompanied by primary fibrino(geno)lysis, as in some cases of acute promyelocytic leukemia, giant cavernous hemangioma, heat stroke, and metastatic carcinoma of the prostate, the use of fibrinolytic inhibitors can be considered if the patient has profuse bleeding that does not respond to replacement therapy and there is evidence of excessive fibrino(geno)lysis. In these situations, it is important to replace depleted blood components, before initiating treatment with fibrinolytic inhibitors.

References

1. Seligsohn U. Disseminated intravascular coagulation. In: Handin RI, Lux SE, Stossel TP, editors. Blood: principles and practice of hematology. Philadelphia: J.B. Lippincott; 2000.
2. Levi M, Seligsohn U. Disseminated intravascular coagulation. In: Kaushansky K, Lichtman M, Beutler E, Kipps T, Prchal J, Seligsohn U, editors. Williams hematology. Philadelphia: McGraw Hill; 2010.
3. Levi M, ten Cate H. Disseminated intravascular coagulation. N Engl J Med. 1999;341:586–92.
4. Levi M. Disseminated intravascular coagulation. Crit Care Med. 2007;35:2191–5.
5. Taylor FBJ, Toh CH, Hoots WK, Wada H, Levi M. Towards definition, clinical and laboratory criteria, and a scoring system for disseminated intravascular coagulation. Thromb Haemost. 2001;86:1327–30.
6. Levi M, Toh CH, Thachil J, Watson HG. Guidelines for the diagnosis and management of disseminated intravascular coagulation. Br J Haematol. 2009;145: 24–33.
7. Maegele M, Schochl H, Cohen MJ. An update on the coagulopathy of trauma. Shock. 2014;41 Suppl 1:21–5.
8. Levi M, van der Poll T. Inflammation and coagulation. Crit Care Med. 2010;38:S26–34.
9. Albert-Weissenberger C, Mencl S, Hopp S, Kleinschnitz C, Siren AL. Role of the kallikrein-kinin system in traumatic brain injury. Front Cell Neurosci. 2014;8:345.
10. Fourrier F, Chopin C, Goudemand J, Hendrycx S, Caron C, Rime A, Marey A, Lestavel P. Septic shock, multiple organ failure, and disseminated intravascular coagulation. Compared patterns of antithrombin III, protein C, and protein S deficiencies. Chest. 1992;101:816–23.
11. Dhainaut JF, Yan SB, Joyce DE, Pettila V, Basson BR, Brandt JT, Sundin D, Levi M. Treatment effects of drotrecogin alfa (activated) in patients with severe sepsis with or without overt disseminated intravascular coagulation. J Thromb Haemost. 2004;2: 1924–33.
12. Levi M, Opal SM. Coagulation abnormalities in critically ill patients. Crit Care. 2006;10:222.
13. Albert-Weissenberger C, Siren AL, Kleinschnitz C. Ischemic stroke and traumatic brain injury: the role of the kallikrein-kinin system. Prog Neurobiol. 2013;101–102:65–82.
14. Esmon CT. The regulation of natural anticoagulant pathways. Science. 1987;235:1348–52.
15. Gerald AG. Update on hemostasis: neurosurgery. Surgery. 2007;142:S55–60.
16. Lippi G, Cervellin G. Disseminated intravascular coagulation in trauma injuries. Semin Thromb Hemost. 2010;36:378–87.
17. Keimowitz RM, Annis BL. Disseminated intravascular coagulation associated with massive brain injury. J Neurosurg. 1973;39:178–80.
18. Hess JR, Lawson JH. The coagulopathy of trauma versus disseminated intravascular coagulation. J Trauma. 2006;60:S12–9.
19. Brohi K, Cohen MJ, Ganter MT, Schultz MJ, Levi M, Mackersie RC, Pittet JF. Acute coagulopathy of trauma: hypoperfusion induces systemic anticoagulation and hyperfibrinolysis. J Trauma. 2008;64:1211–7.
20. Gando S, Nakanishi Y, Tedo I. Cytokines and plasminogen activator inhibitor-1 in posttrauma disseminated intravascular coagulation: relationship to multiple organ dysfunction syndrome. Crit Care Med. 1995;23:1835–42.
21. Roumen RM, Hendriks T, van der Ven-Jongekrijg J, Nieuwenhuijzen GA, Sauerwein RW, van der Meer JW, Goris RJ. Cytokine patterns in patients after major vascular surgery, hemorrhagic shock, and severe blunt trauma. Relation with subsequent adult respiratory distress syndrome and multiple organ failure. Annals of Surgery. 1993;218:769–76.
22. Stein SC, Smith DH. Coagulopathy in traumatic brain injury. Neurocrit Care. 2004;1:479–88.
23. Stein SC, Chen XH, Sinson GP, Smith DH. Intravascular coagulation: a major secondary insult in nonfatal traumatic brain injury. J Neurosurg. 2002; 97:1373–7.
24. Donahue DL, Beck J, Fritz B, Davis P, Sandoval-Cooper MJ, Thomas SG, Yount RA, Walsh M, Ploplis VA, Castellino FJ. Early platelet dysfunction in a rodent model of blunt traumatic brain injury reflects the acute traumatic coagulopathy found in humans. J Neurotrauma. 2014;31:404–10.
25. Lowenberg EC, Meijers JC, Levi M. Platelet-vessel wall interaction in health and disease. Neth J Med. 2010;68:242–51.
26. Levi M, de Jonge E, Meijers J. The diagnosis of disseminated intravascular coagulation. Blood Rev. 2002;16:217–23.
27. Levi M, Meijers JC. DIC: which laboratory tests are most useful. Blood Rev. 2010;24:77–84.
28. Dempfle CE, Borggrefe M. Point of care coagulation tests in critically ill patients. Semin Thromb Hemost. 2008;34:445–50.
29. Levi M, Levy M, Williams MD, Douglas I, Artigas A, Antonelli M, Wyncoll D, Janes J, Booth FV, Wang D,

Sundin DP, Macias WL. Prophylactic heparin in patients with severe sepsis treated with drotrecogin alfa (activated). Am J Respir Crit Care Med. 2007;176:483–90.
30. Abraham E, Reinhart K, Opal S, Demeyer I, Doig C, Rodriguez AL, Beale R, Svoboda P, Laterre PF, Simon S, Light B, Spapen H, Stone J, Seibert A, Peckelsen C, De Deyne C, Postier R, Pettila V, Artigas A, Percell SR, Shu V, Zwingelstein C, Tobias J, Poole L, Stolzenbach JC, Creasey AA. Efficacy and safety of tifacogin (recombinant tissue factor pathway inhibitor) in severe sepsis: a randomized controlled trial. JAMA. 2003;290:238–47.
31. Levi M, de Jonge E, van der Poll T. Rationale for restoration of physiological anticoagulant pathways in patients with sepsis and disseminated intravascular coagulation. Crit Care Med. 2001;29(7 Suppl): S90–4.
32. de Jonge E, van der Poll T, Kesecioglu J, Levi M. Anticoagulant factor concentrates in disseminated intravascular coagulation: rationale for use and clinical experience. Semin Thromb Hemost. 2001; 27(6):667–74.
33. Warren BL, Eid A, Singer P, Pillay SS, Carl P, Novak I, Chalupa P, Atherstone A, Penzes I, Kubler A, Knaub S, Keinecke HO, Heinrichs H, Schindel F, Juers M, Bone RC, Opal SM. Caring for the critically ill patient. High-dose antithrombin III in severe sepsis: a randomized controlled trial. JAMA. 2001;286:1869–78.
34. Levi M. Activated protein C in sepsis: a critical review. Curr Opin Hematol. 2008;15:481–6.
35. Bernard GR, Vincent JL, Laterre PF, LaRosa SP, Dhainaut JF, Lopez-Rodriguez A, Steingrub JS, Garber GE, Helterbrand JD, Ely EW, Fisher CJJ. Efficacy and safety of recombinant human activated protein C for severe sepsis. N Engl J Med. 2001;344(10):699–709.

14 Heparin-Induced Thrombocytopenia (HIT)

Jeanine M. Walenga and M. Margaret Prechel

Introduction

Heparin remains the anticoagulant of choice for many clinical needs. Because heparin is used ubiquitously in the hospital setting, millions of patients are exposed each year. In some patients, heparin therapy elicits formation of antibodies which cause heparin-induced thrombocytopenia (HIT) a severe adverse effect characterized by low platelet count and high risk of thrombotic complications. Healthcare providers must be aware of and understand the clinical diagnosis, laboratory testing, and treatment of HIT because of the devastating clinical consequences of stroke, acute myocardial infarction, pulmonary embolism, limb amputation, and death due to thrombosis with which it is associated.

While much of the work in understanding the pathophysiology, clinical presentation, and treatment of HIT has centered on cardiovascular and orthopedic surgery populations, neurology/neurosurgery patients also have a high frequency of developing HIT (up to 15 % has been reported) [1]. In addition, neurological symptoms are characteristic of HIT making all HIT patients potential neurovascular patients [2, 3]. This chapter summarizes the current practice for the management of patients with HIT (Table 14.1).

J.M. Walenga, Ph.D. (✉)
Departments of Thoracic & Cardiovascular Surgery and Pathology, Stritch School of Medicine, Loyola University Chicago, Maywood, IL 60153, USA
e-mail: jwaleng@luc.edu

M.M. Prechel, Ph.D.
Department of Pathology, Stritch School of Medicine, Loyola University Chicago, Maywood, IL 60153, USA

Development of HIT

Antibodies elicited by heparin therapy are not specifically anti-heparin antibodies. HIT antibodies recognize particular complexes of heparin and the platelet release protein, platelet factor 4 (PF4) [4, 5]. The presence of PF4 is critical to the development (immunogenesis) of HIT antibodies and to their pathogenic function.

PF4 is a positively charged protein that binds to negatively charged heparin and heparin-like molecules. Upon release from activated platelets, PF4 rapidly associates with heparan sulfate on endothelial cells, promoting a procoagulant surface for vascular repair. In the presence of therapeutic heparin, this binding results in large, highly immunogenic PF4-heparin complexes in circulation. In addition to its hemostatic role, PF4 (a member of a highly conserved family of host defense peptides) has both antimicrobial and immune functions. The similarity of PF4 bound to certain pathogens and the conformation of PF4 bound to heparin may explain the immunogenicity of PF4/heparin complexes [6] resulting in the generation of HIT antibodies.

C.M. Loftus (ed.), *Anticoagulation and Hemostasis in Neurosurgery*,
DOI 10.1007/978-3-319-27327-3_14

Table 14.1 Clinical management of heparin-induced thrombocytopenia

• HIT is an immune response to PF4, an activated platelet release protein, bound to heparin
• HIT is a complex syndrome that requires immediate and knowledgeable clinical management
• Patient-dependent variables are associated with a higher risk of developing HIT and poorer outcomes
• Patients with HIT can develop neurological symptoms (thrombosis, but also bleeding from anticoagulant treatment); also the cause of cerebral thrombosis in a neurology patient can be traced back to HIT
• HIT is largely a clinical diagnosis; scoring systems are available to aid in determining the probability that a patient has HIT
• Laboratory tests for HIT help in the diagnosis but they are not optimal and require knowledgeable interpretation of results
• Using a scoring system also helps with lab test ordering (to reduce false positive results)
• An immunoassay is used to screen for HIT antibodies (many false positives); a platelet function assay is the standard to confirm HIT (but sensitivity is low)
• The titer (optical density reading) of the immunoassay for HIT antibodies can be used to follow the clinical progress of a patient
• The first step in managing a patient with HIT is to remove heparin, but until HIT is confirmed consideration for the risk of thrombosis from other causes that dictates anticoagulant protection must be given
• Use intravenous argatroban or bivalirudin, with monitoring, for treatment of acute, severe HIT and HIT thrombosis
• Use bivalirudin for interventional or surgical procedures in patients with HIT; optimal dosing and monitoring protocols are in development
• Be aware of the potential for intracranial bleeding with argatroban and bivalirudin treatment
• Use of fondaparinux for prevention of thrombosis in patients with suspected HIT with no indication for full anticoagulation is gaining favor but not yet approved
• Prevent the occurrence of HIT by limiting exposure to heparin; use LMW heparin, fondaparinux, or other non-heparin anticoagulants in place of heparin where possible; reduce platelet activation

The risk of developing HIT increases with heparin dose and longer treatment duration and is more likely with intravenous than subcutaneous heparin. Still, HIT antibodies can develop from any heparin exposure including incidental amounts from heparin flushes or heparin-coated devices. Due to their smaller molecular size compared to therapeutic heparin, low molecular weight (LMW) heparin and fondaparinux have less ability to bind PF4, alter its configuration, and cause the generation of antibodies.

Immune complexes of HIT IgG bound to PF4-heparin complexes cross-link platelet FcγIIa receptors, resulting in platelet activation with release of additional PF4 and platelet-platelet aggregation. In the presence of heparin, there is continued formation of antigenic complexes, platelet activation and aggregation, and generation of highly procoagulant platelet microparticles. Sustained platelet activation contributes to platelet clearance and thrombin generation that can lead to both thrombocytopenia and HIT-associated thrombosis.

HIT antibodies, once formed, become involved in various hemostatic activation processes beyond platelet activation [7]. These antibodies also recognize PF4 bound to cell membranes via heparan sulfate, which contributes to an inflammatory state whereby macrophages, monocytes, and neutrophils are activated. Antibody and leukocyte binding to activated endothelial cells cause release of tissue factor, plasminogen activator inhibitor-1 (PAI-1), and cytokines, as well as an upregulation of adhesion molecule expression, promoting localized platelet and monocyte binding. The interrelationships of platelets, leukocytes, the endothelium, and the inflammatory state determine the clinical expression of HIT.

The presence of HIT antibodies does not cause thrombocytopenia or thrombosis in the majority of patients. It is when certain HIT antibodies bind PF4, forming immune complexes, that subsequent FcγIIa receptor-mediated platelet activation ensues which can lead to thrombocytopenia and/or thrombosis. Thus, the HIT syndrome depends not only on the presence of HIT antibodies of sufficient *titer* and *specificity* but also on the *presence of PF4* [8].

The availability of PF4 is influenced both by acute and chronic platelet activation and logically plays a role in the risk for generation of PF4-heparin antibodies in the context of anticoagulant therapy. Increased platelet activation and circulating PF4 levels are observed in inflammatory and infectious diseases, diabetes, cardiovascular disease, atherosclerosis, conditions affecting vascular health, and in response to traumatic medical procedures or cardiopulmonary bypass. This suggests an explanation for the common observation that specific patient populations (type of surgery, severity of trauma, age, comorbidities such as renal impairment, low cardiac output, malignancy, critical illness, vascular disease) are known to be at an increased risk of developing HIT antibodies.

Clinical Presentation of HIT

In up to 30 % of patients, administration of heparin is followed by a benign, transient, and self-limited fall in platelet count which occurs through a non-immunological mechanism and resolves within 24–48 h (referred to as HIT Type I). The clinically relevant HIT syndrome discussed herein is immune-mediated HIT (known as HIT Type II) that is associated with thrombocytopenia and an extreme hypercoagulable state.

Immune-mediated HIT is defined as thrombocytopenia or new thrombosis starting 5–10 days after exposure to heparin, in the absence of other explanations for the symptoms [9]. HIT should be suspected on the basis of an unexplained 30–50 % drop in platelet count from baseline in patients being treated or having been recently treated with heparin. No single definition of thrombocytopenia based on platelet count is appropriate in all clinical situations. For example, an abrupt decrease in platelet count that does not result in thrombocytopenia (e.g., platelet count may fall from 450,000 to 225,000/μL) can be HIT. Not all patients with thrombocytopenia experience thrombosis, and thrombotic complications can occur before or in the absence of thrombocytopenia. There can also be variability in the timing of onset of clinical symptoms. Patients with HIT antibodies resulting from heparin exposure within the prior 100–120 days may have an immediate, rapid onset of HIT when restarting heparin [10]. Delayed-onset HIT has been observed with symptoms appearing days to weeks after discontinuation of heparin [11].

There is a wide spectrum of arterial and venous thromboembolic complications associated with HIT, including deep vein thrombosis, pulmonary embolism, ischemic stroke, myocardial infarction, limb ischemia, vein graft occlusion, skin lesions at injection sites, and thrombosis of an extracorporeal circuit. Venous thrombosis predominates 5:1, but arterial thrombosis accounts for the most disturbing symptoms [12]. Mortality among patients with HIT thrombosis that is not effectively treated is 30 %, with 20 % of those who survive requiring a limb amputation [9]. Overall mortality rates of patients with HIT thrombosis approach 10–20 % despite the current practice improvements.

Deep venous thrombosis of the lower limbs and pulmonary embolism commonly occurs; thrombosis in the upper extremities is often associated with a central venous catheter or pacemaker wire. Other less commonly reported events include mesenteric venous thrombosis and adrenal hemorrhagic infarction. Acute limb occlusion is the most common arterial event usually developing in areas of a recent interventional procedure or following trauma.

Stroke was reported in 3 % of all HIT patients and more often in females who tend to experience poorer outcomes [2]. In another study, neurological complications of patients with HIT were reported to be 9 % [3]. Stroke significantly increases the mortality risk [2]. The consideration of HIT in the differential diagnosis when ischemic stroke occurs and of heightened stroke awareness for ≥2 weeks following HIT diagnosis is important.

LMW heparin can also cause HIT but with a tenfold lower rate of occurrence than with heparin. Symptoms are the same but typically appear 8–14 days after exposure to the LMW heparin [13].

Cardiovascular Patients

The cardiovascular patient is at high risk to develop HIT. Patients who undergo percutaneous transluminal angioplasty, percutaneous coronary angioplasty, percutaneous coronary intervention, and coronary artery bypass or vascular surgery appear particularly vulnerable. This is assumed to be due to the repeated and occasionally prolonged exposure to heparin or LMW heparin. When HIT occurs in a post-procedure patient, the presence of an injured vascular intima provides a unique thrombogenic surface that is at a high risk for thrombosis. The increased level of platelet activation and PF4 release is an added reason for the higher incidence of HIT in this population.

The diagnosis of HIT is difficult in post-surgical patients as postoperative thrombocytopenia is frequently present and always present following cardiac surgery using cardiopulmonary bypass. In these patients, HIT should be suspected if the platelet count recovery in the immediate postoperative period is interrupted by a sudden and marked platelet count decrease 5–10 days post-operation (a biphasic platelet count pattern) [14]. However, HIT cannot be definitely excluded in patients with a monophasic pattern of persistent postoperative thrombocytopenia.

Heart failure patients requiring ventricular assist devices who receive anticoagulation during surgery and for extended postoperative periods often develop HIT antibodies but not necessarily HIT thrombosis [15]. These patients have multiple explanations for low platelet counts. No guidelines are yet established for the diagnosis of HIT in this patient group.

Neurovascular Patients

Although there are limited reports of the true frequency of HIT and rate of thrombotic complications in neurosurgical patients, there is good indication of risk in this patient population. HIT should be part of the differential diagnosis.

Heparin is frequently given to acute ischemic stroke patients. A prevalence of 0.5 % of confirmed HIT in this population based on a clinical scoring system and laboratory assay results (2 % prevalence if based on clinical score alone) has been reported [16]. Other less rigorous studies reported higher frequencies. The clinical severity and outcome of acute stroke patients suspected of having HIT were unfavorable.

Subarachnoid hemorrhage (SAH) patients, among neurosurgical patient populations, are exposed to heparin because they are in critical care units, are at risk of venous thrombosis, and have indwelling vascular catheters. In addition, the increase in neurovascular procedures with associated heparinization increases the exposure of patients to heparin. The incidence of HIT in SAH patients at a single center was reported to be as high as 15 % [1]. Other studies reported rates from 2 % to 6 % [17–19]. The SAH patients with HIT had significantly higher rates of thrombotic complications, new hypodensities on head computed tomographic scans, more deaths, and significantly less favorable outcomes.

Other concerns include the relatively common finding of ischemic stroke in all patients first presenting with other symptoms of HIT (discussed above). In addition, the treatment of choice for patients with HIT thrombosis is a direct thrombin inhibitor anticoagulant, yet intracranial hemorrhage can occur from this treatment.

These issues highlight the fact that HIT can be the cause for cerebral thrombosis in neurovascular patients and also that non-neurovascular patients with HIT can develop neurological symptoms from HIT thrombosis or bleeding from treatment of HIT with anticoagulants.

Patients with Mild Thrombocytopenia

Another challenging clinical presentation of HIT is the patient with mild thrombocytopenia receiving heparin or LMW heparin treatment. These patients are to be individually assessed for their risk of HIT considering past exposure to heparin, competing causes for thrombocytopenia, and new thrombosis. The level of risk will determine whether or not to continue heparin/LMW heparin treatment, while laboratory testing is sent to confirm the diagnosis.

Diagnosis and Early Management

The diagnosis of HIT is complicated because patients often do not fit a simple textbook definition. Clinical judgment remains important for directing patient clinical care. Although the diagnosis of HIT can be difficult, it is critical that patients with HIT be identified as soon as possible to initiate early treatment to avoid thrombosis. HIT should be considered in the differential diagnosis of any new thrombosis or extension of an existing thrombus in a patient receiving anticoagulation.

Clinical Scoring Systems

The diagnosis of HIT is based on clinical findings, platelet count, and laboratory testing. It is necessary that causes for thrombocytopenia, a common finding in a hospital setting, other than HIT be ruled out.

Scoring systems, such as the 4Ts [20] or the HEP score (an expanded version of the 4Ts score based on the opinions of 26 HIT experts) [21] to estimate pretest probability of HIT, are useful to risk stratify patients facilitating clinicians' management of patients with suspected HIT. Scoring systems are based on the magnitude and nadir of thrombocytopenia, timing of platelet count fall, thrombosis, other heparin-related reactions, and exclusion of other causes of thrombocytopenia. The 4Ts system is summarized in Table 14.2.

Next Steps

Clinical scores should be determined first on patients suspected of HIT. After this is determined, the decision for laboratory testing is to be made. If clinical suspicion for HIT is low and the clinical score is low, no laboratory testing needs to be performed (to avoid false positives). If the score is intermediate or high, an immunoassay should be performed because it is highly sensitive. If the immunoassay result is positive, a functional assay needs to be performed to confirm the presence of HIT and avoid a false positive (see laboratory test section below). Other likely scenarios of clinical scoring, lab test results, and interpretation are given in Table 14.3. Keep in mind that results of the laboratory tests for HIT do not always coincide with the clinical picture.

Clinical management of HIT at the initial stage must take into consideration the risk of thrombosis from other causes that would dictate anticoagulant protection. Cessation of heparin while waiting for lab test confirmation of HIT needs to be weighed against the need for anticoagulant protection. One simple scoring system (Table 14.4) helps with the decision process of whether or not to immediately discontinue heparin in patients suspected, but not confirmed, of HIT [22]. An immediate switch to argatroban or bivalirudin is costly and carries the risk of hemorrhage.

On the other hand, for patients with a high score by any scoring system for HIT, it is not necessary to wait for laboratory test results to initiate non-heparin anticoagulation therapy. It is important, however, to have laboratory confirmation of HIT, because patients with a history of HIT are at risk for recurrence should they be exposed to heparin in the future. Thus, HIT lab tests should be used to confirm a clinical diagnosis of HIT to guide future therapy.

Table 14.2 The 4Ts clinical scoring system to determine patient's risk of HIT [20, 54]

	2 Points	1 Point	0 Points
Thrombocytopenia	>50 % fall or platelet nadir 20,000–100,000/μL	30–50 % fall or platelet nadir 10,000–19,000/μL	<30 % fall or platelet nadir <10,000/μL
Timing of platelet drop or other sequelae	Onset days 5–10 or <1 day if recent heparin exposure	Onset after day 10 or not clear	Onset ≤4 days without recent heparin exposure
Thrombosis or other sequelae	New thrombosis; skin necrosis at heparin injection site; acute systemic reaction after intravenous heparin bolus	Progressive or recurrent thrombosis; erythematous skin lesions; suspected thrombosis	None
Other causes of thrombocytopenia	None evident	Possible other causes	Definite other causes

Probability: 6–8 = high; 4–5 = intermediate, 0–3 = low
The HEP SCORE [21] is similar with more detail in each category

Table 14.3 Possible laboratory test results for suspected HIT

Clinical suspicion/score	Immunoassay	Functional assay to confirm HIT	Interpretation
Low	Not done	Not done	HIT unlikely
Intermediate	Positive	Positive	HIT likely
Intermediate	Positive	Negative	Indeterminate; repeat testing over the next days
Intermediate	Negative	Not done	Indeterminate; repeat testing over the next days
High	Positive	Not done	HIT likely
High	Negative	Not done	Indeterminate; repeat testing over the next days

This chart illustrates one example of a diagnostic algorithm
The two types of lab test for HIT provide different but complimentary information, which together aid in an accurate diagnosis of HIT. However, limitations of both assays require knowledgeable interpretation of the assay results. The clinical impression remains important for a diagnosis of HIT

Table 14.4 Scoring system to continue or discontinue heparin in suspected HIT [22]

Score	Clinical criteria	Clinical management
0	Heparin therapy not present for 5 days preceding platelet count drop – or – Platelet count did not fall by 30 % – or – Significant competing cause for thrombocytopenia	Continue heparin therapy if clinically indicated while waiting for HIT lab test results
1	On heparin therapy – and – No significant competing cause for thrombocytopenia – and – Platelet count fall by >30 % – or – New thrombosis	Discontinue heparin therapy while waiting for HIT lab test results

Whenever there is a strong clinical suspicion or confirmed diagnoses of HIT, heparin and LMW heparin have to be immediately discontinued. However, cessation of heparin alone is not sufficient to remove the threat of thrombosis from HIT [23]. A non-heparin alternative anticoagulant should be used to treat existing thrombosis from HIT and/or to prevent thrombosis from occurring (see treatment section below). LMW heparin is contraindicated in patients with HIT because this drug class has a high rate of interaction with established HIT antibodies.

Clinical Laboratory Testing for HIT

Platelet Count

During the initial period of heparin and LMW heparin treatment, platelet counts should be performed [9]. If the patient's risk of developing HIT is high, platelet counts should be done more frequently, daily if necessary.

Assays for HIT

There are two different types of specific clinical laboratory tests for the diagnosis of HIT: (1) immunoassays detect the presence of antibodies that bind to PF4/heparin complexes and (2) platelet-based assays that demonstrate whether the antibodies have the functional capacity to cause heparin-dependent platelet activation. Laboratory testing for HIT should only be performed when there is a strong clinical suspicion of HIT to avoid false positive results.

No test for HIT has optimal sensitivity and specificity, and negative test results do not necessarily exclude the diagnosis of HIT [24]. Furthermore, as antibody titers rise, daily testing can turn from negative to positive with repeat testing.

Immunoassays are increasingly common because of the fast turnaround time to result reporting, and this test can be performed in most laboratories. However, certain limitations of result interpretation must be highlighted. These assays are highly sensitive and have a high rate of false positive results. False negative results can also occur. Studies have shown that the presence of HIT antibodies alone is not sufficient to cause the clinical symptoms of HIT (thrombocytopenia and thrombosis) [17, 25]. However, a negative immunoassay in patients with low clinical probability for HIT (low clinical score) has a high negative predictive value. A positive immunoassay has to be reflexed to a platelet function assay to confirm HIT. Antibody levels of ≥1.0 optical density by immunoassay are more likely to be associated with HIT thrombosis [26, 27].

While it is known that IgG-type HIT antibodies are important for platelet activation in HIT, IgM and IgA HIT antibodies may also play a pathophysiological role. Non-IgG HIT antibodies are linked to longer hospital stay, poorer clinical outcome, and poorer rate of survival. Immunoassays that test IgG/A/M HIT antibodies are preferable to IgG-only assays.

Platelet activation functional assays have a lower sensitivity than the immunoassay, but they are specific for HIT antibodies that are associated with clinical symptoms. The serotonin release assay (^{14}C-SRA, SRA) that employs radiolabeled serotonin uptake by the platelets is the reference test. Assays based on light transmission platelet aggregation are also used in many centers. These assays require a skilled and experienced lab to assure accurate results. Platelet activation tests are used to confirm an HIT diagnosis in patients who have an intermediate to high clinical risk assessment for HIT with a positive HIT immunoassay. These tests, while important for confirming a diagnosis of HIT, do have limited sensitivity and can produce false negative results.

Treatment of HIT

Despite the hallmark low platelet count, HIT patients rarely have bleeding complications. Platelet transfusions are contraindicated in patients with HIT but may be considered if there is life-threatening bleeding. The major significance of HIT is the paradoxical risk of thrombosis. HIT antibody positive patients without thrombosis initially have up to 50 % risk of developing thrombosis within the next 30 days if not provided prophylaxis with a non-heparin anticoagulant.

Anticoagulant Treatment for HIT Thrombosis

HIT is characterized by a strong hypercoagulable state with a high risk of thrombosis [9]. It is recommended that all patients with HIT thrombosis be anticoagulated with intravenous administration of a strong acting, non-heparin anticoagulant such as argatroban or bivalirudin [9, 28]. These anticoagulants are direct-acting thrombin inhibitors (DTIs). They are potent anticoagulants that inhibit the high level of thrombin generated in patients with HIT. Because their chemical structure differs from that of heparin, DTIs do not bind to PF4, generate HIT antibodies, or interact with preformed HIT antibodies. DTIs reduce the risk of thrombosis and associated morbidity/mortality in patients with HIT. Death, amputation, and new thrombosis are reduced, and platelet counts recover more rapidly in patients receiving treatment than those not receiving treatment.

Argatroban (Novartis) was the first real solution for effective alternative anticoagulation for patients with HIT. Large clinical studies began in the mid-1990s [29, 30], followed by multiple investigations to assess clinical safety and efficacy in pediatrics and other specific populations [2, 31–37].

Argatroban is a small molecule thrombin inhibitor. It is administered by intravenous infusion. Its use is not recommended in patients with liver failure. Based on clinical experience, dose adjustments to reduce the bleeding risk for argatroban in specific populations have been recommended, including reduced dosing for seriously ill patients [34, 38]. Argatroban has the broadest regulatory approval, i.e., for both prophylaxis and treatment of thrombosis in patients with HIT, as well as for anticoagulation in HIT patients requiring cardiovascular interventional procedures. Argatroban is currently the preferred drug for patients with HIT requiring hemodialysis.

Argatroban therapy reduces the likelihood of new stroke and stroke-associated mortality in HIT [2]. A Japanese study showed that argatroban significantly improved global outcome in patients with acute cerebral thrombosis [39]. High-dose argatroban was shown to be an effective treatment for cerebral infarction including delayed hospitalization after onset [40]. Argatroban in combination with intravenous tissue plasminogen activator in acute stroke was reported to be safe in patients with moderate neurological deficits due to proximal intracranial arterial occlusions [41]. Reports on the use of argatroban, or any DTI, for the treatment of stroke are limited to date. Further studies are needed to better determine safety and efficacy.

Due to an inherent bleeding risk with this potent anticoagulant, argatroban treatment must be monitored. Therapeutic dosages are monitored by the same partial thromboplastin time (PTT) as used for heparin monitoring; higher dosages as used during interventional procedures are monitored by the same activated clotting time (ACT) as used for high-dose heparin monitoring. Argatroban has a substantial effect on the international normalized ratio (INR) [42, 43]; however, monitoring this drug by the INR has not been validated, and it should not be used. Argatroban has an effect on all clot-based assays (e.g., fibrinogen level, coagulation factor assays, protein C assay, etc.) [44]. True values for these coagulation proteins can only be obtained by using a chromogenic-based assay or an immunoassay if testing is to be performed on patients under argatroban treatment.

There is no antidote for argatroban. Given its short half-life of 50 min, the best recourse is to discontinue the infusion to reduce circulating drug levels.

Bivalirudin (Angiomax®; The Medicines Company) is a 20 amino acid synthetic peptide that targets two binding sites within thrombin. It has a very short half-life of 25 min due to enzymatic degradation. Bivalirudin is approved for use as an anticoagulant in cardiovascular interventional procedures in patients with HIT [45, 46]. It is administered intravenously and monitored by the ACT during use. The INR is not to be used for monitoring [42, 43]. As with argatroban, bivalirudin affects all clot-based assays, and it has no antidote.

One of the greatest challenges in the management of patients with HIT is anticoagulation during cardiac surgery where heparin is the drug of choice. Subsequent use of heparin after resolution of HIT can be hazardous, particularly within the first 3 months as rapid onset of the clinical syndrome can erupt. Patients with a previous history of HIT should be tested presurgery for the presence of HIT antibodies. In the absence of antibodies, surgery may be performed using heparin [9, 28]. If HIT antibodies are detectable by immunoassay, it may be reasonable to delay surgery until the antibodies are no longer present. In more urgent situations, surgeries have been successfully performed with heparin in immunoassay positive patients whose antibodies did not cause platelet activation detected by the SRA. In this circumstance standard heparin protocols restricted to the surgery itself can be employed, with a thrombin inhibitor, a factor Xa inhibitor, or warfarin for postoperative care if needed.

Alternative anticoagulation strategies that may be recommended for cardiac surgery use bivalirudin. Anticoagulation with bivalirudin was shown to be feasible in both on-pump (cardiopulmonary bypass pump, CPB) and off-pump (OPCAB) cardiac surgeries [47, 48]. The use of any DTI in cardiac surgery is associated with inherent risks: bleeding can be excessive, standing blood in the pump and devices can clot, and best practice monitoring of the high drug levels is not resolved. Surgical use of bivalirudin remains off-label, yet experience is growing.

Lepirudin had been used for the treatment of HIT thrombosis until recently. This drug has been taken off the market due to hypersensitivity in patients reexposed to the drug. Severe anaphylactic reactions with fatal outcomes have been reported.

Long-Term Anticoagulation

Warfarin is recommended for long-term treatment of HIT-associated thrombosis [9]. Warfarin is not recommended for use in the acute phase of HIT (when platelets are <100,000/μL) due to its potential to intensify the prothrombotic state from a transient protein C deficiency.

Warfarin can be initiated when platelet counts are >100,000/μL or at pre-HIT values starting at a low dose (5 mg warfarin; a loading dose should not be used to avoid possible skin necrosis), while the patient is fully anticoagulated with a DTI and continued for at least 5 days [9]. The DTI can be tapered off when the INR is therapeutic and stable. Warfarin treatment should continue until platelet counts recover to a stable plateau or longer if clinically warranted. These specific dosing guidelines need to be followed to avoid thrombotic complications.

DTIs prolong the prothrombin time (PT)/INR [42, 44, 49]. INRs >5 commonly occur with argatroban-warfarin co-therapy, but this does not correspond with a decrease in coagulation factor levels and bleeding is not enhanced. There is a predictable linear effect on the INR of argatroban doses up to 2 μg/kg/min during warfarin co-therapy, which allows for reliable prediction of the level of oral anticoagulation [49]. If argatroban dosing is higher, guidelines are available for how to proceed with bridging to warfarin.

Anticoagulation for HIT Without Thrombosis

Not all patients with HIT develop the acute stage of the disorder with thrombosis. Many patients develop HIT antibodies, have a mild thrombocytopenia, and have no thrombosis. For these patients the option to treat prophylactically to avoid thrombosis may be prudent knowing the risk of thrombosis and the medical intensity of acute HIT. There are several potential options for thrombosis prophylaxis that are undergoing evaluation.

Fondaparinux (Arixtra®; Mylan) is a synthetic, small molecule factor Xa inhibitor. It mimics the minimum specific saccharide sequence of heparin that binds to antithrombin and factor Xa. Due to its low molecular weight, fondaparinux does not cross-react with preformed HIT antibodies as heparin does. There have been no clinical trials in HIT. There are case reports, small published case series, and one retrospective analysis of 239 patients that show that fondaparinux provides effective anticoagulation of patients with suspected HIT *who have no indication for full anticoagulation* [50].

Although fondaparinux is considered to be a potential second-line agent for the management of patients with suspected HIT, its use in HIT remains off-label. Caution is warranted as there are reported cases of clinical failures.

Desirudin (Iprivask®; Marathon Pharmaceuticals) is a hirudin-based drug and the only DTI approved in the USA for administration by the subcutaneous route. It exhibits predictable pharmacokinetics when administered at a fixed dose and does not require routine monitoring. Desirudin is currently approved for prevention of DVT after orthopedic surgery. This drug has been successfully used in a limited number of patients with HIT [51], and studies to validate desirudin treatment for patients with or at risk for HIT thrombosis are in progress.

New oral anticoagulants are of interest for thrombosis prophylaxis in HIT patients. These synthetic, small molecules inhibit either thrombin (**dabigatran**) or factor Xa (**rivaroxaban, apixaban, edoxaban**). Laboratory studies show that these drugs do not interact with preformed HIT antibodies [52, 53]. Where warfarin has been used for outpatient anticoagulation or for prophylaxis against the development of HIT thrombosis, the new oral anticoagulants may prove useful. It remains to be determined whether these drugs are potent enough to provide sufficient anticoagulation coverage for all phases of the HIT syndrome. Clinical use in HIT is currently off-label, although case reports are appearing.

Other HIT Thrombosis Treatment Options

Certain patients with HIT develop ischemic limbs or organs in which thrombosis is not alleviated with anticoagulant therapy. Adjunct treatment options include thrombolytic agents or surgical removal of life- or limb-threatening thrombi. Plasmapheresis has been used to hasten reduction of antibody load in severely ill patients. These options should be used under the guidance of a clinician experienced in the procedure.

Future Treatment Options

Even with the success of intravenous DTIs for the management of HIT, amputation and death have not been eliminated in this patient population. Considering the pathophysiology of HIT, inhibition of thrombin, while important, likely cannot provide complete medical management of HIT patients. HIT is associated not only with a hypercoagulable state but also with platelet activation, vascular endothelial dysregulation, and inflammation (leukocyte activation, cytokine upregulation).

Thus, optimization of patient management needs to continue. Optimal medical management for HIT patients requires prophylaxis against thrombosis in patients with a mild form of HIT, treatment during the acute active phase of HIT, treatment of HIT thrombosis, and long-term prevention against new thrombosis development—clinical phases that require different potencies of antithrombotic treatment. The use of antiplatelet drugs, anti-inflammatory drugs, new drugs designed to target the specific mechanism of the HIT pathophysiology (i.e., decrease the available PF4), and drug combinations are all future possibilities.

Prevention of HIT

The expanded use of LMW heparins, fondaparinux, and the new oral anticoagulants for the routine management of thrombosis will naturally reduce the development of HIT because these drugs generate HIT antibodies at a far lower frequency than heparin or not at all.

Duration of exposure to heparin, more than dose, is an important consideration. Thus, avoid unnecessary and prolonged exposure to heparin. Be aware that HIT can occur even with prophylactic doses of heparin and heparin from exogenous sources (e.g., heparin flushes, heparin-coated catheters).

If an alternative to heparin can be used, such as saline in indwelling catheters or citrate in devices, exposure to heparin can be eliminated.

Based on the mechanism of action, efforts to reduce platelet activation and the accompanying increased levels of circulating PF4 should also be considered.

References

1. Hoh BL, Aghi M, Pryor JC, Ogilvy CS. Heparin-induced thrombocytopenia type II in subarachnoid hemorrhage patients: incidence and complications. Neurosurgery. 2005;57(2):243–8.
2. LaMonte MP, Brown PM, Hursting MJ. Stroke in patients with heparin-induced thrombocytopenia and the effect of argatroban therapy. Crit Care Med. 2004;32(4):976–80.
3. Pohl C, Harbrecht U, Greinacher A, et al. Neurologic complications in immune-mediated heparin-induced thrombocytopenia. Neurology. 2000;54:1240–5.
4. Greinacher A, Potzsch B, Amiral J, Dummel V, Eichner A, Mueller-Eckhardt C. Heparin-associated thrombocytopenia: Isolation of the antibody and characterization of a multimolecular PF4-heparin complex as the major antigen. Thromb Haemost. 1994;71: 247–51.
5. Rauova L, Poncz M, McKenzie SE, et al. Ultralarge complexes of heparin and PF4 are central to the pathogenesis of heparin-induced thrombocytopenia. Blood. 2005;105:131–8.
6. Prechel MM, Walenga JM. Complexes of platelet factor 4 and heparin activate Toll-like receptor 4. J Thromb Haemost. 2015;13(4):665–70.
7. Walenga JM, Jeske WP, Prechel MM, Bakhos M. Newer insights on the mechanism of heparin-induced thrombocytopenia. Semin Thromb Hemost. 2004;30 Suppl 1:57–67.
8. Prechel MM, Walenga JM. Emphasis on the role of PF4 in the incidence, pathophysiology and treatment of heparin-induced thrombocytopenia. Thromb J. 2013;11(7):1–9.
9. Linkins LA, Dans AL, Moores LK, Bona R, Davidson B, Schulman S, Crowther MA. Treatment and prevention of heparin-induced thrombocytopenia. 9th edition: American College of Chest Physicians evidence-based clinical practice guidelines. Chest. 2012;141 Suppl 2: e495S–530S.
10. Lubenow M, Kempf R, Eichner A, Eichler P, Carlsson LE, Greinacher A. Heparin-induced thrombocytopenia. Temporal pattern of thrombocytopenia in relation to initial use or re-exposure to heparin. Chest. 2002;122:37–42.
11. Rice L, Attisha WK, Drexler A, Francis JL. Delayed-onset heparin-induced thrombocytopenia. Ann Intern Med. 2002;136:210–5.
12. Warkentin TE, Kelton JG. A 14-year study of heparin-induced thrombocytopenia. Am J Med. 1996;101: 502–7.
13. Gruel Y, Pouplard C, Nguyen P, et al. Biological and clinical features of low-molecular-weight heparin-induced thrombocytopenia. Br J Haematol. 2003;121(5):786–92.
14. Pouplard C, May MA, Regina S, Marchand M, Fusciardi J, Gruel Y. Changes in platelet count after cardiac surgery can effectively predict the development of pathogenic heparin-dependent antibodies. Br J Haematol. 2005;128:837–41.

15. Schenk S, El-Banayosy A, Morshuis M, et al. IgG classification of anti-PF4/heparin antibodies to identify patients with heparin-induced thrombocytopenia during mechanical circulatory support. J Thromb Haemost. 2007;5(2):235–41.
16. Kawano H, Toyoda K, Miyata S, Yamamoto H, Okamoto A, Kakutani I, Walenga JM, Naritomi H, Minematsu K. Heparin-induced thrombocytopenia: a serious complication of heparin therapy for acute stroke. Cerebrovasc Dis. 2008;26(6):641–9.
17. Harbrecht U, Bastians B, Kredteck A, Hanfland P, Klockgether T, Pohl C. Heparin-induced thrombocytopenia in neurologic disease treated with unfractionated heparin. Neurology. 2004;62(4):657–9.
18. Kim GH, Hahn DK, Kellner CP, et al. The incidence of heparin-induced thrombocytopenia type II in patients with subarachnoid hemorrhage treated with heparin versus enoxaparin. J Neurosurg. 2009;110(1):50–7.
19. Alaraj A, Wallace A, Mander N, et al. Risk factors for heparin-induced thrombocytopenia type II in aneurysmal subarachnoid hemorrhage. Neurosurgery. 2011;69(5):1030–6.
20. Lo GK, Juhl D, Warkentin TE, Sigouin CS, Eichler P, Greinacher A. Evaluation of pretest clinical score (4T's) for the diagnosis of heparin-induced thrombocytopenia in two clinical settings. J Thromb Haemost. 2006;4:759–65.
21. Cuker A, Arepally G, Crowther MA, et al. The HIT expert probability (HEP) score: a novel pre-test probability model for heparin-induced thrombocytopenia based on broad expert opinion. J Thromb Haemost. 2010;8:2642–50.
22. Messmore HL, Fabbrini N, Bird ML, et al. Simple scoring system for early management of heparin-induced thrombocytopenia. Clin Appl Thromb Hemost. 2011;17(2):197–201.
23. Wallis DE, Workman DL, Lewis BF, Pifarré R, Moran JF. Failure of early heparin cessation as a treatment for heparin-induced thrombocytopenia. Am J Med. 1999;106:629–35.
24. Prechel MM, Walenga JM. Heparin-induced thrombocytopenia: an update. Semin Thromb Hemost. 2012;38(5):483–96.
25. Warkentin TE, Sheppard JA, Moore JC, et al. Laboratory testing for the antibodies that cause heparin-induced thrombocytopenia: how much class do we need? J Lab Clin Med. 2005;146(6):341–6.
26. Ban-Hoefen M, Francis C. Heparin induced thrombocytopenia and thrombosis in a tertiary care hospital. Thromb Res. 2009;124:189–92.
27. Altuntas F, Matevosyan K, Burner J, Shen YM, Sarode R. Higher optical density of an antigen assay predicts thrombosis in patients with heparin-induced thrombocytopenia. Eur J Haematol. 2008;80(5):429–35.
28. Messmore HL, Jeske WP, Wehrmacher WH, Walenga JM. Benefit-risk assessment of treatments for heparin-induced thrombocytopenia. Drug Saf. 2003;26:625–41.
29. Lewis BE, Wallis DE, Berkowitz SD, et al. Argatroban anticoagulant therapy in patients with heparin-induced thrombocytopenia. Circulation. 2001;103(14):1838–43.
30. Lewis BE, Wallis DE, Leya F, Hursting MJ, Kelton JG. Argatroban anticoagulation in patients with heparin-induced thrombocytopenia. Arch Intern Med. 2003;163(15):1849–56.
31. Swan SK, Hursting MJ. The pharmacokinetics and pharmacodynamics of argatroban: effects of age, gender, and hepatic or renal dysfunction. Pharmacotherapy. 2000;20:318–29.
32. Lewis BE, Matthai WH, Cohen M, Moses J, Hursting J, Leya F. Argatroban anticoagulation during percutaneous coronary intervention in patients with heparin-induced thrombocytopenia. Catheter Cardiovasc Interv. 2002;57:177–84.
33. Jang IK, Lewis BE, Matthai WH, Kleiman NS. Argatroban anticoagulation in conjunction with glycoprotein IIb/IIIa inhibition in patients undergoing percutaneous coronary intervention: an open-label, nonrandomized pilot study. J Thromb Thrombolysis. 2004;18:31–7.
34. Gray A, Wallis DE, Hursting MJ, Katz E, Lewis BE. Argatroban therapy for heparin-induced thrombocytopenia in acutely ill patients. Clin Appl Thromb Hemost. 2007;13(4):353–61.
35. Matthai WH, Hursting MJ, Lewis BE, Kelton JG. Argatroban anticoagulation in patients with a history of heparin-induced thrombocytopenia. Thromb Res. 2005;116:121–6.
36. Hursting MJ, Jang IK. Dosing patterns and outcomes in African American, Asian, and Hispanic patients with heparin-induced thrombocytopenia treated with argatroban. J Thromb Thrombolysis. 2009;28:10–5.
37. Madabushi R, Cox DS, Hossain M, et al. Pharmacokinetic and pharmacodynamic basis for effective argatroban dosing in pediatrics. J Clin Pharmacol. 2011;51:19–28.
38. Hursting MJ, Soffer J. Reducing harm associated with anticoagulation: practical considerations of argatroban therapy in heparin-induced thrombocytopenia. Drug Saf. 2009;32(3):203–18.
39. Kobayashi W, Tazaki Y. Effect of the thrombin inhibitor argatroban in acute cerebral thrombosis. Semin Thromb Hemost. 1997;23:531–4.
40. Ishibashi H, Koide M, Obara S, Kumasaka Y, Tamura K. High-dose argatroban therapy for stroke: novel treatment for delayed treatment and the recanalization mechanism. J Stroke Cerebrovasc Dis. 2013;22(5):656–60.
41. Barreto AD, Alexandrov AV, Lyden P, et al. The argatroban and tissue-type plasminogen activator stroke study: final results of a pilot safety study. Stroke. 2012;43(3):770–5.
42. Walenga JM, Drenth AF, Mayuga M, et al. Transition from argatroban to oral anticoagulation with phenprocoumon or acenocoumarol: effect on coagulation factor testing. Clin Appl Thromb Hemost. 2008;14(3):325–31.

43. Gosselin RC, Dager WE, King JH, et al. Effect of direct thrombin inhibitors, bivalirudin, lepirudin, and argatroban, on prothrombin time and INR values. Am J Clin Pathol. 2004;121:593–9.
44. Walenga JM, Fasanella AR, Iqbal O, et al. Coagulation laboratory testing in patients treated with argatroban. Semin Thromb Hemost. 1999;25 Suppl 1:61–6.
45. Mahaffey KW, Lewis BE, Wildermann NM, et al. The anticoagulant therapy with bivalirudin to assist in the performance of PCI in patients with heparin-induced thrombocytopenia (ATBAT) study. J Invasive Cardiol. 2003;15:611–6.
46. Kiser TH, Burch JC, Klem PM. Safety, efficacy, and dosing requirements of bivalirudin in patients with heparin-induced thrombocytopenia. Pharmacotherapy. 2008;28:1115–24.
47. Koster A, Dyke CM, Aldea G, et al. Bivalirudin during cardiopulmonary bypass in patients with previous or acute heparin-induced thrombocytopenia and heparin antibodies: results of the CHOOSE-ON trial. Ann Thorac Surg. 2007;83:572–7.
48. Dyke CM, Aldea G, Koster A, et al. Off-pump coronary bypass with bivalirudin for patients with heparin-induced thrombocytopenia or antiplatelet factor four/heparin antibodies. Ann Thorac Surg. 2007;84:836–40.
49. Hursting MJ, Lewis BE, Macfarlane DE. Transitioning from argatroban to warfarin therapy in patients with heparin-induced thrombocytopenia. Clin Appl Thromb Hemost. 2005;11(3):279–87.
50. Kang M, Alahmadi M, Sawh S, Kovacs MJ, Lazo-Lagner A. Fondaparinux for the treatment of suspected heparin-induced thrombocytopenia: a propensity score-matched study. Blood. 2015;125(6): 924–9.
51. Boyce SW, Bandyk DF, Bartholomew JR, Frame JN, Rice L. A randomized, open-label pilot study comparing desirudin and argatroban in patients with suspected heparin-induced thrombocytopenia with or without thrombosis: PREVENT-HIT Study. Am J Ther. 2011;18(1):14–22.
52. Walenga JM, Prechel M, Jeske WP, Hoppensteadt D, Maddineni J, Iqbal O, Messmore HL, Bakhos M. Rivaroxaban – an oral, direct factor Xa inhibitor – has potential for the management of patients with heparin-induced thrombocytopenia. Br J Haematol. 2008;143(1):92–9.
53. Walenga JM, Prechel M, Hoppensteadt D, Escalante V, Chaudhry T, Jeske W, Bakhos M. Apixaban as an alternate oral anticoagulant for the management of patients with heparin-induced thrombocytopenia. Clin Appl Thromb Hemost. 2013;19:482–7.
54. Crowther MA, Cook DJ, Albert M, et al. Canadian Critical Care Trials Group: the 4Ts scoring system for heparin-induced thrombocytopenia in medical-surgical intensive care unit patients. J Crit Care. 2010;25:287–93.

15 Anticoagulation in Cardiovascular Diseases

Shermeen B. Memon, Lara Bakhos, and Mushabbar A. Syed

Introduction

A 74-year-old Caucasian male presented to the emergency department after an episode of unwitnessed syncope. His wife found him on the floor with a laceration on the back of his head. The patient had no recollection of the event and only remembered waking up on the floor. There was blood on the floor, a broken coffee table, and a knocked down floor lamp. The patient denied headache, chest pain, palpitations, or focal weakness/numbness. Past medical history included atrial fibrillation, coronary artery disease, hypertension, hyperlipidemia, and prostate cancer. His outpatient medications were rivaroxaban, amlodipine, atenolol, atorvastatin, enalapril, tamsulosin, omeprazole, and multivitamins. On examination, he was alert and oriented responding appropriately to questions. There were no significant abnormalities on a neurological examination. He was in atrial fibrillation with heart rate of 120/min, BP was 125/70 mmHg, and the rest of the cardiovascular exam was within normal limits. Head CT in the emergency department showed a small left frontoparietal subdural hematoma without midline shift or herniation (Fig. 15.1a). A repeat head CT later that day showed progression in the size of the subdural hematoma (Fig. 15.1b) and Four-Factor Prothrombin Complex Concentrate (Kcentra) was administered. Subsequent CTs showed a stable hematoma size over the next 48 h. No neurosurgical intervention was performed. Atrial fibrillation was managed with a beta-blocker and digoxin. Patient was subsequently discharged to an inpatient rehabilitation facility 1 week after presentation. He was discharged home from the rehabilitation facility after another week and presented to the emergency department within 24 h with new onset dysphasia. A head CT showed a large acute on chronic subdural hematoma with associated mass effect (Fig. 15.2). An emergent craniotomy was performed and the subdural hematoma was evacuated. The postoperative period was complicated by rapid atrial fibrillation and hypotension, which were successfully managed with IV fluids and IV metoprolol later transitioning to oral regimen. The rest of the hospital course was unremarkable. Management of this patient poses significant challenges including managing the acute intracranial hemorrhage related to a new anticoagulation agent, assessing the risk and benefit for long-term anticoagulation, timing of restarting anticoagulation, and the risk of rebleeding in the future.

S.B. Memon, M.D. • L. Bakhos, M.D. • M.A. Syed, M.D., F.A.C.C. (✉)
Department of Medicine-Cardiology, Heart & Vascular Institute, Loyola University Medical Center, 2160 S. First Ave, Maywood, IL 60153, USA
e-mail: shermeen.memon@gmail.com; larabakhos@gmail.com; masyed@lumc.edu

C.M. Loftus (ed.), *Anticoagulation and Hemostasis in Neurosurgery*,
DOI 10.1007/978-3-319-27327-3_15

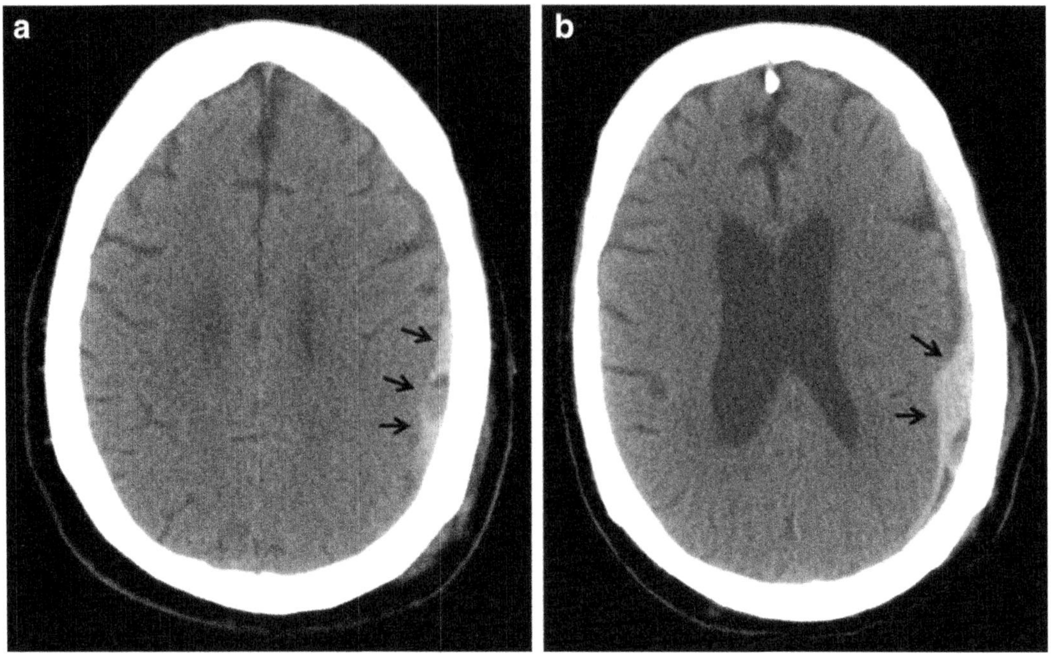

Fig. 15.1 Head CT showing acute subdural hematoma (*black arrows*)

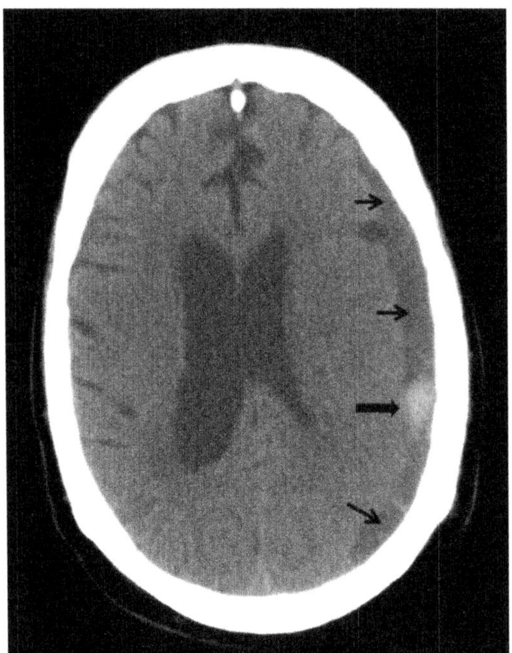

Fig. 15.2 Head CT with subacute (*small arrows*) and acute (*thick arrow*) subdural hematoma with mass effect

In cardiology practice, increasing number of patients are being diagnosed with atrial fibrillation or flutter due to aging of the general population leading to increased use of long term oral systemic anticoagulation. Given the increasing use of these medications, physicians are more likely to see these patients in the emergent, urgent, and elective surgical situations; thus, it is important to understand which cardiac conditions necessitate the use of these agents, the pharmacology of these agents, and the management of such agents in the preoperative, perioperative, and postoperative setting. This chapter aims to summarize these concepts.

Anticoagulation Agents

Short-term anticoagulation is usually achieved by intravenous or subcutaneous use of heparin while long-term use requires oral agents. For a long time warfarin was the only oral agent available in clinical practice; however, recently several novel agents have become clinically available with their unique challenges and limitations (Table 15.1).

Heparin: Unfractionated and Low Molecular Weight Heparins

Unfractionated heparin (UH) is an intravenously available anticoagulant that is used in the management and treatment of stroke prevention in atrial fibrillation, systemic thromboembolic disease, and acute coronary syndromes. UH binds to the enzyme inhibitor antithrombin, resulting in the activation of this enzyme. The activated antithrombin then inactivates thrombin and other proteases involved in blood clotting, most notable factor Xa [1]. Simply put, UH is referred to as an indirect thrombin inhibitor. Although effective for both primary and secondary prevention of stroke in the setting of atrial fibrillation as well as for thromboembolic disease, UH has a number of limitations including the need for intravenous therapy, a narrow therapeutic window, and a highly variable dose–response relation requiring close laboratory monitoring. Monitoring is achieved by following the activated partial thromboplastin time (aPTT) or the activated clotting time (ACT) when high doses of UH are administered. Baseline measures of aPTT and blood counts are made prior to initiation and then monitored every 4–6 h thereafter or after any dose change. The therapeutic level of UH that should be attained within the first 24 h of initiation is 1.5–2 times the upper limit of the control [2]. Failure to promptly achieve a therapeutic aPTT level in patients with venous thromboembolism (VTE) treated with UH has been associated with an increase in the risk of subsequent recurrent thromboembolism [3]. Complications from UH include bleeding, heparin-induced thrombocytopenia, skin lesions/necrosis, and hypersensitivity. Furthermore, given the need for intravenous administration, UH is most commonly used as a bridge to oral anticoagulant therapy.

Low molecular weight heparin (LMWH) is another anticoagulant and is very similar to UH. Unlike antithrombin activated by UH, antithrombin activated by LMWH cannot directly inhibit thrombin but instead inhibits clotting factor Xa. Due to its mechanism of action, the activity of LMWH is monitored by measuring Factor Xa activity as opposed to aPTT or ACT measurements [4]. However, given its predictable anticoagulant properties, most dosing schemes do not require routine laboratory monitoring. Moreover, the duration of the anticoagulant effect is greater than that of UH, allowing for twice a day dosing. The anticoagulant response to LMWH is highly correlated with body-weight and is dosed based on 1 mg/kg dosing; however, the dose may have to be adjusted for patients who are extremely obese or have renal insufficiency. Furthermore, laboratory monitoring is not necessary in non-pregnant patients. LMWH is less likely to induce immune-mediated thrombocytopenia; however, extreme caution must be taken in those individuals with a history of heparin-induced thrombocytopenia as this could still occur. LMWH can also be safely administered in the outpatient setting at is it administered subcutaneously as opposed to intravenously. LMWH provides many advantages over UH and is an effective, viable management and treatment strategy for patients with atrial fibrillation, acute coronary syndrome (ACS), and VTE.

Warfarin

Vitamin K antagonists (VKAs) have been the only oral anticoagulants used in clinical practice for many decades. Warfarin, the most commonly known and used VKA, was initially used as a pesticide for rats and mice. In the 1950s, warfarin was found to be effective and relatively safe for preventing and treating thrombosis in humans, leading to its approval in 1954 [5]. Warfarin's anticoagulant effects are due to its ability to inhibit vitamin K dependent gamma-carboxylation of coagulation factors II, VII, IX,

Table 15.1 Summary of anticoagulation drugs

Medication	Pharmacology	Time to peak action	Route	Dosing	Monitoring	Uses	Reversal agents	Adverse effects
Unfractionated heparin	Indirect thrombin inhibitor	Immediate	IV	IV infusion (weight based dosing per institutional nomogram)	aPTT: 1.5–2× ULN	1. Atrial fibrillation 2. VTE 3. Unstable angina/ NSTEMI 4. Prosthetic valves 5. LV thrombus 6. LVAD	Protamine sulfate	Bleeding Heparin induced thrombocytopenia and thrombosis Skin necrosis
Low molecular weight heparin[a]	Inhibits clotting Factor Xa	3–5 h	SQ	1 mg/kg as twice a day dosing	Factor Xa levels (not routinely monitored)	1. Atrial fibrillation 2. VTE 3. Unstable angina/ NSTEM I 4. LV thrombus	Protamine sulfate	Bleeding Heparin induced thrombocytopenia (less frequent as compared to unfractionated heparin) Skin necrosis Elevation in LFTs
Warfarin	Vitamin K antagonist	24–72 h	Oral	Dosing individualized and guided by INR	PT/INR	1. Atrial Fibrillation (INR goal 2–3) 2. VTE (INR goal 2–3) 3. Prosthetic valves (INR goal 2.5–3.5) 4. LV thrombus 5. LVADs-goal based on specific device	Vitamin K	Bleeding Ecchymosis Skin necrosis Hypersensitivity
Rivaroxaban[a]	Direct factor Xa inhibitor	2–4 h	Oral	1. Nonvalvular atrial fibrillation: 20 mg once daily 2. VTE: 15 mg twice daily for 21 days followed by 20 mg once daily	Non0065	1. Nonvalvular atrial fibrillation 2. VTE	Please see text for details regarding reversal agents	Bleeding Thrombocytopenia Agranulocytosis Hepatitis Elevated LFTs

Apixaban[a]	Direct Factor Xa inhibitor	3–4 h	Oral	1. Nonvalvular atrial fibrillation: 5 mg twice daily[b] 2. VTE: 10 mg twice daily for 7 days followed by 5 mg twice daily	None	1. Nonvalvular atrial fibrillation 2. VTE	Please see test for details regarding reversal agents	Bleeding Hypersensitivity Syncope
Dabigatran[a]	Direct thrombin inhibitor	1 h	Oral	1. Nonvalvular atrial fibrillation: 150 mg twice daily 2. VTE: 150 mg twice daily (after 5–10 of IV anticoagulation)	None	1. Nonvalvular atrial fibrillation 2. VTE	Please see test for details regarding reversal agents	Bleeding Dyspepsia Gastritis Thrombocytopenia
Aspirin	Antiplatelet	~1–2 h	Oral	81–32 mg daily	None	Coronary artery disease Atrial fibrillation	Platelet infusion	Bleeding Gastrointestinal distress
P2Y12 inhibitors (i.e., clopidogrel)	Antiplatelet	Dose dependent	Oral		None	Coronary artery disease		Bleeding

ULN upper limits of normal, *NSTEMI* non-ST elevation myocardial infarction
[a]Medication should be dose reduced for patients with renal insufficiency
[b]Apixiban should be dose reduced in those with any two of the following criteria: Age ≥80 years, body weight ≤60 kg, or serum creatinine ≥1.5 mg/dL, then reduce dose to 2.5 mg twice daily

and X, thereby rendering these proteins inactive [6, 7]. With a high bioavailability, it is rapidly absorbed in the proximal small bowel and metabolically cleared via the hepatic cytochrome P450 [6]. The anticoagulant effects are monitored using the International Normalized Ratio (INR), with a goal of 2.0–3.0 reflecting appropriate anticoagulation in most clinical scenarios for both primary and secondary prevention of thrombosis. The most common clinical indications for warfarin use are atrial fibrillation, artificial heart valves, arterial and venous thromboembolic phenomenon, and hypercoagulable syndromes.

Despite being the most widely prescribed oral anticoagulant, warfarin has many shortcomings. Given that it works by antagonizing vitamin K recycling, patients must have stable dietary habits for vitamin K to allow for proper INR control. Also, numerous drugs interact with warfarin leading to over- or under-anticoagulation. Due to these factors, frequent INR serum assays must be obtained to ensure appropriate anticoagulation, with most algorithms suggesting these measurements be obtained at least every 4 weeks. Despite this, studies have shown only 60 % of patients are maintained within a therapeutic INR range of 2.0–3.0 [8].

Furthermore, patients on warfarin are also at increased risk of bleeding due to its potent anticoagulant effects. Thus, numerous risk scores have been developed to assess this bleeding risk. The HAS-BLED (**H**ypertension, **A**bnormal renal and liver function, **S**troke, **B**leeding tendency/predisposition, **L**abile INRs, **E**lderly with age greater than 65 years, **D**rugs or alcohol) score is a common method utilized to weigh the risk of bleeding versus the benefits of thromboembolic prevention in patients with cardiac disorders such as atrial fibrillation. In the event of a bleed, warfarin's anticoagulant effects can be reversed with the use of vitamin K as well as with replacement of Factors II, VII, IX, and X.

Novel Oral Anticoagulants

Due to the limitations of warfarin's use, options for anticoagulation have steadily been expanding with the introduction of novel oral anticoagulants (NOACs) that target the enzymatic activity of thrombin and factor Xa. Dabigatran extexilate, the only oral direct thrombin inhibitor, is a prodrug that is converted in the liver to dabigatran, which inhibits clot-bound and circulating thrombin [9]. Unlike warfarin, the maximum anticoagulant effects are achieved within 2–3 h of ingestion, absorption is not affected by dietary habits, and monitoring with lab testing is not required [10]. Furthermore, dose changes are generally not required with concomitant administration of cytochrome P450 inducers and inhibitors since dabigatran is renally metabolized; dosing is solely based on clinical indication and renal function. Published in 2009, the RE-LY trial randomized 18,000 patients with moderate to high risk of thromboembolic stroke and nonvalvular AF to dabigatran or warfarin. After a median follow-up of 2 years, dabigatran 150 mg twice daily was shown to be noninferior to warfarin in stroke reduction [11]. Dabigatran has since been approved for use in primary and secondary prevention of venous thromboembolism, treatment of venous thromboembolism, and stroke prevention in atrial fibrillation. Of note, the RE-ALIGN study demonstrated that patients with mechanical aortic or mitral valves receiving dabigatran as opposed to warfarin had increased bleeding and thromboembolic risk [12]. Therefore, dabigatran should not be used in patients with valvular atrial fibrillation or prosthetic heart valves. Moreover, this medication should not be used in pregnant patients as it is associated with an increase in reproductive risks [13]. However, for its approved indications, dabigatran offers a great alternative to warfarin therapy.

The other target used by NOACs is Factor Xa. Factor Xa is a protease that plays a key role in the blood coagulation cascade. Holding a central position that links both the intrinsic and extrinsic pathways to the final common coagulation pathway, factor Xa converts prothrombin to thrombin leading to the formation of thrombus. Rivaroxaban, apixaban, and edoxaban are currently available oral factor Xa inhibitors that block this final common pathway, effectively reducing the risk of thrombus formation.

Rivaroxaban is an orally available factor Xa inhibitor with a half-life of 7–17 h and once a ay dosing. As with dabigatran, rivaroxaban is given at fixed doses without the need for routine monitoring. Dosing is based on a patient's clinical indication and renal function; it is not recommended in those patients with a creatinine clearance less than 30 mL/min or in those with severe hepatic impairment. Rivaroxaban does interact with medications that are inhibitors or inducers of cytochrome P3A4 and P-glycoprotein, such as antifungal agents. In the ROCKET-AF trial, 14,264 patients with nonvalvular atrial fibrillation with at least moderate risk of stroke were randomized to rivaroxaban or warfarin [14]. Rivaroxaban was shown to be noninferior to warfarin in reducing thromboembolic events without increasing bleeding consequences. Rivaroxaban has not been approved for use in pregnant patients, those with prosthetic heart valves, or valvular atrial fibrillation due to the lack of clinical studies. Rivaroxaban provides a practical therapeutic option for use in the primary and secondary prevention of venous thromboembolism, treatment of venous thromboembolism, and stroke prevention in atrial fibrillation.

Apixaban is also an oral factor Xa inhibitor that has a half-life of 5–9 h, requiring a twice a day dosing schedule. Dosing is based on the patient's clinical indication, age, weight, and renal function. As with rivaroxaban, apixaban is generally given at a fixed dose without the need for monitoring and also interacts with medications that are inhibitors or inducers of cytochrome P3A4 and P-glycoprotein. It too is used in the prevention and management of venous thromboembolic disease and stroke prevention in atrial fibrillation. Apixaban's use in nonvalvular atrial fibrillation was evaluated in 18,201 patients in the ARISTOTLE trial, which demonstrated that apixaban was superior to warfarin in reducing stroke and systemic embolism [15]. As with rivaroxaban, apixaban is not approved for use in pregnant patients, those with prosthetic heart valves, or valvular atrial fibrillation.

Edoxaban is another oral factor Xa inhibitor with a half-life of 6–11 h and is typically dosed once a day. As with the previously discussed factor Xa inhibitors, edoxaban is given at a fixed dose without monitoring; dosing is based on a patient's clinical indication and renal function. It is also used in the prevention and management of venous thromboembolic disease and stroke prevention in atrial fibrillation and is similarly contraindicated for use in prosthetic heart valves or during pregnancy.

NOACs offer patients a viable alternative to warfarin therapy in prevention and management of thromboembolic disease. Given their predictable anticoagulant effects, these medications provide reliable anticoagulation in patients at risk for these potentially catastrophic consequences. Although warfarin is more cumbersome for patients due its continued need for monitoring, its numerous drug interactions, and dietary constraints, it remains vital to medical therapy. Its use has been studied in a wider array of medical conditions; warfarin can be prescribed not only in the management of venous thromboembolisms and nonvalvular atrial fibrillation but also in patients with valvular atrial fibrillation, prosthetic heart valves, and various myocardial diseases.

Cardiovascular Indications for Anticoagulation

Atrial Fibrillation

Atrial fibrillation (AF) is the most common sustained cardiac rhythm disturbance and is defined as a supraventricular tachyarrhythmia that results from uncoordinated atrial activity, resulting in ineffective atrial contraction. Rapidly firing ectopic foci, most commonly found in the left atrium and more specifically around the pulmonary veins, bombard the atrioventricular (AV) node, resulting in rapid ventricular rates. These rates and unorganized atrial activity can lead to clinical symptoms or long term consequences such as deterioration in hemodynamic status, increased risk of embolic events, and progressive left ventricular dysfunction.

AF affects between 2.7 million and 6.1 million American adults and is expected to double over the next 25 years [16]. The prevalence of AF increases with age, with up to 12 % of patients between the ages of 75 and 84 and more than one-third of patients over the age of 80 being affected by AF [17]. In addition to advanced age, AF is often associated with structural heart disease and chronic comorbidities, with the most common being hypertension, ischemic heart disease, and heart failure. These comorbidities along with atrial structural abnormalities such as inflammation, fibrosis, dilatation, ischemia, infiltration, and hypertrophy predispose individuals to the development of this arrhythmia [18].

The diagnosis of AF is commonly made by detecting an irregular pulse on physical examination and/or irregular R-R intervals and absence of distinct P-waves with irregularity of the atrial activity on ECG. Clinically, patients can be asymptomatic or present with palpitations, fatigue, dizziness, pre-syncope, and syncope; more severe clinical consequences can result in hospitalizations due to hemodynamic compromise, heart failure, and thromboembolic events. In addition to being a symptomatic burden, AF also is associated with a fivefold increased risk of stroke [19], a threefold increased risk of heart failure [20–22] and twofold increased risk of mortality [19].

Initial evaluation should include ECG documentation, investigation for underlying systemic disease, and evaluation for structural heart disease with a transthoracic echocardiogram (TTE) [18]. TTE evaluates for atrial structural changes such as dilatation and hypertrophy as well as for valvular abnormalities commonly associated with AF such as mitral valve disease. AF related to such valvular disease is referred to as valvular AF.

In addition to understanding the etiology of AF, two principal management decisions must be addressed:

1. The symptom management strategy
2. The need for oral anticoagulation for the reduction in thromboembolic consequences.

Two large clinical trials have compared rate versus rhythm control strategies in patients with AF. The 2002 Atrial Fibrillation Follow-up Investigation of Rhythm Management (AFFIRM) trial was the first and largest study to compare these two strategies. This study randomized 4060 patients with recurrent AF to either rate control or to rhythm control. Enrolled patients had to be ≥65 years of age and/or have other risk factors for stroke or death. Individuals were excluded if patients had contraindications to antiarrhythmic or anticoagulation therapies. After a mean follow-up of 3.5 years, there was no significant difference in the primary end-point of all-cause mortality or composite secondary end points of death, ischemic stroke, anoxic encephalopathy, major bleeding, or cardiac arrest. Moreover, there was no significant difference in functional status or quality of life between the two groups [23]. The RACE (Rate Control versus Electrical Cardioversion for Persistent Atrial Fibrillation) study randomized 522 patients with recurrent persistent AF or atrial flutter of less than 1 year duration who required one or two direct-current cardioversions (DCCV) within the prior 2 years to either rate or rhythm control therapies. After a mean follow-up of 2.3 years, there was no significant difference in primary end-point of composite cardiovascular death, admission for heart failure, thromboembolic event, severe bleeding, pacemaker implantation, or severe side effects from antiarrhythmic medications. As in the AFFIRM trial, there were no significant differences in quality of life between the rate and rhythm control groups [24].

Controlling ventricular rates with medical therapy is an important strategy since attaining rate control can often alleviate a patient's symptoms. Medical therapy for rate control includes beta-blockers, nondihydropyridine calcium channel blockers, digoxin, and certain antiarrhythmic medications, e.g., amiodarone and sotalol. Acutely, beta-blockers such as metoprolol or esmolol are effective when administered intravenously. For chronic management of AF, oral administration of beta-blockers is often used. The nondihydropyridine calcium channel blockers used for ventricular rate control are verapamil and diltiazem; these agents should not be used in patients with decompensated heart failure as they may precipitate further hemodynamic compromise due to their negative inotropic effect. Choice of medication is determined by a patient's symptoms, hemodynamic status, comorbidities, and potential precipitants of AF.

Although digoxin can also be used for rate control, it is usually not first line therapy as it has a slow onset of action and is effective only in controlling heart rates during rest. Furthermore, caution must be used in patients with renal dysfunction, the elderly, and in the presence of other drugs that affect its excretion. Digoxin has a narrow therapeutic window with toxicity manifesting as atrioventricular block, ventricular arrhythmias, and/or aggravation of sinus node dysfunction. Antiarrhythmic drugs, e.g., amiodarone should be avoided for rate control as it can chemically restore sinus rhythm, which could lead to detrimental effects if the patient is not properly anticoagulated.

With regards to heart rate goals, a resting heart rate of less than 80 beats per minute (bpm) is reasonable for symptomatic management of AF (Class IIa) and a lenient goal of less than 110 bpm may be reasonable if the patient remains asymptomatic and left ventricular systolic function is preserved (Class IIb). When medical therapies have proven ineffective in controlling heart rates, referral to an electrophysiologist and invasive procedures can be pursued (class IIa) [18].

Rhythm control is another treatment strategy often employed as a means to restore and/or maintain sinus rhythm. Factors that may favor a rhythm control strategy include inadequate rate control, patient's age (younger being more favorable), first episode of AF, AF precipitated by an acute illness, tachycardia-mediated cardiomyopathy, and patient preference [18]. Antiarrhythmic medications utilized in this strategy include amiodarone, dofetilide, dronedarone, flecainide, propfenone, and sotalol. Medication selection is often times guided by the drug's safety profile and the patient's comorbidities as opposed to the drug efficacy.

In addition to antiarrhythmic medications, DCCV, which involves delivering an electrical shock that is synchronized with the patient's QRS complex, can also be used to restore sinus rhythm and is often times used in conjunction with use of antiarrhythmic drugs.

Finally, a third method of rhythm control is catheter ablation, which provides an alternative to traditional medical therapy. Cardiac ablation is an invasive technique using multiple catheters to localize the foci in the atrium generating these chaotic, irregular impulses. These foci are typically located around the pulmonary veins in the left atrium; however, other foci can be identified with electrophysiologic mapping. Radiofrequency energy or cryotherapy can then be applied to these areas in an attempt to terminate the ectopic electrical activity.

Currently, cardiac catheter ablation is usually considered in patients with symptomatic paroxysmal or persistent AF refractory to or intolerant to at least one class I or class III antiarrhythmic drug (class IIa). In addition, after weighing the risks and benefits with the patient, ablative therapy can be offered to patients with symptomatic paroxysmal or persistent AF prior to a trial of antiarrhythmic therapies (class IIA) [18].

Regardless of the rate or rhythm control strategy, appropriate anticoagulation must be employed to reduce thromboembolic events in both the acute care setting as well as with chronic management of these patients. Due to the uncoordinated atrial activity resulting in ineffective atrial contraction, blood stasis occurs in the "quivering" atria, leading to increased risk of thrombi formation. Dislodgement of such thrombi that are usually found in the left atrium or left atrial appendage, results in ischemic strokes as well as other peripheral thromboembolic events. Due to such devastating consequences, antithrombotic medication is prescribed based on the patient's risk of thromboembolism and irrespective of whether the AF pattern is paroxysmal, persistent, or permanent.

The CHA_2DS_2-VASc scoring system, which has been validated in multiple studies, predicts a patient's risk of thromboembolic events. The components of this scoring system include: **C**ongestive heart failure, **H**ypertension, **A**ge, **D**iabetes mellitus, **S**troke/transient ischemic attack (TIA)/thromboembolic event, **V**ascular disease, **A**ge 65–74, and **S**ex (female gender) (Table 15.2). The higher the score, the higher the thromboembolic risk. This risk is then weighed against the risk of bleeding to determine an individual's need for an antithrombotic agent. For patients with nonvalvular AF and a CHA_2DS_2-VASc of 0, it is reasonable not

Table 15.2 Estimating the risk of thromboembolism in atrial fibrillation

CHA$_2$DS$_2$-VASc scoring system	
Acronym definition	Score
Congestive Heart Failure	1
Hypertension	1
Age ≥75 years	2
Diabetes Mellitus	1
Stroke/Transient Ischemic Attack/ Thromboembolic Event	2
Vascular Disease (prior myocardial infraction, peripheral arterial disease, or aortic plaque)	1
Age 65–74 years	1
Sex (Female gender)	1
Maximum score	9
Stroke risk stratification based on score	
Score	Estimated stroke risk per year (%)
0	0
1	1.3
2	2.2
3	3.2
4	4.0
5	6.7
6	9.8
7	9.6
8	6.7
9	15.2

to initiate anticoagulation (Class IIA). For patients with nonvalvular AF and a CHA$_2$DS$_2$-VASc score of 1, the use of antithrombotic agents or the use of full dose aspirin (325 mg) is left to the patient and physician's discretion (Class IIb). For patients with nonvalvular AF with prior stroke, TIA, or a CHA$_2$DS$_2$-VASc ≥ 2, oral antithrombotic agents are recommended for long-term management (class I) [18]. It is important to recognize that individuals who have had an AV node ablation for rate control still require anticoagulation as deemed appropriate by the CHA$_2$DS$_2$-VASc score since these individuals continue to have uncoordinated atrial activity. It is also important to recognize that CHA$_2$DS$_2$-VASc scoring system does not apply to patients with valvular AF; these individuals require anticoagulation regardless of score.

Another caveat is in those patients undergoing restoration of sinus rhythm with DCCV. Thromboembolism after cardioversion, electrically or chemically, can be due to migration of thrombi present at the time of cardioversion or the formation of subsequent thrombi in the post-cardioversion period while atrial function is still depressed. For patients with AF of less than 48-h duration who are at low thromboembolic risk, anticoagulation or no antithrombotic therapy may be considered for DCCV without the need for post-cardioversion anticoagulation (Class IIB). However, if the duration of the episode exceeds 48 h or if the duration is unknown, patients must be anticoagulated for the preceding 3 weeks and for at least 4 weeks post-DCCV (class I) [18]. Thromboembolic risk after cardioversion is highest in the first 72 h and the majority of events occur within 10 days of cardioversion. If it is not plausible to wait 3 weeks for cardioversion, a transesophageal echocardiogram (TEE) may be performed to look for thrombi in the left atrium and left atrial appendage; if no thrombus is identified and patient has achieved therapeutic anticoagulation, cardioversion can be performed. Following the 4 weeks of anticoagulation in the post-cardioversion setting, the need for chronic anticoagulation is assessed by the CHA$_2$DS$_2$-VASc scoring system.

Antithrombotic agents used for stroke prevention include unfractionated heparin, low-molecular weight heparin, warfarin, direct thrombin inhibitors, and factor Xa inhibitors. The specific antithrombotic agent utilized in stroke reduction in patients with AF is based on the medication's safety profile, the patient's risk factors, and patient preference as discussed earlier in the chapter.

Atrial Flutter

Atrial Flutter (AFL) is another supraventricular tachyarrhythmia that is often times associated with atrial fibrillation. AFL differs in its electrophysiologic properties and is due to a reentry circuit typically localized to the isthmus between the tricuspid valve annulus and inferior vena cava in the right atrium. Despite these differences, atrial flutter is managed in a similar manner to AF. According to the AHA/ACC/HRS Atrial Fibrillation guidelines of 2014, antithrombotic therapy is recommended in AFL according to the same risk profile used for AF (class I) [18].

Valvular Heart Disease

Valvular heart disease (VHD) is defined as damage to or a defect in one or more of the four cardiac valves: aortic, mitral, tricuspid, or pulmonic valves. With the dramatic decline in rheumatic disease, VHD in developed countries is most commonly attributed to degenerative changes and is considered a disease of the elderly. Its prevalence is estimated at 2.5 % in industrialized countries [25]. Valvular defects can result in regurgitation or stenosis of the valve. Progression of these defects can result in irreversible ventricular dysfunction, pulmonary hypertension, stroke, and atrial fibrillation. Some of these valvular abnormalities require anticoagulation, as they are associated with increased risk of thromboembolic events.

Mitral stenosis (MS) results from thickening and immobility of the mitral leaflets and causes an obstruction of blood flow from the left atrium to the left ventricle. MS is most often secondary to rheumatic heart disease or senile calcific disease. Regardless of etiology, the mechanical obstruction causes an increase in pressure in the left atrium, pulmonary vasculature and the right side of the heart leading to symptoms of dyspnea, hemoptysis, and right-sided heart failure. Elevated left atrial pressures results in left atrial dilatation, increasing the risk of developing AF as well as left atrial thrombi. Due to such association, indefinite anticoagulation with warfarin is indicated in all patients with MS and AF, MS and a prior embolic event, or MS and a left atrial thrombus with a goal INR of 2.0–3.0 (Class I) [26]. Because the efficacy of NOACs in preventing embolic events has not been studied in patients with valvular heart disease, warfarin is the only oral anticoagulant recommended in this population.

Progression of valvular regurgitation or stenosis causes significant morbidity and mortality. The purpose of valvular intervention is to improve symptoms, prolong survival, and minimize the risk of irreversible ventricular dysfunction, pulmonary hypertension, stroke, and atrial fibrillation [26]. When a surgical heart valve replacement is warranted, a choice is made between a mechanical or bioprosthetic valve. The choice of valve prosthesis is based on several factors including the patient's age, expected life span, potential risk of lifelong anticoagulation, valve durability, clinical circumstances, and patient preference.

Mechanical valves are durable in patients of any age with a low risk for the need for reoperation; however, these valves require lifelong anticoagulation with warfarin. The goal INR for each patient is based on the mechanical valve position along with a patient's risk factors, which include AF, prior thromboembolism, LV dysfunction, or hypercoagulable states. Three basic types of mechanical valve design are: bileaflet, monoleaflet, and caged ball valves. *Given their risk of thrombosis, anticoagulation with warfarin is recommended for all patients with mechanical valves.* An INR goal of 2.0–3.0 is recommended in patients with a mechanical aortic valve replacement (AVR) with bileaflet mechanical or Medtronic Hall valve and no risk factors for thromboembolism (Class I). Patients with an AVR and any additional risk factor as listed above, those with an older mechanical AVR (Starr–Edwards or disk valves other than Medtronic Hall), or those with a mitral valve replacement (MVR) with any mechanical valve should have a higher goal INR of 2.5–3.5 (Class I). In addition to warfarin, aspirin 75–100 mg/day is recommended in all patients with a mechanical valve prosthesis (Class I) [26].

Bioprosthetic valves are also a viable option for patients with severe valvular disease to avoid the need for lifelong anticoagulation; however, due to their limited life span, patients may require reoperation due to valve degeneration. *Furthermore, despite the use of a bioprosthesis, anticoagulation with warfarin is still considered reasonable in the first 3 months after a bioprosthetic AVR, MVR, or MV repair with a goal INR of 2.0–3.0* [26, 27]. As with mechanical valves, those with bioprosthetic valves in the aortic or mitral valve positions should be considered for aspirin therapy (75–100 mg). Anticoagulation early after the valve implantation is intended to decrease the risk of thromboembolism until the prosthetic valve has completely endothelialized [26]. The risks versus benefits of anticoagulation should be discussed with patients and individualized based on the patient's comorbidities and risk factors.

More recently, patients with aortic stenosis (AS) who are too high risk for surgery have been undergoing transcatheter aortic valve replacement (TAVR). These valves are biological prostheses mounted on an expandable metallic frame. These individuals do not require anticoagulation; however, clopidogrel 75 mg daily is used for the 6 months following the procedure in addition to lifeline aspirin therapy (75–100 mg daily) (Class IIb) [26].

Of note, newer oral antithrombotic agents are not approved in patients with mechanical or bioprosthetic valves. Patients should receive warfarin regardless of whether the anticoagulation is for the valve alone or for the valve in addition to another indication. The RE-ALIGN trial was prematurely stopped as the incidence of stroke, valve thrombosis, and bleeding was all significantly higher in the dabigatran group compared to warfarin [12]. Other NOACs have not been studied in patients with prosthetic heart valves.

Myocardial Diseases

Myocardial Infarction

Myocardial infarction (MI) is defined as acute myocardial ischemia and/or necrosis secondary to coronary plaque rupture resulting in an imbalance of myocardial oxygen supply and demand. With over 700,000 Americans suffering from an MI yearly, these events are a major cause of morbidity and mortality [28]. Clinically, these events are diagnosed when a patients presents with symptoms of ischemia (e.g., chest pain), a rise and/or fall in cardiac biomarkers, new ischemic changes on an electrocardiogram (ECG) (ST-segment changes, left bundle branch block or development of pathologic Q waves), identification of intracoronary thrombus by angiography, or imaging evidence of new loss of viable myocardium or a new regional wall motion abnormality of the left ventricle [29]. The mainstay of therapy for these individuals includes pharmacotherapy in addition to coronary revascularization. Following percutaneous coronary interventions, patients are placed on dual-antiplatelet therapy with aspirin along with a P2Y12 receptor inhibitor such as clopidogrel, prasugrel, or ticagrelor.

Both bare-metal (BMS) and drug-eluting stents (DES) are options during a percutaneous coronary intervention. In patients receiving a drug eluting stent for a non-acute coronary syndrome (ACS) indication, clopidogrel 75 mg daily should be given for at least 12 months if the patient is not at high risk of bleeding. In patients receiving BMS for a non-ACS indication, clopidogrel should be given for a minimum of 1 month and ideally up to 12 months. As noted earlier, a P2Y12 inhibitor and aspirin should be administered for up to 12 months in all patients with ACS who are treated with either an early invasive or ischemia-guided strategy [30].

Balloon angioplasty is an additional option that refers to dilation of coronary stenosis by means of a balloon catheter without stent placement. Although no randomized trials have directly assessed duration of dual antiplatelet therapy in patients undergoing balloon angioplasty, current recommendations suggest 1 month of dual antiplatelet therapy with aspirin and a P2Y12 inhibitor since there is a potential risk of thrombosis caused by iatrogenic plaque rupture [31].

Left ventricular (LV) thrombus is one of the more common complications of myocardial infarctions and varies with infarct location and size. Acute anterior infarction, LV function less than or equal to 35 %, and apical dyskinesia or aneurysm formation are associated with an increased risk in the formation of an LV thrombus [32, 33]. *The risk of embolization in patients with a documented LV thrombus who are not treated with anticoagulant therapy has been estimated at 10–15 %* [34]. *Thus, anticoagulant therapy with a vitamin K antagonist should be considered for patients with acute myocardial infarction and asymptomatic LV mural thrombus (Class IIa)*. Moreover, in patients with an acute myocardial infarction and anterior apical akinesis or dyskinesis without thrombus development, anticoagulant therapy may be considered. Given these patients are also likely to be on dual antiplatelet therapy with aspirin and a P2Y12 receptor inhibitors, a lower INR goal of 2.0–2.5 should be targeted to mitigate the increased risk of bleeding (Class IIB). Treatment can be limited to 3 months in patients with or at risk for LV thrombus formation at which time reevaluation with a TTE may be helpful to guide cessation or prolonged treatment [35]. Of note, NOACs have not been evaluated for use in this context.

Heart Failure

Heart failure (HF) is a common clinical syndrome that results from any structural or functional cardiovascular disorder causing a decrease in systemic perfusion that is inadequate to meet the body's metabolic demands. It is caused by a variety of disorders that affect the pericardium, myocardium, endocardium, cardiac valves, vasculature, or metabolism. Systolic and/or diastolic dysfunction can contribute to a reduced cardiac output and the hallmark symptoms of heart failure, which include dyspnea, fatigue, and fluid retention. Coronary artery disease accounts for approximately two-thirds of patients with LV systolic dysfunction with the remainder of these patients having nonischemic causes such as hypertension, valvular disease, myocarditis, or idiopathic dilated cardiomyopathy [36].

Patients with heart failure and LV systolic dysfunction are at an increased risk of thromboembolic events due to stasis of blood in dilated hypokinetic cardiac chambers and peripheral blood vessels in addition to increased activity in procoagulant factors. This increased risk, however, does not seem to translate to outcomes. Several retrospective analyses have shown that patients with heart failure taking warfarin had similar rates of thromboembolic events when compared to patients not taking anticoagulants. Furthermore, large studies have shown that the risk of thromboembolism in clinically stable patients with depressed ejection fraction (EF) and echocardiographic evidence of intracardiac thrombi is as low as 1–3 % per year [37–39]. Due to such low incidence of events, the risk of anticoagulation may outweigh the benefit; thus, *anticoagulation is not recommended in patients with chronic systolic heart failure without AF, a prior thromboembolic event or a cardioembolic source (Class III)* [36].

Left Ventricular Assist Devices

A subset of patients with advanced systolic heart failure will develop end-stage heart failure refractory to optimal medical therapy, resulting in a very poor prognosis. Cardiac transplantation is a viable option but is only available for a minority of patients due to the lack of suitable donor hearts. The lack of effective therapies for advanced heart failure has led to the development of mechanical circulatory support devices. Initially developed for temporary support in the setting of acute decompensated heart failure, the left ventricular assist device (LVAD) has become a mainstay of therapy for those with end-stage heart failure as a means to "bridge to transplant" as well as for "destination therapy" for those not eligible for transplant. One-fourth of all US heart transplant recipients are supported with these devices prior to transplantation and their use for permanent/destination therapy is increasing [40]. An LVAD allows for the dysfunctional left ventricle to act as a passive conduit through which the mechanical pump fills and provides continuous effective systemic blood flow throughout the cardiac cycle. Though LVADs have become a viable option for numerous patients, such devices introduce a new set of complications including thrombosis and bleeding.

Pump thrombosis causes device obstruction and is clinically suggested by the development of hemolysis and changes in LVAD parameters. To prevent this complication as well as the thromboembolic events associated with it, *patients with LVADs require antiplatelet therapy with aspirin and anticoagulation with warfarin* [41]. INR goals are determined by each device manufacturer.

Despite that, for continuous flow devices, the rate of pump thrombosis ranges from 0.01 to 0.11 per patient [42, 43]. This complication can often times effectively be treated with intensifying anticoagulation. However, if pharmacologic therapy is not effective, immediate pump exchange or heart transplantation is required [41].

Furthermore, these patients are also at increased risk for neurologic complications. Ischemic and hemorrhagic stroke following LVAD placement has been reported to be between 8 and 25 % [44, 45]. Strokes in these patients tend to occur with greater frequency in the right hemisphere, suggestive of a cardioembolic source [46, 47].

Bleeding is the most common complication associated with LVADs, with the incidence of major bleeding being >20 % [43]. This increased risk of bleeding events is not only due to the use of warfarin but also due to the development of acquired von Willebrand disease and gastrointestinal (GI) arteriovenous malformations. In randomized trials comparing different types of LVADs, the leading cause of death in all groups was cerebral hemorrhage [48]. If a hemorrhagic stroke is identified, anticoagulation is discontinued and reversed. In the setting of recurrent GI bleeding with no clear source or a source that is not amenable to therapy, the goal INR or even the use of warfarin all together should be reevaluated [41]. Discontinuation of anticoagulation due to bleeding requires careful monitoring of the LVAD parameters to avoid thrombotic complications and should only be performed under the close supervision of an advanced heart failure specialist.

Left Ventricular Noncompaction

Noncompaction of the ventricular myocardium is classified by the American Heart Association as a primary genetic cardiomyopathy [49]. The prevalence of left ventricular noncompaction (LVNC) has been estimated at 0.05 % of the general population [50]. This cardiomyopathy is thought to be secondary to defects in cardiac embryogenesis resulting in the intrauterine arrest of the compaction of the loose meshwork that makes up the fetal myocardium, resulting in a hypertrabeculated non-compacted layer of myocardium (spongy myocardium). LVNC can be an isolated finding or may be associated with other congenital anomalies such as Ebstein's anomaly, bicuspid aortic valve, and atrial or ventricular septal defects.

The clinical presentation is variable, ranging from asymptomatic to advanced heart failure, ventricular and atrial arrhythmias, and thromboembolic events including stroke. Oechslin et al. described the outcomes of 34 adults with LVNC. Seventy-nine percent of patients reported dyspnea, 35 % presented in New York Heart Association class III or IV heart failure, 41 % experienced ventricular tachycardia, and 24 % were noted to have thromboembolic events [51]. The role of oral anticoagulation for primary prevention is unclear in patients with LVNC particularly with normal LV function and absence of LV hypertrophy [52]. In clinical practice patients with LVNC and systolic dysfunction routinely receive long-term warfarin due to increased risk of thromboembolism.

Venous Thromboembolism/Antiphos pholipid Syndrome

Venous thromboembolism (VTE), which includes deep vein thrombosis (DVT) and pulmonary embolism (PE), has an annual incidence of approximately 0.1–0.27 % [53]. Approximately 20 % of patients with PE die before the diagnosis is made or on the first day following the diagnosis [54]. Risk factors for VTE include but are not limited to immobility due to trauma or surgery, pregnancy, malignancy, use of prothrombotic medications such as hormone replacement therapy, and inherited or acquired hypercoagulable states. When VTE is first diagnosed, the principal objective of therapy is to prevent DVT extension and PE occurrence. Initial treatment requires the use of antithrombotics such as intravenous heparin, subcutaneous low molecular weight heparin, warfarin (INR goal of 2.0–3.0), dabigatran, rivaroxaban, or apixaban, all of which have been approved for this indication. The duration of treatment for VTE/PE should be individualized according to the presence or absence of provoking events, risk factors for recurrence and bleeding, as well as to the individual patient's preferences. A 3-month duration of anticoagulation therapy is recommended for patients with VTE/PE in the postoperative setting, with transient risk factors, and in patients at high risk of bleeding. Consideration can be given to extend or indefinitely continue therapy in patients with unprovoked VTE/PE after weighing the risks and benefits [55].

Management of Anticoagulation and Antiplatelet Therapy in the Perioperative Setting

Millions of individuals receive long-term anticoagulation and/or antiplatelet therapy for the prevention and treatment of thromboembolism due to atrial fibrillation, prosthetic heart valves, myocardial diseases, left ventricular assist devices, and venous thromboembolism. Annually, approximately 10 % of patients taking antithrombotic agents undergo surgical or other invasive procedures that require temporary discontinuation of therapy [56]. The management of anticoagulation in patients undergoing surgery is challenging and requires a balance between reducing the risk of thromboembolism during the interruption of anticoagulation and preventing excessive bleeding associated with the particular invasive procedure. Both of these outcomes adversely affect mortality. Appropriate decision-making should be individualized and requires knowledge of a patient's thrombotic risk, procedure-related bleeding risk, concepts of bridging anticoagulation therapy, and timing of cessation and reinitiation of antithrombotic therapy.

Periprocedural thrombotic risk is generally extrapolated from risks outside the periprocedural period. The risk of thromboembolic events in patients with nonvalvular atrial fibrillation is assessed with the use of the CHA_2DS_2-Vasc score, a higher scoring indicating greater risk as detailed above and in Table 15.2. Risk factors for thromboembolic events in patients with prosthetic heart valves, specifically mechanical heart valves, is determined by the type of valve, the location of the prosthesis, the number of prosthetic valves, and the presence or absence of additional risk factors including atrial fibrillation, severe left ventricular systolic function, prior thromboembolism, and a hypercoagulable state. *Mitral valve prosthesis carries a higher risk of thrombosis than aortic valve prosthesis.* For patients with venous thromboembolism, the risk of recurrent events and embolization is elevated in the first 3 months following the diagnosis and initiation of anticoagulation therapy [55]. If the venous thromboembolism was provoked, the risk of recurrence decreases with resolution of the underlying risk factor. *Patients with coronary artery disease with recent coronary stenting require dual antiplatelet therapy.* Premature discontinuation of dual antiplatelet therapy for an invasive procedure increases the risk of stent thrombosis, potentially precipitating a myocardial infarction with a mortality rate of greater than 50 % [55]. Thromboembolic risk in the perioperative and postoperative period is estimated based on the underlying indication for anticoagulation.

The risk of procedure related bleeding depends on the type of procedure, the residual effects of antithrombotic agents, comorbidities, history of prior bleeding, and timing of reinitiation of anticoagulation. High bleeding risk procedures include coronary artery bypass surgery, neurosurgical procedures, and any procedure lasting greater than 45 min. Low bleeding risk procedures include laparoscopic cholecystectomy, carpal tunnel repair, and endoscopic procedures [57]. Major bleeding is generally defined as bleeding that is fatal, intracranial, requires surgery to correct, lowers hemoglobin by ≥ 2 g/dL, or requires transfusion of ≥ 2 units packed red blood cells [58]. The risk of bleeding is higher for urgent or emergent procedures when compared to elective procedures, as emergent operations do not allow for proper discontinuation of antithrombotic therapy prior to the procedure. Patient factors also contribute to bleeding risk; numerous bleeding risk scores have been developed including the HAS-BLED score. A HAS-BLED risk score of ≥ 3 was found to be the most predictive for bleeding [59]. Evaluation of these risks allows physicians, surgeons, and patients to make informed decisions prior to any invasive procedure.

Once the thromboembolic and bleeding risks have been weighed, the decision can be made to continue, interrupt or bridge anticoagulation therapy. When anticoagulation is discontinued in patients at risk for thromboembolic events, the interval without therapy should be as short as possible. The medication used for antithrombotic therapy as well as renal and hepatic function determines the timing in the cessation of these anticoagulants. For warfarin, an INR range between 2.0 and 3.5 indicates adequate anticoagulation for thromboembolic risk reduction [60]. A relatively normal zone of hemostasis exists when the INR is 1.0–2.0. Approximately 93 % of patients with an INR in the therapeutic range will have an INR of less than 1.5 approximately 5 days after warfarin therapy has been discontinued [61]. An INR of 1.5 or less is considered safe for high-risk procedures, although some surgeons recommend an INR as close to 1.0 for procedures with high bleeding risk. *In patients at high risk for thromboembolic events, anticoagulation bridging is considered standard of care. Bridging therapy with intravenous heparin or subcutaneous low molecular weight heparin is utilized in those patients on warfarin once the INR falls below therapeutic range (<2.0). Intravenous heparin is stopped 4–6 h before the procedure; the last dose of subcutaneous low molecular weight heparin is given 24 h prior to the procedure. Post-procedurally, bridging therapy is resumed once hemostasis has been achieved and warfarin restarted; bridging is continued until the INR has reached the therapeutic range.*

With the use of novel oral anticoagulants that achieve reliable therapeutic levels within a few hours with daily or twice a day dosing, the use of bridging therapy is not needed. The timing for discontinuation of these medications prior to an invasive procedure is based on a patient's creatinine clearance. Dabigatran is held 1–2 days prior to the procedure if the patient has normal renal function (creatinine clearance ≥50 mL/min) and 3–5 days with a creatinine clearance ≤50 mL/min. Rivaroxaban and apixaban, factor Xa inhibitors, are held between 1 and 5 days prior to a procedure and timing is based on a patient's renal function. More conservative approaches are often times recommended in patients undergoing very high-risk surgeries.

Aspirin and P2Y12 receptor inhibitors such as clopidogrel, prasugrel, and ticagrelor are commonly encountered medications in patients with cardiovascular diseases. Aspirin is often used alone as well as in combination with other antiplatelet agents. Low dose aspirin alone does not substantially increase the risk of clinically significant bleeding after an invasive procedure but is often times stopped prior to very high-risk procedures [62]. Aspirin along with P2Y12 receptor inhibitors are typically suspended 5–7 days prior to surgery. Appropriate timing in the cessation of antithrombotic and antiplatelet medications provides thromboembolic risk reduction without increasing the risk of periprocedural bleeding for an elective procedure.

Urgent and emergent procedures do not allow physicians the luxury of time when making decisions regarding holding anticoagulation therapy. The administration of reversal agents, if available, may be considered if the risk of bleeding outweighs the risk of thrombotic events. For warfarin, the INR can be reliably reversed within 24–48 h by administering vitamin K. Fresh frozen plasma is usually used to rapidly reverse the INR for a short duration. Prothrombin complex concentrates (PCC) are also used in cases of significant bleeding. PCC contains a combination of blood clotting factors II, VII, IX, X and proteins C and S. For patients receiving direct thrombin or factor Xa inhibitors, there is no specific antidote available for reversal as vitamin K for warfarin. For patients taking dabigatran who have life threatening bleeding, hemodialysis or charcoal hemoperfusion can be considered. Oral activated charcoal can be used to remove the unabsorbed prodrug from the gastrointestinal tract if the last dose was within the previous 2 h. PCC can also be used in life threatening bleeding; however, PCC is not considered standard of care for the management of dabigatran associated bleeding due to the prothrombotic risks as well as lack of evidence from clinical studies. Likewise, reversal with PCC can also be used for those patients with life-threatening bleeds taking rivaroxaban or apixaban. Again, given the risk of thrombosis as well as the lack of clinical studies evaluating its effectiveness, PCC is only considered appropriate in an imminent life-threatening bleed. Administration of an antifibrinolytic agent such as tranexamic acid or ε-aminocaproic acid can also be utilized in these situations.

Postoperatively, anticoagulant and antiplatelet therapy should be resumed once appropriate hemostasis has been achieved and deemed safe from the surgical perspective. In most instances, patients with a high-risk of thromboembolic events are restarted on warfarin and are bridged with heparin or low molecular weight heparin until therapeutic INRs are achieved. The novel oral anticoagulants are initiated without the need of bridging therapy due to their effectiveness of achieving adequate anticoagulation within a short duration. Resumption of antithrombotic therapy is dictated by achieving proper postoperative hemostasis in order to reduce the risk of postoperative bleeding.

For patients receiving long-term antithrombotic therapy, the approach to periprocedural use of these agents is individualized. Physicians must consider the patient's thromboembolic risk, the procedure's bleeding risk, and the urgency of the procedure to determine the need for possible bridging therapy as well as the appropriate timing for possible cessation of therapy. Emergencies require knowledge regarding possible reversible agents and their risks associated with administration.

Anticoagulation Issues with Mechanical Prosthetic Valves

Given the need for anticoagulation to prevent thrombosis in patients with mechanical prosthetic heart valves, physicians and surgeons are often faced with the important question of anticoagulation management in the setting of various types of procedures. Warfarin with a therapeutic INR is recommended in patients with mechanical heart valves undergoing minor procedures such as dental extractions or cataract removal, where bleeding is easily controlled. *For more invasive surgical procedure, temporary interruption of warfarin without bridging agents is recommended in patients with a bileaflet mechanical aortic valve prosthesis and no other risk factors for thrombosis. But, in patients with a mechanical aortic valve and any thromboembolic risk factor or an older generation mechanical aortic valve, IV UH or subcutaneous LMWH is recommended when the INR is subtherapeutic prior to surgery* [26].

Emergent procedures in this subset of patients require a balance between decreasing a patient's risk of bleeding as well as preventing valve thrombosis. *Fresh frozen plasma or prothrombin complex concentrate (see above) is reasonable in these patients who have uncontrollable bleeding or require emergency surgery* [26]. Following these procedures, patients should immediately be started on parenteral anticoagulation followed by warfarin when appropriate hemostasis has been achieved as deemed by the surgical team.

Anticoagulation in the Setting of Dual Antiplatelet Therapy

With expanding population with myocardial infarction, atrial fibrillation, prosthetic valves etc., *the concomitant use of dual antiplatelet therapy and oral anticoagulation, referred to as triple therapy, is increasing*. However, triple therapy should be used cautiously in these patients, many of them elderly, to balance the benefits with the risk of bleeding. Therefore, triple therapy with warfarin, aspirin, and a P2Y12 should be restricted to specific situations in which the risk of venous thromboembolism or stent thrombosis is considered to exceed the risk of bleeding [35]. It is estimated that between 5 and 10 % of patients scheduled to undergo percutaneous coronary intervention are also on oral anticoagulation [63]. For such patients, the avoidance of drug eluting stents is strongly preferred to limit the duration of triple therapy. Moreover, consideration may be given to lower the target INR goal to 2.0–2.5 (Class IIb) [35]. According to the European Society of Cardiology guidelines, the type of stent utilized, bare metal versus drug eluting stent, as well as the context of the coronary event, elective versus urgent, also dictates the duration of triple therapy. *Patients who have a low risk of bleeding and are undergoing elective procedures with the use of bare metal stents are recommended to receive triple therapy for 1 month followed by up to 12 months of antiplatelet therapy with clopidogrel or aspirin in addition to warfarin. In these same patients who receive drug-eluting stents, triple therapy should be extended to 3 months followed by 12 months of warfarin and either clopidogrel or aspirin.* For emergent procedures in patients with high risk of bleeding, 4 weeks of triple therapy should be prescribed [35]. Of note, the use of NOACs has not been evaluated in this context.

Conclusion

With an ever-growing population requiring the use of oral anticoagulation, physicians are likely to encounter patients taking these medications in both the inpatient and outpatient settings. To provide appropriate care to these patients, it is imperative to understand the clinical indications for prescribing anticoagulation, the pharmacology of these agents as well as the management of such medications in the elective, urgent, and emergent situations.

References

1. Bjork I, Lindahl U. Mechanism of the anticoagulant action of heparin. Mol Cell Biochem. 1982;48(3):161–82.
2. Hirsh J, Bauer KA, Donati MB, et al. Parenteral anticoagulants: American College of Chest Physicians evidence-based clinical practice guidelines (8th edition). Chest. 2008;133(6):141–59.
3. Hull RD, Raskob GE, Brant RF, et al. Relation between the time to achieve the lower limit of the APTT therapeutic range and recurrent venous thromboembolism during heparin treatment for deep vein thrombosis. Arch Intern Med. 1997;157:2562–8.
4. Hirsh J, Raschke R. Heparin and low-molecular-weight heparin: the Seventh ACCP Conference on Antithrombotic and Thrombolytic Therapy. Chest. 2004;126:188S–203.
5. Pirmohamed M. Warfarin: almost 60 years old and still causing problems. Br J Clin Pharmacol. 2006;62(5):509–11.
6. Ansell J, Hirsh J, Hylek E, et al. Pharmacology and management of the vitamin K antagonists: American College of Chest Physicians evidence-based clinical practice guidelines (8th edition). Chest. 2008;133(6 Suppl):160S–98.
7. Freedman MD. Oral anticoagulants: pharmacodynamics, clinical indications and adverse effects. J Clin Pharmacol. 1992;32:196–209.
8. Makris M, van Veen JJ, McLean R. Warfarin anticoagulation reversal: management of the asymptomatic and bleeding patient. J Thromb Thrombolysis. 2010;29:171–81.
9. Hauel NH, Nar H, Priepke H, et al. Structure-based design of novel potent nonpeptide thrombin inhibitors. J Med Chem. 2002;45:1757–66.
10. van Ryn J, Stangier J, Haertter S, et al. Dabigatran etexilate—a novel, reversible, oral direct thrombin inhibitor: interpretation of coagulation assays and reversal of anticoagulant activity. Thromb Haemost. 2010;103(6):1116–27.
11. Connolly SJ, Ezekowitz MD, Yusuf S, et al. Dabigatran versus warfarin in patients with atrial fibrillation. N Engl J Med. 2009;361(12):1139–51.
12. Eikelboom JW, Connolly SJ, Bruekmann M, et al. Dabigatran versus warfarin in patients with mechanical heart valves. N Engl J Med. 2013;369(13):1206–14.
13. Bates SM, Greer IA, Middeldorp S, et al. VTE, thrombophilia, antithrombotic therapy, and pregnancy: antithrombotic therapy and prevention of thrombosis: American College of Chest Physicians evidence-based clinical practice guidelines (9th edition). Chest. 2012;141:e691S–736.
14. Patel MR, Mahaffey KW, Garg J, et al. Rivaroxaban versus warfarin in nonvalvular atrial fibrillation. N Engl J Med. 2011;365(10):883–91.
15. Granger CB, Alexander JH, McMurray JJ, et al. Apixaban versus warfarin in patients with atrial fibrillation. N Engl J Med. 2011;365(11):981–2.
16. Go AS, Mozaffarian D, Roger VL, et al. Heart disease and stroke statistics—2014 update: a report from the American Heart Association. Circulation. 2014;129:e28–292.
17. Wolf PA, Benjamin EJ, Belanger AJ, et al. Secular trends in the prevalence of atrial fibrillation: the Framingham Study. Am Heart J. 1996;131:790–5.
18. January CT, Wann LS, Alpert JS, et al. 2014 AHA/ACC/HRS guideline for the management of patients with atrial fibrillation: a report of the American College of Cardiology/American Heart Association Task Force on practice guidelines and the Heart Rhythm Society. J Am Coll Cardiol. 2014;64(21):2246–80.
19. Kannel WB, Wolf PA, Benjamin EJ, et al. Prevalence, incidence, prognosis, and predisposing conditions for atrial fibrillation: population-based estimates. Am J Cardiol. 1998;82:2N–9.
20. Wang TJ, Larson MG, Levy D, et al. Temporal relations of atrial fibrillation and congestive heart failure and their joint influence on mortality: the Framingham Heart Study. Circulation. 2003;107:2920–5.

21. Krahn AD, Manfreda J, Tate RB, et al. The natural history of atrial fibrillation: incidence, risk factors, and prognosis in the Manitoba follow-up study. Am J Med. 1995;98:476–84.
22. Stewart S, Hart CL, Hole DJ, et al. A population-based study of the long-term risks associated with atrial fibrillation: 20-year follow-up of the Renfrew/Paisley study. Am J Med. 2002;113:359–64.
23. Wyse DG, Waldo AL, DiMarco JP, et al. A comparison of rate control and rhythm control in patients with atrial fibrillation. N Engl J Med. 2002;347:1825–33.
24. Van Gelder IC, Hagens VE, Bosker HA, et al. A comparison of rate control and rhythm control in patients with recurrent persistent atrial fibrillation. N Engl J Med. 2002;347:1834–40.
25. Iung B, Vahanian A. Epidemiology of acquired valvular heart disease. Can J Cardiol. 2014;30:962–70.
26. Nishimura RA, Otto CM, Bonow RO, et al. 2014 AHA/ACC guideline for the management of patients with valvular heart disease: a report of the American College of Cardiology/American Heart Association Task Force on Practice Guidelines. J Thorac Cardiovasc Surg. 2014;148:e1–132.
27. Vahanian A, Alfieri O, Andreotti F, et al. Guidelines on the management of valvular heart disease: the Joint Task Force on the Management of Valvular Heart Disease of the European Society of Cardiology (ESC) and the European Association for Cardio-Thoracic Surgery (EACTS). Eur J Cardiothorac Surg. 2012;42:S1–44.
28. Mozaffarian D, Benjamin EJ, Go AS, et al. Heart disease and stroke statistics—2015 update: a report from the American Heart Association. Circulation. 2015;131:e29–322.
29. Thygesen K, Alpert JS, Jaffe AS, et al. Third universal definition of myocardial infarction. Circulation. 2012;126:2020–35.
30. Levine GN, Bates ER, Blankenship JC, et al. 2011 ACCF/AHA/SCAI guideline for percutaneous coronary intervention: a report of the American College of Cardiology Foundation/American Heart Association Task Force on Practice Guidelines and the Society for Cardiovascular Angiography and Interventions. J Am Coll Cardiol. 2011;58(24):e44–122.
31. Vandvik PO, Lincoff AM, Gore JM, et al. Primary and secondary prevention of cardiovascular disease: Antithrombotic therapy and prevention of thrombosis, 9th ed: American College of Chest physicians evidence-based clinical practice guidelines. Chest. 2012;141:e637S–68.
32. Nihoyannopoulos P, Smith GC, Maseri A, et al. The natural history of left ventricular thrombus in myocardial infarction: a rationale in support of masterly inactivity. J Am Coll Cardiol. 1989;14:903–11.
33. Weinreich DJ, Burke JF, Pauletto FJ. Left ventricular mural thrombi complicating acute myocardial infarction. Long-term follow-up with serial echocardiography. Ann Intern Med. 1984;100:789–94.
34. Stratton JR, Resnick AD. Increased embolic risk in patients with left ventricular thrombi. Circulation. 1987;75:1004–11.
35. O'Gara PT, Kushner FG, Ascheim DD, et al. 2013 ACCF/AHA guideline for the management of ST-elevation myocardial infarction: a report of the American College of Cardiology Foundation/American Heart Association Task Force on Practice Guidelines. J Am Coll Cardiol. 2013;61:e78–140.
36. Yancy WC, Jessup M, Bozkurt B, et al. Guideline for the management of heart failure. Circulation. 2013;128:e240–327.
37. Dunkman WB, Johnson GR, Carson PE, et al. Incidence of thromboembolic events in congestive heart failure: the V-HeFT VA Cooperative Studies Group. Circulation. 1993;87(6 Suppl):VI94–101.
38. Dunkman WB. Thromboembolism and antithrombotic therapy in congestive heart failure. J Cardiovasc Risk. 1995;2:107–17.
39. Katz SD. Left ventricular thrombus and the incidence of thromboembolism in patients with congestive heart failure: can clinical factors identify patients at increased risk? J Cardiovasc Risk. 1995;2:97–102.
40. Stehlik J, Edwards LB, Kucheryavaya AY, et al. The Registry of the International Society for Heart and Lung Transplantation: twenty-seventh official adult heart transplant report—2010. J Heart Lung Transplant. 2010;29:1089–103.
41. Feldman D, Pamboukian SV, Teuteberg JJ, et al. The 2013 International Society for Heart and Lung Transplantation Guidelines for mechanical circulatory support: executive summary. J Heart Lung Transplant. 2013;32(2):157–87.
42. Starling RC, Moazami N, Silvestry SC, et al. Unexpected abrupt increase in left ventricular assist device thrombosis. N Engl J Med. 2014;370:1466–7.
43. Eckman PM, John R. Bleeding and thrombosis in patients with continuous-flow ventricular assist devices. Circulation. 2012;125:3038–47.
44. Tsukui H, Abla A, Teuteberg JJ, et al. Cerebrovascular accidents in patients with a ventricular assist device. J Thorac Cardiovasc Surg. 2007;134:114–23.
45. Kato TS, Schulze PC, Yang J, et al. Pre-operative and post-operative risk factors associated with neurologic complications in patients with advanced heart failure supported by a left ventricular assist device. J Heart Lung Transplant. 2012;31:1–8.
46. Korn-Lubetzki I, Oren A, Asher E, et al. Strokes after cardiac surgery: mostly right hemispheric ischemic with mild residual damage. J Neurol. 2007;254:1708–13.
47. Kato TS, Ota T, Schulze PC, et al. Asymmetric pattern of cerebrovascular lesions in patients after left ventricular assist device implantation. Stroke. 2012;43:872–4.
48. Slaughter MS, Rogers JG, Milano CA, et al. Advanced heart failure treated with continuous-flow left ventricular assist device. N Engl J Med. 2009;361:2241–51.
49. Maron BJ, Towbin JA, Thiene G, et al. Contemporary definitions and classification of the cardiomyopathies: an American Heart Association Scientific Statement from the Council on Clinical Cardiology, Heart Failure and Transplantation Committee; Quality of

Care and Outcomes Research and Functional Genomics and Translational Biology Interdisciplinary Working Groups; and Council on Epidemiology and Prevention. Circulation. 2006;113:1807.
50. Petersen SE, Selvanayagam JB, Wiesmann F, et al. Left ventricular non-compaction: insights from cardiovascular magnetic resonance imaging. J Am Coll Cardiol. 2005;46:101–5.
51. Oechslin EN, Attenhofer Jost CH, Rojas JR, et al. Long-term follow-up of 34 adults with isolated left ventricular noncompaction: a distinct cardiomyopathy with poor prognosis. J Am Coll Cardiol. 2000;36:493–500.
52. Arbustini E, Weidemann F, Hall JL. Left ventricular noncompaction: a distinct cardiomyopathy or a trait share by different cardiac diseases? J Am Coll Cardiol. 2014;64(17):1840–50.
53. Carrier M, Le Gal G, Wells PS, Rodger MA. Systematic review: case-fatality rates of recurrent venous thromboembolism and major bleeding events among patients treated for venous thromboembolism. Ann Intern Med. 2010;152(9):578–89.
54. Heit JA, Silverstein MD, Mohr DN, et al. Predictors of survival after deep vein thrombosis and pulmonary embolism: a population-based, cohort study. Arch Intern Med. 1999;159(5):445–53.
55. Kearon C, Akl EA, Comerota AJ, et al. American College of Chest Physicians. Antithrombotic therapy for VTE disease: Antithrombotic therapy and prevention of thrombosis, 9th ed: American College of Chest Physicians evidence-based clinical practice guidelines. Chest. 2012;141(2 Suppl):e419S–94.
56. Douketis JD, Spyropoulos AC, Spencer FA, et al. Perioperative management of antithrombotic therapy: antithrombotic therapy and prevention of thrombosis: American College of Chest Physicians evidence-based clinical practice guidelines (9th edition). Chest. 2012;141:e326S–50.
57. Spyropoulos AC, Douketis JD. How I treat anticoagulated patients undergoing an elective procedure or surgery. Blood. 2012;120:2954–62.
58. Mehran R, Rao SV, Bhatt DL, et al. Standardized bleeding definitions for cardiovascular clinical trials: a consensus report from the Bleeding Academic Research Consortium. Circulation. 2011;123:2736–47.
59. Omran H, Bauersachs R, Rübenacker S, et al. The HAS-BLED score predicts bleedings during bridging of chronic oral anticoagulation. Results from the national multicentre BNK Online bRiDging REgistRy (BORDER). Thromb Haemost. 2012;108:65–73.
60. Dzik WS. Reversal of drug-induced anticoagulation: old solutions and new problems. Transfusion. 2012;52 Suppl 1:45S–55.
61. Schulman S, Elbazi R, Zondag M, O'Donnell M. Clinical factors influencing normalization of prothrombin time after stopping warfarin: a retrospective cohort study. Thromb J. 2008;16:15.
62. Atwell TD, Smith RL, Hesley GK, et al. Incidence of bleeding after 15,181 percutaneous biopsies and the role of aspirin. Am J Roentgenol. 2010;194:784–9.
63. Schömig A, Sarafoff N, Seyfarth M. Triple antithrombotic management after stent implantation: when and how? Heart. 2009;95:1280.

Workup and Treatment of Pulmonary Embolus

16

Agnieszka A. Ardelt

Introduction

Neurosurgical patients present a special challenge in the diagnosis and treatment of venous thromboembolism (VTE) and pulmonary embolism (PE). First, neurosurgical patients are generally at high risk of VTE/PE due to factors related to malignancy, immobilization, or the postoperative state. Second, medical VTE prophylaxis and treatment with systemic anticoagulation are sometimes contraindicated in neurosurgical patients. In general, there is little data to inform decision-making in specific difficult patient scenarios.

Definitions and Classifications

VTE consists of deep venous thrombosis (DVT) and PE. DVT typically occurs in the veins of the pelvis, lower extremities, or upper extremities, and a PE is a thrombus which originates elsewhere in the body, such as within the deep veins of the pelvis or lower extremity, and lodges in the pulmonary artery and/or its branches. Specifically, the iliac, femoral, or popliteal veins are the most common sites of PE origin, although in certain patient populations, such as those with malignancy, a PE source in the extremities or pelvis may not necessarily be demonstrated [1]. With respect to DVTs in the calf veins, approximately a third will progress proximally resulting in a concomitant increase in the likelihood of embolization [2, 3].

Pulmonary emboli may be classified as acute, subacute, or chronic depending on the timing and type of symptoms. In acute PE, symptoms referable to pulmonary artery obstruction develop immediately, while in chronic PE, patients may develop pulmonary hypertension over time. Acutely, a PE may result in impairment of gas exchange, pulmonary infarcts, right heart dysfunction, and hypotension (SBP <90 mmHg). The occurrence of hypotension is an important clinical sign because it has important prognostic and therapeutic consequences, i.e., it portends a poor prognosis and may require emergent thrombolysis or mechanical embolectomy. The severity of the clinical presentation is also sometimes used to classify patients into those with massive, submassive, or nonmassive PE [4].

Additional classifications refer to the location of the PE within the pulmonary artery and branches. This is of importance specifically

A.A. Ardelt, M.D., Ph.D., F.A.H.A. (✉)
Department of Neurology, The University of Chicago, Chicago, IL, USA

Department of Surgery (Neurosurgery), The University of Chicago, Chicago, IL, USA
e-mail: aardelt@neurology.bsd.uchicago.edu

C.M. Loftus (ed.), *Anticoagulation and Hemostasis in Neurosurgery*,
DOI 10.1007/978-3-319-27327-3_16

because proximal localization (i.e., within the pulmonary artery trunk or at the bifurcation, the so-called saddle PE) is more likely to result in hemodynamic dysfunction and poor outcome.

Epidemiology of VTE

In the United States, the incidence of DVT has been reported as 422/100,000 [5]. The incidence of PE averages approximately 100/100,000 depending on the data source, and some sources have reported that up to 40 % of patients diagnosed with DVT experience PE [6]. Mortality in acute PE in the United States varies from 1 to 10 % of patients diagnosed with PE depending on the study and whether all-cause mortality was included [7]. Among patients with hemodynamic dysfunction, 30-day mortality may be >15 % [8]. In the long term, chronic thromboembolic pulmonary hypertension (CTEPH) may increase the overall PE-associated mortality to >40 %. Factors which correlate with mortality in PE are age >70, malignancy, congestive heart failure, chronic lung disease, hypotension, tachypnea, and right heart dysfunction on echocardiography [7].

Risk Factors for VTE

General risk factors for VTE and PE include acute medical illness, immobilization, trauma, postoperative state, malignancy, age >65, obesity, metabolic syndrome, cigarette smoking, hypertension, oral contraceptives, hormone replacement, pregnancy, and inherited thrombophilias. A specific cause of VTE is frequently not found despite extensive evaluation. Pathophysiologically, inflammation, hypercoagulability, stasis, and endothelial injury underlie VTE risk.

In neurosurgical patients, a retrospective analysis of the American College of Surgeons NSQIP database comprising >1.7 million patients showed that ventilator dependence, immobilization, malignancy, chronic treatment with steroids, and sepsis were factors independently correlating with VTE [9].

Prevention of VTE in General

Mechanical and Medical Thromboprophylaxis

Intermittent compression devices (ICD) and/or medical thromboprophylaxis can be utilized for prevention of VTE in patients who are at risk, and several professional societies such as the American College of Chest Physicians (ACCP) have periodically published detailed guidelines on thromboprophylaxis [10]. The 8th edition of the ACCP guidelines was updated in 2012, and the recommendations from the current 9th edition were recently reviewed in detail [11]. There are several medications approved by the Federal Drug Administration (FDA) for thromboprophylaxis (unfractionated heparin, dalteparin, enoxaparin, rivaroxaban, fondaparinux, and warfarin), and the guidelines suggest approaches to thromboprohylaxis in specific patient populations and scenarios [11]. In general, ICD are used in isolation only in patients at risk for bleeding and, thus, ineligible for medical thromboprophylaxis. In some populations, e.g., patients with an active malignancy, the combination of ICD and medical prophylaxis may be more effective than either method alone [12].

The main concern limiting the use of medical prophylaxis in neurosurgical patients is hemorrhage. A meta-analysis of 30 studies including a total of 7,779 neurosurgical patients showed that ICD were superior to placebo in DVT prevention, and that low molecular weight heparin was superior to compression stockings [13]. Patients not treated with prophylaxis experienced a DVT rate of 15.5 %, and patients treated with ICD, unfractionated heparin, or low molecular weight heparin experienced reduced DVT rates of 1.9 %, 0.9 %, and 4.1 %, respectively [13]. In the majority of studies in this meta-analysis, medical thromboprophylaxis was administered prior to surgery, intraoperatively, or within the first 24 h postoperatively. Intracranial hemorrhage rates for patients receiving unfractionated heparin versus low molecular weight heparin were 0.35/1000 and 1.5/1000, respectively [13]. Caution should be used in interpretation of any meta-analysis due to variability in study design of the included studies, and no conclusions should be drawn beyond that mechanical and medical prophylaxis reduced the rate of DVT formation in neurosurgical patients with medical prophylaxis incurring a relatively low, although perhaps not negligible, rate of intracranial hemorrhage.

Prevention of PE in the Setting of DVT

Anticoagulation

The first-line therapy for DVT and prevention of subsequent PE is systemic anticoagulation, which is discussed further in the section on treatment of PE.

While there is little controversy regarding anticoagulation for a proximal DVT, there are some nuances in the treatment of isolated distal DVT [11]. Distal DVT solely involves the veins of the calf, i.e., the peroneal, tibial, soleal, or gastrocnemius veins. The risk of embolization from distal DVT is generally lower than from a proximal DVT, but a distal DVT may extend proximally over time resulting in increased risk of PE [14]. If the patient does not harbor risk factors which correlate with DVT extension, the distal DVT may be followed with serial lower extremity ultrasonography, e.g., once every week for 2 weeks [11]. If the DVT does not extend during this time, the risk of subsequent expansion and/or embolization is thought to be low. If the DVT is observed to extend, anticoagulation should be commenced. Patients who are thought to be at high risk of distal DVT extension, however, should be anticoagulated [11, 14]. Factors correlating with extension include involvement of multiple veins, prior DVT/PE, active malignancy, or recent surgery or hospitalization.

Thrombosis of the upper extremity deep veins (subclavian, innominate, brachial, or axillary) may occur in patients with indwelling venous catheters. Anticoagulation is generally recommended for these patients [11].

Inferior Vena Cava Filters

There are currently two types of devices, permanent or retrievable filters, which can be inserted into the vena cava in order to prevent a piece of lower extremity or pelvic vein thrombus from lodging in the lung. While placement of an IVCF for this purpose makes intuitive sense, there are no studies in which patients were randomized to IVCF versus anticoagulation, and a Cochrane review failed to show support for the idea [6]. In the PREPIC trial, patients received anticoagulation with or without an IVCF [15]. In long-term follow-up, there was no mortality benefit of anticoagulation with IVCF versus anticoagulation without IVCF, but the rate of PE was initially lower (4.8 vs. 1.1 % at 12 days), while the rate of symptomatic DVT was higher at 2 years (20.8 vs. 11.6 %) with IVCF.

Due to the paucity of data, the indications for IVCF placement are diverse and vary among society guidelines [6]. While most agree that an IVCF is indicated in patients in whom anticoagulation is absolutely contraindicated, either temporarily or permanently, in order to decrease the risk of PE, some also advocate for IVCF placement in patients who had a recurrent PE despite therapeutic anticoagulation [16] and for other indications [6].

In patients in whom contraindications to anticoagulation are transient and/or the DVT is thought to have been caused by a temporary condition, retrievable filters can be used and subsequently removed [6].

Clinical Presentation of PE

There is a wide spectrum of presentations of PE, from no symptoms to sudden death, and some have observed that the majority of patients who die from PE do so before the diagnosis is made [8]. This observation requires that physicians should always have a high index of suspicion for PE when dealing with at-risk patient populations. Common symptoms and signs of PE include dyspnea, pleuritic chest pain, sinus tachycardia, as well as local extremity symptoms and signs associated with DVT. Hemoptysis which is relatively specific for PE occurs only in approximately 10 % of patients, whereas lower extremity swelling which is relatively specific for DVT occurs in 42 % of patients [8].

Evaluation for PE

Clinical Probability

The evaluation for PE in hemodynamically stable patients is centered on the determination of clinical probability of PE. Several clinical scores of PE probability have been developed for this purpose. The Wells score and the revised Geneva score are frequently used (Tables 16.1 and 16.2).

Table 16.1 Wells score for PE in patients admitted to the hospital [17]

Clinical signs of DVT	3
Alternative diagnosis less likely	3
Prior DVT or PE	1.5
Heart rate >100 bpm	1.5
Recent surgery or immobilization	1.5
Hemoptysis	1
Cancer	1
Low probability: 0–1	
Intermediate probability: 2–6	
High probability: ≥7	
Dichotomized scoring	
PE unlikely: 0–4	
PE likely: >4	

Table 16.2 Revised Geneva score [18]

Heart rate >94 bpm	2
Pain on leg palpation and edema	1
Prior DVT or PE	1
Unilateral leg pain	1
Heart rate 75–94 bpm	1
Active malignancy	1
Surgery (GA) or fracture (LE)	1
Hemoptysis	1
Age >65 years old	1
Dichotomized scoring	
PE unlikely: 0–2	
PE likely: >2	

Once the clinical probability of PE is determined, further dedicated testing is done (Fig. 16.1). Blood testing for the fibrin degradation product, D-dimer, lower extremity compression ultrasound (CUS), and computed tomographic pulmonary angiography (CTPA) are currently frequently utilized in the evaluation of patients for PE.

D-Dimer

Depending on the specific assay used, a negative D-dimer result rules out acute VTE in most patients with low or intermediate probability of PE [7]. The D-dimer ELISA has a sensitivity of >93 % and specificity of 39 % and a high negative predictive value in the setting of low clinical probability of PE [7, 19]. D-dimer testing is less reliable in patients with conditions leading to an inflammatory response including traumatic injury, surgery, or pregnancy as well as in patients with high clinical probability of PE [7]. D-dimer levels may be above threshold in hospitalized patients and in individuals older than 65. Therefore, an elevated D-dimer level has a low positive predictive value and should generally be followed by CTPA. In summary, if clinical probability is low, a negative D-dimer rules out PE while an elevated D-dimer may warrant CTPA, while if clinical probability is high, only CTPA is indicated (Fig. 16.1).

Postoperative neurosurgical patients are expected to have an elevated D-dimer level due to causes other than VTE. One study prospectively evaluated D-dimer levels in 101 patients who underwent elective craniotomy primarily for tumors [19]. The D-dimer test used in the study used 0.5 mg/L as the normal cutoff, which had a 99.4 % sensitivity and a 38.2 % specificity for VTE in an outpatient population. In post-craniotomy patients, on day 3 postoperatively, patients without VTE had mean D-dimer levels of 1.59 mg/L, while those with VTE had mean D-dimer levels of 5.49 mg/L. The authors determined the value of 2 mg/L as a reasonable cutoff for VTE prediction with this particular test in postoperative patients who had undergone an elective craniotomy. The positive predictive value

Fig. 16.1 Workup of PE based on clinical probability. *PE* pulmonary embolism, *CTPA* computed tomography pulmonary angiogram

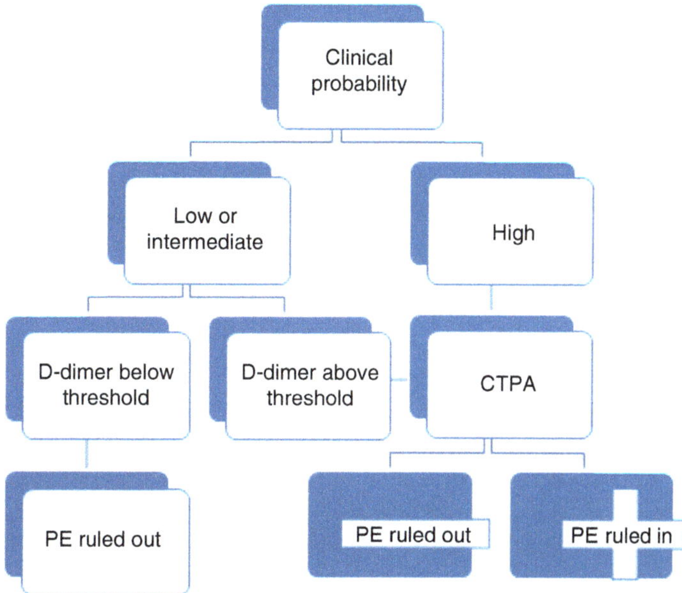

was 73.2 %, and the negative predictive value was 95.6 %. In the study, patients who had a D-dimer level >4 mg/L were diagnosed with PE.

Imaging

Two invasive tests are considered the gold standard of PE and DVT diagnosis: conventional pulmonary angiography and venography, respectively. As these two tests are invasive, they are used only in highly selected patients, while noninvasive tests are utilized in the majority [7]. Although ventilation-perfusion scanning had been used in the past to make the diagnosis of PE, the high likelihood of a non-diagnostic scan (up to 50 %) has resulted in decreased use for the acute diagnosis of PE [8]. In the majority of cases, pulmonary CTPA has supplanted ventilation-perfusion scanning and compares favorably with invasive pulmonary angiography in the acute diagnosis of PE [7].

Since in patients with low clinical probability of PE a negative D-dimer effectively rules out a PE, CTPA is not indicated. Despite this, CTPA use has increased during the past decade, and a large percentage is being utilized in patients with low clinical probability of PE [20]. As part of the Choosing Wisely campaign, the goal of which is to identify and discourage tests or treatments that are used inappropriately in patients, the American Thoracic Society and the ACCP recommended that CTPA not be used in patients with low clinical probability duc to unnecessary exposure to radiation and contrast. Additional consequences of performing CTPA in patients with low clinical probability of PE include incidental findings requiring additional tests and detection of small (sub-segmental) PE of unclear clinical significance.

In symptomatic patients with high clinical probability of PE, those with high D-dimer levels, and those with contraindications to CTPA, lower extremity CUS showing acute proximal thrombus is sufficient for diagnosis of PE [7]. CT venography is not routinely used in combination with CTPA due to concerns for radiation exposure and contrast load. Magnetic resonance pulmonary angiography and magnetic resonance venography have not replaced CTPA due to the high likelihood (approximately 52 %) of a non-diagnostic scan [7].

In hemodynamically unstable patients in whom CTPA may be impractical and/or unsafe, the clinical diagnosis of PE may be supported with findings on EKG (sinus tachycardia, right bundle branch block, S1Q3T3) [21], bedside transthoracic echocardiography [TTE; right ventricular (RV) dysfunction (RV end-diastolic volume >30 mm; interventricular septal paradoxical motion and/or flattening; RV/LV ratio >0.9; pulmonary artery systolic pressure >30 mmHg; and tricuspid regurgitation] [4, 22], and/or CUS positive for acute thrombus.

Treatment of PE

Severity Score

Initial treatment of patients with PE begins with resuscitation and determination of disease severity [23]. Clinical prognostic models have been developed to estimate the risk of mortality in PE. The Pulmonary Embolism Severity Index (PESI) and its shortened version stratify patients into categories of risk of death by 30 days based on clinical variables [24, 25] (Table 16.3). Patients at high risk of death should be evaluated for thrombolysis and admitted to the hospital, while low-risk patients could conceivably be treated with anticoagulation as outpatients [7].

Table 16.3 PE severity index [24, 25]

Age >80 years/old	Age in years
Altered mental status	60
History of cancer	30
SBP <100 mmHg	30
heart rate ≥110 bpm	20
Respiratory rate ≥30 mmHg	20
Temperature <36 °C	20
PaO_2 <90 %	20
Male sex	10
History of heart failure	10
History of chronic lung disease	10
Class 1 ≤65 points	
Class 2 66–85 points	
Class 3 86–105 points	
Class 4 106–125 points	
Class 5 >125 points	
Dichotomized scoring	
Class 1 and 2: low risk	
Class 3–5: high risk	

Thrombolysis

Patients at high risk for death based on clinical score; presence of hemodynamic instability, RV dilatation, or dysfunction on TTE; and/or elevation of troponin or brain natriuretic peptide require rapid consideration of medical thrombolysis followed by systemic anticoagulation [26]. Some reserve medical thrombolysis for hemodynamically unstable patients with PE, but more recently medical thrombolysis, was suggested for patients with high risk of mortality who are hemodynamically stable and have a low risk of bleeding [26]. For example, a meta-analysis showed that hemodynamically stable patients with PE who exhibited RV dysfunction on TTE experienced a 2.29 times increase in short-term mortality [27].

Thrombolysis is most effective when administered within 48 h of onset, but retains some benefit for up to 14 days [4]. Contraindications to thrombolysis include recent trauma, bleeding, ischemic stroke, intracranial hemorrhage, major surgery, coagulopathy, or pregnancy [4]. Some have advocated thrombolysis despite the presence of contraindications after informed decision-making in moribund patients with massive PE [28].

Embolectomy

Patients with massive central PE at high risk of death in whom thrombolysis is contraindicated or those who have not responded to thrombolysis, i.e., those who continue to exhibit RV dysfunction, warrant consideration of surgical, or catheter embolectomy [4]. The goal of either procedure is to decrease clot burden in order to improve RV function. In the case of catheter embolectomy, catheter-delivered thrombolytic agents can further attenuate clot size [4].

Anticoagulation

Rapid anticoagulation is the mainstay of therapy in patients with PE. Decision-making regarding systemic anticoagulation focuses on determination of suitability for anticoagulation, choice of drug, and length of therapy. Drugs currently approved by the FDA for the treatment of PE include unfractionated heparin, enoxaparin, dalteparin, fondaparinux, warfarin, and rivaroxaban (Table 16.4) [11].

Generally, prior to the availability of the novel oral anticoagulants (factor Xa inhibitors and thrombin inhibitors), the standard approach was to treat patients with PE with unfractionated heparin, enoxaparin, dalteparin, or fondaparinux followed by transition to a vitamin K antagonist with a target international normalized ratio (INR) of 2.0–3.0. For example, in a hypothetical patient with a history 2 weeks prior to a deep intracerebral hemorrhage due to hypertension presenting with a PE, anticoagulation with an intravenous unfractionated heparin drip as a bridge to warfarin is a reasonable treatment strategy given the short half-life of unfractionated heparin, as well as the complete reversibility of unfractionated heparin (with protamine) and warfarin (with vitamin K, prothrombin complex concentrates, or plasma) if the patient were to have recurrent bleeding despite adequate blood pressure control. Since two novel oral anticoagulant drugs, dabigatran etexilate and rivaroxaban, have been studied in the context of DVT and PE, and rivaroxaban is approved for use in this setting, a new therapeutic strategy for VTE has become available. Despite the ease of use of these drugs (unadjusted oral dosing, no routine laboratory monitoring, generally low hemorrhage risk in clinical studies), the lack of specific robust reversal strategies until recently limited their use in neurosurgical patients with DVT or PE in the acute postoperative or post-hemorrhage period. In October 2015, the FDA approved idarucizumab, a specific reversal agent for dabigatran etexilate. Future development of reversal strategies for the other novel agents may increase their utilization in patients at risk for hemorrhage, including neurosurgical patients.

Table 16.4 Drugs approved by the FDA for anticoagulation in VTE [11]

Drug Name	Dose	Monitoring
Unfractionated heparin	IV 80 U/kg bolus[a], then gtt	aPTT; goal 1.5–2.5
Enoxaparin	SQ 1 mg/kg q12h or 1.5 mg/kg q24h	
Dalteparin	SQ 200 U/kg q24h	
Fondaparinux	SQ, adjusted by weight	
Rivaroxaban	Oral 15 mg q12h for 21 days followed by 20 mg q24h	
Warfarin	Oral, titrated to INR	INR; goal 2.0–3.0

FDA Federal Drug Administration, *IV* intravenous, *U* units, *gtt* IV drip, *aPTT* activated partial thromboplastin time, *SQ* subcutaneous, *INR* international normalized ratio
[a]If intravenous unfractionated heparin is used in neurosurgical patients at a moderate risk for hemorrhage, the bolus dose may be avoided and slower anticoagulation commenced with the drip

Specific drugs may be preferred or avoided in certain conditions, for example, in patients with heparin-induced thrombocytopenia, heparins should be avoided; in patients with renal failure, low molecular weight heparins may accumulate; in patients with malignancy, heparins are preferred; and in pregnant patients, warfarin is contraindicated [10]. In neurosurgical patients at risk for bleeding in the setting of systemic anticoagulation, the treatment strategy and choice of drug should depend in part on the availability and effectiveness of agents for anticoagulant effect reversal.

Acutely, the goal of anticoagulation is active treatment, i.e., prevention of extension of the existing thrombus and embolization. Studies investigating different durations of treatment found that, in general, increased VTE recurrence was observed when anticoagulation was discontinued prior to 3 months, suggesting that 3 months is required to stabilize the thrombus [29]. There may be patients in whom a longer duration of treatment may appear reasonable, e.g., those with a large, proximal thrombus and a PE, but studies have not provided evidence that this is the case. Although some patients with small, distal thrombi which were provoked by a transient event such as surgery may not require the full 3-month treatment duration, it is reasonable to use 3 months as a guide given the uncertainty of the effects of shorter treatment durations. In summary, anticoagulation should be continued for 3 months after the index VTE, at which time determination of stopping therapy versus continuing indefinitely should be made [29].

After 3 months, the goal of anticoagulation changes from active treatment to prevention of subsequent new episodes of VTE. Decision-making centers on determination of the risk of new VTE versus the risk of hemorrhage: in patients with low risk of new VTE, anticoagulation should be stopped at 3 months, and in those at high risk, it should be continued indefinitely unless the risk of hemorrhage is higher [29]. The risk of recurrence of VTE depends on the factors that provoked the first episode. Transient, reversible factors such as surgery are associated with a 1 % VTE risk, whereas persistent factors such as active cancer may be associated with a rate as high as 20 %, within the year of anticoagulation discontinuation [29].

If the first VTE episode was unprovoked, D-dimer levels obtained 1 month after cessation of anticoagulation may aid in decision-making. Although the following results require confirmation, one study found that a woman with a negative D-dimer has a 5 % chance of VTE in the first year; a woman with a positive D-dimer, 10 %; a man with a negative D-dimer, 8 %; and a man with a positive D-dimer, 16 % [29]. Aspirin started after cessation of anticoagulation further decreases the risk of VTE recurrence in patients at low risk of recurrence [29].

Complications of VTE

Post-Thrombotic Syndrome

Post-thrombotic syndrome (PTS) typically affects the lower extremity and consists of edema, pigmentation, and ulceration [7]. While the syndrome is common—some state that it develops in up to half of patients with properly treated DVT—it is usually mild. Approximately 5–10 % of patients develop severe manifestations (ulceration) by 6 years after DVT [30].

Pathophysiologically, PTS is due to consequences of inflammatory damage to venous valves resulting in valvular reflux and, in combination with thrombus-related obstruction, venous hypertension [30]. A meta-analysis and a Cochrane review suggested that the use of elastic compression stockings (ECS) for up to 2 years after a proximal DVT may be effective at preventing the development of PTS [30]. Several other treatment modalities (surgical and procedural) are currently being investigated, but no firm recommendations can be made at this time.

Chronic Thromboembolic Pulmonary Hypertension

CTEPH develops in up to 4 % of patients with PE and is characterized by mean pulmonary artery pressure >25 mmHg 6 months after PE diagnosis. The main debilitating symptom is dyspnea which may occur at rest as well as with exertion. CTEPH is a risk factor for right heart failure and sudden death and, therefore, accounts for a percentage of PE-related mortality [7].

The main screening test for CTEPH is the ventilation-perfusion (VQ) scan, as, in contradistinction to the acute setting, CTPA is less sensitive than the VQ scan for chronic disease: VQ 96 % and CTPA 51 % [31]. In cases of suspected CTEPH based on screening, right-heart catheterization and conventional pulmonary angiography are necessary to properly assess risk/benefit of pulmonary endarterectomy, which is the recommended treatment for CTEPH [31]. Alternatives for CTEPH treatment including percutaneous approaches are currently being investigated, and no firm recommendations can be made at this time.

Patients who are not candidates for surgery, or patients in whom surgery did not eliminate pulmonary hypertension, may be candidates for medical therapy. Riociguat, a soluble guanylate cyclase stimulator, has been approved by the FDA for the treatment of pulmonary arterial hypertension and CTEPH specifically [32]. Additionally, lung transplantation may be an option in selected patients [31].

Summary

Neurosurgical patients are frequently at risk for VTE due to malignancy, immobility, and the post-surgical state. Testing for PE should be performed based on the assessment of clinical probability of PE. Treatment options include systemic anticoagulation, thrombolysis, and/or thromboembolectomy with selection of specific treatments based on clinical severity. PTS and CTEPH are two potentially serious complications of VTE.

References

1. Schwartz T, Hingorani A, Ascher E, et al. Pulmonary embolism without deep venous thrombosis. Ann Vasc Surg. 2012;26:973–6.
2. Kearon C. Natural history of venous thromboembolism. Circulation. 2003;107:I22–30.
3. Monreal M, Ruiz J, Olazabal A, Arias A, Roca J. Deep venous thrombosis and the risk of pulmonary embolism. A systematic study. Chest. 1992;102:677–81.
4. Moorjani N, Price S. Massive pulmonary embolism. Cardiol Clin. 2013;31:503–18. vii.
5. Deitelzweig SB, Johnson BH, Lin J, Schulman KL. Prevalence of clinical venous thromboembolism in the USA: current trends and future projections. Am J Hematol. 2011;86:217–20.
6. Weinberg I, Kaufman J, Jaff MR. Inferior vena cava filters. J Am Coll Cardiol Intv. 2013;6:539–47.
7. Goldhaber SZ, Bounameaux H. Pulmonary embolism and deep vein thrombosis. Lancet. 2012;379:1835–46.
8. Meyer G. Effective diagnosis and treatment of pulmonary embolism: Improving patient outcomes. Arch Cardiovasc Dis. 2014;107:406–14.
9. Rolston JD, Han SJ, Bloch O, Parsa AT. What clinical factors predict the incidence of deep venous thrombosis and pulmonary embolism in neurosurgical patients? J Neurosurg. 2014;121:908–18.
10. Kearon C, Kahn SR, Agnelli G, et al. Antithrombotic therapy for venous thromboembolic disease: American College of Chest Physicians Evidence-Based Clinical Practice Guidelines (8th Edition). Chest. 2008;133:454S–545.
11. Pollak AW, McBane 2nd RD. Succinct review of the new VTE prevention and management guidelines. Mayo Clin Proc. 2014;89:394–408.
12. Kuderer NM, Lyman GH. Guidelines for treatment and prevention of venous thromboembolism among patients with cancer. Thromb Res. 2014;133 Suppl 2:S122–7.
13. Collen JF, Jackson JL, Shorr AF, Moores LK. Prevention of venous thromboembolism in neurosurgery: a metaanalysis. Chest. 2008;134:237–49.
14. Palareti G. How I treat isolated distal deep vein thrombosis (IDDVT). Blood. 2014;123:1802–9.
15. Group PS. Eight-year follow-up of patients with permanent vena cava filters in the prevention of pulmonary embolism: the PREPIC (Prevention du Risque d'Embolie Pulmonaire par Interruption Cave) randomized study. Circulation. 2005;112:416–22.
16. Jaff MR, McMurtry MS, Archer SL, et al. Management of massive and submassive pulmonary embolism, iliofemoral deep vein thrombosis, and chronic thromboembolic pulmonary hypertension: a scientific statement from the American Heart Association. Circulation. 2011;123:1788–830.
17. Wells PS, Anderson DR, Rodger M, et al. Derivation of a simple clinical model to categorize patients probability of pulmonary embolism: increasing the models utility with the SimpliRED D-dimer. Thromb Haemost. 2000;83:416–20.
18. Le Gal G, Righini M, Roy PM, et al. Prediction of pulmonary embolism in the emergency department: the revised Geneva score. Ann Intern Med. 2006;144:165–71.
19. Prell J, Rachinger J, Smaczny R, et al. D-dimer plasma level: a reliable marker for venous thromboembolism after elective craniotomy. J Neurosurg. 2013;119:1340–6.
20. Wiener RS, Ouellette DR, Diamond E, et al. An official American Thoracic Society/American College of Chest Physicians policy statement: the Choosing Wisely top five list in adult pulmonary medicine. Chest. 2014;145:1383–91.
21. Brown G, Hogg K. Best evidence topic report. Diagnostic utility of electrocardiogram for diagnosing pulmonary embolism. Emerg Med J. 2005;22:729–30.
22. Perera P, Lobo V, Williams SR, Gharahbaghian L. Cardiac echocardiography. Crit Care Clin. 2014;30:47–92. v.
23. Torbicki A, Perrier A, Konstantinides S, et al. Guidelines on the diagnosis and management of acute pulmonary embolism: the Task Force for the Diagnosis and Management of Acute Pulmonary Embolism of the European Society of Cardiology (ESC). Eur Heart J. 2008;29:2276–315.
24. Aujesky D, Obrosky DS, Stone RA, et al. Derivation and validation of a prognostic model for pulmonary embolism. Am J Respir Crit Care Med. 2005;172:1041–6.
25. Jimenez D, Aujesky D, Moores L, et al. Simplification of the pulmonary embolism severity index for prognostication in patients with acute symptomatic pulmonary embolism. Arch Intern Med. 2010;170:1383–9.
26. Squizzato A, Ageno W. The 8(th) American College of Chest Physicians Guidelines—a perspective on venous thromboembolism guidelines. Thromb Haemost. 2009;101:31–5.
27. Cho JH, Kutti Sridharan G, Kim SH, et al. Right ventricular dysfunction as an echocardiographic prognostic factor in hemodynamically stable patients with acute pulmonary embolism: a meta-analysis. BMC Cardiovasc Disord. 2014;14:64.
28. Bottinor W, Turlington J, Raza S, et al. Life-saving systemic thrombolysis in a patient with massive pulmonary embolism and a recent hemorrhagic cerebrovascular accident. Tex Heart Inst J. 2014;41:174–6.

29. Kearon C, Akl EA. Duration of anticoagulant therapy for deep vein thrombosis and pulmonary embolism. Blood. 2014;123:1794–801.
30. Baldwin MJ, Moore HM, Rudarakanchana N, Gohel M, Davies AH. Post-thrombotic syndrome: a clinical review. J Thromb Haemost. 2013;11: 795–805.
31. Kim NH, Delcroix M, Jenkins DP, et al. Chronic thromboembolic pulmonary hypertension. J Am Coll Cardiol. 2013;62:D92–9.
32. Mielniczuk LM, Swiston JR, Mehta S. Riociguat: a novel therapeutic option for pulmonary arterial hypertension and chronic thromboembolic pulmonary hypertension. Can J Cardiol. 2014;30:1233–40.

Part 3

Coagulation Issues Specific to Neurosurgery

Classes of Drugs and Blood Products for Acute Reversal of Anticoagulant Effect

17

Christopher D. Witiw, Laureen D. Hachem, and Michael G. Fehlings

Abbreviations

VKAs	Vitamin K antagonists
INR	International normalized ratio
PCC	Prothrombin complex concentrates
aPCC	Activated prothrombin complex concentrate
FFP	Fresh frozen plasma
ICH	Intracerebral hemorrhage
uFH	Unfractionated heparin
LMWH	Low molecular weight heparin
aPTT	Activated partial thromboplastin time
TT	Thrombin time
CEA	Carotid endarterectomy
TSOACs	Target-specific oral anticoagulants
rFVIIa	Recombinant activated factor VII

C.D. Witiw, M.D.
Division of Neurosurgery, Department of Surgery, University of Toronto, Toronto, ON, Canada
e-mail: christopher.witiw@mail.utoronto.ca

L.D. Hachem
Faculty of Medicine, University of Toronto, Toronto, ON, Canada
e-mail: laureen.hachem@mail.utoronto.ca

M.G. Fehlings, M.D., Ph.D. (✉)
Division of Neurosurgery, Department of Surgery, University of Toronto, Toronto, ON, Canada

Toronto Western Hospital, University Health Network, Toronto, Ontario, Canada
e-mail: Michael.Fehlings@uhn.on.ca

Expeditious and safe reversal of anticoagulation is a primary tenet in the effective management of anticoagulated patients with bleeding of the central nervous system or the need for emergency neurosurgical intervention. Classically, the iatrogenic anticoagulant effect was induced by either warfarin or heparin and most practicing neurosurgeons possessed a commensurate armamentarium of effective strategies for reversal of these anticoagulants for nearly all clinical scenarios.

The recent introduction of target-specific oral anticoagulants (TSOACs) has ushered in a new era of anticoagulation. The growth in popularity of these novel TSOACs has greatly outpaced the rate of investigation into the reversal of their anticoagulant effect. This concerning discord is well recognized and is an area of active research. However, the neurosurgeon practicing in this continuously developing field is faced with a perpetual influx of data pertaining to the reversal of the new agents in addition to updated and optimized strategies for reversal of classic anticoagulants. A sound understanding of all classes of drugs and blood products that are currently available for acute reversal of the anticoagulant effect is needed to navigate this ever-changing landscape.

The aim of this chapter is to provide a framework to facilitate clinical decision-making when cessation of bleeding and reversal of anticoagulation is of paramount importance for preservation of life. Each reversal option will be reviewed in a

C.M. Loftus (ed.), *Anticoagulation and Hemostasis in Neurosurgery*,
DOI 10.1007/978-3-319-27327-3_17

structured manner including mechanism of action, onset and duration of action, means of administration, potential adverse effects, and the evidence for efficacy in reversal of specific anticoagulants. Furthermore, we will describe the novel agents that have reached the early stages of clinical study that hold promise for effective reversal of the new TSOACs. This chapter is not meant to represent a comprehensive compilation of all available evidence for anticoagulant reversal. Instead the key features and considerations have been highlighted and will serve to facilitate communication with other specialists and appraisal of forthcoming evidence in this ever-changing landscape.

Vitamin K

Vitamin K is a fat soluble vitamin, necessary for the hepatic synthesis of clotting factors II, VII, IX, X, and proteins C and S which are essential components of normal hemostasis. Vitamin K antagonists (VKAs), most notably Warfarin, are the most common form of anticoagulant therapy and act by inhibiting the generation of vitamin K in the liver and thus, vitamin K is a first-line therapy for reversal of VKA-induced anticoagulation.

Mechanism of Action

Vitamin K is converted to its reduced (active) form by vitamin K reductase in the liver. Reduced vitamin K is a co-factor in the carboxylation reaction that activates the precursors of vitamin K-dependent clotting factors. During this reaction, reduced vitamin K is converted to vitamin K epoxide which must be recycled back to vitamin K through the action of vitamin K epoxide reductase [1]. By inhibiting vitamin K epoxide reductase, VKAs effectively prevent the regeneration of vitamin K and decrease the levels of activated clotting factors in the blood. Administration of exogenous vitamin K provides an alternative substrate for the carboxylation reaction needed to activate vitamin K-dependent clotting factors (Fig. 17.1).

Onset and Duration of Action

The action of vitamin K on reversal of anticoagulation is delayed by the requirement of de novo synthesis of clotting factors by the liver. While a decrease in INR may be seen 4 h after IV vitamin K administration, this is largely due to an early elevation in factor VII that precedes the rise in factor II necessary for normal hemostasis [2, 3]. Thus full therapeutic effect is generally not reached until 12 h after IV or 24 h after oral administration [4]. Consequently, in the acute setting where rapid anticoagulant reversal is required, vitamin K should always be supplemented with vitamin K-dependent coagulation factors in the form of blood products like PCC or FFP [4].

Administration

Vitamin K can be administered orally, intravenously, subcutaneously, or intramuscularly. Subcutaneous and intramuscular administrations should be avoided because of delayed onset of action and unreliable absorption. The reliable delivery and rapid onset of action afforded by IV administration make it the route of choice in the setting of a life-threatening bleed. Despite the advantage of rapid normalization of INR with IV vitamin K, similar degrees of INR correction have been noted at 24 h when IV and oral administration are compared [3]. This makes oral administration an appropriate choice for situations where semi-urgent surgery is required or for asymptomatic patients with a supratherapeutic INR.

Dosing

In the setting of life-threatening bleeding or the need for emergency neurosurgical intervention doses of 5–10 mg are generally recommended at an intravenous infusion rate of 0.5–1.0 mg/min [5–7]. In patients requiring urgent reversal in the absence of major bleeding, as in cases of urgent surgery or severely elevated INR, high-dose oral vitamin K (5–10 mg) may replace the IV

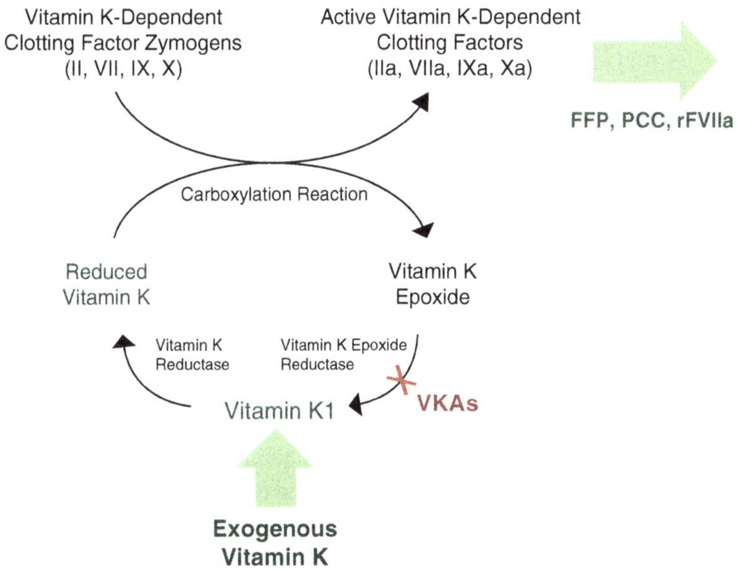

Fig. 17.1 Reversal of anticoagulant effects of vitamin K antagonists by administration of exogenous vitamin K and vitamin K-dependent factor replacement (FFP, PCC, rFVIIa). VKAs inhibit vitamin K epoxide reductase and thus reduced vitamin K is unavailable for the carboxylation reaction that activates vitamin K-dependent clotting factors. Exogenous administration of vitamin K bypasses the blockage at vitamin K epoxide reductase and allows for the carboxylation reaction to proceed. Administration of FFP, PCC or rFVIIa provides a direct source of activated vitamin K-dependent clotting factors and bypasses the need for de novo synthesis. *FFP* fresh frozen plasma, *PCC* prothrombin complex concentrate, *rFVIIa* recombinant activated factor VII, VKA vitamin K antagonist

route [7, 8]. Low-dose oral vitamin K (1–2.5 mg) is reserved for nonurgent situations of an elevated INR in asymptomatic patients.

Potential Adverse Events

IV administration has been associated with rare but severe anaphylactic reactions (3 out of 10,000 doses) [9], and for this reason, the IV route should be reserved for life-threatening situations [6, 7]. This reaction is thought to be due to the presence of polyethoxylated castor oil in older formulations of vitamin K. Since most new formulations do not contain this agent, the risk of developing a severe reaction is likely much lower than previous estimates. Vitamin K administration may lead to thromboembolic complications, especially in patients with mechanical heart valves or a recent history of thrombosis, but the rate of such events is low [10, 11]. In most acute settings, the benefits of reversing the anticoagulant effect to halt life-threatening bleeding or allow urgent surgery outweigh the potential thromboembolic risks.

Considerations for Specific Anticoagulant Reversal

Vitamin K is a mainstay of therapy for reversal of VKAs. It is not indicated for the acute reversal of any other anticoagulant agent.

Vitamin K Antagonists

Life-threatening bleeding associated with VKAs should be managed with intravenous vitamin K in combination with coagulation factor replacement [6, 7]. The primary role for vitamin K in the setting of acute VKA reversal is maintenance of anticoagulant reversal as the effect of coagulation factors weans. In a study of patients with intracerebral hemorrhage, PCC administered without vitamin K led to significant rebound increases in INR after 12–24 h and was associated with hematoma enlargement, while patients receiving PCC supplemented with vitamin K sustained INR normalization past 24 h [12]. The importance of combining vitamin K with a fast-acting coagulation factor replacement is underscored by findings from a retrospective study comparing the efficacy of different anticoagulant reversal regimens in patients experiencing VKA-associated ICH. Huttner et al. found that patients receiving vitamin K monotherapy required more than 12 h to achieve sufficient INR reduction and experienced a significantly higher frequency of hematoma growth compared to those receiving PCC (either alone, or supplemented with FFP or vitamin K) [13].

Box 17.1: Pearls and Pitfalls of Vitamin K for Anticoagulant Reversal

Pearls

- Vitamin K should be administered via the intravenous route when emergency anticoagulant reversal is needed.
- At high INRs, small changes in clotting factors produce relatively larger decreases in INR while relatively larger doses are required to achieve incremental decreases in INR once less than 2.

Pitfalls

- While vitamin K is available as oral, intravenous, intramuscular, and subcutaneous formulations, the latter two routes should be avoided due to unreliable absorption.
- Vitamin K has a delayed onset of action and therefore must be used in combination with faster acting agents for emergency reversal of the anticoagulant effect of VKAs.

Plasma and Prothrombin Complex Concentrates

Fresh frozen plasma (FFP), prothrombin complex concentrates (PCC), and activated prothrombin complex concentrate (aPCC) are all sources of vitamin K-dependent clotting factors that can be used for reversal of the anticoagulant effect for patients taking oral anticoagulants. FFP is inexpensive and readily available at most centers; however a substantial body of evidence has emerged to support the use of PCC over FFP if available and evidence is mounting that aPCCs may have a role in the reversal of TSOACs.

Table 17.1 Prothrombin complex concentrates by coagulation factor composition

	Coagulation factors				
	II	VII	VIIa	IX	X
FFP[a]	✓	✓		✓	✓
3 Factor PCC	✓			✓	✓
4 Factor PCC	✓	✓		✓	✓
Activated PCC	✓		✓	✓	✓

FFP fresh frozen plasma, *PCC* prothrombin complex concentrate

[a]FFP contains all vitamin K-dependent clotting factors only at concentrations that are approximately 25 times less than PCCs

Mechanism of Action

FFP is plasma that has been isolated from a unit of whole blood or collected directly by apheresis and frozen below −18 °C within 8 h of collection. It contains all clotting factors in addition to fibrinogen, proteins C and S, and antithrombin in nonconcentrated form [14]. Often FFP is used interchangeably with plasma that was isolated and frozen between 8 and 24 h and plasma that has been thawed and stored at refrigerator temperatures for up to 5 days. All of these products are considered to have equivalent clinical efficacy for anticoagulant reversal.

PCCs contain a mixture of vitamin K-dependent clotting factors derived from pooled plasma by ion-exchange chromatography and cryoprecipitation [15]. These products fall into one of three categories (Table 17.1); three factor PCC (3PCC), four factor PCC (4PCC), and activated PCC (aPCC). 3PCCs contain significant concentrations of inactive factors II, IX, and X, while 4PCCs contain these inactivate factors in addition to inactive factor VII. aPCC differs from 4PCC by inclusion of activated factor VII. All of these act to rapidly replace factors that are deficient secondary to impaired production blocked by VKAs or rendered inactive by TSOCAs.

Onset and Duration of Action

Although FFP provides an immediate source of clotting factors, it requires a significantly longer time to correct INR compared to PCC/aPCCs due to the lower concentration of clotting factors and the time needed to safely transfuse larger volumes [16, 17]. While most studies report a mean time to INR reversal with FFP between 2 and 12 h [18–21], complete correction can take upwards of 24 h due to the extended time needed for administration [22, 23]. A recent randomized, phase IIIb comparison of 4PCC to FFP enrolling 202 patients found that patients in the 4PCC group achieved INR correction more rapidly than those in the plasma group [24]. One hour after the start of infusion, 68 patients (69 %) in the 4PCC group had an INR ≤ 1.3 while none in the plasma group reached this target. The median INR remained significantly lower in the 4PCC group until 12 h after the start of infusion (Fig. 17.2a). At the 24 h

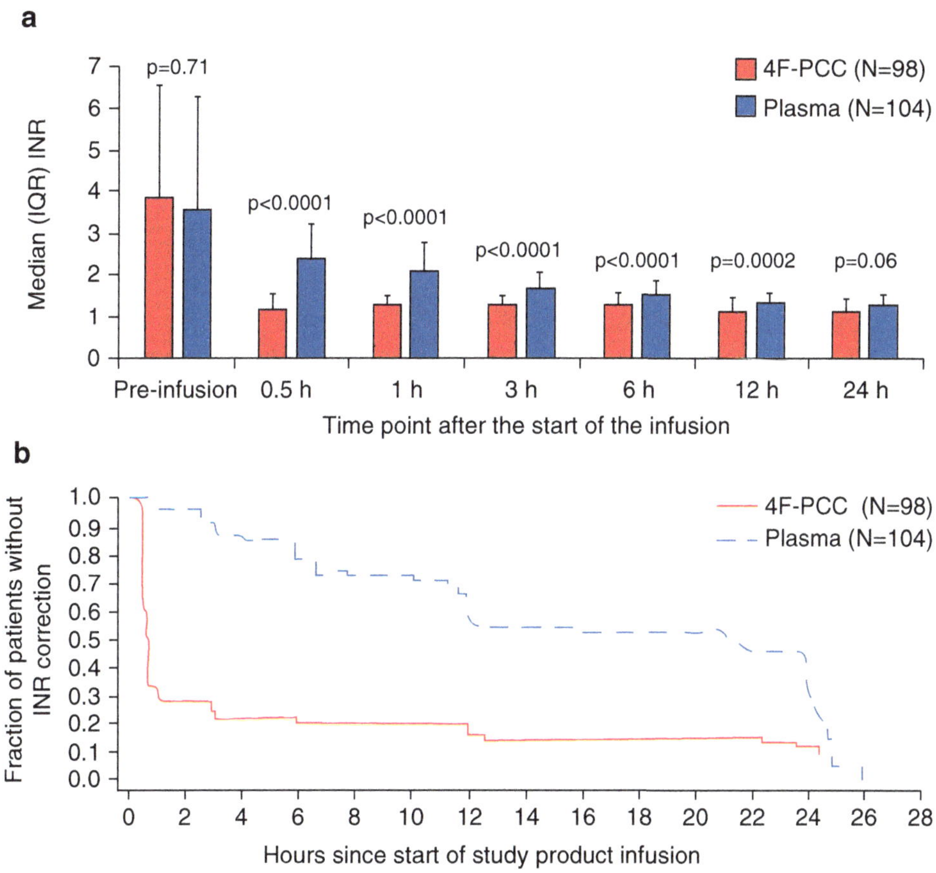

Fig. 17.2 Comparison of time to target INR with 4PCC vs. FFP administration. Results of a multicenter, prospective, randomized trial for reversal of the anticoagulant effect in patients receiving VKA therapy with an elevated INR (≥2.0 within 3 h before study treatment). (**a**) Comparison of median INR by time point. (**b**) Time to reach target INR (≤1.3). Patients in the 4PCC group reached target INR more rapidly than those in the plasma group and the trend continued out to 24 h and the median INR was significantly lower in the 4PCC group until 12 h after the start of treatment. Figure adapted from Sarode et al. Circulation. 2013 Sep 10;128(11):1234–43. *INR* international normalized ratio, *4F-PCC* 4 factor prothrombin complex concentrate, *IQR* interquartile range, *VKA* vitamin K antagonist

Table 17.2 Considerations for administration of FFP vs. PCC

	PCC	FFP
Route of administration	Intravenous	Intravenous
Blood type matching required	No	Yes
Preparation time	<10 min	30–45 min
Infection risk	Yes	Yes
Infusion volume	0.2 L	1–3 L

FFP fresh frozen plasma, *PCC* prothrombin complex concentrate

Table 17.3 PCC dosing options for reversal of warfarin anticoagulation

INR-based dosing [27]		Factor IX-based dosing [28]	
Initial INR	Dose to attain target INR < 1.3 (IU/kg)	Initial factor IX level[a]	Dose to attain target factor IX level of 50 % (IU/kg)
2.0–3.9	25	10 % (INR 2–3)	40
4.0–6.0	35	5 % (INR 3–4)	45
>6.0	50	1 % (INR >4)	49

INR international normalized ratio, *IU* international units
[a]Factor levels are based upon initial INR

time mark, 88 % of patients receiving 4PCC had reached an INR ≤ 1.3 compared with only 58 % of patients receiving FFP (Fig. 17.2b).

Administration

Several administration-related factors make PCC advantageous to FFP (Table 17.2). The concentration of clotting factors in PCC is approximately 25 times higher than FFP and thus a much smaller volume is required and can be given over a much shorter time period. No blood type matching is required, as it is for FFP because of the presence of isohemagglutinins. PCC can be reconstituted from its lyophilized storage powder in minutes while FFP can take up to 30–45 min for thawing.

Dosing of FFP

While the optimal dose of FFP depends on the degree of INR elevation, a volume of 15 mL/kg (which equates to a total transfusion volume of approximately 1050 mL for an average 70 kg patient) is commonly administered [25, 26]. Standard units of FFP have a volume of 200–250 cc. Larger volumes may be necessary to correct severely elevated INR and dosing should be based upon repeat measurement of INR after administration of an initial dose. The optimal infusion rate will be dictated by the patient's ability to tolerate the additional volume and a range of 1–3 ml/kg/h is often used.

Dosing of PCC

The concentration of PCC/aPCCs is standardized by the concentration of factor IX, and the recommendations for dosing are based upon the quantity of factor IX administered. Numerous regimes have been reported and these vary from institution to institution. Most recommendations fall within 25–50 IU/kg and are often based upon initial INR but others rely on differences between target and current serum factor levels (Table 17.3). It is reasonable to expect a 1 % increase in factor XI for each 1 IU/kg infusion. An upper limit for the rate of infusion has yet to be established and a rate of up to 210 IU/min was well tolerated in healthy volunteers [29].

Potential Adverse Events

As with all blood products, the administration of FFP and PCC/aPCC carries a small risk of transmitting blood-borne viral infection. Furthermore, the presence of anti-leukocyte antibodies in FFP can cause immune-mediated transfusion-related acute lung injury [26, 30]. FFP must be transfused intravenously at a slow infusion rate in order to reduce the risk of transfusion-associated circulatory overload [30]. The risk of thrombotic complications for administration of PCCs is concerning, but the overall rate has been observed to be low [31].

Considerations for Specific Anticoagulant Reversal

Traditionally, FFP in combination with vitamin K was considered the standard of care for rapid VKA reversal in the setting of life-threatening bleeding; however the evidence now favoring PCC has mounted to such an extent that it has become the new standard for acute reversal of VKAs, and FFP should be used only when PCC is unavailable [6, 7, 26]. Furthermore, evidence is now emerging to suggest that PCC/aPCCs may have a role in the reversal of target-specific oral anticoagulants.

Vitamin K Agonist Reversal

Among patients with VKA-induced ICH, FFP has consistently been shown to require significantly longer times to correct INR compared to PCC [18, 21, 22], and in many cases failed to achieve complete reversal [17, 18, 32]. The prolonged time to reversal has also been associated with significantly poorer bleeding control and higher rates of hematoma growth [13, 21, 23]. Recent evidence has also emerged linking FFP to worse long-term clinical outcomes. Among patients with ICH requiring VKA reversal, the use of FFP was associated with a greater risk of continued hemorrhage and a 3-month increased risk of severe disability and death compared to PCC [33]. The protracted time necessary to correct INR using FFP can significantly delay surgical intervention and worsen clinical outcome. Yanamandala et al. found that among patients requiring urgent VKA reversal prior to emergency neurosurgery, the average time from patient presentation to operation was significantly longer among patients receiving FFP compared to PCC (307 min versus 159 min, $P<0.05$) [19].

Concern has been expressed that 3PCCs may be suboptimal to 4PCCs because of the lack of Factor VII. Some have suggested co-administration of FFP or rFVIIa with 3PCC to provide a source of exogenous factor VII [34]. The evidence remains controversial and many believe that 3PCC and 4PCCs are equivalent when INR is less than 4.5 (which reflects an intrinsic concentration of factor VII that is less than 15 %), and it may only be once INR is greater than this mark that additional factor VII is needed [35]. However, in 2013 the FDA approved Kcentra (CSL Behring, King of Prussia, PA), the first 4PCC for use in the United States, for urgent reversal of anticoagulation in adults with major bleeding. In the face of controversial evidence we support the use of 4PCCs over 3PCCs, if available, for acute reversal of the anticoagulant effect of VKAs.

Direct Thrombin Inhibitors

Animal experimental models have demonstrated promising findings for the role of FFP and PCC in the management of life-threatening bleeding from the anticoagulant effect of direct thrombin inhibitors. Excess intracerebral hematoma expansion was found to be prevented in a mouse model on high-dose dabigatran with treatment with PCC and FFP (albeit less consistently) compared with saline [36]. Bleeding induced by high doses of dabigatran has been shown to be significantly reduced in a rat tail bleeding model by the administration of PCC [37].

Results from a study of administration of 4PCC to healthy volunteers demonstrated no influence on the anticoagulant action of dabigatran [38]; however an ex vivo study of aPCC on healthy patients taking dabigatran showed encouraging effect on the reversal of impaired thrombin generation [39, 40]. A recently published case series of three patients with life-threatening intracranial bleeds demonstrated potential for the reversal of the anticoagulant effect of dabigatran with the use of aPCC [41]. Without data from well-designed trials providing evidence for clinical efficacy in humans we favor aPCC administration over PCC if available for reversal of dabigatran.

Factor Xa Inhibitors

PCC has been demonstrated to prevent expansion of intracerebral hematoma in a mouse model treated with rivaroxaban, and normalization of laboratory coagulation parameters has been shown for rabbits treated with apixaban and then given PCC [42, 43]. In a study of healthy subjects taking rivaroxaban, normalization of a prolonged PT was attained at a dose of 50 IU/kg [38]. As with direct thrombin inhibitors, PCC remains an option for reversal of anticoagulation for patients who are taking factor Xa inhibitors and present with life-threatening neurosurgical conditions, but further data from trials evaluating clinical efficacy in humans is desperately needed.

Box 17.2: Pearls and Pitfalls of Plasma and Prothrombin Complex Concentrates for Anticoagulant Reversal

Pearls

- If FFP is administered for anticoagulant reversal, careful clinical monitoring for evidence of fluid overload is critical as doses may exceed 2 l depending on the clinical scenario.
- The evidence is limited for reversal of direct thrombin inhibitors but the authors favor aPCC over PCC or FFP if cessation of life-threatening bleeding is needed.

Pitfalls

- When emergency reversal of anticoagulation induced by a VKA is needed, FFP should only be used when PCC is unavailable and the authors prefer 4PCCs rather than 3PCCs if both are available.
- 3PCC lacks factor VII and if ongoing bleeding is a concern, co-administration of FFP or rFVIIa may be necessary to provide adequate clotting factor replacement.

Recombinant Factor VIIa

Recombinant factor VIIa (rFVIIa) is a vitamin K-dependent glycoprotein consisting of 406 amino acid residues that is structurally similar to human-derived factor VII and approved by the FDA in the United States for the treatment of hemophilia A and B and for the treatment of congenital factor VII deficiency. It is used off-label to treat severe life-threatening bleeding as a reserve strategy when other conventional therapy is ineffective.

Mechanism of Action

The administration of rFVIIa enhances thrombin generation; however the exact mechanism remains to be elucidated. It likely mediates thrombin formation via a complex of factor VIIa and tissue factor on the surface of tissue factor bearing cells, and once tissue factor has been consumed mediates formation on the surface of activated platelets leading to accelerated fibrin clot formation localized to the site of vascular injury [44].

Onset and Duration of Action

The true onset of action of rFVIIa remains unknown because presently there is no laboratory test available that correlates with the clinical efficacy of rFVIIa. Administration of rFVIIa to healthy patients taking a VKA normalized the INR in less than 1 h; however concerns have been expressed that an INR that has been normalized by rFVIIa may not represent successful reversal of anticoagulation [45, 46]. There is little data to guide the duration of therapy and in general the dosing can be stopped when the practitioner can be assured that bleeding has ceased.

Administration

rFVIIa is administered intravenously and shares the comparative advantages of PCC versus FFP. There is no need for blood type matching and preparation time is negligible. The primary disadvantage of rFVIIa is cost. Pricing for NovoSeven RT (Novo Nordisk, Inc., Princeton, NJ) is $2.20 USD per μg. The smallest vial available is 1 mg, at a cost of $2200.

Dosing

There is currently no optimal dosing established for anticoagulant reversal by rFVIIa. Ranges vary widely from one institution to another. The dosing in initial studies was in keeping with ranges recommended for treatment of hemophilia (90 μg/kg). However, subsequent studies demonstrated that effective reversal can be accomplished with notably lesser doses. Many case series have reported successful normalization of INR using much smaller non-weight-based single doses of 1200–1400 μg [47, 48].

Potential Adverse Events

A substantial amount of concern has been expressed regarding the potential for administration of rFVIIa to incite thromboembolic events.

A meta-analysis of 4468 subjects from 35 randomized clinical trials using rFVIIa off-label to treat life-threatening bleeding found the rate of venous thromboembolic events was not significantly different compared with placebo (5.3 % vs. 5.7 %) but the rate of arterial thromboembolic events was elevated significantly for patients receiving rFVIIa (5.5 % vs. 3.2 %, $P=0.003$) [49]. The volume of administration is negligible mitigating any of the risks of circulatory overload seen with FFP and there is no risk of transmission of blood-borne infection as there is with FFP and PCC.

Considerations for Specific Anticoagulant Reversal

With the exception of reversal of VKAs, the current evidence for anticoagulant reversal with rFVIIa is limited to animal models, studies of coagulation parameters and thrombin generation assays based on administration to healthy volunteers, and case reports of administration in an attempt to halt life-threatening bleeding.

Vitamin K Antagonists

The best evidence for off-label use of rFVIIa in anticoagulant reversal is in the setting of VKAs. In a small retrospective study, Nishijima et al. found that in patients taking warfarin who presented with traumatic intracranial hemorrhage the time to normalization of INR was significantly less if 1.2 mg of rFVIIa was administered in addition to standard care [50]. Similar results were found in another retrospective trial where patients receiving co-administration of rFVIIa with conventional therapy required significantly less FFP and attained target INR in a much shorter period of time [51]. However, it is critical to note that the effect of rFVIIa on INR values may be far greater than its actual effect on in vivo hemostasis and until further evidence of clinical efficacy is available for its use in VKA reversal, many suggest avoiding routine administration for this indication [52].

Direct Thrombin Inhibitors

rFVIIa was found to be ineffective in preventing excess intracerebral hematoma expansion caused by dabigatran in a murine model. Furthermore, rFVIIa failed to correct the endogenous thrombin potential of dabigatran in ex vivo plasma samples from healthy volunteers and affected thrombin generation indices to a lesser extent than PCC and aPCC [39, 53]. Further study is needed to delineate the role of rFVIIa in management of life-threatening bleeding in patients anticoagulated with direct thrombin inhibitors but given the present literature it is likely that stronger consideration should be given to upfront management with PCC or aPCC before rFVIIa.

Factor Xa Inhibitors

In vitro animal studies have demonstrated variable effects of rFVIIa on coagulation parameters and thrombin generation indices. rFVIIa corrected PT prolongation and reduced bleeding time in rats treated with rivaroxaban but only reduced PT prolongation and not bleeding time in rivaroxaban-treated primates [54]. An ex vivo human study demonstrated that rFVIIa added to plasma from healthy volunteers receiving rivaroxaban reversed prolonged PT, clotting time, and thrombin generation lag time to a greater extent than both PCC and aPCC [55].

Low Molecular Weight Heparin Reversal

The ineffectiveness of protamine sulfate for reversal of LMWH has driven a search for an alternative to mange bleeding in the setting of LMWH. Recombinant factor VIIa has emerged as a potential option. Promise has been demonstrated in animal model bleeding induced by LMWH [56]. Furthermore, clinical reports have documented safe and effective control of LMWH-associated clinically significant bleeding with administration of rFVIIa at concentrations of 20–120 μg/kg [57, 58].

Pentasaccharide Reversal

The lack of efficacy of protamine sulfate to reverse the effects of pentasaccharide anticoagulants has led to attempts at utilizing rFVIIa. Normalization of coagulation times and thrombin generation has been demonstrated in healthy volunteers taking fondaparinux and then given a 90 μg/kg dose of rFVIIa [59]. In the setting of life-threatening bleeding in a patient with pentasaccharide anticoagulation, administration of rFVIIa is a reasonable consideration.

Box 17.3: Pearls and Pitfalls of Activated Recombinant Factor VII for Anticoagulant Reversal

Pearls

- rFVIIa should be considered as a reserve strategy for reversal of the anticoagulant effect of LMWH in patients who have ongoing life-threatening bleeding despite administration of protamine sulfate.

Pitfalls

- There is currently no laboratory test that correlates with the clinical efficacy of rFVIIa. An INR that has been normalized by rFVIIa may not represent successful reversal of anticoagulation and decision-making regarding further efforts at reversal of anticoagulation should be driven by clinical evidence of bleeding.
- rFVII may increase the risk of arterial thromboembolic events especially at high doses.

Protamine Sulfate

Protamine sulfate is a small synthetic cationic polypeptide. It is the only agent currently approved for rapid reversal of heparin anticoagulation—both unfractionated heparin (uFH) and low molecular weight heparin (LMWH).

Mechanism of Action

Binding of protamine sulfate to uFH forms an inactive salt complex that completely neutralizes both the antithrombin and anti-factor Xa activities of uFH. While protamine sulfate also binds LMWH, it only partially neutralizes its anti-factor Xa activity. Although the exact mechanisms underlying this interaction are not well defined, the differential effect of protamine sulfate on these two agents is likely due to reduced sulfate charge density in LMWH compared with uFH [60].

Onset and Duration of Action

Following IV administration of protamine sulfate, neutralization of heparin occurs within 5–10 min as indicated by a reversal of activated partial thromboplastin time (aPTT), thrombin time (TT), and anti-factor Xa activity. Complete correction of aPTT and TT with protamine sulfate is seen in both uFH and LMWH. Anti-factor Xa activity, while completely reversed in uFH, is reduced by only 60 % in LMWH [60–62]. A "heparin rebound" phenomenon has been reported in patients receiving protamine sulfate for heparin reversal where a reappearance of coagulopathy occurs within hours of complete reversal. This has been postulated to occur due to sequestration of heparin by plasma proteins which can lead to a delayed release of heparin following degradation of protamine sulfate [63].

Administration

Protamine sulfate is administered intravenously at a maximum rate of 5 mg per minute. Rapid infusion can lead to histamine release resulting in hypotension and bronchoconstriction and should be avoided.

Dosing

For the reversal of uFH, a dosing regimen of 1 mg protamine sulfate per 100 U of uFH received in the last 2 h is recommended. To reverse LMWH, 1 mg protamine sulfate should be administered for every 100 anti-Xa units given in the last 8 h. If bleeding continues, a subsequent dose of half of the original should be delivered [64]. Since protamine itself has anticoagulant properties, careful attention should be made not to exceed the recommended dose of 50 mg (Table 17.4).

Potential Adverse Events

Protamine sulfate may cause hypotension, bradycardia, and bronchoconstriction if administered too quickly. Because of its intrinsic anticoagulant activity, high doses can lead to increased bleeding

Table 17.4 Protamine sulfate dosing for reversal of anticoagulation induced by uFH or LMWH

Agent	Protamine sulfate dose[a]
uFH	1 mg/100 U μFH received in the last 2 h
Enoxaparin	1 mg/1 mg enoxaparin received in last 8 h
Dalteparin	1 mg/100 U dalteparin received in last 8 h
Tinzaparin	1 mg/100 U tinzaparin received in last 8 h

uFH unfractionated heparin, *LMWH* low molecular weight heparin
[a]Maximum total dose is 50 mg

[65, 66]. Protamine sulfate may also cause an allergic response in individuals previously exposed to protamine although the risk is small [64, 67].

Considerations for Specific Anticoagulant Reversal

Protamine sulfate is currently the only agent recommended for urgent reversal of uFH and LMWH. Because protamine sulfate has been considered the standard of care for heparin reversal and due to the rare incidence and acute nature of heparin-induced bleeding events, evidence for anticoagulant reversal with protamine sulfate is limited to experimental models, studies in nonurgent settings, and case reports of emergency reversal.

Unfractionated Heparin Reversal

Protamine sulfate is the gold standard treatment for reversal of uFH as it provides complete correction of aPTT, TT, and anti-factor Xa activity [61, 62]. Since heparin is commonly administered in the setting of endovascular treatments to avoid thrombotic events, protamine sulfate should be administered if urgent heparin reversal is necessary. This is especially indicated in the case of intraprocedural aneurysmal rupture [68]. There are conflicting reports, however, on the utility of protamine sulfate for heparin reversal in the absence of intraprocedural bleeding in the setting of carotid endarterectomy (CEA), due to the potential risk of thrombosis [69]. Recently, a large retrospective study among 4587 CEAs (46 % used protamine, 54 % did not) found that protamine sulfate decreased the rate of reoperation for bleeding (0.64 % vs. 1.66 %, $P=0.001$) and was not associated with an increased risk of myocardial infarction, stroke, or death [70].

Low Molecular Weight Heparin Reversal

Although protamine sulfate is the sole agent approved for reversal of LMWH, it neutralizes approximately 60 % of the anti-factor Xa activity and therefore does not fully correct coagulopathy [60, 61]. Among the LMWHs, tinzaparin may achieve the most effective reversal with protamine sulfate compared with dalteparin and enoxaparin due to the presence of more sulfate charge densities (Fig. 17.3) [60]. However, protamine sulfate is an unreliable option when urgent correction is needed—among 12 patients with active bleeding who received protamine sulfate for urgent reversal of enoxaparin or tinzaparin, only 8 achieved bleeding cessation [71]. Furthermore, a number of case reports demonstrate that protamine sulfate is ineffective in correcting enoxaparin-induced intracranial bleeding [72, 73].

Pentasaccharide Reversal

Despite the structural similarities between the pentasaccharide fondaparinux and uFH or LMWH, protamine sulfate does not bind to fondaparinux and has therefore shown no effect in its reversal. While there are experimental reports in animal models suggesting protamine sulfate may reduce bleeding induced by a synthetic anti-factor Xa pentasaccharide, this was not associated with neutralization of anti-factor Xa activity and there are no other reports demonstrating the utility of protamine sulfate for pentasaccharide reversal [74, 75].

Box 17.4: Pearls and Pitfalls of Protamine Sulfate for Anticoagulant Reversal

Pearls

- Ongoing clinical evidence of bleeding in the setting of prior administration of subcutaneous uFH or LMWH may require repeated dosing of protamine sulfate owed to the slow release of the subcutaneous formulation.

continued

Box 17.4 (continued)

- Monitor closely for the clinical triad of hypotension, bradycardia, and broncho-constriction suggestive of protamine-induced histamine release caused by a rapid infusion rate or an allergic reaction.

Pitfalls

- Protamine sulfate does not completely reverse the anticoagulant effects of LMWH or pentasaccharides.
- Overdosing of protamine sulfate can exacerbate bleeding and therefore careful dosing is essential. This should be guided by ongoing clinical evidence of bleeding and coagulation studies.

Novel Agents in Early Clinical Study

There is presently a compelling search ongoing of agents that may effectively act to reverse the anticoagulant effects of the novel TSOACs. Three of these have reached the early stages of clinical trials. None of these have demonstrated clinical efficacy for cessation of the hemorrhage and only Idarucizumab has reached this stage of clinical efficacy testing; nonetheless the early results of normalization of bleeding parameters in healthy volunteers are highly encouraging.

Andexanet alpha (PRT064445)

Andexanet alfa (PRT064445; Portola Pharmac euticals, San Francisco, USA) is a recombinant factor Xa derivative without catalytic activity but with retained binding affinity, which allows it to act as a decoy for oral factor Xa inhibitors [76]. The results of a phase II study in healthy volunteers receiving rivaroxaban demonstrated decreased anti-Xa activity and reduced concentrations of free rivaroxaban compared to placebo [77]. Preliminary results of a phase III double-blind, placebo-controlled study in older individuals taking apixaban demonstrated reversal of apixaban-induced anti-FXa activity and restoration of thrombin generation compared with placebo [78].

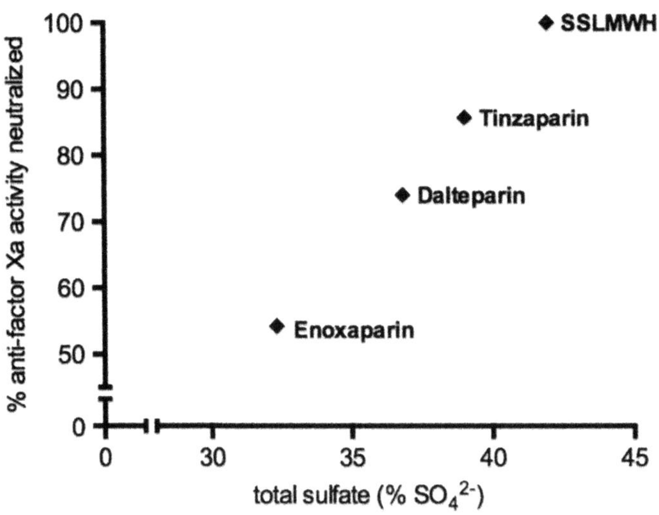

Fig. 17.3 Percentage of anti-factor Xa activity neutralized by protamine sulfate in various LMWHs. Neutralization of anti-factor Xa activity correlates with total sulfate content (r^2=0.92). Tinzaparin appears to achieve the most effective reversal of commonly used LMWHs. Figure derived from the data of *Crowther* et al. Br J Haematol. 2002 Jan;116(1):178–86 [60]. *LMWH* low molecular weight heparin, *SSLMWH* super sulfonated low molecular weight heparin

Aripazine (PER977)

Aripazine (PER977; Perosphere, Bedford, New York, USA) is currently undergoing development as a nonspecific agent for reversal of the anticoagulant effect of TSOACs. It is a small synthetic, water-soluble molecule that has been shown to bind through noncovalent hydrogen bonding and charge–charge interactions to oral factor Xa inhibitors and direct thrombin inhibitors. Aripazine demonstrated restoration of baseline hemostasis within 10–30 min after administration to healthy volunteers treated with edoxaban [79]. The encouraging results have led to further clinical investigation and a phase II study of aripazine in volunteers receiving edoxaban is underway.

Idarucizumab

Idarucizumab (anti-Dabi-Fab; Boehringer Ingelheim, Biberach, Germany) is a monoclonal antibody with a high affinity for dabigatran. This dabigatran antidote achieves a 350 times stronger affinity for dabigatran than its affinity for thrombin and has demonstrated rapid reversal of the anticoagulant activity of dabigatran in vivo in a rat model of anticoagulation [80]. In a phase I human clinical trial, idarucizumab reversed the anticoagulant effect of dabigatran in healthy male volunteers [81]. A phase III clinical trial to assess the efficacy of idarucizumab for reversal of the anticoagulant effect of dabigatran in patients who have uncontrolled bleeding or require emergency surgery is currently underway.

Summary

The ongoing influx of new anticoagulant agents into medical practice has led to an unprecedented level of complexity in the field of antithrombotic therapy. Moreover, data continues to emerge regarding optimization of reversal of classic anticoagulants and promising options for reversal of the novel agents. This has led to ever-increasing challenges for those tasked with anticoagulant reversal as a means of preserving life and providing optimal outcomes. As such, it is imperative that the practicing neurosurgeon maintain a framework of the classes of drugs and blood products available for this purpose (Table 17.5).

Table 17.5 Summary of drug and blood product options for reversal of currently available anticoagulants

Anticoagulant	Target	Classes of drugs or blood products available for reversal
Vitamin K antagonists	Vitamin K epoxide reductase	Vitamin K Must be coadministered with factor replacement (FFP, PCC) if emergency reversal required PCC Standard of care for emergency reversal FFP Only if PCC is unavailable
Unfractionated heparin	Antithrombin, factors Xa and IIa	Protamine sulfate Standard of care for emergency reversal
Low molecular weight heparin	Predominantly factor Xa	Protamine sulfate Only partially corrects anti-Xa activity rFVIIa Salvage strategy for ongoing bleeding despite protamine sulfate administration
Pentasaccharides	Predominantly factor Xa	rFVIIa Normalization of clotting parameters in healthy volunteers
Direct thrombin inhibitors	Factor IIa	aPCC Encouraging results from animal models and case reports
Factor Xa inhibitors	Factor Xa	PCC/aPCC An option based on results from animal models and healthy volunteers rFVIIa Variable results in animal models but greater effect on clotting parameters in healthy volunteers than PCC/aPCC

FFP fresh frozen plasma, *PCC* prothrombin complex concentrate, *aPCC* prothrombin complex concentrate with activated factor VII, *rFVIIa* recombinant activated factor VII

The specifics will likely change quickly, but a solid conceptual foundation serves as a basis for effective incorporation of new evidence as it emerges.

References

1. Hirsh J, Fuster V, Ansell J, Halperin JL. American Heart Association/American College of Cardiology Foundation guide to warfarin therapy. Circulation. 2003;107(12):1692–711.
2. Vigue B. Bench-to-bedside review: optimising emergency reversal of vitamin K antagonists in severe haemorrhage - from theory to practice. Crit Care (London, England). 2009;13(2):209.
3. Watson HG, Baglin T, Laidlaw SL, Makris M, Preston FE. A comparison of the efficacy and rate of response to oral and intravenous Vitamin K in reversal of over-anticoagulation with warfarin. Br J Haematol. 2001;115(1):145–9.
4. Vigue B, Ract C, Tremey B, et al. Ultra-rapid management of oral anticoagulant therapy-related surgical intracranial hemorrhage. Intensive Care Med. 2007;33(4):721–5.
5. Beshay JE, Morgan H, Madden C, Yu W, Sarode R. Emergency reversal of anticoagulation and antiplatelet therapies in neurosurgical patients. J Neurosurg. 2010;112(2):307–18.
6. Keeling D, Baglin T, Tait C, et al. Guidelines on oral anticoagulation with warfarin - fourth edition. Br J Haematol. 2011;154(3):311–24.
7. Ansell J, Hirsh J, Hylek E, Jacobson A, Crowther M, Palareti G. Pharmacology and management of the vitamin K antagonists: American College of Chest Physicians Evidence-Based Clinical Practice Guidelines (8th Edition). Chest. 2008;133(6 Suppl):160s–98.
8. Pabinger I, Brenner B, Kalina U, Knaub S, Nagy A, Ostermann H. Prothrombin complex concentrate (Beriplex P/N) for emergency anticoagulation reversal: a prospective multinational clinical trial. J Thromb Haemost. 2008;6(4):622–31.
9. Riegert-Johnson DL, Volcheck GW. The incidence of anaphylaxis following intravenous phytonadione (vitamin K1): a 5-year retrospective review. Ann Allergy Asthma Immunol. 2002;89(4):400–6.
10. Lousberg TR, Witt DM, Beall DG, Carter BL, Malone DC. Evaluation of excessive anticoagulation in a group model health maintenance organization. Arch Intern Med. 1998;158(5):528–34.
11. Patel RJ, Witt DM, Saseen JJ, Tillman DJ, Wilkinson DS. Randomized, placebo-controlled trial of oral phytonadione for excessive anticoagulation. Pharmacotherapy. 2000;20(10):1159–66.
12. Yasaka M, Sakata T, Minematsu K, Naritomi H. Correction of INR by prothrombin complex concentrate and vitamin K in patients with warfarin related hemorrhagic complication. Thromb Res. 2002;108(1):25–30.
13. Huttner HB, Schellinger PD, Hartmann M, et al. Hematoma growth and outcome in treated neurocritical care patients with intracerebral hemorrhage related to oral anticoagulant therapy: comparison of acute treatment strategies using vitamin K, fresh frozen plasma, and prothrombin complex concentrates. Stroke. 2006;37(6):1465–70.
14. Benjamin RJ, McLaughlin LS. Plasma components: properties, differences, and uses. Transfusion. 2012;52 Suppl 1:9s–19.
15. Bershad EM, Suarez JI. Prothrombin complex concentrates for oral anticoagulant therapy-related intracranial hemorrhage: a review of the literature. Neurocrit Care. 2010;12(3):403–13.
16. Schulman S, Bijsterveld NR. Anticoagulants and their reversal. Transfus Med Rev. 2007;21(1):37–48.
17. Makris M, Greaves M, Phillips WS, Kitchen S, Rosendaal FR, Preston EF. Emergency oral anticoagulant reversal: the relative efficacy of infusions of fresh frozen plasma and clotting factor concentrate on correction of the coagulopathy. Thromb Haemost. 1997;77(3):477–80.
18. Cartmill M, Dolan G, Byrne JL, Byrne PO. Prothrombin complex concentrate for oral anticoagulant reversal in neurosurgical emergencies. Br J Neurosurg. 2000;14(5):458–61.
19. Yanamadala V, Walcott BP, Fecci PE, et al. Reversal of warfarin associated coagulopathy with 4-factor prothrombin complex concentrate in traumatic brain injury and intracranial hemorrhage. J Clin Neurosci. 2014;21(11):1881–4.
20. Hickey M, Gatien M, Taljaard M, Aujnarain A, Giulivi A, Perry JJ. Outcomes of urgent warfarin reversal with frozen plasma versus prothrombin complex concentrate in the emergency department. Circulation. 2013;128(4):360–4.
21. Fredriksson K, Norrving B, Stromblad LG. Emergency reversal of anticoagulation after intracerebral hemorrhage. Stroke. 1992;23(7):972–7.
22. Woo CH, Patel N, Conell C, et al. Rapid Warfarin reversal in the setting of intracranial hemorrhage: a comparison of plasma, recombinant activated factor VII, and prothrombin complex concentrate. World Neurosurg. 2014;81(1):110–5.
23. Lee SB, Manno EM, Layton KF, Wijdicks EF. Progression of warfarin-associated intracerebral hemorrhage after INR normalization with FFP. Neurology. 2006;67(7):1272–4.
24. Sarode R, Milling Jr TJ, Refaai MA, et al. Efficacy and safety of a 4-factor prothrombin complex concentrate in patients on vitamin K antagonists presenting with major bleeding: a randomized, plasma-controlled, phase IIIb study. Circulation. 2013;128(11):1234–43.
25. Hanley JP. Warfarin reversal. J Clin Pathol. 2004; 57(11):1132–9.
26. Tran HA, Chunilal SD, Harper PL, Tran H, Wood EM, Gallus AS. An update of consensus guidelines for warfarin reversal. Med J Aust. 2013;198(4):198–9.
27. Preston FE, Laidlaw ST, Sampson B, Kitchen S. Rapid reversal of oral anticoagulation with warfarin

by a prothrombin complex concentrate (Beriplex): efficacy and safety in 42 patients. Br J Haematol. 2002;116(3):619–24.
28. Boulis NM, Bobek MP, Schmaier A, Hoff JT. Use of factor IX complex in warfarin-related intracranial hemorrhage. Neurosurgery. 1999;45(5):1113–8. discussion 1118–9.
29. Ostermann H, Haertel S, Knaub S, Kalina U, Jung K, Pabinger I. Pharmacokinetics of Beriplex P/N prothrombin complex concentrate in healthy volunteers. Thromb Haemost. 2007;98(4):790–7.
30. Pandey S, Vyas GN. Adverse effects of plasma transfusion. Transfusion. 2012;52 Suppl 1:65–79.
31. Leissinger CA, Blatt PM, Hoots WK, Ewenstein B. Role of prothrombin complex concentrates in reversing warfarin anticoagulation: a review of the literature. Am J Hematol. 2008;83(2):137–43.
32. Bartal C, Freedman J, Bowman K, Cusimano M. Coagulopathic patients with traumatic intracranial bleeding: defining the role of recombinant factor VIIa. J Trauma. 2007;63(4):725–32.
33. Frontera JA, Gordon E, Zach V, et al. Reversal of coagulopathy using prothrombin complex concentrates is associated with improved outcome compared to fresh frozen plasma in warfarin-associated intracranial hemorrhage. Neurocrit Care. 2014;21(3): 397–406.
34. Baker RI, Coughlin PB, Gallus AS, Harper PL, Salem HH, Wood EM. Warfarin reversal: consensus guidelines, on behalf of the Australasian Society of Thrombosis and Haemostasis. Med J Aust. 2004;181(9):492–7.
35. Makris M, Van Veen JJ. Three or four factor prothrombin complex concentrate for emergency anticoagulation reversal? Blood Transfus. 2011;9(2):117–9.
36. Zhou W, Schwarting S, Illanes S, et al. Hemostatic therapy in experimental intracerebral hemorrhage associated with the direct thrombin inhibitor dabigatran. Stroke. 2011;42(12):3594–9.
37. van Ryn J, Schurer J, Kink-Eiband M, Clemens A. Reversal of dabigatran-induced bleeding by coagulation factor concentrates in a rat-tail bleeding model and lack of effect on assays of coagulation. Anesthesiology. 2014;120(6):1429–40.
38. Eerenberg ES, Kamphuisen PW, Sijpkens MK, Meijers JC, Buller HR, Levi M. Reversal of rivaroxaban and dabigatran by prothrombin complex concentrate: a randomized, placebo-controlled, crossover study in healthy subjects. Circulation. 2011;124(14):1573–9.
39. Marlu R, Hodaj E, Paris A, Albaladejo P, Cracowski JL, Pernod G. Effect of non-specific reversal agents on anticoagulant activity of dabigatran and rivaroxaban: a randomised crossover ex vivo study in healthy volunteers. Thromb Haemost. 2012;108(2):217–24.
40. Khoo TL, Weatherburn C, Kershaw G, Reddel CJ, Curnow J, Dunkley S. The use of FEIBA(R) in the correction of coagulation abnormalities induced by dabigatran. Int J Lab Hematol. 2013;35(2):222–4.
41. Schulman S, Ritchie B, Goy JK, Nahirniak S, Almutawa M, Ghanny S. Activated prothrombin complex concentrate for dabigatran-associated bleeding. Br J Haematol. 2014;164(2):308–10.
42. Zhou W, Zorn M, Nawroth P, et al. Hemostatic therapy in experimental intracerebral hemorrhage associated with rivaroxaban. Stroke. 2013;44(3):771–8.
43. Martin AC, Le Bonniec B, Fischer AM, et al. Evaluation of recombinant activated factor VII, prothrombin complex concentrate, and fibrinogen concentrate to reverse apixaban in a rabbit model of bleeding and thrombosis. Int J Cardiol. 2013;168(4):4228–33.
44. Lisman T, De Groot PG. Mechanism of action of recombinant factor VIIa. J Thromb Haemost. 2003; 1(6):1138–9.
45. Erhardtsen E, Nony P, Dechavanne M, Ffrench P, Boissel JP, Hedner U. The effect of recombinant factor VIIa (NovoSeven) in healthy volunteers receiving acenocoumarol to an International Normalized Ratio above 2.0. Blood Coagul Fibrinolysis. 1998;9(8):741–8.
46. Skolnick BE, Mathews DR, Khutoryansky NM, Pusateri AE, Carr ME. Exploratory study on the reversal of warfarin with rFVIIa in healthy subjects. Blood. 2010;116(5):693–701.
47. Roitberg B, Emechebe-Kennedy O, Amin-Hanjani S, Mucksavage J, Tesoro E. Human recombinant factor VII for emergency reversal of coagulopathy in neurosurgical patients: a retrospective comparative study. Neurosurgery. 2005;57(5):832–6. discussion 832-836.
48. Stein DM, Dutton RP, Hess JR, Scalea TM. Low-dose recombinant factor VIIa for trauma patients with coagulopathy. Injury. 2008;39(9):1054–61.
49. Levi M, Levy JH, Andersen HF, Truloff D. Safety of recombinant activated factor VII in randomized clinical trials. N Engl J Med. 2010;363(19):1791–800.
50. Nishijima DK, Dager WE, Schrot RJ, Holmes JF. The efficacy of factor VIIa in emergency department patients with warfarin use and traumatic intracranial hemorrhage. Acad Emerg Med. 2010;17(3):244–51.
51. Ilyas C, Beyer GM, Dutton RP, Scalea TM, Hess JR. Recombinant factor VIIa for warfarin-associated intracranial bleeding. J Clin Anesth. 2008;20(4):276–9.
52. Rosovsky RP, Crowther MA. What is the evidence for the off-label use of recombinant factor VIIa (rFVIIa) in the acute reversal of warfarin? ASH evidence-based review. Hematol Am Soc Hematol Educ Program. 2008;2008:36–8.
53. Herrmann R, Thom J, Wood A, Phillips M, Muhammad S, Baker R. Thrombin generation using the calibrated automated thrombinoscope to assess reversibility of dabigatran and rivaroxaban. Thromb Haemost. 2014;111(5):989–95.
54. Perzborn E, Gruber A, Tinel H, et al. Reversal of rivaroxaban anticoagulation by haemostatic agents in rats and primates. Thromb Haemost. 2013;110(1):162–72.
55. Perzborn E, Heitmeier S, Laux V, Buchmuller A. Reversal of rivaroxaban-induced anticoagulation with prothrombin complex concentrate, activated prothrombin complex concentrate and recombinant activated factor VII in vitro. Thromb Res. 2014;133(4):671–81.
56. Chan S, Kong M, Minning DM, Hedner U, Marder VJ. Assessment of recombinant factor VIIa as an antidote

for bleeding induced in the rabbit by low molecular weight heparin. J Thromb Haemost. 2003;1(4):760–5.
57. Firozvi K, Deveras RA, Kessler CM. Reversal of low-molecular-weight heparin-induced bleeding in patients with pre-existing hypercoagulable states with human recombinant activated factor VII concentrate. Am J Hematol. 2006;81(8):582–9.
58. Wang CH, Chen YC, Tsao CW, Yang SS. Dalteparin-associated catastrophic retroperitoneal hematoma successfully treated with recombinant factor VIIa. Int Urol Nephrol. 2012;44(4):1091–5.
59. Bijsterveld NR, Moons AH, Boekholdt SM, et al. Ability of recombinant factor VIIa to reverse the anticoagulant effect of the pentasaccharide fondaparinux in healthy volunteers. Circulation. 2002;106(20): 2550–4.
60. Crowther MA, Berry LR, Monagle PT, Chan AK. Mechanisms responsible for the failure of protamine to inactivate low-molecular-weight heparin. Br J Haematol. 2002;116(1):178–86.
61. Holst J, Lindblad B, Bergqvist D, et al. Protamine neutralization of intravenous and subcutaneous low-molecular-weight heparin (tinzaparin, Logiparin). An experimental investigation in healthy volunteers. Blood Coagul Fibrinolysis. 1994;5(5):795–803.
62. Wolzt M, Weltermann A, Nieszpaur-Los M, et al. Studies on the neutralizing effects of protamine on unfractionated and low molecular weight heparin (Fragmin) at the site of activation of the coagulation system in man. Thromb Haemost. 1995;73(3):439–43.
63. Teoh KH, Young E, Bradley CA, Hirsh J. Heparin binding proteins. Contribution to heparin rebound after cardiopulmonary bypass. Circulation. 1993;88(5 Pt 2):Ii420–5.
64. Hirsh J, Bauer KA, Donati MB, Gould M, Samama MM, Weitz JI. Parenteral anticoagulants: American College of Chest Physicians Evidence-Based Clinical Practice Guidelines (8th Edition). Chest. 2008;133(6 Suppl):141s–59.
65. Ni Ainle F, Preston RJ, Jenkins PV, et al. Protamine sulfate down-regulates thrombin generation by inhibiting factor V activation. Blood. 2009;114(8):1658–65.
66. Bolliger D, Szlam F, Azran M, et al. The anticoagulant effect of protamine sulfate is attenuated in the presence of platelets or elevated factor VIII concentrations. Anesth Analg. 2010;111(3):601–8.
67. Nybo M, Madsen JS. Serious anaphylactic reactions due to protamine sulfate: a systematic literature review. Basic Clin Pharmacol Toxicol. 2008;103(2): 192–6.
68. Li MH, Gao BL, Fang C, et al. Prevention and management of intraprocedural rupture of intracranial aneurysm with detachable coils during embolization. Neuroradiology. 2006;48(12):907–15.
69. Fearn SJ, Parry AD, Picton AJ, Mortimer AJ, McCollum CN. Should heparin be reversed after carotid endarterectomy? A randomised prospective trial. Eur J Vasc Endovasc Surg. 1997;13(4):394–7.
70. Stone DH, Nolan BW, Schanzer A, et al. Protamine reduces bleeding complications associated with carotid endarterectomy without increasing the risk of stroke. J Vasc Surg. 2010;51(3):559–564, 564.e551.
71. van Veen JJ, Maclean RM, Hampton KK, et al. Protamine reversal of low molecular weight heparin: clinically effective? Blood Coagul Fibrinolysis. 2011;22(7):565–70.
72. Makris M, Hough RE, Kitchen S. Poor reversal of low molecular weight heparin by protamine. Br J Haematol. 2000;108(4):884–5.
73. Olson S, Rossato R, Guazzo E. Acute subdural haematomas and enoxaparin. J Clin Neurosci. 2002;9(3): 256–9.
74. Bernat A, Herbert JM. Protamine sulphate inhibits pentasaccharide (SR80027)-induced bleeding without affecting its antithrombotic and anti-factor Xa activity in the rat. Haemostasis. 1996;26(4): 195–202.
75. Bernat A, Hoffmann P, Herbert JM. Antagonism of SR 90107A/Org 31540-induced bleeding by protamine sulfate in rats and mice. Thromb Haemost. 1996;76(5):715–9.
76. Lu G, DeGuzman FR, Hollenbach SJ, et al. A specific antidote for reversal of anticoagulation by direct and indirect inhibitors of coagulation factor Xa. Nat Med. 2013;19(4):446–51.
77. Crowther M, Vandana M, Michael K, et al. A phase 2 randomized, double-blind, placebo-controlled trial demonstrating reversal of rivaroxaban-induced anticoagulation in healthy subjects by andexanet alfa (PRT064445). An antidote for Fxa inhibitors. Blood. 2013;122(21):3636.
78. Crowther M, Levy GG, Lu GM, et al. ANNEXA (TM)-A: A phase 3 randomized, double-blind, placebo-controlled trial, demonstrating reversal of Apixaban-induced anticoagulation in older subjects by Andexanet alfa (PRT064445), a universal antidote for factor Xa (fXa) inhibitors. Circulation. 2014; 130(23):2116–7.
79. Ansell JE, Bakhru SH, Laulicht BE, et al. Use of PER977 to reverse the anticoagulant effect of edoxaban. N Engl J Med. 2014;371(22):2141–2.
80. Schiele F, van Ryn J, Canada K, et al. A specific antidote for dabigatran: functional and structural characterization. Blood. 2013;121(18):3554–62.
81. Glund S, Stangier J, Schmohl M, et al. A specific antidote for dabigatran: immediate, complete and sustained reversal of dabigatran induced anticoagulation in healthy male volunteers. Circulation. 2013;128(22):2.

Rescue Strategies to Facilitate Emergency Neurosurgery in Patients on Antiplatelet or Anticoagulant Agents

18

Erinç Aktüre, Andrew Goodwin, and Bruce Tranmer

The management of neurosurgical emergencies in patients on antiplatelet agents or anticoagulants poses a real challenge for the neurosurgeon. The central nervous system resides in a closed space with a fixed volume encased by cranial and spinal bones. The equilibrium and relationship of the contents in this space—blood, CSF, and brain tissue—is explained by Monro-Kellie doctrine. Due to this fine balance as well as the delicacy of the brain tissue and its susceptibility to sustained increased intracranial pressures, a neurosurgeon's tolerance of poor hemostasis and bleeding is less than other disciplines in medicine. This poses a challenge in both managing these patients and applying the literature and data originating from other disciplines in medicine.

Current and novel oral anticoagulant (NOAC) medications and antiplatelet medication result in reduced hemostatic control in patients requiring a neurosurgical procedure. As the population ages, an increasing number of patients meet the requirements for some type of anticoagulation. Common indications for anticoagulation include treatment of a thrombotic stroke, prevention of thrombus formation in the setting of cardiac arrhythmias and valvular disease, and management of hypercoagulable states. Also, the use of antiplatelet medications has significantly increased, partly due to the use of cardiac, vascular, and cerebral stents. As these newer NOAC and antiplatelet medications emerge, proven reversal strategies to improve hemostasis are lacking, and thus, the concern for significant morbidity and mortality has prompted many surgery centers to develop their own reversal strategies.

The need for rapid reversal of antiplatelet agents and anticoagulants is not an uncommon emergency for the neurosurgeon. With an intracranial hemorrhage that is expanding, the neurosurgeon only has precious hours to get the patient to the operating room to evacuate the clot. In a patient on an antiplatelet agent or an anticoagulant with an intracranial bleed and a deteriorating neurological condition, there will be a necessary delay while reversing the medication's effect because neurosurgery cannot be performed on a patient with impaired hemostasis, and this delay may result in significant morbidity and mortality—"Time is Brain." These emergency patients with hemorrhages not uncommonly have poorly controlled anticoagulation values. Furthermore, these patients have been on the drug for a longer period than necessary, and sometimes the patients even have forgotten why they were being treated with the medication.

E. Aktüre, M.D. • B. Tranmer, M.D. (✉)
Division of Neurosurgery, University of Vermont, Burlington, VT, USA
e-mail: Bruce.tranmer@uvm.edu; Bruce.tranmer@vtmednet.org

A. Goodwin, M.D.
Department of Pathology, University of Vermont, Burlington, VT, USA

C.M. Loftus (ed.), *Anticoagulation and Hemostasis in Neurosurgery*, DOI 10.1007/978-3-319-27327-3_18

The use of anticoagulants increases risk for spontaneous intracranial hemorrhage as well as the risk for hematoma expansion. The risk of intracranial bleeding in a patient on chronic anticoagulation is as high as 1–2 % per year [17]. In a patient over 65 with a traumatic intracerebral hemorrhage on warfarin, the mortality rate is extremely high. The need for reversal of anticoagulants may be necessary in various emergent neurosurgical scenarios including traumatic brain injury, spontaneous subdural hematomas, aneurysmal subarachnoid hemorrhage, as well as spine emergencies requiring emergent neurosurgery just to name a few. Aggressive reversal of anticoagulation will be necessary in those neurosurgical emergencies requiring surgical intervention to stabilize the patient before surgery and to reduce intraoperative morbidity and mortality as well as reducing postoperative bleeding complications. Emergency reversal of anticoagulants can also be vital for nonoperative neurosurgical emergencies as means of preventing secondary injury from an expanding hematoma and preventing the need for surgical intervention. Regardless of the indication, the need for reversal protocols for antiplatelet agents and anticoagulants in neurosurgical patients is required.

Different strategies for reversing various anticoagulant agents will be discussed in this chapter. The different types of medications to be discussed include (Table 18.1):

1. Antiplatelet agents such as Aspirin and Plavix.
2. Parenteral anticoagulants such as Heparin and Lovenox.
3. Oral anticoagulants such as Warfarin.
4. Novel oral anticoagulants (NOAC) such as Eliquis and Pradaxa.

The first step in managing a coagulopathy in a neurosurgical emergency is performing a proper patient history, which must include an accurate medication list. The patient's current medication(s), the timing of the last dose, and the indication for anticoagulation carry crucial importance in the management of these patients.

The second step for managing these patients is determining and quantifying the effects of the anticoagulant. It is important to note that many of the NOAC used today lack a reliable means for monitoring. Results of coagulation parameters can dictate the dose and means of reversal.

The final step is to determine the reversal strategy. This step depends on many different factors such as the extent of the bleeding and the need for emergent neurosurgery or bedside procedure versus nonoperative management. Also, patient wishes, goals of care, and predicted patient outcome should be considered before mobilizing resources for anticoagulant reversal. It is important to note that not all anticoagulants have a reliable specific reversal agent and some have multiple reversal strategies.

Current methods for determining the degree of the effect of the antiplatelet agent or anticoagulant are discussed in Table 18.2.

Table 18.1 List of antiplatelet agents and anticoagulants

Antiplatelet drugs
Acetyl salicylic acid (Aspirin)
Thienopyridines (clopidogrel/Plavix®, ticlopidine/Ticlid®, and prasugrel/Effient®)
Ticagrelor (Brilinta®)
Dipyridamole (Persantine®, Aggrenox®—aspirin combination)
Vorapaxar
Atopaxar
GPIIb/IIIa antagonists (parenteral) (Abciximab, Eptifibatide, and Tirofiban)
Anticoagulants
Parenteral anticoagulants
Unfractionated heparin
Low-molecular-weight heparins (Enoxaparin/Lovenox®, Dalteparin/Fragmin®, Tinzaparin/Innohep®)
Fondaparinux (Arixtra®)
Parenteral direct thrombin inhibitors (desirudin, argatroban, and bivalirudin)
Oral anticoagulants
Vitamin K antagonists
Warfarin
Phenprocoumon
Acenocoumarol
Novel oral anticoagulants (NOACs)
Dabigatran etexilate/Pradaxa™
Apixaban/Eliquis™
Rivaroxaban/Xarelto™
Edoxaban

Table 18.2 List of blood tests used to monitor effects of antiplatelet agents and anticoagulants

Assay	UFH	LMWH and fondaparinux	Vitamin K antagonists	Direct thrombin inhibitors	Xa inhibitors
aPTT	Prolonged	Variable; no effect to prolonged	No effect in short term, prolonged with stable therapy	Prolonged	Prolonged
PT/INR	No effect with therapeutic dose, potential prolongation with supratherapeutic dose	No effect with therapeutic dose, potential prolongation with supratherapeutic dose	Prolonged	Prolonged	Prolonged
Thrombin clot time	Prolonged	Prolonged	No effect	Prolonged	No effect
Fibrinogen	May be falsely low	No effect	No effect	May be falsely low	No effect
PTT 50:50 mixing study (nonincubated)	Incomplete correction (inhibitor)	Incomplete correction (inhibitor)	Correction into reference range	Incomplete correction (inhibitor)	Incomplete correction (inhibitor)
PT 50:50 mixing study (nonincubated)	Often not indicated	Often not indicated	Variable; long-term therapy may show incomplete correction	Incomplete correction (inhibitor)	Incomplete correction (inhibitor)
Chromogenic anti-Xa activity	Increased anti-Xa activity	Increased anti-Xa activity	Not clinically indicated	No anti-Xa activity	Increased anti-Xa activity

Table 18.3 List of agents used to reverse effects of antiplatelet agents and anticoagulants. (Adapted with permission from 2011 Clinical Practice Guide on Anticoagulant Dosing and Management of Anticoagulant Associated Bleeding Complications in Adults. Mary Cushman, MD, MSc Wendy Lim, MD, MSc, FRCPC, Neil A Zakai, MD, MSc. American Society of Hematology)

Agent	Dosing	Comments
Vitamin K	1–10 mg IV/PO, not SQ or IM	• Infusion reactions rare; administer over 20–30 min • Takes 6 (IV) to 24 (PO) hours to reverse warfarin • Large doses can cause warfarin resistance on resumption • Repeat every 12–24 h as needed
Protamine sulfate	12.5–50 mg IV	• Full reversal of unfractionated heparin • 60–80 % reversal of LMWH • No reversal of fondaparinux
Platelets	1 apheresis unit 5–8 whole blood units	• Raise platelet count by 30 × 109/L • Goal platelet count 50–100 × 109/L (indication dependent) • No clear recommendation on dosing on antiplatelet reversal
Fresh frozen plasma (FFP)	10–30 mL/kg (1 U = ~250 ml)	• Replaces all coagulation factors, but cannot fully correct • Hemostasis usually requires factor levels ~30 % • Factor IX may only reach 20 % • May need repeat dose after 6 h • Large volume, takes hours to thaw and infuse
Prothrombin complex concentrates (PCC)	25–50 U/kg IV	• Rapid INR correction in warfarin patients • Small volume infusion over 10–30 min • Risk of thrombosis especially with previous thrombosis history • Contraindicated with history of HIT • May need repeat dose after 6 h with regular PT checks • Needs concomitant vitamin K administration for prolonged INR reversal • Consider adding FFP if 3-factor PCC used
Recombinant factor VIIa (rFVIIa)	15–90 U/kg	• Rapid infusion of small volume • Rapid INR correction of warfarin, but may not correct bleeding because only restores FVIIa • Risk of thrombosis 5–10 % • May need repeat dose after 2 h
Desmopressin	0.3 mcg/kg diluted in saline and infused slowly over 15–30 min	• Can be used in conjunction with other reversal agents for reversal of many different drugs (i.e., heparin, hirudin, antiplatelet agents, dextran, streptokinase) • Increases in the plasma levels of factor VIII and vWF, shortens prolonged aPTT and bleeding time • Can cause hypotension

The various strategies for the emergent reversal of the neurosurgical patient on antiplatelet agents or anticoagulants will also be discussed in this chapter and are summarized in Table 18.3.

Reversal of Antiplatelet Agents

The two most commonly used antiplatelet agents in the United States are acetyl salicylic acid (aspirin) and clopidogrel (Plavix) [3]. However, there is a whole array of other antiplatelet agents available in the market.

Aspirin

The main effect of Aspirin on platelets is irreversible inhibition of cyclooxygenase 1 (COX-1) in platelets by acetylation, thus inhibiting synthesis of thromboxane A2, a potent platelet aggregator and vasoconstrictor [16]. Non-enteric coated aspirin exerts antiplatelet effects as soon as 15 min after administration. Enteric coating delays its absorption and delays the antiplatelet effect. Aspirin has an elimination half-life of 15–20 min in the plasma in normal dosing regimen. A single dose of 100 mg Aspirin inhibits all COX 1 function in all platelets in healthy individuals [16, 37].

Since the platelets cannot regenerate COX 1 function, all circulating platelets are affected for the duration of their life (approximately 10 days) [6]. However, the body replenishes platelets by a rate of approximately 10 % a day [6, 16]. Normal hemostasis may be maintained by as little as 20 % platelets with intact COX1 function, which is achievable in 2 days. Aspirin has no specific antidote and the main reversal strategy is platelet transfusion.

Various studies and meta-analyses report that 15–25 % people lack anticipated antiplatelet response when taking aspirin [36]. Aspirin effect on platelet function can be measured with point of care tests Platelet Function Analyzer (PFA)-100/200®, VerifyNow®, PlateletWorks®, Multiplate, as well as Thromboelastography Platelet Mapping®. *These testing strategies have been discussed in detail in the chapter by Li et al. elsewhere in this book.*

Thienopyridines (Clopidogrel, Ticlopidine, and Prasugrel)

The thienopyridines are all structurally related drugs and include clopidogrel, ticlopidine, and prasugrel. These drugs selectively inhibit ADP-induced platelet aggregation by irreversibly blocking P2Y12 [6]. All three drugs are prodrugs that must be metabolized by the hepatic cytochrome P450 (CYC) enzyme system to their active forms. Two percent of white, 4 % of black, and 14 % of Asian populations carry loss of function alleles in their CYP systems and therefore are resistant to clopidogrel [36]. The half-life of clopidogrel is 6 h and half-life of the active metabolite is about 30 min. These drugs also have no active specific antidotes. Due to long half-life, platelet transfusion is less reliable in reversing or reducing antiplatelet effects of these drugs. TEG platelet mapping or VerifyNow can be used to assess platelet function with ADP receptor blockers.

Other Antiplatelet Drugs

Ticagrelor, also a direct inhibitor of P2Y12, belongs to cyclopentyl-triazolopyrimidine class. Unlike thienopyridines, Ticagrelor is not an irreversible inhibitor of P2Y12 and it does not require activation to exert its antiplatelet effect [15, 37]. However, Ticagrelor also has an active metabolite. Half-life of this drug is 7 and 9 h for the active metabolite [15].

Dipyridamole is a weak antiplatelet agent which inhibits phosphodiesterase, and blocks the breakdown of cyclic adenosine monophosphate (cAMP). Increased levels of cAMP reduce intracellular calcium and inhibit platelet activation. Dipyridamole also blocks the uptake of adenosine by platelets and other cells. This produces a further increase in local cAMP levels because the platelet adenosine A2 receptor is coupled to adenylate cyclase. Dipyridamole is usually used in combination with aspirin and this drug is marketed with the trade name of Aggrenox.

GP IIb/IIIa Inhibitors

Abciximab, eptifibatide, and tirofiban are three GPIIb/IIIa antagonists currently available in the United States. All are parenteral drugs. The GPIIb/IIIa receptor is one of the most abundant receptors in platelets. Its function is to bind to adhesion molecules like fibrin and von Willebrand factor [6]. Abciximab is an irreversible inhibitor of this enzyme, whereas eptifibatide and tirofiban are reversible inhibitors. Half-life of abciximab is 10 min and a second phase half-life of about 30 min, eptifibatide is 2.5 h, and tirofiban is 2 h [37]. The main use for these drugs is for patients undergoing percutaneous coronary interventions, especially with ST-segment elevation acute myocardial infarction. Tirofiban and eptifibatide are also used in high-risk patients with unstable angina. These drugs, especially abciximab, can also be used by neurointerventionalists during nonplanned/emergency intracranial stent placement (i.e., stent-assisted aneurysm coiling) where the patient has not been loaded by oral antiplatelet agents or after intraprocedural thrombosis complications. VerifyNow IIb/IIIa Test® can detect antiplatelet effects of abciximab, eptifibatide, and tirofiban.

Measuring Platelet Function

Historically, the bleeding time was used to evaluate platelet function, yet literature clearly indicates the bleeding time test does not accurately predict the risk of intraoperative bleeding [20, 23, 29]. In addition, the bleeding time test has been identified in the Choosing Wisely Campaign as an assay that lacks clinical benefit. Also the bleeding time test does not meet the College of American Pathologist laboratory accreditation standards due to lack of available proficiency testing. For these reasons, the bleeding time test should not be used to predict the impact of antiplatelet medications.

The TEG® and ROTEM® analyzers have the capacity to investigate the effect of antiplatelet medications [8]. For example, TEG® platelet mapping assays utilize different platelet activators including arachidonic acid (AA) and adenosine diphosphate (ADP) [1]. The activated platelets will contribute to clot formation, and using a combination of information, the overall clot strength is determined and reported as maximum amplitude (MA) for each individual platelet agonist. In a patient who appropriately responds to antiplatelet medication, the inhibited platelet function can be identified on the TEG® platelet mapping assay. These results (percent inhibition and maximum clot strength (MA)) demonstrate the antiplatelet effect from medications used to block cyclooxygenase, ADP receptors, or glycoprotein IIb/IIIa receptors. It is essential to review both the percent inhibition and MA when understanding platelet function. The standard kaolin-activated thrombelastography assay is not sensitive to the effect of antiplatelet medications, and thus, the TEG® platelet mapping assay is required. Studies comparing the TEG® platelet mapping assay to the gold standard light transmission aggregometry report good correlation for detection of reduced platelet function [19].

In patients using the ADP receptor blocker clopidogrel, the TEG® platelet mapping assay is useful when evaluating the bleeding risk in patients preparing for coronary bypass surgery (CABG). The 2012 TARGET-CABG study evaluated timing for surgery based on preoperative platelet function testing with TEG® platelet mapping [25]. The results of this study showed no increased bleeding for the clopidogrel-treated patients compared to the clopidogrel-naïve patient when specific timing strategy was used. Furthermore, in comparison to the current guidelines in clopidogrel-treated patients, a 50 % shorter waiting time was achieved when the TEG® platelet mapping assay was used to evaluate platelet function [25]. It is unclear if the data from this study applies to other patient populations such as the neurosurgical patient.

Additional assays such as VerifyNow®, PFA-100/200®, multiplate impedance aggregometry, flow cytometry, and light transmission/impedance platelet aggregometry are available to evaluate the antiplatelet effects in patients [19]. While the VerifyNow® and PFA-100/200® tests are often readily available, the remaining tests such as flow cytometry and platelet aggregation require specialized technical training and often are not available in all laboratories. The sensitivity of all platelet function assays varies greatly and is impacted by many variables including the quality of the phlebotomy, delays in testing, other non-specific, antiplatelet medications (e.g., serotonin reuptake inhibitors, histamine blockers, lipid lowering medications), food stuff (e.g., high doses of vitamin E, fish oil), and technical ability/experience of the laboratory [5]. Many of these assays, including the TEG® platelet mapping, require an evaluation of the graphical results of the platelet function to ensure that known artifactual abnormalities are excluded and not used when reported numerical values. For example, with TEG® platelet mapping, the phenomenon "growing MA" results in certain clinical situations, including thrombin breakthrough, pregnancy, and antithrombin III deficiency. If the "growing MA" tracing is not recognized, incorrect management decisions will result based on the inaccurate percent inhibition calculation.

A complete blood count, particularly the hematocrit and platelet count, should be considered when evaluating a patient's overall hemostasis. Thrombocytopenia will increase the risk for procedural-related bleeding complications, and a platelet count of 100 K/cmm is desired for neurosurgical procedures. Improved hemostasis is reported in patients who have a hematocrit greater than 30 % due to increased viscosity and platelet adhesion [32]. Transfusion support may be required to achieve the appropriate platelet count and/or hematocrit. Additionally, some of the platelet function analyzers are impacted by both thrombocytopenia and anemia. Prolonged closure times with the PFA-100/200® can occur when the platelet count is less than 135 K/cmm or the hematocrit is less than 35 %.

Reversal Strategies for Antiplatelet Drugs: Table 18.4

Reversal of Thienopyridines (clopidogrel, ticlopidine, and prasugrel) may require multiple platelet transfusions for several days to achieve reliable hemostasis [22]. One of the proposed regimens is 10–20 U followed by 10 U every 12 h for 48 h [2, 37]. Continuous slow transfusion of platelets can be considered for patients undergoing emergency neurosurgery on clopidogrel [2, 4, 14]. Desmopressin is used to increase platelet activity in patients treated with antiplatelet drugs by releasing a greater number of von Willebrand factor and factor VIII [26]. Desmopressin can be considered in the acute phase with life-threatening bleeding to supplement platelet transfusion [26]. The use of recombinant activated factor VII (rFVIIa, NovoSeven®) has been postulated in the reversal of aspirin and aspirin plus clopidogrel dual antiplatelet therapy with promising initial results [34].

Before reversing the antiplatelet drugs, one should investigate the medical reason behind the antiplatelet therapy. History taking for recently placed stents (coronary, carotid, intracranial etc.) is vital. Freshly placed stents will pose risk for thrombosis if antiplatelet agents are reversed. A multidisciplinary approach with risk-benefit analysis in reversing antiplatelet therapy in these patients is recommended.

In summary the main strategy for emergency reversal of antiplatelet drugs still remains platelet transfusion. While platelet transfusion can successfully reverse the effects of aspirin, for the drugs with longer half-life and active metabolites like clopidogrel, platelet transfusion is not as reliable. Multiple platelet transfusions for a prolonged period of time may be required to achieve adequate clotting. Desmopressin can be considered in aiding hemostasis in patients on antiplatelet agents. Activated factor VII can be used in life-threatening emergencies especially in dual antiplatelet therapy. However, risk of thrombotic complications should be taken in account.

Reversal Strategies for Parenteral and Oral Anticoagulants: Table 18.4

There is a wide array of anticoagulants a neurosurgeon encounters in the emergency room. Main parenteral anticoagulants include heparin, low-molecular-weight heparin (LMWH) enoxaparin, and fondaparinux. The oral anticoagulants include

Table 18.4 Rescue strategies for commonly used antiplatelet agents and anticoagulants

Antiplatelet agents	• Platelet transfusion is mainstay • Prolonged platelet transfusion may be needed for agents with long half-life or with active metabolites like clopidogrel (Plavix) • Desmopressin can be considered for acute life-threatening bleeding • Activated factor VII can be used in life-threatening emergencies especially in dual antiplatelet therapy
Vitamin K antagonists (Warfarin)	• Vitamin K and fresh frozen plasma are the traditional reversal method • Four factor prothrombin complex concentrate (PCC) (Kcentra) is an FDA-approved alternative. • Vitamin K needs to be administered with "**K**"centra • Activated factor VII is another alternative, it is associated with a higher thrombotic complication rate, and duration of action is shorter.
Heparins	• Protamine is the mainstay reversal agent for both heparin and low-molecular-weight heparins • Activated factor VII can be used in life-threatening emergencies
Novel oral anticoagulants (NOACs)	• No specific antidote yet • Multiple rescue strategies with limited success • For Apixaban and Rivaroxaban four factor PCC can be given • For Dabigatran activated factor VII can be considered. • Hemodialysis is an option for Dabigatran

the vitamin K antagonists—phenprocoumon, warfarin, and acenocoumarol, of which warfarin is the agent most often used. There are also newer agents (NOAC) that target thrombin (dabigatran etexilate) or factor Xa (rivaroxaban and apixaban). Emergence of these NOAC irreversible agents, without reliable means of monitoring their anticoagulant effects, poses a new challenge for neurosurgeons.

Regardless of the agent, the management remains the same. The first goal is to identify the agent and the reason for anticoagulation, second, to try to measure the effect of the anticoagulant if feasible, and third to reverse the agent by either an antidote or coagulation factors to achieve safe hemostasis.

Parenteral Anticoagulants

Unfractionated heparin and low-molecular-weight heparins (LMWHs) (i.e., Enoxaparin, Dalteparin, Tinzaparin) are polysaccharides that bind to antithrombin (AT) and potentiate its inhibitory effect on thrombin (FIIa) and activated factor X (FXa). While unfractionated heparin predominantly works on anti-IIa activity, LMWHs predominantly potentiate anti-Xa activity [6]. This property plays an important role in monitoring the anticoagulant effects of these drugs. Monitoring the effects of unfractionated heparin can be achieved by using the activated partial thromboplastin time (aPTT) or anti-factor Xa level, with the aPTT test being the more commonly used. Activated clotting time (ACT) can be used in interventional OR suites for monitoring effects of heparin and it can be utilized in monitoring reversal of heparin in intraprocedural emergencies (i.e., aneurysmal rupture while coiling). Its use in emergency room is limited due to requiring a baseline comparison to interpret the results. Up to 25 % of heparin-treated patients with venous thromboembolism are considered heparin resistant. It may be useful to measure anti-factor Xa levels in these patients because many will have a therapeutic anti-factor Xa level despite a subtherapeutic aPTT. This occurs because elevated plasma levels of fibrinogen and factor VIII, both of which are acute-phase proteins, shorten the aPTT but have no effect on anti-factor Xa levels. In these patients requiring emergent neurosurgical care, obtaining anti-factor Xa levels as well as aPTT to monitor heparin effect and response to treatment is advisable.

Since most LMWH preparations have little effect on the aPTT, anti-factor Xa levels must be measured in monitoring the anticoagulation effect of these drugs.

The main reversal agent for parenteral anticoagulants is Protamine (Table 18.5) [18]. Protamine sulfate is a basic protein that displaces AT and neutralizes heparin by forming a complex with it. It is also a partial antagonist for LMWH, and it can reverse 60–80 % effect of LMWHs [18]. However, it should be noted that in the absence of heparin, protamine sulfate shows an anticoagulant effect. Therefore, it is important to know the timing and amount of last dose of the heparin or LMWH before a reversal attempt is made. It should be noted that the maximum dose for protamine is 50 mg. Half-life of heparin is 1–2 h. 1 mg protamine per 90–100 U heparin given in previous 2–3 h is a reasonable heparin reversal strategy. Different LMWH preparations have different

Table 18.5 Use of protamine for the reversal of parenteral anticoagulants. (Adapted with permission from 2011 Clinical Practice Guide on Anticoagulant Dosing and Management of Anticoagulant Associated Bleeding Complications in Adults. Mary Cushman, MD, MSc Wendy Lim, MD, MSc, FRCPC, Neil A Zakai, MD, MSc. American Society of Hematology)

Agent	Half-life (h)	Protamine sulfate dosing for reversal
All		Maximum dose is 50 mg
Heparin	1–2	1 mg/90–100 U heparin given in previous 2–3 h
Enoxaparin	4.5	1 mg/1 mg Enoxaparin in previous 8 h
Dalteparin	2.2	1 mg/100 U Dalteparin in previous 8 h
Tinzaparin	3.9	1 mg/100 U Tinzaparin in previous 8 h
Fondaparinux	17–21	No specific reversal

Half-life is longer with subcutaneous administration for all agents so may require monitoring with PTT (heparin) or anti-Xa level (LMWH) every 3 h with repeat protamine (0.5 mg per indicated amount of LMWH or heparin) if bleeding continues half-lives (Enoxaparin 4.5 h, Dalteparin 2.2 h, Tinzaparin 3.9 h) and dosing standards. For Enoxaparin, 1 mg protamine can be given per 1 mg Enoxaparin in previous 8 h. For Dalteparin and Tinzaparin, 1 mg protamine per 100 U of these drugs in previous 8 h can be given. It should be noted that half-life of these agents is longer with subcutaneous administration so aPTT (heparin) or anti-Xa level (LMWH) should be monitored every 3 h with repeat protamine (0.5 mg per indicated amount of LMWH or heparin) if bleeding continues. Smaller doses of protamine sulfate can be administered if the time since LMWH administration is longer than 8 h. In life-threatening bleeding with unfractionated heparin, LMWHs, and fondaparinux, rVIIa can be considered. It should be noted that rVIIa in case of fondaparinux lasts for 2–6 h and half-life of this drug is 17–21 h. Multiple dosing strategies may be required in life-threatening bleeding. There is no specific reversal agent available for fondaparinux.

In summary, the reversal of these parental agents includes the use of protamine and possibly Factor VII in life-threatening emergencies [18]. While protamine can reverse heparin completely, it partially reverses LMWHs (60–80 %). Action of heparin can be monitored with aPTT for patients on LMWHs, anti-Xa level should be measured. Consider obtaining anti-Xa levels in trauma patients on heparin since increased fibrinogen and factor VIII factor can lower an increased aPTT.

Parenteral Direct Thrombin Inhibitors

Direct thrombin inhibitors bind directly to thrombin and block its function unlike heparin and LMWH, which are indirect inhibitors of thrombin which exert their effects through antithrombin. Currently approved parenteral direct thrombin inhibitors are desirudin, argatroban, and bivalirudin. All these agents have short half-lives (argatroban 50 min, bivalirudin 25 min) except for desirudin which has a half-life of 2 h. Lepirudin and argatroban are licensed for the treatment of heparin-induced thrombocytopenia (HIT). Bivalirudin is approved as an alternative to heparin in patients undergoing percutaneous coronary interventions. Desirudin is licensed for thromboprophylaxis after elective hip replacement surgery and dosed twice daily subcutaneously. Argatroban and bivalirudin are infused parenterally. All these agents affect aPTT and their action can be monitored using aPTT. All these agents affect PT and INR with Argatroban having the greatest effect followed by bivalirudin. There is no specific antidote for these agents. rVIIa can be used to reverse the effects of these drugs in life-threatening bleeding. Blood products such as fresh frozen plasma can be tried. Antifibrinolytic drugs such as Amicar can be used. Also desmopressin can be considered. Modified ultrafiltration and hemodialysis can eliminate 45–69 % of bivalirudin, depending on the filter type. The elimination of argatroban is less effective or unclear. Hemodialysis decreases the plasma concentration of bivalirudin by only 25 % [37]. Argatroban is not eliminated by dialysis [37].

In summary rapid reversal of these agents is problematic. The use of FFP or PCC may be tried as well as antifibrinolytics but will not be very effective. Factor VII or antifibrinolytics will also be likely unsuccessful. Hemodialysis may be the way to eliminate some of these drugs from the patient; however, special filters may be required.

Oral Anticoagulants

Vitamin K Antagonists

Vitamin K antagonists are oral anticoagulation drugs that generate the same effect as a vitamin K deficiency. They include phenprocoumon, warfarin, and acenocoumarol, with warfarin being the most widely used one. Warfarin works by inhibiting the vitamin K-dependent synthesis of biologically active forms of the calcium-dependent clotting factors II, VII, IX, and X, as well as the regulatory factors protein C, protein S, and protein Z by γ-carboxylation of select glutamic acid residues in the N-terminus of these peptides. The coagulant activity of these proteins in plasma declines depending on their half-lives. Half-lives of factors VII, IX, and X and prothrombin are 6, 24, and 40 and 60 h, respectively [6]. Although 1–2 days of warfarin prolongs the PT assay (because of the rapid decrease in factor VII concentration), therapeutic anticoagulation requires at least 4–5 days. The anticoagulation effect of Warfarin is typically followed by PT which measures three vitamin K-dependent coagulation factors VII, X, and prothrombin. The PT is more sensitive to factor VII than other factors. International normalized ratio (INR) is a result of a method that standardizes PT assays by using reference thromboplastin preparation accepted as a standard by the World Health Organization (WHO). Each PT test system is calibrated using the WHO standard.

Warfarin use increases the risk of primary ICH by 2–5 % [2]. Of all spontaneous ICH cases 15–20 % are anticoagulated by warfarin. Risk of ICH for patient taking Warfarin is approximately 1 % per year. The incidence of ICH and the size of ICH on presentation increase as the INR increases. Anticoagulated patients also have increased risk of hematoma expansion. Also it is not uncommon to encounter trauma patients on warfarin presenting with acute subdural hematomas, parenchymal contusions, as well as subarachnoid hemorrhage patients on warfarin.

Traditionally, reversal of warfarin in life-threatening bleeding was primarily achieved with stopping the drug, giving vitamin K and replenishing the vitamin K-dependent coagulation factors by means of fresh frozen plasma (FFP). However, this approach has several limitations. The patient should be ABO matched before beginning infusion. FFP is stored at 4 °C and needs thawing before administration. Infusing the desired volume takes significant time. FFP is traditionally given 2 U at a time and a repeat INR is obtained in between. A retrospective study by Lee et al. found that a median time of 6.5 h was needed to infuse 5 U of FFP to patients who suffered from warfarin-induced ICH. Considering that most modern ICH studies use the 6 h mark for repeat CT scan to assess stability of the hematoma, and the inverse relationship between hematoma size and patient outcome, the time required for the reversal of warfarin with FFP is suboptimal in managing neurosurgical emergencies. Other limitations of FFP are, as with all blood products, FFP carries a risk of pathogen transmission and the varying levels of coagulation factors seen in FFP may result in a partial or insufficient reversal of INR. Considering each unit of FFP carries 250 ml volume, the total volume required to reverse this particular patient population with significant cardiopulmonary morbidities carries a significant risk. Transfusion-related acute lung injury is another concern for FFP. While the incidence of TRALI is rare (1 per 5000 transfusions), it requires mechanical ventilation in 70 % of cases and is fatal in 6–9 % of cases. Finally, FFP also cannot lower INR below 1.6.

Vitamin K also is used widely for the reversal of warfarin. Administration of vitamin K turns on the endogenous activation of coagulation factors. Vitamin K can be administered subcutaneously, orally, or intravenously. Subcutaneous vitamin K is not effective correcting INRs. Although both oral and intravenously administered vitamin K are effective at correcting supratherapeutic INRs at 24 h, intravenous vitamin K can correct the INR as few as 4–6 h. It should be noted that IV vitamin K has been associated with severe anaphylactic reactions (3 in 10,000 administrations) [31].

In recent years prothrombin complex concentrates (PCC) and recombinant factor VIIa have emerged as alternatives for warfarin reversal [35]. Currently most institutions in the United States have replaced FFP with either or both of these preparations in their emergency warfarin reversal protocols. There are some available 3-factor PCCs approved for bleeding in hemophilia patients which have been used off label in warfarin reversal. These preparations do not have factor VII or have nontherapeutic levels (i.e., profilnine SD). These products were used in combination with FFP or recombinant factor VIIa. Recombinant factor VIIa also has been used in reversal of warfarin. It should be noted that INR reversal effect of factor VIIa is 2–6 h and activated coagulation factors have been associated with increased risk for thromboembolism. In 2013 the FDA approved a 4-factor PCC, Kcentra, for reversal of warfarin. This drug has been in use in Europe for over a decade. Kcentra is purified, heat-treated, nanofiltered, lyophilized, nonactivated 4F-PCC made from pooled human plasma. It contains factors II, VII, IX, and X, and the antithrombotic Proteins C and S. It is 25 times more concentrated than plasma in factors II, VII, IX, and X levels. Kcentra does not require thawing or ABO typing and it is stored at room temperature, which facilitates faster administration times. It is more reliable compared to FFP in the content of vitamin K-dependent factors. Kcentra can reduce INR faster and more reliably compared to FFP; 55–62 % of patients achieve INR of less than 1.3 in 30 min compared to 10 % achieved by FFP [12, 30]. Kcentra is dosed depending on the INR and body weight. Kcentra contains 8–40 U of heparin per 500 U vial.

It should be noted that effects of PCCs are limited by the duration of coagulation factors they contain. Therefore it is recommended that PCCs should be administered with vitamin K and repeat INR should be obtained (i.e., every 6 h). Repeat dosing may be necessary if INR starts to rise. Currently, we recommend the use of 4-factor PCC (Kcentra) in reversal of Warfarin in neurosurgical emergencies along with IV vitamin K. Vitamin K can be redosed in 12 h after the initial dose and INR should be monitored regularly possibly beyond the 24 h mark. PCCs can be redosed if INR starts to climb. The patients and the families should be informed about the possible thromboembolism after warfarin reversal, especially in those patients with previous history of thromboembolism [12, 30].

The safe INR to perform neurosurgery has been long debated and there is no consensus on the matter among neurosurgeons or institutions. Some studies suggest that surgical bleeding complications are not present at INR < 1.7 [9]. There is not clear evidence of increased surgical risk in INR < 1.7. The decision making is on a case by case basis and depends on the nature of the surgical intervention and the experience and comfort level of the surgeon.

In summary, reversal of warfarin anticoagulation can involve the use of vitamin K, FFP, and PCC. Currently four-factor PCC (Kcentra) is an FDA-approved alternative to FFP.

Reversal Strategies for Novel Oral Anticoagulants (NOACs): Table 18.6

These drugs exert their effects on either thrombin or factor Xa. They have rapid onset of action, few drug interactions, and favorable pharmacokinetics and pharmacodynamics. They do not require monitoring of their anticoagulant action and they are reliable anticoagulants at given doses. These properties make these drugs attractive alternatives to warfarin in the eyes of prescribing physicians and patients. However, to neurosurgeons, the names dabigatran etexilate (Pradaxa™), Apixaban (Eliquis™), and Rivaroxaban (Xarelto™) have been associated with high anxiety and desperation in neurosurgical emergencies mainly because of lack of specific antidotes or real means of reversing or monitoring these drugs.

Dabigatran: Pradaxa

Dabigatran etexilate is a direct inhibitor of thrombin and is a prodrug; once absorbed, the drug is rapidly biotransformed by esterases to dabigatran, the levels of which peak 1–2 h after oral administration. Dabigatran has a half-life of 14–17 h. About 80 % of the drug is excreted unchanged by the kidneys. Dabigatran targets the active site of thrombin and

Table 18.6 Pro-hemostatic agents and their potential role in NOAC-associated bleeding. (Adapted with permission from http://www.thrombosiscanada.ca/)

Agent	Dabigatran	Rivaroxaban or Apixaban
4-Factor Prothrombin Complex Concentrate (PCC; Beriplex, Octaplex)	Possibly beneficial	Probably beneficial
3-Factor Prothrombin Complex Concentrate	No available evidence	No available evidence
Activated 4-Factor Prothrombin Complex Concentrate (FEIBA)	Probably beneficial	Probably beneficial
Recombinant activated Factor VII (NovoSeven, Niastase)	Possibly beneficial	Possibly beneficial
Fresh frozen plasma	Probably ineffective	Probably ineffective
Cryoprecipitate	Probably ineffective	Probably ineffective

blocks its procoagulant activities. Dabigatran inhibits both free and fibrin-bound thrombin. It is approved in patients with nonvalvular atrial fibrillation use to reduce the risk of stroke and systemic embolism; for the treatment of deep vein thrombosis and pulmonary embolism in patients who have been treated with a parenteral anticoagulant for 5–10 days and to reduce the risk of recurrence of deep vein thrombosis and pulmonary embolism in patients who have been previously treated.

Rivaroxaban: Xarelto

Rivaroxaban is an oral factor Xa inhibitor, which binds to the active site of factor Xa even when the enzyme is incorporated in the prothrombinase complex. Plasma levels peak 2–3 h after drug administration and the half-life is 7–11 h, and one-third of the drug is cleared unchanged by the kidneys. The remainder is metabolized in the liver; half is cleared by the kidneys as inactive metabolites, and the rest is excreted in the feces. It is indicated in reduction of risk of stroke and systemic embolism in nonvalvular atrial fibrillation and for prophylaxis of deep vein thrombosis.

Apixaban: Eliquis

Apixaban also targets the active site of free factor Xa or factor Xa incorporated in the prothrombinase complex. Plasma levels peak 3–4 h after drug administration. The half-life of apixaban is 8–14 h. Apixaban is metabolized in the liver via CYP3A4/5-dependent and independent pathways. About 25 % of the drug is cleared unchanged by the kidneys, and the remainder is excreted in the feces. Apixaban is approved for treatment and secondary prophylaxis of DVT and PE.

Betrixaban is another direct factor Xa inhibitor, currently under development.

Monitoring the Effects of NOACs

Because of the NOACs' predictable pharmacokinetics and pharmacodynamics, regular laboratory monitoring is not required. These medications received FDA approval for patient care, yet readily available, accurate, and precise laboratory tests are often not available. While clinical coagulation laboratories understand the qualitative (i.e., normal vs. abnormal) impact of these medications on routine coagulation screening tests, reliable quantitative values (i.e., drug concentrations) are often only available at highly specialized laboratories offering laboratory-developed assays using calibrators deemed as "research use only."

Should a patient sustain significant trauma while on a NOAC medication, reversal of the medication is critical to achieve adequate hemostasis. In an editorial to the *New England Journal of Medicine*, three trauma surgeons comment on the increasing number of hemorrhagic complications in severely injured patients [7]. They comment that the lack of readily available laboratory methods to determine the degree of anticoagulation in combination with the lack of evidence-based reversal methods proves as a major challenge in properly caring for these patients. They urge the FDA to require more pragmatic trials studying the hemorrhagic complications and mortality resulting from traumas as part of the routine surveillance of the newly approved NOAC.

During the laboratory investigation of a patient on NOAC mediations, health care providers must clearly understand how medications can impact plasma-based coagulation assays. A thorough review describing many coagulation tests and their performance with a variety of anticoagulation medications is available. Table 18.2, a modified version from this thorough review, provides general information regarding expected effects from heparins, vitamin K antagonists, and NOAC medications. However, plasma-based screening assay systems such as prothrombin time, partial thromboplastin time, and thrombin time have varied sensitivity to the NOAC medications; health providers should inquire with their laboratory(s) regarding their specific analyzer/reagent combination response with each NOAC medication.

Whole blood assay systems such as thromboelastography (TEG®) and rotational thromboelastometry (ROTEM®) are reportedly sensitive to the effects of NOAC medications. However, the predictive value for potential procedural related bleeding in the neurosurgical patient population is unclear with these assays. Many protocols utilize the TEG® and ROTEM® assays when assessing and managing bleeding patients secondary to trauma or acute hemorrhage [33]. These whole blood assays are rapid and have the added advantage of global assessment of coagulation including (1) Enzymatic coagulation cascade (secondary hemostasis); (2) Overall clot strength due to stable fibrin formation and platelet function; and (3) Fibrinolytic activity. In vitro, plasma-based coagulation assays measure the time to form a fibrin clot without influence from other cellular components such as platelets. The whole blood assays measure the viscoelastic properties of a blood clot, which is impacted by other cellular components; theoretically, these assays are more representative of the in vivo process of coagulation [28].

Standard coagulation tests are not reliable in monitoring the NOAC drugs [11]. Rivaroxaban can increase PT/INR, Apixaban has minimal effect on PT/INR, Dabigatran has variable effects on PT/INR, and INR is usually <2. Dabigatran increases PTT; Rivaroxaban and Apixaban have dose-dependent effects on PTT. Specific rivaroxaban and apixaban calibrators are required to measure these drugs' effect on anti-factor Xa level which may not be available in many institutions and in emergency situations. Dabigatran has no effect on anti-factor Xa level. History taking becomes an important part of management of patients on NOACs due to limitation of laboratory tests monitoring their actions.

Currently there are no approved antidotes for the reversal of these agents. Data is limited on the use of prothrombin complex concentrate (PCC), activated prothrombin complex concentrate (aPCC), or recombinant factor VIIa [10, 21, 24, 27]. However, we would recommend using four-factor PCC in life-threatening situations with Apixaban and Rivaroxaban. Recombinant factor VIIa administration and hemodialysis can be considered for dabigatran. Tranexamic acid can also be considered in active bleeding with these agents. Andexanet alfa is a new antidote for anti-Xa anticoagulants (Rivaroxaban and Apixaban) currently under development [13]. *The chapter by Jeske in this book elaborates on TSOAC antidotes in development.*

In summary, there is no specific antidote for reversal of these agents. There are some specific reversal agents currently under development. We recommend using four-factor PCC in case of Apixaban and Rivaroxaban. Hemodialysis is an option for dabigatran.

References

1. Agarwal S, Coakley M, Coakely M, et al. Quantifying the effect of antiplatelet therapy: a comparison of the platelet function analyzer (PFA-100) and modified thromboelastography (mTEG) with light transmission platelet aggregometry. Anesthesiology. 2006;105:676–83.
2. Beshay JE, Morgan H, Madden C, et al. Emergency reversal of anticoagulation and antiplatelet therapies in neurosurgical patients. J Neurosurg. 2010;112:307–18. doi:10.3171/2009.7.JNS0982.
3. Campbell PG, Sen A, Yadla S, et al. Emergency reversal of antiplatelet agents in patients presenting with an intracranial hemorrhage: a clinical review. World Neurosurg. 2010;74:279–85. doi:10.1016/j.wneu.2010.05.030.
4. Campbell PG, Yadla S, Sen AN, et al. Emergency reversal of clopidogrel in the setting of spontaneous intracerebral hemorrhage. World Neurosurg. 2011;76:100–4. doi:10.1016/j.wneu.2011.02.010. discussion 59–60.
5. Chandler WL, Ferrell C, Trimble S, Moody S. Development of a rapid emergency hemorrhage panel. Transfusion (Paris). 2010;50:2547–52. doi:10.1111/j.1537-2995.2010.02753.x.
6. Colman RW, editor. Hemostasis and thrombosis: basic principles and clinical practice, 5th ed. Philadelphia, PA: Lippincott Williams & Wilkins; 2006.
7. Cotton BA, McCarthy JJ, Holcomb JB. Acutely injured patients on dabigatran. N Engl J Med. 2011;365:2039–40. doi:10.1056/NEJMc1111095.
8. Craft RM, Chavez JJ, Bresee SJ, et al. A novel modification of the Thrombelastograph assay, isolating platelet function, correlates with optical platelet aggregation. J Lab Clin Med. 2004;143:301–9. doi:10.1016/j.lab.2004.01.011.
9. Davis JW, Davis IC, Bennink LD, et al. Placement of intracranial pressure monitors: are "normal" coagulation parameters necessary? J Trauma. 2004;57:1173–7.
10. Eerenberg ES, Kamphuisen PW, Sijpkens MK, et al. Reversal of rivaroxaban and dabigatran by prothrombin complex concentrate: a randomized, placebo-controlled, crossover study in healthy subjects. Circulation. 2011;124:1573–9. doi:10.1161/CIRCULATIONAHA.111.029017.
11. Funk DMA. Coagulation assays and anticoagulant monitoring. Hematol Am Soc Hematol Educ Program.2012;2012:460–5.doi:10.1182/asheducation-2012.1.460.

12. Goldstein JN, Refaai MA, Milling TJ, et al. Four-factor prothrombin complex concentrate versus plasma for rapid vitamin K antagonist reversal in patients needing urgent surgical or invasive interventions: a phase 3b, open-label, non-inferiority, randomised trial. Lancet. 2015. doi:10.1016/S0140-6736(14)61685-8.
13. Gomez-Outes A, Suarez-Gea ML, Lecumberri R, et al. Specific antidotes in development for reversal of novel anticoagulants: a review. Recent Pat Cardiovasc Drug Discov. 2014;9:2–10.
14. Gordon JL, Fabian TC, Lee MD, Dugdale M. Anticoagulant and antiplatelet medications encountered in emergency surgery patients: a review of reversal strategies. J Trauma Acute Care Surg. 2013;75:475–86. doi:10.1097/TA.0b013e3182a07391.
15. Hobl E-L, Derhaschnig U, Firbas C, et al. Reversal strategy in antagonizing the P2Y12-inhibitor ticagrelor. Eur J Clin Invest. 2013;43:1258–61. doi:10.1111/eci.12168.
16. Hoffman R, editor. Hematology: basic principles and practice. 6th ed. Philadelphia, PA: Saunders; 2013.
17. James RF, Palys V, Lomboy JR, et al. The role of anticoagulants, antiplatelet agents, and their reversal strategies in the management of intracerebral hemorrhage. Neurosurg Focus. 2013;34:E6. doi:10.3171/2013.2.FOCUS1328.
18. Kaatz S, Kouides PA, Garcia DA, et al. Guidance on the emergent reversal of oral thrombin and factor Xa inhibitors. Am J Hematol. 2012;87 Suppl 1:S141–5. doi:10.1002/ajh.23202.
19. Karon BS, Tolan NV, Koch CD, et al. Precision and reliability of 5 platelet function tests in healthy volunteers and donors on daily antiplatelet agent therapy. Clin Chem. 2014;60:1524–31. doi:10.1373/clinchem.2014.226332.
20. Lehman CM, Blaylock RC, Alexander DP, Rodgers GM. Discontinuation of the bleeding time test without detectable adverse clinical impact. Clin Chem. 2001; 47:1204–11.
21. Levine M, Goldstein JN. Emergency reversal of anticoagulation: novel agents. Curr Neurol Neurosci Rep. 2014;14:471. doi:10.1007/s11910-014-0471-7.
22. Li C, Hirsh J, Xie C, et al. Reversal of the anti-platelet effects of aspirin and clopidogrel. J Thromb Haemost. 2012;10:521–8. doi:10.1111/j.1538-7836.2012.04641.x.
23. Lind SE. The bleeding time does not predict surgical bleeding. Blood. 1991;77:2547–52.
24. Liotta EM, Levasseur-Franklin KE, Naidech AM. Reversal of the novel oral anticoagulants dabigatran, rivaroxaban, and apixaban. Curr Opin Crit Care. 2015;21:127–33. doi:10.1097/MCC.0000000000000181.
25. Mahla E, Suarez TA, Bliden KP, et al. Platelet function measurement-based strategy to reduce bleeding and waiting time in clopidogrel-treated patients undergoing coronary artery bypass graft surgery: the timing based on platelet function strategy to reduce clopidogrel-associated bleeding related to CABG (TARGET-CABG) study. Circ Cardiovasc Interv. 2012;5:261–9. doi:10.1161/CIRCINTERVENTIONS.111.967208.
26. Mannucci PM. Desmopressin (DDAVP) in the treatment of bleeding disorders: the first 20 years. Blood. 1997;90:2515–21.
27. Marlu R, Hodaj E, Paris A, et al. Effect of non-specific reversal agents on anticoagulant activity of dabigatran and rivaroxaban: a randomised crossover ex vivo study in healthy volunteers. Thromb Haemost. 2012;108:217–24. doi:10.1160/TH12-03-0179.
28. Monroe DM, Hoffman M, Roberts HR. Platelets and thrombin generation. Arterioscler Thromb Vasc Biol. 2002;22:1381–9.
29. Peterson P, Hayes TE, Arkin CF, et al. The preoperative bleeding time test lacks clinical benefit: College of American Pathologists' and American Society of Clinical Pathologists' position article. Arch Surg (Chic Ill 1960). 1998;133:134–9.
30. Quinlan DJ, Eikelboom JW, Weitz JI. Four-factor prothrombin complex concentrate for urgent reversal of vitamin K antagonists in patients with major bleeding. Circulation. 2013;128:1179–81. doi:10.1161/CIRCULATIONAHA.113.005107.
31. Riegert-Johnson DL, Volcheck GW. The incidence of anaphylaxis following intravenous phytonadione (vitamin K1): a 5-year retrospective review. Ann Allergy Asthma Immunol. 2002;89:400–6. doi:10.1016/S1081-1206(10)62042-X.
32. Schmid-Schönbein H. Microrheology of erythrocytes, blood viscosity, and the distribution of blood flow in the microcirculation. Int Rev Physiol. 1976; 9:1–62.
33. Schöchl H, Nienaber U, Maegele M, et al. Transfusion in trauma: thromboelastometry-guided coagulation factor concentrate-based therapy versus standard fresh frozen plasma-based therapy. Crit Care (Lond Engl). 2011;15:R83. doi:10.1186/cc10078.
34. Skolnick BE, Shenouda M, Khutoryansky NM, et al. Reversal of clopidogrel-induced bleeding with rFVIIa in healthy subjects: a randomized, placebo-controlled, double-blind, exploratory study. Anesth Analg. 2011;113:703–10. doi:10.1213/ANE.0b013e318228c690.
35. Tanaka KA, Mazzeffi M, Durila M. Role of prothrombin complex concentrate in perioperative coagulation therapy. J Intensive Care. 2014;2:60. doi:10.1186/s40560-014-0060-5.
36. Tantry US, Gesheff M, Liu F, et al. Resistance to antiplatelet drugs: what progress has been made? Expert Opin Pharmacother. 2014;15:2553–64. doi:10.1517/14656566.2014.968126.
37. Marcucci C, Schoettker P. Perioperative hemostasis: coagulation for anesthesiologists. New York: Springer; 2014.

Considerations for Coagulation in the Multi-trauma Patient

19

Craig Rabb and Allison Williams

Introduction

Anticoagulation in the trauma patient with traumatic brain injury and spinal cord injury is a common and complex issue. Per year, there are over 1.7 million brain injuries, 365,000 emergency room visits, 275,000 hospitalizations, and 52,000 deaths from traumatic brain injuries [1]. Per year, there are approximately 12,000 cases of spinal cord injury [2]. The primary issues of concern in the injured patient that relate to anticoagulation include reversal of preexisting anticoagulation in the acute phase, and administration of these agents for prophylaxis of deep vein thrombosis (DVT).

In an age when pharmaceutical companies continue to develop anticoagulants with different mechanisms of action, knowledge of reversal agents is key to saving lives. Patients on anticoagulation at the time of arrival are at risk of death if anticoagulation is not reversed in a timely matter. As a result, intimate familiarity with these contemporary agents and potential reversal agents is critical.

Patients with traumatic brain injury and spinal cord injury have an increased risk of developing venous thromboembolism with prolonged immobilization in hospital beds and hypercoagulable states after trauma. The rate of venous thromboembolism has been reported to be as high as 25 % in patients with isolated traumatic brain injury. Thromboembolism risk is quoted as 2 % in all trauma patients and 18 % in high-risk trauma patients [3]. The incidence of venous thromboembolism has been reported to be as high as 54 % among patients with major head injury not treated by mechanical or pharmacological prophylaxis [4]. Thus, early anticoagulation is key to prevent the complications associated with venous thromboembolism in patients with traumatic brain injury.

If anticoagulants are not started soon after injury, patients risk venous thromboembolism and further complications. However, starting anticoagulants too soon increases the risk of intracerebral hemorrhage progression in patients with traumatic brain injury. An expansion in cerebral hemorrhage may result in further morbidity and mortality. To that end, it is vital to have an understanding of available literature that helps elucidate what is known about the optimal window of opportunity to initiate chemoprophylaxis.

C. Rabb, M.D. (✉) • A. Williams, M.D.
Neurosurgery Department, OU Medical Center, 1000 N. Lincoln Blvd, Suite 400, Oklahoma City, OK 73104, USA
e-mail: Craig-Rabb@ouhsc.edu; Allison-Strickland@ouhsc.edu

C.M. Loftus (ed.), *Anticoagulation and Hemostasis in Neurosurgery*, DOI 10.1007/978-3-319-27327-3_19

Anticoagulation: Identification and Reversal in the Patient with Acute Traumatic Brain Injury

Initial Assessment

The initial assessment of the patient in the trauma bay is critical. The patient with traumatic brain injury must be identified early on in evaluation. Once the patient has been stabilized, the patient should be sent for CT scan, and basic labs checking coagulation status should be drawn immediately.

The anticoagulation status of the patient must be determined early so that reversal agents and medications can be administered. During the secondary survey, the provider should identify the patient's past medical history, home medications, surgical scars, and medical alert bracelets [5].

Laboratory Studies

Assessment of coagulation status in the trauma patient often includes prothrombin time (PT), activated partial thromboplastin time (aPTT), international normalized ratio (INR), and platelet count. The prothrombin time measures the time it takes plasma to clot after addition of tissue factors. The prothrombin time is a measure of the extrinsic pathway of coagulation. Prothrombin time measures factors I (fibrinogen), II (prothrombin), V, VII, and X. The normal reference range is typically 12–13 s, but is dependent on the analytical method used. Prolongations in the prothrombin time (PT) can be a result of vitamin K deficiency, warfarin therapy, and intestinal malabsorption of vitamin K.

The activated partial thromboplastin time (aPTT) measures the time it takes plasma to clot after phospholipid, an activator (silica, celite, kaolin, ellagic acid), and calcium are mixed into a plasma sample. The activated partial thromboplastin time (aPTT) is a measure of the intrinsic and common coagulation pathways. The normal reference range is typically 30–50 s. A normal activated partial thromboplastin time (aPTT) requires normal amounts of coagulation factors: I, II, V, VIII, IX, X, XI, and XII. Prolongations in activated partial thromboplastin time (aPTT) can result from use of Heparin, antiphospholipid antibody, coagulation factor deficiency, antibody to coagulation factors, and coagulation factor consumption in severe illness such as sepsis.

The international normalized ratio (INR) was developed to standardize the results of the prothrombin time. The international normalized ratio (INR) is the ratio of the patient's prothrombin time to a normal control. The normal reference range is 0.8–1.2. The goal of patients on warfarin therapy is typically 2.0–3.0 and may be higher for patients with mechanical heart valves.

Platelet count is the number of platelets in the blood. The normal range of platelets in the blood is 150,000–400,000 platelets per microliter (mcL).

Vitamin K antagonists are usually readily assessed by prothrombin time (PT), activated partial thromboplastin time (aPTT), international normalized ratio (INR), and platelet count. However, the level of anticoagulation and drug activity of newer agents such as direct thrombin and Xa inhibitors are not readily assessed by these lab tests. Thromboelastography (TEG) and rotational thromboelastometry (ROTEM) are being used to assess coagulation status for these newer drugs. These assays test the speed and strength of clot formation. The assays test the activity of the plasma coagulation system, platelet function, and fibrinolysis. Four values for clot formation are determined by this test: the reaction time (*R* value), the *K* value, the angle, and the maximum amplitude (MA). Reaction time (*R*) is the time until first evidence of clot. The angle also offers information for speed of clot formation. The *K* value (*K*) is the speed of clot formation. The maximum amplitude (MA) is reflection of clot strength. A mathematical formula is then used with these four variables to determine the Coagulation Index (CI) which gives an overall assessment of coagulability.

The P2Y12 assay is an additional test that can estimate the inhibition of platelet function for patients on clopidogrel (Plavix). Clopidogrel works by irreversibly blocking the binding of ADP to the platelet P2Y12 receptor. The assay works by injecting a sample of whole blood into a cartridge with two reaction channels. One channel has fibrinogen-coated beads, the platelet agonist ADP, and Prostaglandin E1. Prostaglandin E1 decreases nonspecific platelet aggregation via a second ADP P2Y1 receptor that is not blocked by clopidogrel. This channel measures the effect of clopidogrel on P2Y12-mediated platelet aggregation. The number of activated platelets is equal to the number of fibrinogen-coated beads that aggregate in whole blood. The results are reported in P2Y12 Reaction Units (PRU) and are equal to the amount of residual P2Y12 receptor mediated aggregation. A lower PRU indicates a good response to clopidogrel and a higher PRU indicates a less than optimal response to clopidogrel. In the trauma patient on clopidogrel, a higher PRU suggests a lower amount of drug or response to drug in a patient.

Common Anticoagulants and Reversal Agents

Antiplatelet Agents

Aspirin and Plavix are antiplatelet agents that are often given to patients with coronary artery disease, after stroke, and after placement of stents. Aspirin is classified as an antiplatelet drug that works by irreversible inhibition of the enzyme cyclooxygenase-1 (COX-1). Cyclooxygenase-1 is an enzyme in the inflammatory pathway. Aspirin works by acting as an inhibitor to this enzyme. Inhibition of the enzyme inhibits platelet aggregation for the life of the platelet. It takes 36 h after the last dose of aspirin until 20 % new circulating platelet volume is present. Potential reversal agents for aspirin include platelet transfusions, desmopressin (DDAVP), and recombinant factor VIIa (rFVIIa, brand name Novoseven) (Fig. 19.1).

Traditionally, aspirin reversal has been treated with administration of nonacetylated platelets. Restoration of platelet activity has been shown with transfusion of platelets to patients on low-dose aspirin 75–81 mg per day [6, 7]. However, transfusion of platelets to patients on aspirin 325 mg per day has shown failure to halt progression of intracerebral hemorrhage [6, 7]. Recent studies suggest that patients with small intracerebral hemorrhages should be treated with five platelet concentrate units [5].

Clopidogrel, brand name Plavix, works as an adenosine diphosphate (ADP) receptor antagonist that inhibits platelet function. Platelet function returns to baseline approximately 5–7 days after discontinuation of the drug. A newer, related agent is Prasugrel (trade name Effient). Platelets, desmopressin (DDAVP), and recombinant factor VIIa (rFVIIa, brand name Novoseven) work as potential reversal agents for clopidogrel or prasugrel. Recent evidence suggests that patients on clopidogrel with small intracerebral hemorrhages should be treated with ten platelet concentrate units [5].

For patients on clopidogrel with severe intracerebral hemorrhage, studies recommend addition of desmopressin and serial platelet transfusions every 12 h for 48 h [5]. The exact mechanism of desmopressin is unknown. The drug is thought to increase Von Willebrand factor and factor VIII levels by three- to fivefold. Intravenous, subcutaneous, and intranasal routes are available for administration. The dose is 0.3 μg/kg, and intravenous and subcutaneous routes are preferred.

Additional platelet transfusions may be required for up to 5 days for patients on clopidogrel due to the active metabolite of the drug. Recombinant factor VIIa (rFVIIa, brand name Novoseven) works to promote hemostasis by activating the extrinsic pathway of the coagulation cascade. Recombinant factor VIIa, Novoseven, is structurally similar to human plasma-derived Factor VIIa and functions by a similar mechanism.

Additional antiplatelet medications that may be encountered include nonsteroidal anti-inflammatory drugs. Nonsteroidal anti-inflammatory drugs (NSAIDs) work through reversible cyclooxygenase-1 (COX-1) inhibition. Common nonsteroidal anti-inflammatory drugs include: diclofenac, diflunisal, etodlac, fenoprofen, ibuprofen, indomethacin, ketoprofen, ketorolac, meclofenamate, meloxicam, nabumetone, naproxen, oxaprozin, piroxicam, sulindac, and tolmetin. The effect of nonsteroidal anti-inflammatory drugs lasts 36 h after the last dose. Platelets and desmopressin (DDAVP) are potential reversal agents.

Medication	Mechanism of Action	Duration of Effect	Potential Reversal Agents
Antiplatelets			
Aspirin	Irreversible COX-1 inhibition	Inhibition lasts for the life of the platelet; 36 hours after last dose until 20% new circulating platelet volume	Platelets, DDAVP, rFVIIa
Clopidogrel (Plavix) Prasugrel (Effient)	ADP receptor antagonist on platelets	Platelet aggregation returns to baseline 5 days after discontinuation	Platelets, DDAVP, rFVIIa
NSAIDs*	COX-1 inhibition	36 hours after last dose	Platelets, DDAVP
Cilostazol	PDE-III inhibitor	48-96 hours after last dose	Platelets, DDAVP
Vitamin K Antagonist			
Warfarin (Coumadin)	Inhibit vitamin K dependent clotting factors (II, VII, IX, X)	INR will return to baseline 4 to 10 days after last dose	Phytonidione (vitamin K1), FFP, PCC, cryoprecipitate, rFVIIa
Antithrombin III			
Heparin	Facilitates AT-III binding to and inactivation of Factor IIa, IXa, and Xa	6-8 hours after last subcutaneous injection	Protamine
Enoxaparin, Dalteparin, Tinzeparin	Facilitates AT-III binding to and inactivation of Factor Xa and IIa	12-24 hours after last subcutaneous injection	Protamine, rFVIIa
Fondaparinux (Arixtra)	Facilitates selective AT-III binding to Factor Xa	Approximately 60 hours after last dose	rFVIIa

Fig. 19.1 Common anticoagulants

Direct Thrombin Inhibitors			
Argatroban	Direct thrombin inhibitor	Hepatic clearance in 60-90 minutes	No effective reversal agent identified
Bivalirudin (Angiomax)	Reversible direct thrombin inhibitor	Enzymatic clearance in blood in 25-45 minutes	rFVIIa
Dabigatran (Pradaxa)	Direct inhibitor of free thrombin, fibrin-bound thrombin, and thrombin-induced platelet aggregation	14-17 hours and renal clearance	APCC, PCC, hemodialysis
Direct Factor Xa Inhibitors			
Rivaroxaban (Xarelto)	Direct active inhibitor of activated factor X (factor Xa)	5-13 hours and clearance both hepatic and renal	APCC, PCC, rFVIIa
Apixaban (Eliquis)	Direct active inhibitor of activated factor X (factor Xa)	9-14 hours and clearance both hepatic and renal	APCC, PCC, rFVIIa

*NSAIDs include the following: diclofenac, diflunisal, etodlac, fenoprofen, ibuprofen, indomethacin, ketoprofen, ketorolac, meclofenamate, meloxicam, nabumetone, naproxen, oxaprozin, piroxicam, sulindac, and tolmetin

Abbreviations:

APCC: Activated Prothrombin Complex Concentrate, brand name (FEIBA)

AT-III: Antithrombin III

DDAVP: Desmopressin

NSAIDs: Non-steroidal anti-inflammatory drugs

PCC: Prothrombin Complex Concentrate

PDE-III: Phosphodiesterase III

rFVIIa: Recombinant Activated Factor Seven (Novoseven)

Fig. 19.1 (continued)

A less common agent, Cilostazol, acts as an inhibitor to phosphodiesterase III (PDE-III) and increases cyclic adenosine monophosphate (cAMP). An increase in cAMP results in an increase in protein kinase A (PKA) which inhibits platelet aggregation. The effect of the drug lasts for 48–96 h. Platelets and desmopressin (DDAVP) work as potential reversal agents.

Vitamin K Antagonist

Warfarin, brand name Coumadin, acts by inhibiting vitamin K dependent clotting factors. These factors include II, VII, IX, and X. The duration of effect of warfarin lasts for 4–10 days after the last dose. The drug has hepatic clearance. Patients with atrial fibrillation, mechanical valves, ventricular devices, deep vein thrombosis, or pulmonary embolism are often on warfarin to prevent thrombosis.

Approximately 3 % of patients presenting to Level 1 Trauma Centers are anticogulated with warfarin [8]. Studies have shown a threefold increase in mortality in this group compared to those not taking warfarin or antiplatelet agents [8]. Warfarin therapy is typically monitored with the international normalized ratio (INR). Patients on Coumadin with INR greater than 1.6 require immediate reversal after traumatic brain injury. Patients with traumatic intracerebral hemorrhage should begin therapy to correct their INR to less than 1.6 within 2 h of arrival, and INR should be corrected to INR again of less than 1.6 within 4 h [9]. Early reversal of warfarin effect reduces progression of intracerebral hemorrhage and reduces mortality [10].

Potential warfarin reversal agents include phytonidione (vitamin K1), fresh frozen plasma, prothrombin complex concentrate (PCC, brand name KCentra), cryoprecipitate, and recombinant factor VIIa (rFVIIa, brand name Novoseven). Fresh frozen plasma (FFP) has been the traditional reversal agent. However, fresh frozen plasma is frozen, takes time to thaw, and must be cross-matched. Administration can result in transfusion reactions and often requires multiple doses. The large fluid volumes of multiple units of FFP often cannot be tolerated in patients with congestive heart failure and low cardiac reserves.

A newer reversal agent is prothrombin complex concentrate (PCC, KCentra). The agent contains multiple coagulation factors that aid reversal of warfarin. There are 3-factor (factors II, IX, and X) and 4-factor (factors II, VII, IX, and X) forms. Prothrombin complex concentrate has low risk of infection, no cross matching is required, is contained in a small volume, and can be infused quickly within 15–30 min.

As alternative strategies, cryoprecipitate is a frozen blood product acquired from plasma that contains fibrinogen, factor VIII, von Willebrand factor, and factor XIII. There is limited evidence for use of recombinant activated VII (Novoseven) to reverse vitamin K antagonists. It can be used when first line agents are not available. There is significant risk of thrombosis when administering Novoseven due to the activated component of factor VII. There is less risk of thrombosis when giving prothrombin complex concentrate because the factors are not activated.

Antithrombin III Antagonism

Heparin acts by facilitating antithrombin III (AT-III) binding to and inactivation of Factor IIa, IXa, and Xa. The effect of Heparin lasts for 6–8 h after the last subcutaneous dose. Unfractionated heparin has hepatic clearance, and low molecular weight heparin has renal clearance. Protamine acts as a potential reversal agent.

Enoxaparin, Dalteparin, and Tinzeparin act by facilitating antithrombin III (AT-III) binding to and inactivation of Factor Xa and IIa. The effect of these medications lasts for 12–24 h. Protamine, recombinant factor VIIa (rFVIIa, brand name Novoseven), and activated prothrombin complex concentrate (aPCC, brand name FEIBA) act as potential reversal agents. FEIBA provides factors II (prothrombin), IX, and X in the non-activated form and factor VII in the activated form. Factor VIII coagulant antigen is also present to promote hemostasis. Protamine sulfate exhibits partial, temporary reversal of anti-factor IIa activity [5]. Anticoagulant activity may return 3 h after reversal [5]. Ongoing administration is often required [5] (Fig. 19.2).

Fondaparinux acts by facilitating selective antithrombin III (AT-III) binding to Factor Xa. The effect lasts for approximately 60 h after

Reversal Agent/Antidote	Mechanism of Action
FEIBA: activated prothrombin complex concentrate (aPCC)	Contains factors II (prothrombin), IX, and X in the non-activated form, factor VII in the activated form, factor VIII coagulant antigen which promote hemostasis within the coagulation cascade
KCentra: prothrombin complex concentrate (PCC)	Contains four coagulation factors within the coagulation cascade: factors II, VII, IX, and X which promote clotting
NovoSeven: recombinant factor VIIa (rFVIIa)	Promotes hemostasis by activating the extrinsic pathway of the coagulation cascade through administration of chemically engineered factor VIIa; structurally similar to human plasma-derived Factor VIIa and functions by a similar mechanism

Fig. 19.2 Reversal agents for anticoagulants

the last dose. The drug has renal clearance. Recombinant factor VIIa (rFVIIa, brand name Novoseven) acts as a potential reversal agent.

New Anticoagulants

Direct Thrombin Inhibitors

Argatroban acts as a direct thrombin inhibitor. The liver clears this medication in 60–90 min. The drug has hepatic clearance. No effective means has been established to reverse the effects of Argatroban.

Bivalirudin, bran name Angiomax, acts as a reversible direct thrombin inhibitor. Bivalirudin is cleared enzymatically in the blood within 25–45 min. Recombinant factor VIIa (rFVIIa, brand name Novoseven) acts as a potential reversal agent.

Dabigatran, brand name Pradaxa, is a direct inhibitor of free thrombin, fibrin-bound thrombin, and thrombin-induced platelet aggregation. The drug is approved for prevention of deep vein thrombosis, stroke, and embolism in patients with nonvalvular atrial fibrillation [5]. The duration of effect is 14–17 h. The drug has renal clearance.

Potential reversal agents are activated prothrombin complex concentrate (aPCC, brand name FEIBA), prothrombin complex concentrate (PCC, brand name KCentra), and hemodialysis. The manufacturer of direct thrombin inhibitors recommends fresh frozen plasma to restore circulating coagulation factors, but fresh frozen plasma is unlikely to reverse the drug effect based on its mechanism [11, 12]. Case reports and animal models recommend prothrombin complex concentrate (PCC, KCentra), activated prothrombin complex concentrate (aPCC, brand name FEIBA), and recombinant factor VIIa (rFVIIa, Novoseven) [13, 14]. Currently, a true antidote, anti-Dabi Fab, is under development. The antibody would function as a high-affinity complex inhibitor to dabigatran [15]. The drug of choice for reversal of direct thrombin inhibitors in patients with intracerebral hemorrhage is prothrombin complex concentrate (PCC, KCentra).

Direct Factor Xa Inhibitors

Rivaroxaban, brand name Xarelto, acts as a direct inhibitor of activated factor 10 (factor Xa). The duration of effect is 5–13 h. The drug has both hepatic and renal clearance. Activated prothrombin complex concentrate (aPCC, brand name

FEIBA), prothrombin complex concentrate (PCC, brand name KCentra), and recombinant factor VIIa (rFVIIa, brand name Novoseven), are potential reversal agents. Fresh frozen plasma does not reverse the drug, but helps maintain coagulation factors during ongoing hemorrhage.

High doses of prothrombin complex concentrate (PCC, KCentra) have been shown to normalize bleeding times in animal models [16]. The dose of prothrombin complex concentrate is approximately twice the amount needed for vitamin K Antagonists [17]. The dose of FEIBA needed for reversal is 8–25 U/kg.

Apixaban, brand name Eliquis, acts as a direct inhibitor of activated factor 10 (factor Xa). The duration of effect is 9–14 h. The drug has both hepatic and renal clearance. Activated prothrombin complex concentrate (aPCC, brand name FEIBA), prothrombin complex concentrate (PCC, brand name KCentra), and recombinant factor VIIa (rFVIIa) (Novoseven) are potential reversal agents.

Safety of DVT Prophylaxis in Post-traumatic Brain Injury Patients and Spinal Cord Injury Patients

The risk and benefits of anticoagulation after trauma and the type of anticoagulant to use must be carefully weighed. Deep vein thrombosis can be silent; however, symptoms can present themselves. Common symptoms included leg swelling and pain behind the calf muscle. There is a 25 % incidence of deep vein thrombosis in traumatic brain injury patients after trauma. Deep vein thrombosis is present in 16–17 % of spinal cord injury patients. One to five percent of traumatic brain injury patients will have a pulmonary embolism. Pulmonary embolism is reported in 4–5 % of spinal cord injury patients [18]. The formation of an embolism usually takes 72 h. Patients with pulmonary emboli typically present with shortness of breath, tachycardia, and decrease in oxygenation saturations.

Deep vein thrombosis is diagnosed by physical exam, impedance plethysmography, and ultrasound. CT chest angiogram is the gold standard for patients suspected of having pulmonary embolism. Risk factors for venous thromboembolism include immobility, extremity or pelvic fractures, and morbid obesity. In trauma patients, patients with traumatic brain injury have a higher incidence of venous thromboembolism [19].

Mechanical prophylaxis and pharmacologic prophylaxis are key to preventing deep vein thrombosis in patients with traumatic brain injury. TED Hose and pneumatic intermittent compression devices for the calves help prevent deep vein thrombosis. TED Hose and pneumatic intermittent compression devices are probably equivalent in efficacy. Pneumatic intermittent compression devices reduce risk from 23 to 6 % in traumatic brain injury patients. Pharmacologic prophylaxis is important in spinal cord injury patients who are immobile. A case series of spinal cord injury patients showed that 43 % of paralyzed patients developed deep vein thrombosis when treated with intermittent compression devices [20].

In the Cochrane analysis for thromboprophylaxis in trauma patients with traumatic brain injury, there was no strong evidence that either mechanical or pharmacological interventions reduced death or pulmonary embolisms. The evidence showed that mechanical and pharmacological interventions prevent formation of deep vein thrombosis in the legs [21]. Level three evidence suggests that compression stockings or intermittent pneumatic compression stockings are recommended unless lower extremity injury prevents their use. The stockings should be used until the patient is ambulatory [22]. Vena cava filters are recommended for patients who do not respond to anticoagulation or who are not candidates for anticoagulation therapy or mechanical devices [23]. Routine use of vena cava filters in spinal cord injury is not indicated unless there is an associated long bone fracture that increases risk of deep vein thrombosis [24].

There is controversy as to the specific agents that should be used for prophylaxis in traumatic brain injury. Low molecular weight heparin (LMWH) or low dose unfractionated heparin should be used in combination with mechanical prophylaxis. However, there is an increased risk for expansion of intracranial hemorrhage. There is insufficient evidence to support recommendations regarding the preferred agent, dose, or timing of pharmacologic prophylaxis for deep vein thrombosis.

Venous ultrasounds should be used to screen for deep vein thrombosis in patients with multisystem trauma, complex extremity or pelvic fractures, and patients with severe traumatic brain injury. For patients with traumatic brain injury, recommendations are to perform venous ultrasounds at 48 h after trauma. Repeat scans should be performed 7–10 days after trauma [25]. For patients with spinal cord injuries, weekly screening for deep vein thrombosis during the first 13 weeks after injury detects most of the asymptomatic events within this population [18].

Class three evidence suggests reduced incidence of DVT and no increase in worsening traumatic brain injury in patients started on unfractionated heparin within 72 h of injury [26]. Enoxaparin was studied in a group of 150 traumatic brain injury patients. Enoxaparin was given 24 h after admission. Six patients on Enoxaparin had worsening of their injury on CT Head after prophylaxis for deep vein thrombosis. The study concluded Enoxaparin can be safe 24 h after injury [27].

A further study compared unfractionated heparin and Enoxaparin. 159 patients received Enoxaparin and 171 received unfractionated heparin. Deep vein thrombosis and pulmonary embolism was increased in the group receiving unfractionated heparin. Patients on unfractionated heparin had more events of worsening intracerebral hemorrhage [28].

For patients with spinal cord injury, no particular agent was found to be superior when comparing low molecular weight heparin versus unfractionated heparin and Dalteparin versus Enoxaparin [29, 30]. It is recommended that administration of anticoagulation in spinal cord injury be initiated within 72 h of injury. When surgical intervention is needed, anticoagulation should be held the morning of surgery, and resumed within 24 h after surgery.

Conclusions

There is no standard of care guideline for the use of anticoagulants post-traumatic brain injury. The guideline for management of severe traumatic brain injury cites level III evidence for using low-molecular weight heparin or low-dose unfractionated heparin (UFH) in combination with mechanical prophylaxis [31]. The guideline provides no recommendation with regard to which subgroups of traumatic brain injury patients might benefit more from prophylactic anticoagulation as well as the preferred agent, timing, and dose [31].

A review of the literature suggests that prophylactic anticoagulation can be safe in traumatic brain injury patients with stable head CT. Prophylactic anticoagulation in traumatic brain injury patients with stable or improved head CT scans after 24 h of injury reduced incidence of deep vein thrombosis without increasing risk of intracerebral hemorrhage progression [32]. Studies suggest that there is no prophylactic agent of choice for anticoagulation, there is no significant difference in rate or hemorrhage based on agent chosen, and there is no significant difference in rate of deep vein thrombosis [28, 33].

With respect to spinal cord injury, prophylactic pharmacologic anticoagulation is recommended in patients with severe motor deficits. Low-dose heparin in combination with pneumatic compression stockings, electrical stimulation, or rotating beds is recommended. Duplex Doppler Ultrasound, impedance plethysmography, and venography are recommended for use as diagnostic tests for deep vein thrombosis in the spinal cord-injured patient population. A 3-month duration of prophylactic treatment for deep venous thrombosis and pulmonary embolism is recommended. Vena cava filters are recommended for patients who do not respond to anticoagulation or who are not candidates for anticoagulation therapy or mechanical devices [23].

Thus, further studies are needed to guide the use of anticoagulants post-traumatic brain injury and spinal cord injury. Mechanical and pharmacological prophylaxis is key and patients should be followed with surveillance ultrasounds checking for deep vein thrombosis. Thus, initiation of anticoagulation is ultimately the decision of the practicing provider. Risks and benefits of anticoagulation must be weighed. In the end, each physician must factor in his or her own risk tolerance into this decision.

References

1. Faul MXL, Wald MM, Coronado VG. Traumatic brain injury in the United States: emergency department visits, hospitalizations and deaths 2002–2006. Atlanta, GA: Centers for Disease Control and Prevention; 2010.
2. National Spinal Cord Injury Statistical Center (2014) Birmingham, Alabama. https://www.nscisc.uab.edu. Accessed 1 Mar 2015.
3. Denson K, Morgan D, Cunningham R, et al. Incidence of venous thromboembolism in patients with traumatic brain injury. Am J Surg. 2007;193(3):380–3. discussion 383–4.
4. Geerts WH, Code KI, Jay RM, Chen E, Szalai JP. A prospective study of venous thromboembolism after major trauma. N Engl J Med. 1994;331(24):1601–6.
5. McCoy CC, Lawson JH, Shapiro ML. Management of anticoagulation agents in trauma patients. Clin Lab Med. 2014;34:563–74.
6. Taylor G, Osinski D, Thevenin A, et al. Is platelet transfusion efficient to restore platelet reactivity in patients who are responders to aspirin and/or clopidogrel before emergency surgery? J Trauma Acute Care Surg. 2013;74(5):1367–9.
7. Nishijima DK, Zehtabchi S, Berrong J, et al. Utility of platelet transfusion in adult patients with traumatic intracranial hemorrhage and preinjury antiplatelet use: a systematic review. J Trauma Acute Care Surg. 2012;72(6):1658–63.
8. Bonville DJ, Ata A, Jahraus CB, et al. Impact of preinjury warfarin and antiplatelet agents on outcomes of trauma patients. Surgery. 2011;150(4):861–8.
9. Calland JF, Ingraham AM, Martin N, et al. Evaluation and management of geriatric trauma: an Eastern Association for the Surgery of Trauma practice management guideline. J Trauma Acute Care Surg. 2012;73(5 Suppl 4):S345–50.
10. Ivascu FA, Howells GA, Junn FS, et al. Rapid warfarin reversal in anticoagulated patients with traumatic intracranial hemorrhage reduces hemorrhage progression and mortality. J Trauma. 2005;59(5):1131–7 (discussion: 1137–9).
11. Van Ryn J, Stangier J, Haertter S, et al. Dabigatran etexilate—a novel, reversible, oral direct thrombin inhibitor: interpretation of coagulation assays and reversal of anticoagulant activity. Thromb Haemost. 2010;103(6):1116–27.
12. Boehringer Ingelheim Pharmaceuticals (2013) Pradaxa prescribing information. http://bidocs.boehringer-ingelheim.com/BIWebAccess/ViewServlet.ser?docBase=rent&folderPath=/Prescribing%20Information/Pls/Pradaxa/Pradaxa.pdf. Accessed 28 Feb 2015.
13. Faust AC, Peterson EJ. Management of dabigatran-associated intracerebral and intraventricular hemorrhage: a case report. J Emerg Med. 2014;46(4):525–9.
14. Dumkow LE, Voss JR, Peters M, et al. Reversal of dabigatran-induced bleeding with a prothrombin complex concentrate and fresh frozen plasma. Am J Health Syst Pharm. 2012;69(19):1646–50.
15. Schiele F, van Ryn J, Canada K, et al. A specific antidote for dabigatran: functional and structural characterization. Blood. 2013;121(18):3554–62.
16. Perzborn E, Gruber A, Tinel H, et al. Reversal of rivaroxaban anticoagulation by haemostatic agents in rats and primates. Thromb Haemost. 2013;110(1):162–72.
17. CSL Behring GmbH. Kcentra prescribing information. 2013. Available at: http://www.kcentra.com/prescribing-information.aspx. Accessed 28 Feb 2015.
18. Furlan JC, Fehlings MG. Role of screening tests for deep venous thrombosis in asymptomatic adults with acute spinal cord injury: an evidence-based analysis. Spine. 2007;32(17):1908–16.
19. Reiff DA, Harichan RN, Bullington NM, Griffin RL, McGwin G, Rue LW, et al. Traumatic brain injury associated with the development of deep vein thrombosis independent of pharmacologic prophylaxis. J Trauma. 2009;66(5):1436–40.
20. Chung SB, Lee SH, Kim ES, et al. Incidence of deep vein thrombosis after spinal cord injury: a prospective study in 37 consecutive patients with traumatic or nontraumatic spinal cord injury treated by mechanical prophylaxis. J Trauma. 2011;71:867–71.
21. Barrera M, Perel P, Ker K, et al (2013) Thromboprophylaxis for trauma patients. Cochrane Database Syst Rev. http://researchonline.lshtm.ac.uk/856572/. Accessed 28 Feb 2015.
22. Brain Trauma Foundation (2007) J Neurotrauma 24(1). http://online.liebertpub.com/doi/abs/10.1089/neu.2007.9999. Accessed 27 Feb 2015.
23. Hadley MN, Walters BC, Grabb PA, Oyesiku NM, Przybylski GJ, Resnick DK, Ryken TC. Deep venous thrombosis and thromboembolism in patients with cervical spinal cord injuries. Neurosurgery. 2002;50:S73–80.
24. Maxwell RA, Chavarria-Aguilar M, Cockerham WT, et al. Routine prophylactic vena cava filtration is not indicated after acute spinal cord injury. J Trauma. 2002;52:902–6.
25. Cothren CC, Smith WR, Moore EE, et al. Utility of once daily dose of low-molecular-weight heparin to prevent venous thromboembolism in multi-system trauma patients. World J Surg. 2007;31:98–104.
26. Kim J, Gearhart MM, Zurick A, et al. Preliminary report on the safety of heparin for deep venous throm-

bosis prophylaxis after severe head injury. J Trauma. 2002;53:38–43.
27. Norwood SH, McAuley CE, Berne JD, Vl V, Kerns DB, Grahm TW, et al. Prospective evaluation of the safety of Enoxaparin prophylaxis for venous thromboembolism in patients with intracranial hemorrhagic injuries. Arch Surg. 2002;137:696–702.
28. Minshall CT, Eriksson EA, et al. Safety and efficacy of heparin or enoxaparin prophylaxis in blunt trauma patients with a head abbreviated injury score >2. J Trauma. 2011;71(2):396–400.
29. Worley S, Short C, Pike J, Anderson D, Douglas JA, Thompson K. Dalteparin vs low-dose unfractionated heparin for prophylaxis against clinically evident venous thromboembolism in acute traumatic spinal cord injury: a retrospective cohort. J Spinal Cord Med. 2008;31(4):379–87.
30. Slavik CRS, Gorman E, et al. Dalteparin versus Enoxaparin for venous thromboembolism prophylaxis in acute spinal cord injury and major orthopedic trauma patients: "DETECT" trial. J Trauma. 2007; 62:1075–81 (discussion 1081).
31. Bratton SL, Chestnut RM, Ghajar J, et al. Guidelines for the management of severe traumatic brain injury, part v: deep vein thrombosis prophylaxis. J Neurotrauma. 2007;24 Suppl 1:S32–6.
32. Scudday T, Brasel K, Webb T, et al. Safety and efficacy of prophylactic anticoagulation in patients with traumatic brain injury. J Am Coll Surg. 2011;213(1): 148–53. discussion 153–4.
33. Dudley RR, Aziz I, Bonnici A. Early venous thromboembolic event prophylaxis in traumatic brain injury with low-molecular weight heparin: risks and benefits. J Neurotrauma. 2010;27(12):2165–72.

Cerebral Venous Sinus Thrombosis

20

William W. Ashley Jr

Introduction

Cerebral venous sinus thrombosis (CVST) is a relatively rare but potentially devastating entity that mainly affects young adults and children and represents between 0.5 and 1 % of all strokes [1]. Despite significant improvements in outcomes [2], CVST is a heterogeneous stroke subtype that can be challenging to diagnose and effectively treat and, as a result, is still a significant cause of death and disability [2, 3]. Anticoagulation is currently the mainstay of treatment [4–6] but a multidisciplinary) approach is usually required to achieve optimal outcomes. Expertise in neurologic diagnosis, medical/surgical management of intracranial hypertension and cerebral edema, neuro-endovascular therapy and critical care, often places the neurosurgeon at the center of this multidisciplinary team. And as an integral part of this team, modern neurosurgeons must have an excellent understanding of this complex and interesting stroke subtype. The purpose of this chapter is to provide a basic review of CVST and its treatment with a focus on the role of systemic anticoagulation as a part of the overall treatment methodology. The specific objectives are to

1. Review the epidemiology and clinical significance of CVST.
2. Discuss the pathophysiology of CVST and its relation to clinical subtypes and potential treatments.
3. Provide evidence based review of modern treatment options for CVST with a focus on anticoagulation.
4. Offer a clinical algorithm for care of the CVST patient.
5. Highlight future directions.

Epidemiology

CVST is reported to have been initially described as early as 1825 by French physician Ribes [7, 8]. However, due to a combination of poor diagnostic/imaging techniques and a highly variable clinical presentation, CVST was historically only diagnosed at autopsy [5]. Therefore, it is likely that its true incidence was underestimated. Widespread access to advanced, modern imaging techniques has lead to the ability to diagnose CVST more accurately and at earlier, more benign stages of presentation. As expected the overall incidence of CVST has increased accordingly. Currently, CVST is estimated to occur in three to four people per million in adults and between six and seven million in children and neonates [4, 5, 9]. Using data from Portugal, Hong Kong, Mexico, and Iran, the incidence has

W.W. Ashley Jr , M.D., Ph.D., M.B.A. (✉)
Loyola University Medical Center,
2160 S. First Avenue, Maywood, IL 60153, USA
e-mail: washley72@yahoo.com

C.M. Loftus (ed.), *Anticoagulation and Hemostasis in Neurosurgery*,
DOI 10.1007/978-3-319-27327-3_20

been estimated at 0.2–1.23 per 100,000. Most recently a Dutch population study looking at 9270 patients over a 2-year period found an incidence of approximately 1.32 per 100,000 in the general population [10, 11].

As mentioned, CVST is a disease of young adults and children. Indeed, based on the International Study on Cerebral Venous and Dural Sinuses Thrombosis (ISCVT), the largest cohort study to date, 78 % of those affected were less than 50 years of age [1, 3]. Similarly, in a retrospective analysis of the National Inpatient Sample (NIS) data for 11,400 patients older 15 years of age admitted to US hospitals (2001–2008), the mean age was 38 years old and 78 % of the patients were between the ages of 15 and 49 years old [1, 3, 12].

CVST also preferentially affects women. Nearly 75 % of adult CVST patients are women. This predilection for women is based on gender specific issues including pregnancy, puerperium, oral contraceptive pill (OCP) use (especially third generation), and hormone supplementation [9]. The incidence of CVST in female population is reported to be as high as 2.78 per 100,000 in certain groups [10]. Pregnancy/puerperium related cases alone account for between 5 and 20 % of all CVST in developed countries [6]. When controlling for gender specific factors, the incidence in women is similar to that of their male counterparts. This has been demonstrated in studies that have shown that rates of CVST in female children and elderly women are the same as in men. Moreover, a significant rise in the incidence of CVST in women occurred in the 1970s coincident with the introduction and widespread adoption of the OCP [9]. Interestingly, the presentation and outcomes associated with CVST can vary with gender as well [13, 14]. Women with gender-specific causes tend to have better outcomes as compared to their male counterparts [14].

Outcomes

Historically, CVST was associated with mortality rates as high as 40–50 % and was usually diagnosed upon the patient's death. Recent studies have demonstrated that the prognosis has improved and current mortality is 2–6 % [3, 9, 11, 12]. A recent review of the literature highlights a significant reduction in mortality over the last 2 decades that can be linked to four main factors. *Hospital care*, including ICU and critical care, has significantly improved over the last several decades leading to improved outcomes for a variety of disease processes. The second major factor is *improved imaging*. Major improvements in the ability to diagnose CVST occurred with the advent of invasive catheter cerebral angiography. The utility of catheter angiography was limited by the fact that the technique was slow, required technical expertise and had significant risks. It was, and continues to be, somewhat cumbersome to use invasive angiography as an initial diagnostic or screening tool. Thus even further improvement occurred with the widespread adoption of noninvasive techniques such as magnetic resonance imaging (MRI), magnetic resonance venography (MRV), and CT venography (CTV) that, with some limitations, allowed safe and efficient diagnosis of CVST. In the future molecular based imaging techniques may yield further advances [15]. *Shifts in risk factors* have also contributed to overall decline in mortality from CVST. Indeed over the last decades the incidence of traumatic and infectious CVST has been on the decline. As will be discussed, these subtypes are associated with worse outcomes. Conversely, the relative incidence of CVST associated with gender specific causes, such as OCP use, has been increasing. In general, these subtypes have relatively lower risk profiles [3, 13]. Finally, the ability *to treat CVST has improved*. And although still controversial, the use of intravenous heparin or subcutaneous low molecular weight heparin (LMWH) is the recommended first line therapy and seems to be associated with lower mortality and improved outcomes. Other measures such as hemicraniectomy or endovascular techniques have also been shown to improve outcomes in certain cases. The combination of these factors and improved awareness of CVST has lead to marked improvements in mortality.

Currently, CVST is associated with good outcomes in over 85 % of patients and has an overall mortality of about 2–6 % and a rare recurrence rate of about 3 % [2, 3, 9, 12]. Despite improvement there are several factors that have been associated with poor outcomes. Some examples are: malignancy as a cause of the CVST, CNS infection, seizures, associated brain hemorrhage, GCS <9 on admission and/or altered mental status, hemiparesis, male gender, age over 37 years, and CVST affecting the straight sinus or deep venous system [3].

The best outcomes can be achieved when CVST is recognized and treated in a timely *and* appropriate manner. Indeed, delay in diagnosis and treatment is a significant problem with CVST. Data from the ISCVT study showed in the ISCVT, the median delay from onset of symptoms to hospital admission was 4 days. Further it took an additional 3 days in the hospital for the diagnosis of CVST to be made. Thus, the median delay from initial symptom to diagnosis was about 1 week [16]. Patients presenting with visible parenchymal or hemorrhagic lesions, seizures, or mental status changes, are usually diagnosed most quickly. While patients presenting without visible lesions on imaging and only symptoms of elevated intracranial pressure (usually headache) alone are a diagnostic challenge and face greater delays in diagnosis and initial of treatment. Interestingly men are also subject to relative diagnostic delay [16].

Pathophysiology

CVST is a stroke subtype that is characterized by thrombo-occlusion of major cerebral veins and/or dural venous sinuses. In general, these two broad interrelated pathophysiologic mechanisms contribute to the findings that characterize CVST. Thrombosis of major cerebral veins leads to local blockage of normal venous outflow pathways. In turn this contributes to the development of venous hypertension and cerebral edema. Gross and micropathologic examination reveals engorged thrombotic veins, ischemic neurons, edema, and microhemorrhages. Intracellular cytotoxic edema develops as a result of ischemia which damages the cellular Na/K pumps [9, 17, 18]. This is followed by development of reversible interstitial vasogenic edema that results from secondary disruption of the blood brain barrier. Venous infarction and/or hemorrhage are common sequelae [9, 18] (Fig. 20.1). Elevated intracranial pressure (ICP) and, sometimes, herniation can develop as a result of malignant edema or mass effect from large hemorrhagic lesions. The nature and viability of collateral venous drainage is an important consideration. Those with robust alternative venous drainage may be able to tolerate thrombosis for longer periods of time.

The next mechanism is intracranial hypertension that results from reduction of CSF reabsorption. As venous outflow is impaired, the gradient for CSF reabsorption via the arachnoid granulations is interrupted. As a result, patients develop signs and symptoms of intracranial hypertension such as headache or papilledema. Despite the presence of elevated intracranial pressure, CVST is not usually associated with ventricular dilatation or hydrocephalus. These two mechanisms usually occur in concert with each other leading to the more common clinical presentations associated with CVST. Isolated intracranial hypertension without cortical venous thrombosis occurs in about 20 % of patients presenting with CVST [3, 9].

In accordance with the Virchow triad of blood stasis, changes in the vessel wall and changes in the composition of the blood, CVST usually occurs in the setting of an inherited thrombophilia or an acquired prothrombotic state or condition. In the ISCVT study a thrombophilia was documented in 34 % of patients [3, 19]. Multiple specific predisposing conditions have been identified and are presented in Table 20.1 [3]. In many cases there is a double hit type of phenomenon and CVST occurs as a result of an antecedent prothrombotic cause in the setting the setting of a preexisting underlying thrombophilia (Fig. 20.2). As will be discussed, an important part of therapy for CVST is the identification and treatment of modifiable factors. Unfortunately, a likely risk factor for CVST can only be identified in only 85 % of cases [9].

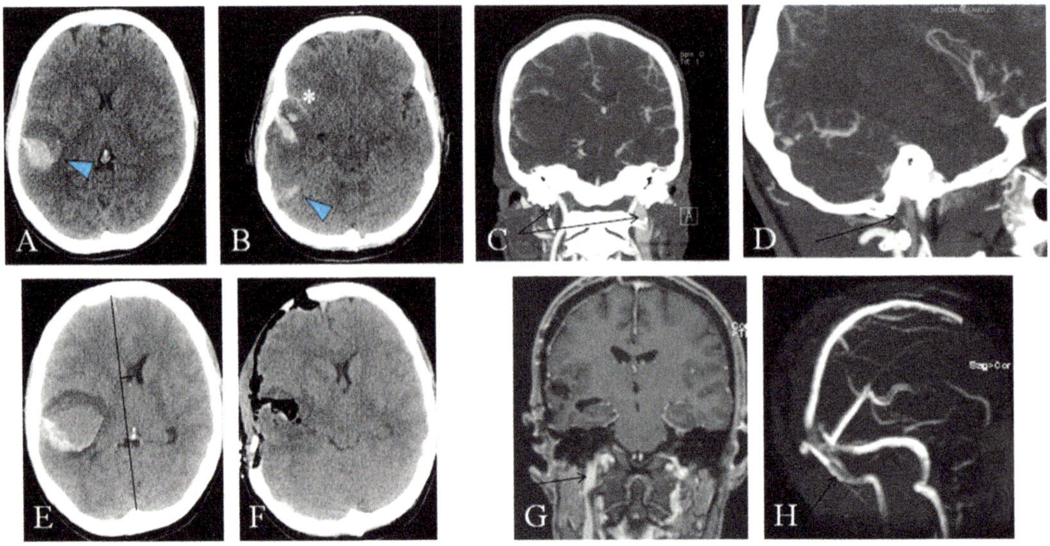

Fig. 20.1 Case I: A young woman with hemorrhagic CVST in setting of OCP use. A 49-year-old right-handed woman with unremarkable medical history presented with acute confusional state. While at work, she began having difficulties with naming and became disoriented. Her initial head CT (A&B) showed an approximately 3×3 cm intraparenchymal hematoma (**a**—*arrowheads*) in the right frontal lobe with adjacent subarachnoid hemorrhage in the right sylvian fissure and overlying the right frontotemporal lobes (**b**—*asterisk*). There was significant surrounding edema but no significant mass effect or midline shift. There was hyperdensity at the right transverse sigmoid sinus (**b**—*arrowhead*). Further history from family revealed a 2-month history of intermittent right occipital headaches (worse over the last 2 weeks) and retroauricular pain. She had been given a diagnosis of mastoiditis and treated with augmentin. She had been taking oral contraceptive pills for many years. Her history and imaging (hyperdensity at the right transverse sinus) were concerning for CVST. She could not tolerate MRI due to her confusion and agitation. So a CTA/CTV (C&D) was obtained. It showed no evidence cerebral aneurysm on CTA. CTV showed dural venous sinus thrombus extending from the proximal right transverse sinus through the sigmoid sinus and into the proximal jugular vein (**c** and **d**—*arrows*). She was initially admitted and followed on the neurology service with serial CT scans showing stable intraparenchymal hemorrhage, and started on a therapeutic heparin drip for 3 days and subsequently started on coumadin (received one dose). On the fourth day she was noted to be progressively more confused and developed worsened LUE weakness. Repeat CT (**e**) head showed progressive midline shift and increased mass effect from IPH with early uncal herniation. Neurosurgery was consulted and she was taken for decompressive hemicraniectomy (**f**). She stabilized and made some improvement while in the hospital. She was discharged to rehab with mild language apraxia. She was restarted on LMWH and coumadin 10 days after surgery. She was continued on anticoagulation for 6 months total. Repeat MRI/MRV was obtained at 6 month follow-up and showed that normal contrast and flow related enhancement are demonstrated throughout the major dural sinuses and proximal internal jugular veins without occlusive filling defect with no evidence of sinus occlusion (**g** and **h**—*arrows*)

Historically, post-infectious CVST was common. However, recently this has been on the decline as a risk factor for most patients with CVST. However, it is more common as a risk in male patients, pediatric patients and in patients from developing countries [11, 13, 20–23]. Other less common but notable risk factors include lumbar puncture with intracranial hypotension [24], intracranial trauma, and neurosurgical procedures. These can present significant treatment challenges due to the inherent risk of bleeding when considering using anticoagulation for treatment following trauma or surgery. In a recent study of over 900 patients (ages 1–77, mean 36.1) admitted to a US University Hospital with skull fractures, over 10 % had a skull fracture associated with a cerebral venous sinus and, of those, over 34 % had an associated thrombus involving at least one venous sinus [25].

Table 20.1 Shows common risk factors for CVST. No underlying risk factor is identified in up to 15 % of patients with CVST

Thrombophilia	
	Deficiencies of antithrombin, protein C, and protein S
	Factor V Leiden mutation
	Prothrombin gene mutation 20210
	Antiphospholipid antibodies
	Hyperhomocysteinemia
Female Gender-Specific Risks	
	Pregnancy
	Postpartum state
	Hormonal contraceptive or replacement therapy
Infection	
	Localized infections such as otitis, mastoiditis, sinusitis
	Meningitis
	Systemic infectious disorders
Chronic inflammatory diseases	
	Vasculitides
	Inflammatory bowel disease
Cancer	
	Hypercoagulable state
	Chemotherapy
	Local venous compression
Hematologic disorders	
	Polycythemia
	Essential thrombocytosis
	Paroxysmal nocturnal hemoglobinuria
Trauma/Mechanical	
	Head trauma
	Local injury to cerebral sinuses or veins
	Jugular venous cannulation
	Neurosurgical procedures
	Lumbar puncture
	Nephrotic syndrome
Other	
	Dehydration
	Dural arteriovenous fistula[a]

[a]dAVF is rare but of interest to the neurosurgeon

Presentation and Clinical Subtypes

The presentation of CVST varies widely and largely depends on the location of thrombosis, chronicity of presentation, presence of intraparenchymal lesions, and the underlying pathophysiology (Fig. 20.3, Table 20.2). Those with involvement of dural sinuses with cortical venous thrombosis may present with only features of elevated intracranial pressure such as headache or papilledema. CVST can present in an acute, subacute, and chronic time course. 90 % of patients present with headache [6, 9]. It is the initial symptom in nearly 80 % and the only symptom in 15–25 % of patients [1, 6, 26, 27]. Thus a high index of suspicion must be maintained in patients with isolated headache and risk factors for CVST. The type of headache is also quite variable but is often gradual, diffuse and subacute in nature. Rarely CVST can present with sudden, severe headache pattern similar to that usually associated with aneurysmal subarachnoid hemorrhage. Conversely, 5–30 % of patients have been reported to present without headache [28]. These patients tend to be older, male and show a trend towards worse clinical outcomes [28].

Focal neurologic deficits can be seen and usually correspond to the locale of intraparenchymal lesions [3, 9], while marked alterations in consciousness or coma are associated with deep venous thrombosis with associated thalamic involvement. In general focal deficits or coma as a presenting feature portend poor outcomes [1, 3, 9].

Seizure is also a common presenting feature and has been reported as a presenting feature in nearly 40 % of patients with CVST [29]. Logistic-regression analysis showed that CVST presenting with seizure was associated with supratentorial lesions, cortical vein thrombosis, sagittal sinus thrombosis and puerperal CVST. In patients at higher risk for seizure, prophylactic antiepileptic medical therapy may be considered [1, 29]. Seizures are much more common in CVST as compared to arterial stroke subtypes. Indeed, seizures with suspicious imaging findings should raise suspicion for CVST [1, 30].

Finally, there are variations based on demographic subgroups. As mentioned, women with gender specific causes usually present acutely with headache and seem to have better outcomes as compared to men. Subgroup analysis from ISCVT study showed that 81 % of women presenting with CVST had a complete recovery versus only 71 % of men [14]. The elderly often

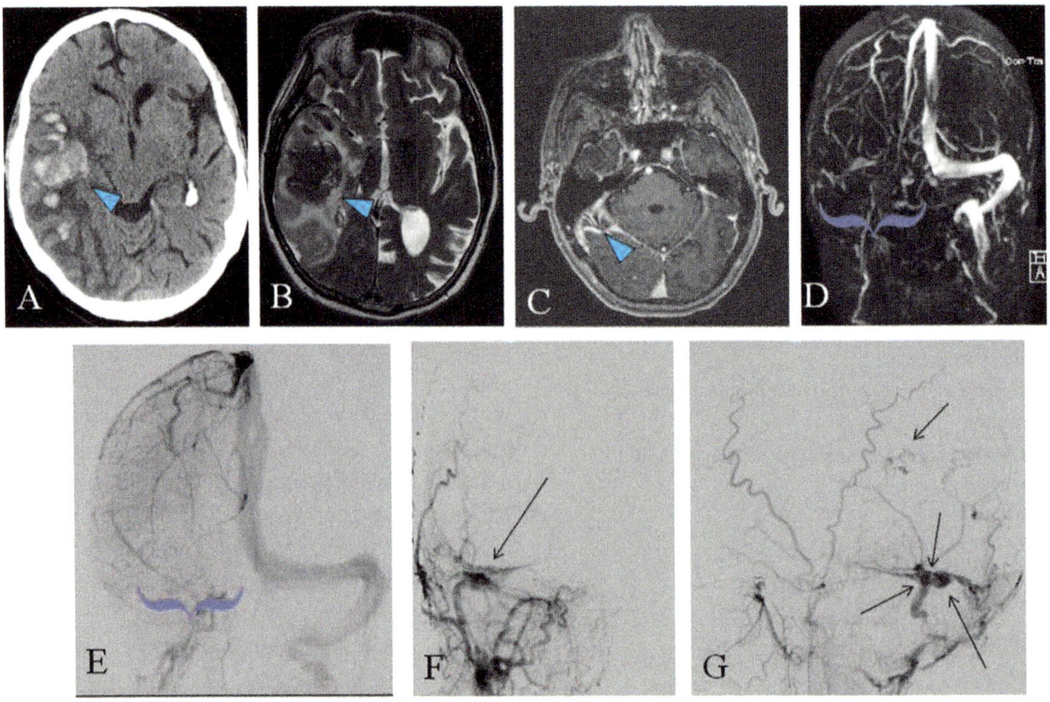

Fig. 20.2 Case II: A man with recent dehydration and underlying history of malignancy with CVST and dAVF. A 66-year-old male with a history of CML s/p bone marrow transplant on immunosuppression who presents after obtaining MRI brain this evening for workup of pulsatile tinnitus which incidentally showed hemorrhagic conversion of a area of stroke. He reported being on a hiking trip 3 weeks ago and dehydrated after significant exertion. At that time he had a severe 10/10 headache with dizziness that lasted for the day, and resolved by the following day. He did not seek medical care at that time. He did, however, start to take daily ASA since he thought his symptoms may be related to an MI. He reports only a couple of mild headaches since that time. He did have one episode of vomiting after dinner 1 week ago, but none since then. He has noted a "wooshing" sound in his R ear which was worked up by his primary care physician and ENT who recommended an MRI/MRA. He denied any diplopia, blurry vision, visual field disturbance, seizures, weakness/numbness/tingling. His initial non-contrast CT head (**a**—*arrowhead*) showed an approximately 7 cm area of non-confluent intraparenchymal hemorrhage and edema in the right temporal-occipital region with associated mass effect and midline shift, the MRI/MRA showed diffuse abnormal signal intensity involving the right temporal lobe with heterogeneous T2 signal intensity centrally consistent with blood products and surrounding edema (**b**—*arrowhead*). There is some thickening of the overlying cortex with mass effect causing effacement of the right lateral ventricle, midline shift from left to right, and minimal uncal herniation into the suprasellar cistern. It appeared to be consistent with hemorrhagic transformation of an ischemic event. There was concern for CVST and/or dAVF based on his history of cancer, dehydration, and tinnitus/swooshing in the ear. A dedicated MRI/MRV (**c** and **d**) was then obtained. Post-contrast images (**c**) demonstrated branched vascular enhancement (**c**—*arrowhead*) throughout most of the right temporal, occipital and inferior parietal lobes. This enhancement appears to converge on the anterior superior margin of the medial right tentorium cerebelli. These findings were concerning for dAVF. There was a large tubular filling defect within the transverse sinus, sigmoid sinus and visualized proximal internal jugular vein is consistent with a near occlusive venous thrombosis. This was well seen on the 3D reconstruction (**d**—*bracket*). Digital subtraction angiography (**e**–**g**) confirmed a high grade dAVF filling mainly from arterial feeders arising from the occipital artery as well as to a lesser extent the superficial temporal artery. There was egress into a venous pouch in the region of the transverse sigmoid sinus (**f** and **g**—*arrows*). There was marked retrograde reflux into the cortical veins. There was no obvious filling from the right internal carotid and the right-sided venous system in the region of the transverse sigmoid appears to be occluded (**e**—*bracket*). It is not clear whether the sinus thrombosis or the dAVF was the initial event. The dAVF was treated for cure using staged endovascular embolization. The patient made an excellent neurologic recovery and no longer has tinnitus

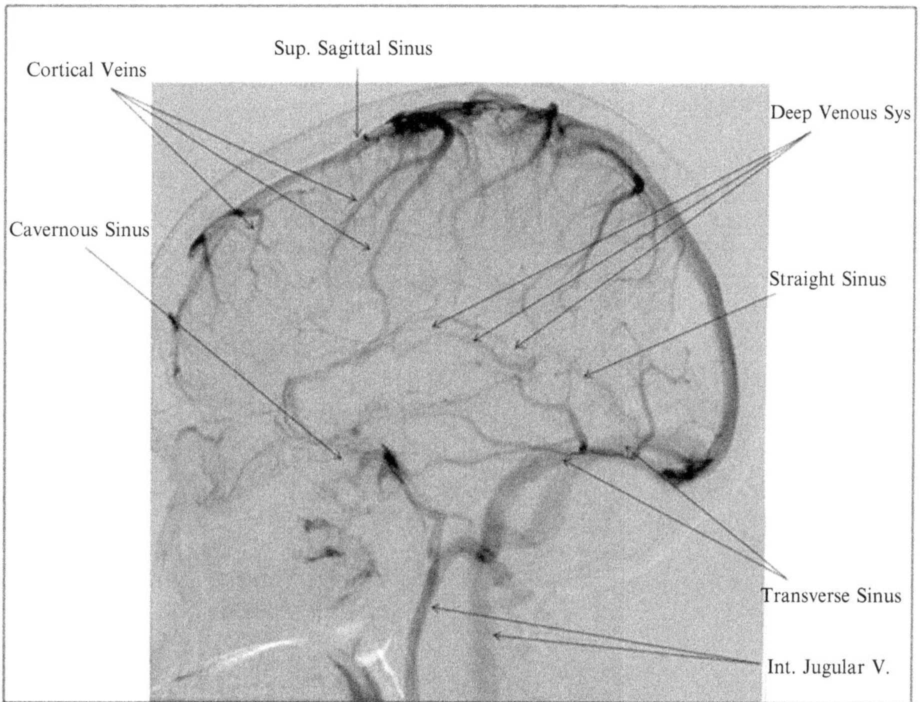

Location of CVST	Frequency (%)	Common Associated Clinical Syndrome
Cortical Veins	17	Sensorimotor deficits (unilateral), seizures
Superior Sagittal Sinus	62	Sensorimotor deficits (bilateral), seizures
Straight Sinus	18	Motor deficits, mental status changes (thalamic)
Deep venous system	11	Motor deficits, mental status changes (thalamic)
Transverse Sinus (left or right)	86	Isolated intracranial hypertension (headache), aphasia (usually left)
Jugular Vein	12	Neck pain, tinnitus, cranial nerve palsy
Cavernous Sinus	1	Ocular Signs-orbital pain, chemosis, proptosis, oculomotor palsy

Fig. 20.3 Shows a venous phase, oblique projection of a digital subtraction cerebral angiogram labeled with relevant venous anatomy

present with mental status changes and depressed consciousness. They have poor outcomes relative to younger patients. Only 49 % of the elderly (age >65 years old) make a complete recovery versus 82 % of younger patients and the elderly have a mortality of more than 25 % [31]. Children have unique characteristics. In a recent study, 55 % of children ages 0–12 years old were less than 6 months of age at presentation. Common presenting features included seizures (59 %), coma (30 %), motor weakness (21 %), and headache (18 %). Over half were found to have decreased level of consciousness. The most common risk factor was infection which was notable as a cause in over 40 %. In this study 13 % of children died and 46 % had a neurologic deficit at discharge [20].

Diagnosis

Clinical

As discussed above the presentation of CVST is highly variable and, as a result, clinical diagnosis can be quite challenging. The main stay of diagnosis is a thorough history and physical examination. Practitioners must maintain a high level of suspicion for CVST in high risk groups. With that in mind the clinical evaluation must be focused on uncovering and treating risk factors for CVST including significant past medical history, recent trauma, recent use of OCPs or pregnancy, infection, dehydration, or other clues as discussed above.

Table 20.2 Lists common sites of thrombus, frequency of involvement and common associated clinical syndromes

Location of CVST	Frequency (%)	Common associated syndrome
Cortical veins	17	Sensorimotor deficits (unilateral), seizures
Superior sagittal sinus	62	Sensorimotor deficits (bilateral), seizures
Straight sinus	18	Motor deficits, mental status changes (thalamic)
Deep venous system	11	Motor deficits, mental status changes (thalamic)
Transverse Sinus (left or right)	86	Isolated intracranial hypertension (headache), aphasia (usually left)
Jugular vein	12	Neck pain tinnitus, cranial nerve palsy
Cavernous sinus	1	Ocular signs—orbital pain, chemosis, proptosis, oculomotor palsy

Laboratory

Focused laboratory investigations can be of benefit in patients in whom CVST is suspected. According to the AHA/ASA guidelines, a complete blood count, chemistry panel, sedimentation rate, prothrombin time, and activated partial thromboplastin time may be useful in uncovering occult infection, or underlying coagulopathy [1].

Measurement of the fibrin breakdown product, D-dimer, can also be useful in laboratory diagnosis of CVST but should be considered in combination with an estimation of clinical suspicion. Studies have reported that positive D-dimer levels (>500 μg/ml) have been shown to be highly sensitive (94–97 %) for detection of CVST but less specific (90 %) [1]. Indeed, D-dimer is highly associated with CVST in patients with positive D-dimer levels *and* neurological deficit. False negatives were most common in patients presenting with isolated headache. The AHA/ASA guidelines point out some controversy in the use of D-dimer and further recommend that normal D-dimer level according to a sensitive immunoassay or rapid enzyme-linked immunosorbent assay (ELISA) may also be useful to help identify patients with low probability of CVST [1, 6, 32]. Thus it seems that D-dimer is best used to establish a positive diagnosis of CVST in patients with high clinical suspicion, a negative diagnosis in patients with low clinical suspicion, but is not as useful to rule out CVST in patients with high clinical suspicion. In general lab evaluation is not used as the sole or primary means of diagnosis. Imaging is the mainstay of modern diagnosis.

Imaging

Computed Tomography (Figs. 20.1, 20.2, and 20.4)

Although not the test of choice for diagnosis of CSVT, standard non-contrast head CT (Figs. 20.1a, b, e, f, 20.2a, and 20.4a) is often the first imaging study obtained in a patient presenting acutely with headache. It is helpful to rule out other more common intracranial pathologies but is only positive in about 30 % of known CVST cases [1]. There are findings on CT that can raise suspicion of CVST. These include hyperdensity of a cortical vein or dural sinus, a dense delta sign involving the posterior sagittal sinus, and ischemic lesions in a non-arterial pattern at or near a dural sinus that are sometimes associated with a characteristic fluffy appearing hemorrhage. Although rare, subarachnoid blood can be noted and is usually along the convexity and not in basilar cisterns or within the sylvian fissure [33]. Contrast enhanced CT may show a filling defect within the sinus. The addition of **CT venography** significantly improves the sensitivity of CT (Figs. 20.1c, d, 20.2a, and 20.4b, c, f) With an overall sensitivity of about 95 % and specificity of 91 %, CTV with multiplanar reconstruction is about as reliable as MRI with MR venography [34]. It can be obtained quickly, is noninvasive and is tolerated well by patients and is most useful for subacute and chronic thrombosis. It has an overall accuracy of 90–100 % and is best for detection of major dural sinus thrombosis.

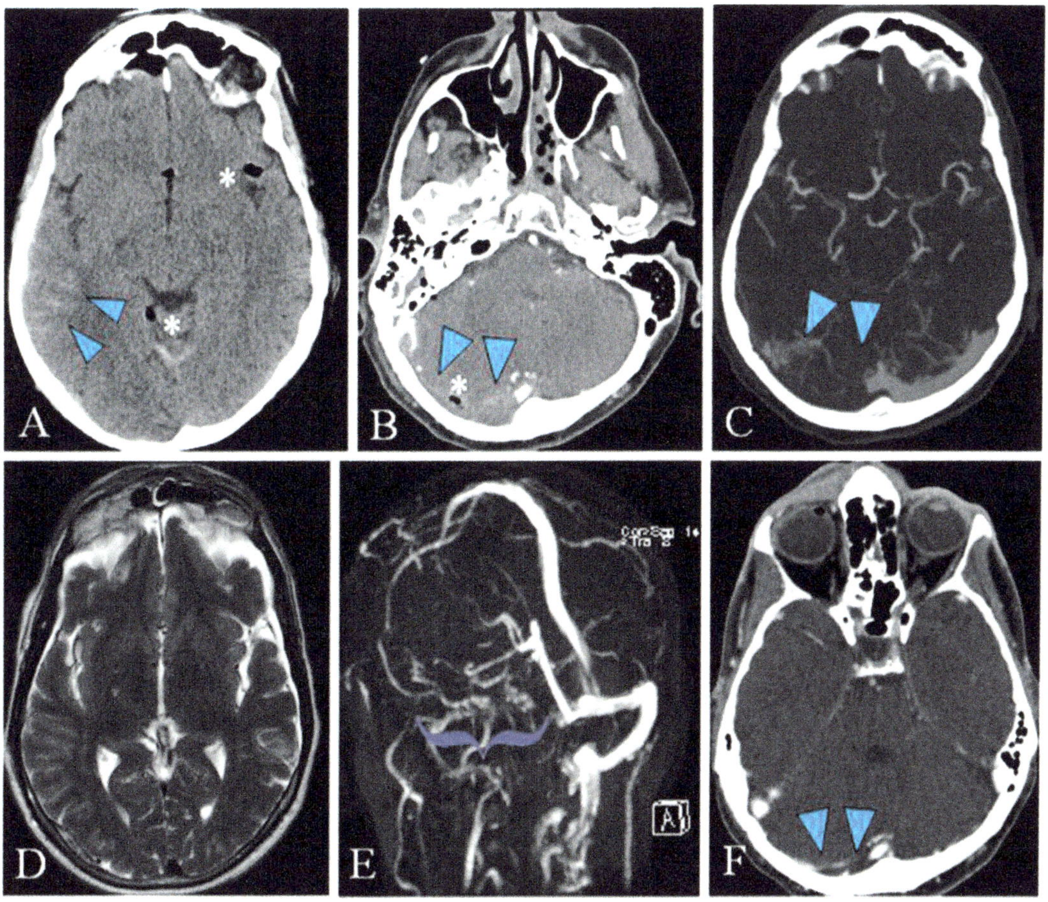

Fig. 20.4 Case III: A man with a history of seizures, CVST and a recent trauma. A 54-year-old left-handed male presented after a fall from standing 1 day prior to admission. He was amnestic to the event but thinks he may have slipped on some gravel. He hit the back of his head on the ground. He was neurologically intact on presentation but had right posterior parieto-occipital scalp bruising and bilateral racoon eyes (R>L) and right Battle's sign. He reports headache but denied nausea, vomiting, or confusion. He did have a generalized tonic-clonic seizure 2 weeks prior. An initial non-contrast head CT head (**a** and **b**) obtained for rapid evaluation in the setting of trauma. It showed trace right temporal-parietal subarachnoid hemorrhage (**a**—*arrowheads*), a transverse fracture of the right temporal bone with extensive pneumocephalus (**a**—*asterisk*) intracranially as well along the right transverse and sigmoid sinuses (**b**—*arrowheads* and *asterisk*) as well as the right jugular fossa. These findings were concerning for sinus involvement and a CTA/CTV confirmed associated thrombosis of the right transverse sinus and sigmoid sinus (**c**—*arrowheads*) as well as non-occlusive thrombosis of the right jugular vein. One day later an MRI (**d**) with MRV (**e**) was performed which confirmed the findings on CTV. 3D reconstruction demonstrates thrombosis in the transverse/sigmoid sinus (**e**—*bracket*). He was admitted to the ICU with trauma evaluation as well as neurology, ENT and ophthalmology consults. He was started on seizure prophylaxis. He remained stable with stable CT head. He was started on an IV heparin drip on post-trauma day 2. In the setting of trauma, no bolus was given and he had a goal PTT of 50–70. Serial CT head evaluation was stable and he was transitioned to coumadin for INR of 2–3 on post trauma day 5. Follow-up CT venogram 8 weeks later showed improved flow through a partially recanalized right transverse sinus (**f**—*arrowheads*). He remained clinically stable without neurologic deficit until the completion of coumadin therapy

Evaluation of cortical venous thrombosis and thrombosis of the deep venous system is relatively poor using CTV. Other drawbacks include relatively poor accuracy for visualization of smaller parenchymal lesions, radiation exposure and need for contrast in those with allergies, significant kidney dysfunction, or other contraindications [1, 19, 34].

Magnetic Resonance

The AHA/ASA 2011 guidelines recommend MR with T2-weighted imaging and **MR venography** as the imaging test of choice for evaluation of suspected CVST (Figs. 20.1g, h, 20.2b–d, and 20.4d, e) MRI/MRV provides excellent visualization of cortical veins and deep and superficial venous systems, and shows good tissue detail including micro-hemorrhagic lesions and developing cerebral edema. MRI does not expose patients to ionizing radiation but takes longer, and is difficult for patients unable to tolerate closed spaces or those with defibrillators or ferrous metal in the body. Moreover, chronic venous thrombosis, anatomic variation and slow-flow states can confound the diagnosis of CVST using MR. Using a combination of static and dynamic MR imaging techniques has been shown to improve accuracy in these cases [1, 35–37].

Digital Subtraction Angiography

Intra-arterial digital subtraction angiography (DSA) is the gold standard for visualization of CVST. However, due to the invasive, time consuming and relatively risky nature of DSA and because reliable noninvasive alternatives are readily available, DSA is no longer the recommended first choice for initial diagnosis. Its use is reserved for cases in which CTV or MR/MRV is contraindicated or cannot provide a certain diagnosis. It can provide particularly useful visualization of cortical and deep venous thrombosis. DSA is also used if endovascular therapy is under consideration (Figs. 20.2 and 20.3e, g) [1, 9].

Other

Direct venous angiography has also been used but is rarely necessary. Advanced imaging techniques such as PET or perfusion studies are rarely used in the initial diagnosis of CVST. However, there is recent interest in the use of CT perfusion as a way to follow the progression of CVST after diagnosis and initiation of treatment using systemic anticoagulation [38] or endovascular [39] techniques. There are no large well designed studies evaluating CTP, so more work needs to be done establish its clinical value and justify its widespread use in evaluation of CVST after treatment .

Treatment

Approach

As discussed above CVST is complex and presents significant diagnostic challenges. Similarly, effective treatment of CVST is also complex and often requires a multidisciplinary team within a specialized environment. Neurosurgeons are uniquely qualified because of their experience with making neurological diagnosis, dealing with critical care issues and because of their expertise in surgical and endovascular techniques. However, involvement of other specialists including neurologists, neuroradiologists, hematologists, emergency medicine practitioners, pediatricians, obstetrician/gynecologists, and others is paramount to achieve optimal outcomes.

The goal of treatment is to stabilize the patient, eliminate any treatable thrombophilic conditions, reduce clot burden/revascularize to improve venous outflow and to prevent death and disability. Thus after stabilization of the comatose or critically ill patients, the initial phase of treatment entails discovery of any conditions, such as dehydration, that can be treated. In addition, after acute CVST treatment, long-term treatment of underlying thrombophilic conditions must be considered.

Anticoagulation

Treatment of CVST with anticoagulation is somewhat controversial but there is no true equipoise [1, 40]. The consensus in the literature supports the use of anticoagulation therapy for treatment of acute CVST in adults and children [9, 20, 26, 30]. Moreover, the AHA/ASA guideline [1], and the EFNS guidelines [5] and the EPNS/SFNP guidelines for children and neonates [41], recommend therapeutic dosing of IV heparin or low molecular weight heparin (LMWH) as the primary therapy for acute CVST in most adult and pediatric patients. The controversy stems from a logical concern about hemorrhagic complications after use of anticoagulation to treat

CVST—especially those presenting with hemorrhage and the fact that there are only two well-designed randomized, controlled trials comparing anticoagulation to placebo in the general adult population. These two trials evaluate the use of IV unfractionated heparin (UFH) or subcutaneous LMWH (nandroparin) in 20 and 59 patients respectively. Meta analysis of these small trials revealed a nonsignificant trend toward reduction (−13 %) in absolute risk of death and severe disability with heparin treatment [4]. Importantly, there was no symptomatic ICH in either group after use of anticoagulation. A third randomized controlled trial of anticoagulation for CVST was performed in pregnancy-related CVST and demonstrated a benefit of UFH over no anticoagulation therapy in these women [26]. Much of the data regarding CVST comes from observational studies and in particular from the **ISCVT** which is the largest study of its kind. In this study 624 patients from 89 centers were enrolled. Most (>80 %) were treated with anticoagulation and the mortality was about 8 % at 16 months and nearly 80 % had complete recovery. *These and other studies indicate that use of PTT adjusted IV heparin or body weight adjusted LMWH is safe and effective for treatment of CVST even in the setting of hemorrhage.* Data from ISCVT indicates a range of risks for ICH after anticoagulation for CVST from 0 to 5.4 % [3]. In general treatment of CVST using IV heparin or LMWH has similar outcomes. However, a small number of small studies suggest that there may be a slight advantage of LMWH in terms of effectiveness and risk of hemorrhage [1, 6, 42]. In patients that may need surgical treatment; IV heparin may be advantageous due to the relatively short ½ life of IV heparin and ability to effectively reverse IV heparin if needed. In cases where a direct cause can be identified, stable patients should be converted to oral therapy using oral vitamin K antagonists such as warfarin and treatment continued for 3–6 months. In patients without an identifiable cause, long term oral therapy should be continued for 6–12 months. In cases of recurrence, CVST at additional sites or CVST in setting of severe underlying prothrombotic states (i.e., antithrombin deficiency), lifetime oral anticoagulation may be considered [5, 26, 43]. Newer generation oral anticoagulation agents, such as dabigatran or direct factor Xa inhibitors, have been tried with some success in case series but no high quality data is available to support the widespread use of these medications [44, 45]. In addition to prevention of progressive or recurrent CVST, long-term oral anticoagulation therapy is also aimed at preventing venous thromboembolism in the lung or other extracranial sites. Consultation with a hematologist for management of complex cases may be of benefit [1].

Endovascular Therapy

Anticoagulation therapy acts mainly to prevent extension of thrombosis and has significantly improved the prognosis associated with CVST. , However, 9–13 % of CVST patients have poor outcomes despite being adequately anticoagulated. High risk patients, especially those with large clot burdens and persistent underlying prothrombotic conditions, are more likely to fail anticoagulation treatment. This is often due to incomplete or partial recanalization that can occur in greater than 50 % of patients treated with anticoagulation alone. In patients that deteriorate or progress despite anticoagulation, endovascular measures including direct local thrombolysis or mechanical thrombectomy and others may be considered [1]. These therapies have the benefit of dissolving the thrombus leading to more rapid recanalization. There have been multiple small reports composed of case reports and series that have shown benefit of endovascular therapies in selected patients but no large randomized controlled studies have been performed. A recent review of the literature on mechanical thrombectomy for treatment of CVST reports on a total of 64 patients from case reports and case series. IV heparin use was reported in 60 patients, not used in one patient and not reported in three patients. 48 % of patients had a hemorrhage at presentation. There were nine reported complications and after a mean follow-up period of about 28 weeks nine patients had died. After the same follow-up period, 62 % had good outcome with documented MRS of 0–2 [46]. In the ISCVT study 38 % of patients treated using thrombolysis (local or systemic) died. There is a great deal of potential bias in the reports about thrombolysis for CVST. The patients usually have a more severe clinical condition but there is also publication bias for positive findings.

Several possible endovascular techniques have been reported. These include direct catheter thrombolysis, balloon assisted thrombectomy/thrombolysis, catheter based thrombectomy/thrombolysis, stenting or stent based thrombus retrieval. Further evaluation must be done to determine which among these techniques provides a meaningful benefit [47–50]. Endovascular therapy seems to be a safe and effective option and some have even suggested its use as a first line treatment [51]. However, at this time, endovascular therapy can only be recommended in cases of failed anticoagulation therapy [1, 52]. In a prospective case series of 20 patients with CVST, patients with large hemorrhagic infarcts did not benefit from endovascular thrombolysis. This may be due in part to the potential for increase in size of the lesion and the associated increased risk of herniation [6, 53].

The *Thrombolysis or anticoagulation for cerebral venous thrombosis* (TO-ACT) trial opened in 2011 and is currently ongoing with 50 patients enrolled (http://www.to-act-trial.org/). The TO-ACT trial is a multicenter, prospective, randomized, open-label, blinded endpoint trial designed to determine if ET improves the functional outcome of patients with a severe form of CVST Patients are included if they have a radiologically proven CVST, a high probability of poor outcome (defined by presence of one or more of the following risk factors: mental status disorder, coma, intracranial hemorrhagic lesion, or thrombosis of the deep cerebral venous system), and if the responsible physician believes that there is clinical equipoise between endovascular thrombolysis or standard anticoagulant treatment. One hundred sixty four patients (82 in each treatment arm) will be included to detect a 50 % relative reduction (from 40 to 20 %) of poor outcomes [54].

Systemic thrombolysis has also been used in limited cases. There are no randomized clinical trials, but a recent meta-analysis reports on a total of 26 patients from 16 reports. In this group of patients, most regained independence with 88 % achieving MRS 0–2 [55]. However, there were three serious bleeding events and two deaths. The results of systemic thrombolysis were similar to local thrombolysis noted in other studies. As with other therapies, there is a serious risk of hemorrhagic complication and more work needs to be done to establish the role and safety of systemic thrombolysis. But it may represent an additional tool for treatment of patients who fail anticoagulation therapy. It has the advantage of being non-invasive and potentially more widely available than local thrombolysis using endovascular techniques.

Surgery

As endovascular techniques have improved, the need for direct surgical treatment of CVST has nearly disappeared. On the rare occasion that indirect transvenous access cannot be obtained, surgical exposure of a dural sinus may be used to provide direct access for endovascular therapy.

Hemicraniectomy

The main cause of death in patients with CVST is transtentorial herniation due to a unilateral lesion or diffuse edema from multiple intraparenchymal lesions [56]. In recent studies as many as 4.3 % of patients die in the acute phases of CVST. In patients that fail medical and/or endovascular treatments, **hemicraniectomy** has been demonstrated to be an effective and life saving measure in patients with malignant edema, large space occupying lesions and/or clinical evidence of herniation (Fig. 20.1) [1, 57–60]. There are no well designed studies to evaluate the clinical effectiveness of hemicraniectomy for CVST, but in small patient series, despite more severe clinical presentations, most patients demonstrate good or excellent outcomes at follow-up [58, 59, 61, 62].

Treatment of Associated Problems

Seizures

Seizures are common in CVST occurring in 37 % of adults, 48 % of children, and 71 % of neonates [1, 29]. Seizures can be dangerous due to the increased risk of anoxic damage. Therefore treatment of documented seizure with appropriate antiepileptic medications is recommended to reduce the risk of further seizures [1, 5]. Prophylactic use of AEDs is controversial because there is a paucity of data to support its use. Despite this the EFNS suggests that prophylactic antiepileptic therapy may be a therapeutic option in patients deemed high risk for seizure such as those with focal neurological deficits and supratentorial lesions on admission CT/MRI [5], whereas the AHA/ASA guidelines states that in the absence of seizure, routine prophylactic use of AEDs is not recommended [1].

Intracranial Hypertension

Intracranial hypertension is common in CVST but frank hydrocephalus is not. However, in patients with persistently elevated intracranial pressures and associated problems such as severe headache, papilledema or vision loss, altered level of consciousness or cranial nerve palsy, specific measures to manage elevated ICP can be instituted. Reasonable measures include lumbar puncture, use of acetazolamide, ventriculostomy, or even shunting if indicated [1, 63, 64]. However, recent subgroup analysis of 15 patients from the ISCVT study suggests that CSF diversion may not be effective in preventing death from herniation [63]. Ophthalmologic consultation should be considered to evaluate for possible optic nerve fenestration in the setting of intractable intracranial hypertension.

Steroids

Steroids are not recommended [1]

Sequelae

The current prognosis of CVST is good. Over 85 % are reported to have good outcomes (MRS <2) at 16 month follow-up and only about 10 % were dead or severely disabled [3]. Despite this some patients experience chronic headaches (50 %), late seizures (5 %), visual problems recurrence (4 %), or VTE in extracranial sites (5.5 %) [1]. Other more rare problems such as dural arteriovenous fistulae are also noted (Fig. 20.2). dAVF may also be causative in some cases of CVST.

Special Groups

Special consideration must be taken when treating pregnant women or children. Specialty consultation with obstetrics/gynecology and pediatrics or neonatology would be recommended. The clinical characteristics and presentations are similar but do have some important variations as mentioned above. The incidence ranges from 1 in 2500 to 1 in 10,000 during pregnancy. As much as 73 % of all CVST in women occur during pregnancy. It is most likely during the last trimester and first postpartum month. Treatment principles are similar in pregnant women and anticoagulation is the mainstay of therapy. *However unfractionated heparin is teratogenic and warfarin is associated with fetal embryopathy and bleeding. Thus, LMWH is the treatment of choice and should be continued throughout the entire pregnancy followed by LMWH or warfarin in the postpartum period.* In women with a history of CVST, future pregnancy is not contraindicated but prophylaxis with LMWH during the pregnancy may be advisable [1].

In children, neonatal CVST has the highest incidence. Outcomes are worse in neonates as compared to older children and adults. Forces on the child's head during birth and a lack of circulating anticoagulant factors put neonates at increased risk. Careful monitoring must be undertaken because this population cannot easily communicate problems. Surveillance for visual disturbances and papilledema is recommended. Continuous EEG is advisable for comatose patients. Investigation for underlying thrombophilia should be undertaken [1, 41]. Anticoagulation for 3–6 months with UFH or LMWH followed by warfarin is the recommended treatment for children greater than 28 weeks old even in the presence of hemorrhage. The data regarding use of anticoagulation in neonates is not clear. The EPNS/SFNP guidelines suggest that anticoagulation for neonates with acute CVST may be safe and effective but that it must be evaluated on a case by case basis. If chosen, anticoagulation should be continued for a shorter period of 6–12 weeks [1, 41].

Clinical Care Algorithm (Fig. 20.5)

A potential clinical care algorithm is presented in Fig. 20.5.

Conclusion and Future Directions

CVST is a relative rare stroke subtype that preferentially affects the young. There are wide variations in clinical presentation that make timely diagnosis and effective treatment challenging. Fortunately, as a result of modern imaging and treatment paradigms, the prognosis for CVST has been improving. As study of this interesting problem continues, it is likely that the prognosis will continue to improve. Additional study needs to be undertaken to evaluate endovascular therapy for use in high risk patients and/or in patients after failing standard anticoagulation treatment. It is also being considered for use as a first line

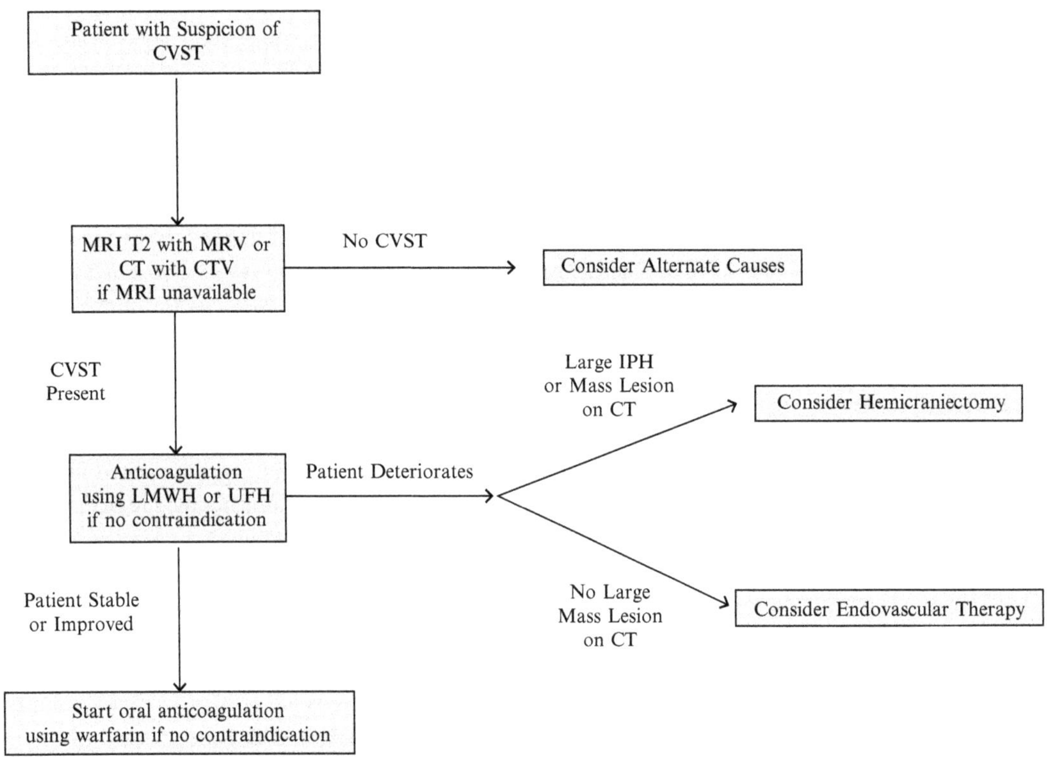

Fig. 20.5 Proposed clinical algorithm for CVST. It is not comprehensive and each patient must be considered on a case-by-case basis. This takes into account current data but may change as more information becomes available especially regarding newer treatments including novel anticoagulants and endovascular therapies. In addition to above patients must be evaluated and stabilized if necessary. Patients should also receive necessary treatment for associated conditions including intracranial hypertension, visual changes, seizures, and coma. Oral anticoagulation therapy should be continued for at least 3 months in adults depending on the underlying cause

approach. The ongoing TO-ACT trial will hopefully address some of these issues. Laboratory investigation of molecular signaling and associated molecular imaging may lead to the ability to diagnose CVST even earlier. Screening in high risk groups could be considered in certain circumstances. Indeed, prevention along with screening, counseling or other methodologies will be an essential element in the overall "treatment" of CVST. As awareness improves and more is known about how and why CVST affects certain groups, more can be done to prevent or eliminate CVST. The neurosurgeon is an integral part of the modern multidisciplinary approach to CVST and thus must maintain a high clinical awareness for CVST and be familiar with the use of anticoagulation and other treatment options for CVST.

References

1. Saposnik G, et al. Diagnosis and management of cerebral venous thrombosis: a statement for healthcare professionals from the American Heart Association/American Stroke Association. Stroke. 2011;42(4):1158–92.
2. Coutinho JM, Zuurbier SM, Stam J. Declining mortality in cerebral venous thrombosis: a systematic review. Stroke. 2014;45(5):1338–41.
3. Ferro JM, et al. Prognosis of cerebral vein and dural sinus thrombosis: results of the International Study on Cerebral Vein and Dural Sinus Thrombosis (ISCVT). Stroke. 2004;35(3):664–70.
4. Coutinho J et al. Anticoagulation for cerebral venous sinus thrombosis. Cochrane Database Syst Rev. 2011(8):CD002005.
5. Einhaupl K, et al. EFNS guideline on the treatment of cerebral venous and sinus thrombosis in adult patients. Eur J Neurol. 2010;17(10):1229–35.
6. Weimar C. Diagnosis and treatment of cerebral venous and sinus thrombosis. Curr Neurol Neurosci Rep. 2014;14(1):417.
7. Ribes M. Des recherches faites sur la phlebite. Rev Med Franc Etrang. 1825;3:5–41.
8. Yakovlev SB, et al. Endovascular treatment of acute thrombosis of cerebral veins and sinuses. Neuroradiol J. 2014;27(4):471–8.
9. Stam J. Thrombosis of the cerebral veins and sinuses. N Engl J Med. 2005;352(17):1791–8.
10. Coutinho JM, et al. The incidence of cerebral venous thrombosis: a cross-sectional study. Stroke. 2012;43(12):3375–7.
11. Ruiz-Sandoval JL, et al. Cerebral venous thrombosis in a Mexican multicenter registry of acute cerebrovascular disease: the RENAMEVASC study. J Stroke Cerebrovasc Dis. 2012;21(5):395–400.
12. Borhani Haghighi A, et al. Mortality of cerebral venous-sinus thrombosis in a large national sample. Stroke. 2012;43(1):262–4.
13. Hinnell C, et al. Sex differences in adult cerebral venous sinus thrombosis: a 10-year experience. Can J Neurol Sci. 2012;39(1):74–7.
14. Coutinho JM, et al. Cerebral venous and sinus thrombosis in women. Stroke. 2009;40(7):2356–61.
15. Stracke CP, et al. Molecular MRI of cerebral venous sinus thrombosis using a new fibrin-specific MR contrast agent. Stroke. 2007;38(5):1476–81.
16. Ferro JM, et al. Delay in the diagnosis of cerebral vein and dural sinus thrombosis: influence on outcome. Stroke. 2009;40(9):3133–8.
17. Pfefferkorn T, et al. Clinical features, course and outcome in deep cerebral venous system thrombosis: an analysis of 32 cases. J Neurol. 2009;256(11):1839–45.
18. Filippidis A, et al. Cerebral venous sinus thrombosis: review of the demographics, pathophysiology, current diagnosis, and treatment. Neurosurg Focus. 2009; 27(5):E3.
19. Piazza G. Cerebral venous thrombosis. Circulation. 2012;125(13):1704–9.
20. Wasay M, et al. Cerebral venous sinus thrombosis in children: a multicenter cohort from the United States. J Child Neurol. 2008;23(1):26–31.
21. Narayan D, et al. Risk factors, clinical profile, and long-term outcome of 428 patients of cerebral sinus venous thrombosis: insights from Nizam's Institute Venous Stroke Registry, Hyderabad (India). Neurol India. 2012;60(2):154–9.
22. Sidhom Y, et al. Cerebral venous thrombosis: clinical features, risk factors, and long-term outcome in a Tunisian cohort. J Stroke Cerebrovasc Dis. 2014;23(6):1291–5.
23. Hedlund GL. Cerebral sinovenous thrombosis in pediatric practice. Pediatr Radiol. 2013;43(2):173–88.
24. Kate MP, Thomas B, Sylaja PN. Cerebral venous thrombosis in post-lumbar puncture intracranial hypotension: case report and review of literature. F1000Res. 2014;3:41.
25. Rivkin MA, Saraiya PV, Woodrow SI. Sinovenous thrombosis associated with skull fracture in the setting of blunt head trauma. Acta Neurochir (Wien). 2014;156(5):999–1007. discussion 1007.
26. Thorell SE, et al. Cerebral venous thrombosis-A primer for the haematologist. Blood Rev. 2015;29(1):45–50.
27. Gameiro J, et al. Prognosis of cerebral vein thrombosis presenting as isolated headache: early vs. late diagnosis. Cephalalgia. 2012;32(5):407–12.
28. Coutinho JM, et al. Cerebral venous thrombosis in the absence of headache. Stroke. 2015;46(1):245–7.
29. Ferro JM, et al. Early seizures in cerebral vein and dural sinus thrombosis: risk factors and role of antiepileptics. Stroke. 2008;39(4):1152–8.
30. Kernan WN, et al. Guidelines for the prevention of stroke in patients with stroke and transient ischemic attack: a guideline for healthcare professionals from the American Heart Association/American Stroke Association. Stroke. 2014;45(7):2160–236.

31. Ferro JM, et al. Cerebral vein and dural sinus thrombosis in elderly patients. Stroke. 2005;36(9):1927–32.
32. Dentali F, et al. D-dimer testing in the diagnosis of cerebral vein thrombosis: a systematic review and a meta-analysis of the literature. J Thromb Haemost. 2012;10(4):582–9.
33. Panda S, et al. Localized convexity subarachnoid haemorrhage--a sign of early cerebral venous sinus thrombosis. Eur J Neurol. 2010;17(10):1249–58.
34. Wetzel SG, et al. Cerebral veins: comparative study of CT venography with intraarterial digital subtraction angiography. AJNR Am J Neuroradiol. 1999;20(2):249–55.
35. Meckel S, et al. Cerebral venous thrombosis: diagnostic accuracy of combined, dynamic and static, contrast-enhanced 4D MR venography. AJNR Am J Neuroradiol. 2010;31(3):527–35.
36. Idbaih A, et al. MRI of clot in cerebral venous thrombosis: high diagnostic value of susceptibility-weighted images. Stroke. 2006;37(4):991–5.
37. Ihn YK, Jung WS, Hwang SS. The value of T2*-weighted gradient-echo MRI for the diagnosis of cerebral venous sinus thrombosis. Clin Imaging. 2013;37(3):446–50.
38. Gupta RK, et al. Prognostic indices for cerebral venous thrombosis on CT perfusion: a prospective study. Eur J Radiol. 2014;83(1):185–90.
39. Lin N, et al. Reversible changes in diffusion- and perfusion-based imaging in cerebral venous sinus thrombosis. BMJ Case Rep. 2015. doi:10.1136/bcr-2014-011447.
40. Cundiff DK. Evidence-basis for anticoagulants for cerebral sinus venous thrombosis? Stroke. 2013;44(6):e67.
41. Lebas A, et al. EPNS/SFNP guideline on the anticoagulant treatment of cerebral sinovenous thrombosis in children and neonates. Eur J Paediatr Neurol. 2012;16(3):219–28.
42. Coutinho JM, et al. Unfractionated or low-molecular weight heparin for the treatment of cerebral venous thrombosis. Stroke. 2010;41(11):2575–80.
43. Caprio F, Bernstein RA. Duration of anticoagulation after cerebral venous sinus thrombosis. Neurocrit Care. 2012;16(2):335–42.
44. Geisbusch C, et al. Novel factor xa inhibitor for the treatment of cerebral venous and sinus thrombosis: first experience in 7 patients. Stroke. 2014;45(8):2469–71.
45. Mendonca MD, et al. Oral direct thrombin inhibitor as an alternative in the management of cerebral venous thrombosis: a series of 15 patients. Int J Stroke. 2015;10(7):1115–8.
46. Haghighi AB, et al. Mechanical thrombectomy for cerebral venous sinus thrombosis: a comprehensive literature review. Clin Appl Thromb Hemost. 2013;20(5):507–15.
47. Khan IS, et al. Endovascular thrombolysis for pediatric cerebral sinus venous thrombosis with tissue plasminogen activator and abciximab. J Neurosurg Pediatr. 2014;13(1):68–71.
48. Choudhri O, et al. Endovascular management of cerebral venous sinus thrombosis. Neurosurg Focus. 2014;37(1 Suppl):1.
49. Coutinho JM, Middeldorp S, Stam J. Advances in the treatment of cerebral venous thrombosis. Curr Treat Options Neurol. 2014;16(7):299.
50. Shaikh H, et al. Combined use of Solitaire FR and Penumbra devices for endovascular treatment of cerebral venous sinus thrombosis in a child. BMJ Case Rep. 2014. doi:10.1136/bcr-2013-011088.
51. Dashti SR, et al. Mechanical thrombectomy as first-line treatment for venous sinus thrombosis: technical considerations and preliminary results using the AngioJet device. J Neurointerv Surg. 2013;5(1):49–53.
52. Coutinho JM, et al. Mechanical thrombectomy cannot be considered as first-line treatment for cerebral venous thrombosis. J Neurointerv Surg. 2013;5(6):621–2.
53. Stam J, et al. Endovascular thrombectomy and thrombolysis for severe cerebral sinus thrombosis: a prospective study. Stroke. 2008;39(5):1487–90.
54. Coutinho JM, et al. Thrombolysis or anticoagulation for cerebral venous thrombosis: rationale and design of the TO-ACT trial. Int J Stroke. 2013;8(2):135–40.
55. Viegas LD, et al. Systemic thrombolysis for cerebral venous and dural sinus thrombosis: a systematic review. Cerebrovasc Dis. 2014;37(1):43–50.
56. Canhao P, et al. Causes and predictors of death in cerebral venous thrombosis. Stroke. 2005;36(8):1720–5.
57. Ferro JM, et al. Decompressive surgery in cerebrovenous thrombosis: a multicenter registry and a systematic review of individual patient data. Stroke. 2011;42(10):2825–31.
58. Aaron S, et al. Decompressive craniectomy in cerebral venous thrombosis: a single centre experience. J Neurol Neurosurg Psychiatry. 2013;84(9):995–1000.
59. Raza E, et al. Decompressive surgery for malignant cerebral venous sinus thrombosis: a retrospective case series from Pakistan and comparative literature review. J Stroke Cerebrovasc Dis. 2014;23(1):e13–22.
60. Theaudin M, et al. Should decompressive surgery be performed in malignant cerebral venous thrombosis? A series of 12 patients. Stroke. 2010;41(4):727–31.
61. Zuurbier SM, et al. Decompressive hemicraniectomy in severe cerebral venous thrombosis: a prospective case series. J Neurol. 2012;259(6):1099–105.
62. Mohindra S, et al. Decompressive craniectomy for malignant cerebral oedema of cortical venous thrombosis: an analysis of 13 patients. Br J Neurosurg. 2011;25(3):422–9.
63. Lobo S, et al. Shunting in acute cerebral venous thrombosis: a systematic review. Cerebrovasc Dis. 2014;37(1):38–42.
64. Canhao P, et al. Safety of lumbar puncture in patients with cerebral venous thrombosis. Eur J Neurol. 2013;20(7):1075–80.

Coagulation Studies in Preoperative Neurosurgery Patients

21

Hugh J.L. Garton

Introduction

This chapter focuses on the preoperative coagulation assessment of patients undergoing cranial and spinal neurosurgery. Although it has been common, even standard, practice to obtain preoperative laboratory assessment of the platelet count, prothrombin time (PT)/international standardized ratio (INR), and activated partial thromboplastin time (aPTT) in adult patients in preoperative neurosurgical settings, the value of this practice has been questioned and the published evidence on this topic suggests that the routine use of these studies neither reliably identifies patients who will suffer surgical bleeding complications nor safely excludes those who will not. As a result, a variety of alternative laboratory assessments like bleeding time (BT), and platelet function tests such as the PFA-100 have sparked interest. Similarly, clinical assessment tools to formalize preoperative history taking with respect to coagulation issues have also been developed and continue to be refined. However, as of this writing none have clearly demonstrated a high sensitivity and specificity for the outcomes of interest. Nevertheless, understanding the various available laboratory tests and clinical assessment tools provides the basis for informed decision making with respect to patient care in this area.

The Coagulation Cascade

The standard teaching of the coagulation cascade as divided into an extrinsic, intrinsic, and common pathway has been of value in understanding how particular coagulation assays work in the laboratory. However understanding in vivo coagulation requires a blurring of these two pathways. Davies et al. and Macfarland described the "waterfall" sequence of enzymes that are sequentially activated following exposure to a triggering bleeding event [1, 2]. Exposure of blood to glass in a laboratory resulted in activation of the intrinsic (contact-activated) enzyme cascade including factors XII, XI, IX, and VIII. Exposure of blood to calcium, phospholipid, and tissue factor resulted in activation of the extrinsic (tissue factor) pathway, including primarily factor VII. The products of either pathway lead to the activation of factor X which cleaves prothrombin to thrombin (IIa) which in turn converts fibrinogen to the fibrin that forms the actual clot. Fibrin is further acted upon by Factor XIII to cross-link the fibrin clot [3] (Fig. 21.1—Intrinsic, Extrinsic, and Common pathways). In vivo, the extrinsic, tissue factor pathway is the more important primary mechanism, while the intrinsic pathway performs

H.J.L. Garton, M.D., M.H.Sc. (✉)
Department of Neurosurgery, University of Michigan, Ann Arbor, MI, USA
e-mail: hgarton@umich.edu

C.M. Loftus (ed.), *Anticoagulation and Hemostasis in Neurosurgery*, DOI 10.1007/978-3-319-27327-3_21

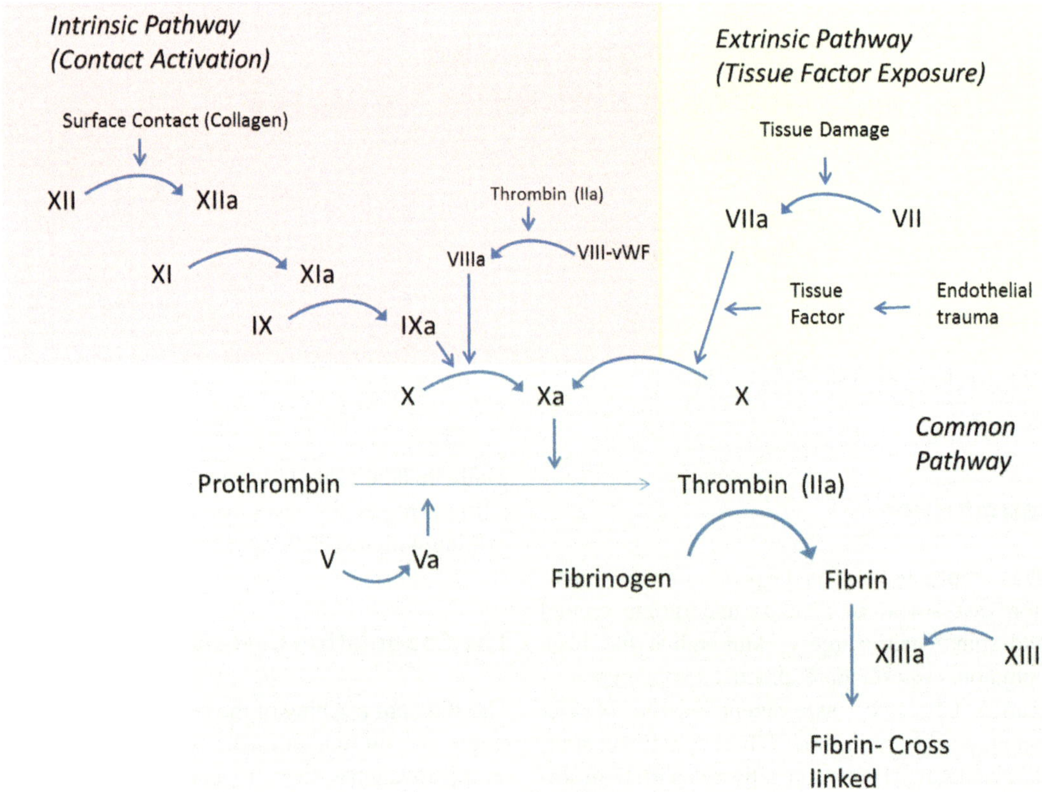

Fig. 21.1 Coagulation cascade, fibrinolytic and pathway inhibitors such as Protein C, S, Antithrombin III omitted for simplicity

a secondary role in the normal state. The current, cell-based model of blood clotting blurs the lines between these two separate pathways, focusing instead on phases of the coagulation process, namely initiation, amplification, propagation, stabilization, and finally attenuation. Blood clotting begins with the exposure of subendothelial von Willebrand's Factor (vWF) and collagen, resulting in platelet adhesion. Adhered platelets subsequently undergo degranulation to become activated and release several coagulation cascade proteins (V, VIII) and stimulate production of thromboxane A2 (TxA2). TxA2 with ADP helps aggregate additional platelets to form the platelet plug. Coincident with the platelet process and interconnected with it, the initiation phase of coagulation begins with the exposure of circulating factor VII to tissue factor (TF) in the subendothelium forming an activated FVIIa-TF complex. This cleaves/activates Factor X to Xa, which generates thrombin (IIa) by a similar cleavage. However, this initial phase creates only a modest amount of thrombin. To form a robust clot, a second "amplification" stage is needed, in which thrombin from the initiation stage binds to platelets, promoting the release and activation of factors VIII and V from platelet granules. Subsequently, in the propagation phase, these factors significantly enhance the conversion of Factor X to Xa (tenase complex, on the surface of activated platelets, using FIXa, FVIIIa) and prothrombin to thrombin (prothrombinase complex, on the surface of activated platelets, using FXa, Va) in the propagation stage. Finally, the forming clot is stabilized as thrombin catalyzes factor XIII to XIIIa, which, as noted above, cross-links the Fibrin [3–6]. A fourth "attenuation" phase is often also included to describe the regulatory components that prevent excessive thrombosis (Fig. 21.2: Coagulation cascade—cell-based model).

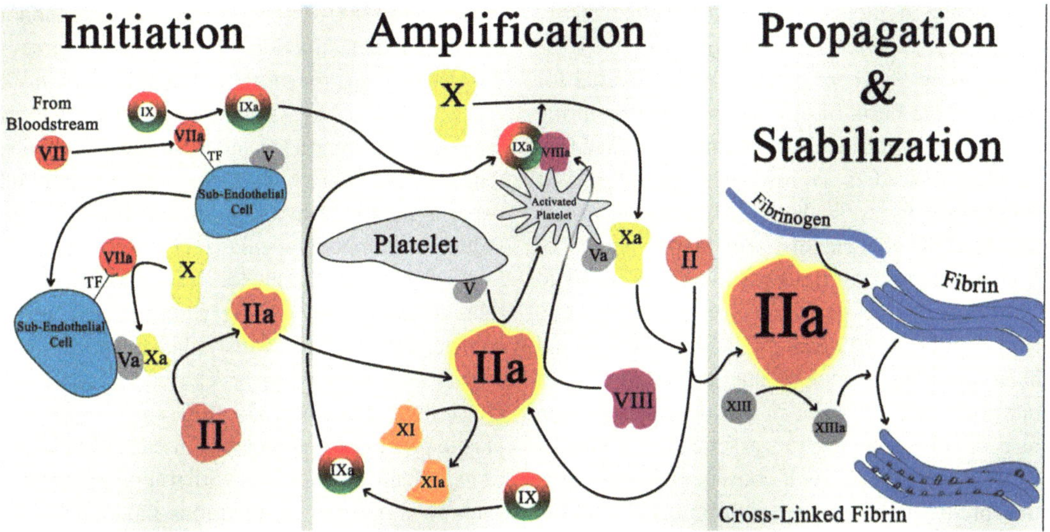

Fig. 21.2 Cell-based model of coagulation, illustrated by T. Garton, based on: [3, 5, 6]

Preoperative Screening Guidelines

No formal guidelines on preoperative coagulation testing specific to neurosurgery patients exist. General guidelines relating to surgical patients have however appeared from a number of mostly European medical societies. *The British Committee for Standards in Haematology published guidelines in 2008. The primary recommendation were as follows: one, routine use of presurgical laboratory screening in unselected patients was not recommended; two, a personal and family bleeding history and identification of consumed antithrombotic medications should be performed in all patients; three, in the face of a negative bleeding history no further laboratory studies are necessary; four, a positive history or observed clinically concerning condition such as liver failure necessitates a comprehensive assessment* [7]. The evidentiary basis for these recommendations was limited by the rarity of high-quality prospective studies, such that these recommendations were all grade B or C recommendations, supported by level III or IV evidence. *Conversely, the Italian Society for Hemostasis and Thrombosis recommended that aPTT, PT, and platelet count should be obtained in both adult and pediatric patients even in the face of a negative bleeding history.* The evidence at the time of publication (2009) was essentially the same for both groups, but the Italian society specifically noted that they viewed the potential for failing to identify an avoidable bleeding complication as paramount and the cost of testing as less important [8]. The possible adverse medical consequences of falsely positive screening studies were not addressed directly. French and German Anesthetic societies published recent guidelines similar to the British guidelines [9, 10]. *Specific to children, the Italian Society of Pediatric and Neonatal Anesthesia and Intensive Care recommended that children undergo a standardized questionnaire assessment and that coagulation tests be reserved for positive history or in cases with a specifically high risk of bleeding* [11]. *The American Society of Anesthesiologists advises that preoperative tests not be ordered routinely, but should be selectively used when clinical characteristics suggest a bleeding disorder, renal dysfunction, or liver dysfunction and "depending on the type and invasiveness of the procedure"* [12].

The utility of preoperative screening depends in part on the frequency or prevalence of abnormalities. Considering the general presurgical patient, the incidence of laboratory abnormality on unselected patients ranges from 0.5 % to 16 % vs. up to 40 % where patients were selected for study on the basis of clinical history [9]. In the pediatric population, the incidence of congenital bleeding disorders is low. For example, Von Willebrand disease is the most frequent congenital bleeding abnormality with a prevalence of approximately 1:500; however only 1 in 10 to 1 in 20 of these patients are symptomatic. Hemophilia A (Factor VIII deficiency) and hemophilia B (Factor IX deficiency) occur at rates of 1 in 5000 and 1 in 25,000 male children respectively, reducing the practicality of preoperative testing [13]. As a consequence, the positive predictive values of abnormal coagulation studies (the % of patient with a positive test who actually have a bleeding disorder) in the general preoperative setting are low, ranging from a high of 22 %, to more commonly <10 % in nine studies identified in one guideline review [7].

When initial tests are abnormal, often, testing conditions rather than patient pathology are to blame. One study looking at pediatric patients undergoing routine testing prior to tonsillectomy noted that 0.1 % of 1600 patients had abnormal PT, PTT, or BT on initial screening, but in half of these repeat testing was normal [14].

Despite the aforementioned guidelines, preoperative hemostatic testing remains a common practice. It has been argued that laboratory studies could play an important role when preoperative history taking is inadequate either based on limitations of the provider to ask or the patient to provide the necessary information. Pediatric patients, particularly young pediatric patients, may not have had sufficient life exposure to hemorrhage inducing events. Or patients may recently have acquired a bleeding diathesis, as in the case of acquired von Willebrand disease in aortic valve stenosis [15].

Individual Hematologic Tests

Platelet Count

The platelet count measures the quantity of platelets in a cubic mm of whole blood. The normal range is 150,000–400,000/mm^3. The test cannot assess platelet function. *Neurosurgical procedural thresholds for platelets have typically been 100,000/mm^3* [16]. Because heparin use is extremely common in neurosurgical patients, repeat assessment of platelet count for patient on heparin therapy is important in detecting heparin-induced thrombocytopenia (HIT), with the absolute value of the count less important than the relative change [17]. Falsely thrombocytopenic values can occur with platelet clumping. Thrombocytopenia can be caused by processes that reduce platelet production, such myelodysplastic processes and their treatments, viral infections, splenic enlargement with trapping platelets, such as may occur in infectious mononucleosis, and platelet consumption as occurs in sepsis, thrombocytic thrombocytopenic purpura (TTP), and autoimmune processes such as HIT.

Platelet Function Assays

Platelet function assays attempt to recreate platelet aggregation in vitro. The PFA-100 is one common example of this type of testing. Whole blood is tested for the rate at which it occludes an aperture in a testing membrane coated with either epinephrine or adenosine diphosphate. Normal closing times are <120 s. The study is frequently used to assess the impact of aspirin on platelet function, to which it is quite sensitive [18]. It has also been used to assess for von Willebrand disease. A recent meta-analysis suggests it performs well as a screening tool for this disorder in the setting of a specialty pediatric hematology clinic [13]. The test is, however, also sensitive to anemia, thrombocytopenia, and other pharmacological agents affecting platelet function.

The PFA-100 is not useful for assessing the degree of platelet inhibition from alternative agents such as clopidogrel. Clopidogrel is a commonly used antiplatelet thienopyridine that functions by blocking the P2Y12 receptor for ADP on the platelet surface. This blocks both platelet activation and limits the participation of platelets in fibrin cross-linking [19]. The extent to which P2Y12 inhibitors successfully block platelet activity is variable and the concept of Clopidogrel resistance or nonresponsiveness has been aggressively pursued in the cardiovascular medicine. Because agents like Clopidogrel also have an important role in neuroendovascular procedures, preoperative assessments of the extent of P2Y12 inhibition are becoming more common. The P2Y12 platelet function test, known commercially by names like Verify Now P2Y12, measures the effect of clopidogrel on platelet function by comparing the degree of aggregation caused by attempting to stimulate the P2y12 receptor pathway with adenosine diphosphate/prostacyclin E1 and comparing this to the degree of platelet aggregation caused by stimulation of the thrombin receptor activating peptide (TARP), which bypasses the P2Y12 pathway and serves as a baseline for comparison. Results are reported in both arbitrary units related to the change in optical properties of the specimen or as a ratio, or percentage of inhibition comparing the two parts of the assay. Whether using a thrombin-based platelet activation test as a baseline value is accurate is debated, and on/off clopidogrel testing may be more accurate [20].

The screen filtration pressure method (SFP) of platelet aggregation assessment is another alternative procedure in common use. This method assesses the changes in back pressure as blood is forced through a screen with openings 20–40 μm square [21]. To assess platelet aggregation, whole blood is mixed with ADP.

aPTT

The activated partial thromboplastin time (aPTT) tests the "contact" or intrinsic clotting pathway factors including factors XII, XI, and IX and to a lesser extent common pathway factors X, V, II, and fibrinogen. The patient's serum is mixed with phospholipid (which lacks tissue factor, hence the *partial* thromboplastin time), and calcium against a contact surface such as silica or kaolin [7]. The formation of a clot is tracked usually by light transmission and the time measured in seconds. Normal values are between 20 and 35 s. Importantly, the aPTT does not assess factor VII, which is part of the extrinsic pathway [5]. As a clinical tool, it screens for factor deficiencies of >50 % in VII, IX, and XI [9]. *Importantly aPTT is sensitive to inhibition of thrombin, and hence is used to monitor therapy with unfractionated heparin, but is relatively insensitive to alterations in Factor Xa levels and so insensitive to the effects of Xa inhibitors (see below).* The aPTT will be prolonged in the presence of other inhibitors such as the lupus anticoagulant and fibrin split products, such as is seen in disseminated intravascular coagulation.

PT/INR

The prothrombin time measures the primary tissue factor-driven or extrinsic coagulation pathway. Thus it assesses factor VII and the common factors of II, V, X and Fibrinogen. Citrated plasma, calcium, and tissue thromboplastin (containing tissue factor) are combined and clot formation typically measured optically. Normal values are typically 10–15 s. *The PT is prolonged in Vitamin K deficiency, Factor VII deficiencies, and, of course, warfarin therapy, for which the INR is usually followed* [5, 7].

The International Normalized Ratio (INR) was introduced to standardize the PT time, given that there was some variability in the thromboplastin reagents used in the reaction. The $INR = (\text{Patient PT/mean normal PT})^{ISI}$. ISI is a value assigned to the specific reagents used. Normal values are 0.9–1.2 [22]. However, increases in reagent sensitivity mean that higher concentrations of factor VII are typically present at higher INR values than was previously the case. Matevosyan and colleague noted that in 25 neurosurgery patients with INR 1.3–1.7, the plasma concentrations of the important factors II, VII, and VII were all above generally accepted surgical thresholds and argued against correcting for INR values at these levels [23].

The level at which an elevated prothrombin time (PT) should be considered clinically relevant in neurosurgical patients has been debated. INR values were developed to assess patients taking Vitamin K antagonists, specifically Coumadin. *It is common practice to see preoperative treatment initiated for INR > 1.3. West and colleagues surveyed the literature and concluded that patients with INR 1.5 or less, in the absence of clinical bleeding, should not be treated for this with FFP preoperatively* [24].

Bleeding Time (BT)

Bleeding time should be the ideal tool for assessing the likelihood of excessive surgical bleeding, since it would appear to assess all aspects of the clotting process, recreating surgical tissue trauma in a controlled fashion. It is generally considered to be an assay of platelet function more than other aspects of the clotting pathway, and is used in assessing von Willebrand disease (vWD), as well as other disorders of platelet-vessel wall interactions. However, practically, the bleeding time has not been shown to correlate with clinically important surgical hemorrhage outcomes and is not widely used [25]. The test is conducted by making a standardized small laceration to the forearm while a blood pressure cuff is inflated on the upper arm to 40 mmHg. Normal range is usually <10 min [5].

Thrombin Time (TT)

Thrombin time measures the rate of clot formation, typically measured by changes in light transmission. Thrombin is added to patient plasma. Time to clot formation is typically 10–20 s. As noted below, this test can be important in assessing whether a patient has activity from a direct thrombin inhibitor such as dabigatran. Other factors raising the TT include fibrin split products, heparin, and quantitative or qualitative fibrinogen loss [5].

Fibrinogen

Fibrinogen as the final factor in the clotting cascade can be directly measured. Levels less than 150 mg/dL are abnormal. In preoperative settings, causative factors include liver impairment and malnutrition, as well as inherited factor deficiency. Consumption of factor such as in DIC and surgical or traumatic blood loss and transfusion therapy can also lead to low levels.

ACT

The activated clotting time (ACT) is primarily used as a rapid assessment tool for measuring the degree of anticoagulation achieved by unfractionated heparin for bypass and angiographic procedures. Both the pre- and post-heparinization values are needed. The normal range is from 80 to 160 s. The test measures the function of the intrinsic coagulation pathway and has many similarities with aPTT testing; however it not sensitive to low levels of anticoagulation and is not a typical preoperative lab test.

Other Assays

Anti-Xa levels are measured to assess the effect of direct Xa inhibitors including enoxaparin. *Fibrin split products (FSP)* or fibrin degradation products are measured to evaluate for excessive fibrinolysis such as seen in disseminated intravascular coagulation. *Reptilase* is a snake enzyme that functions like thrombin but is not sensitive to inactivation by antithrombin III, the enzyme heparin promotes to achieve its anticoagulant effects. In the heparinized patient, Reptilase times (RT) will still be normal, while patient with factors that interfere with fibrin polymerization, like FSP, will show elevated RTs.

Viscoelastic Measures of Coagulation

Viscoelastic measures of coagulation assess the physical properties of a developing clot as it arises out of whole blood. The appeal is that this assesses the interaction between platelets and clotting cascade, and by following clot formation over time, can assess the various stages of the

Table 21.1 Impact of hematological conditions on screening coagulation tests

Condition	Platelet count	PT	aPTT	Alternative test
Unfractionated heparin use	NL	NL	$\Uparrow$	aPTT
Newer oral anticoagulants				
Rivaroxaban				Xa level
Dabigatran	NL		+/−$\Uparrow$	Thrombin time
Apixaban		NL	NL	
Von Willebrand disease	NL	NL	+/−$\Uparrow$	Ristocetin-induced platelet aggregation study or Platelet Function Assay (PFA-100)
Vitamin K deficiency and Coumadin use	NL	$\Uparrow$	NL	INR
Hemophilia (A or B)	NL	NL	$\Uparrow$	Specific factors studies
Aspirin	NL	NL	NL	PFA-100
Disseminated intravascular coagulation	$\Downarrow$	$\Uparrow$	$\Uparrow$	Fibrin split products

clotting process noted above. The test measures the changing physical properties of the blood sample over time as it is rotated, while a clot forms. Four values are produced by the test: the R value indicated the time to first clot formation, akin to the initiation phase; the K value represents the time to a set clot expansion, and is focused on clot amplification; the MA value measures the strength of the clot, assessing the stabilization phase; and the Coagulation Index (CI) is a calculated summary measure [26]. Neurosurgical experience with this modality is limited and not conclusive and includes trauma, endovascular procedures, and stroke care [27–29].

The impact of a variety of clinical conditions on common preoperative laboratory tests is given in Table 21.1.

Effect of Newer Anticoagulation Agents on Coagulation Tests

While older antiplatelet and anticoagulant agents such as heparin, coumadin, and clopidogrel are familiar to neurosurgeons, a variety of "single target" or newer oral anticoagulants and antiplatelet agents have come into widespread use. These include direct thrombin inhibitors such as dabigatran, and factor Xa inhibitors including rivaroxaban and apixaban. Unlike Warfarin, which can be properly monitored by PT/INR, single-target agents cannot reliably be followed in a similar fashion. A normal INR does not exclude treatment effect with Dabigatran, for example [30]. Dabigatran effect should elevate aPTT and will certainly elevate Thrombin Time (TT) [19]. Rivaroxaban, as a Factor Xa inhibitor, will show an increase in PT, but not always at the dosing trough, when anticoagulant activity will still be present. Similarly, aPTT is not sensitive to low drug concentrations [19]. Apixaban effect is not assessed by either PT or aPTT. Anti-Xa levels should be informative in these later two agents, given their mechanism, but published experience is limited [31]. At least one paper has assessed TEG in the management of a subdural hematoma in a patient on Dabigatran whose TT was prolonged [32].

Structured Clinical History

As noted above for general presurgical guidelines, and below for specific studies in neurosurgical patients, the predictive values of preoperative laboratory tests for adverse bleeding outcomes are limited. Assessment of bleeding risk by clinical history of both the patient and family, by contrast, is generally recommended in published guidelines [7–10, 12, 33]. However, clinical studies assessing the accuracy of clinical history to predict operative bleeding show variable predictive values. Houry et al. evaluated 3242 general surgical patients with a 3.2 % underlying prevalence rate of hematoma formation. Using a standardized, but nonvalidated questionnaire 951 (28 %) reported affirmative answers. Of these, 38 (PPV=4 %) developed postoperative hematoma. The negative predictive value (NPV) of the screen was 97 %; thus 2.8 % with a negative screen still had bleeding complications, not much lower than the underlying prevalence. Laboratory assessments of bleeding risk did not perform better [34]. Gabriel et al. studied 1479 children undergoing tonsillectomy. Again, using a previously described but nonvalidated instrument, 13 (1 %) reported an abnormal bleeding history. Three of these had excessive intraoperative or postoperative bleeding as assessed by surgeon (PPV=23 %). Of 1466 patients with a negative bleeding screen, 148 had bleeding complication, giving a negative predictive value (NPV) of 90 %, but meaning that 10 % of those with a negative bleeding screen still experienced increased bleeding. Again, laboratory assessment did not more accurately predict bleeding risk [35].

Validated questionnaires do exist for von Willebrand disease, and in particular, the Pediatric Bleeding Questionnaire has been assessed in a number of publications [36]. The questionnaire focuses on epistaxis, cutaneous bruising, bleeding from minor wounds, oral cavity bleeding, including dental extraction, gastrointestinal bleeding, prior surgical bleeding, menorrhea, and postpartum hemorrhage, where applicable, muscle hematomas and hemarthrosis. The full questionnaire can be found at the World Federation of Hemophilia web site at http://www.wfh.org/en/resources/bleeding-assessment-tool-pediatric-bleeding, as of this writing. However, this tool has been validated only in the setting of specialized coagulation clinics for the detection of Von Willebrand disease, and not in the general adult or pediatric operative population and not in neurosurgery patients specifically [13, 36]. Absent a validated instrument for the preoperative setting, suggestions for specific history questions are identified in Table 21.2 [9, 37]. A partial list of medications that can raise the risk of bleeding complications is given in Table 21.3, as an aid to history taking.

Table 21.2 History taking for bleeding risk assessment

General questions:
Do you bruise easily?
Do small wounds incurred in daily life bleed excessively?
Have you had significant blood loss with dental extractions or other minor procedures?
Do you have frequent nosebleeds?
Have you ever had bleeding into a joint or muscle?
Have you ever had blood in your stool?
Do you have liver or kidney disease?
Do you have a history of kidney, liver, or myeloproliferative disease
Is there malnutrition?
Is there a family history of bleeding disorders?
Additional for women:
Do you bleed profusely with menstruation?
Have you had major bleeding after childbirth?
Additional for young children/infants:
Was there a cephalohematoma or unusual umbilical stump bleeding at birth?

Table 21.3 Selected medications at risk for affecting surgical bleeding

Platelet inhibitors	Anticoagulants—parenteral
Aspirin	Argatroban (Acova)
Abciximab (ReoPro)	Dalteparin (Fragmin)
Clopidogrel (Plavix)	Enoxaparin (Lovenox)
Dipyridamole (Persantine)	Heparin
Eptifibatide (Integrilin)	Anticoagulants—Enteral
Ticlopidine (Ticlid)	Dabigatran (Pradaxa)
NSAIDs (examples)	Rivaroxaban (Xarelto)
Celebrex	Warfarin (Coumadin)
Ibuprofen	Vitamins, Herbal Supplements
Meloxicam (Mobic)	Feverfew
Naprosyn (Aleve)	Garlic=high dose
Salsalate (Disalcid)	Ginger—high dose
Sulindac (Clinoril)	Ginseng
Piroxicam (Feldene)	Gingko
Anticonvulsants	Omega 3 fatty acids
Valproic acid (Depakote)	Saw Palmetto
	Vitamin E—high dose

See also: https://www.facs.org/~/media/files/education/patient%20ed/medicationsform.ashx

Neurosurgery-Specific Studies

A modest body of literature deals specifically with preoperative testing in neurosurgery patients. Schramm et al. reported on 1211 patients undergoing cranial (56 %), spinal (33 %), and other (11 %) neurosurgical procedures. Three quarters of patients underwent preoperative coagulation testing and 7.2 % of these had either low platelet count, or prolonged PT or aPTT. Postoperative bleeding was predicted by preoperative elevated aPTT, but not PT or platelet count, and most of 14 patients with both elevated aPTT and postoperative bleeding had an identifiable risk factor on clinical history [38]. Dutzmann and colleagues sought to evaluate whether preoperative assessment of prothrombin time (PT) was essential in routinely planned neurosurgical procedures [39]. They studied 4310 consecutive patients undergoing elective cranial and spinal procedures. Considering a PT of >1.28 as abnormal, 1.8 % (78 patients) were found to have an abnormally elevated PT preoperatively, but all but five of these had obvious causes for the PT elevation such as coumadin use or liver disease. Thus the sensitivity of history for elevated PT was 93.5 %. Of the five with unexpectedly elevated PTs, two were given replacement factor, three were not, and none had hemorrhagic complications. Among the >4000 patient cohort, 33 patients (0.77 %) suffered a bleeding complication requiring reoperation and 31 patients of these had a normal pre-op PT. Of the two patients who had abnormal PTs and suffered bleeding complications, both had concerning histories (cancer, recent Warfarin use, and hepatocellular carcinoma). The authors noted a positive predictive value (PPV) of preoperative elevated PT to indicate hemorrhage was 2.5 % (2/78), although this rate appears to discount that many or most patients in this study who had preoperatively elevated PTs were treated with factor replacement [39].

The largest analysis of preoperative coagulation testing in neurosurgery, by number of patients included, also assessed the relative utility of preoperative history for bleeding risk vs. preoperative coagulation studies using the National Surgical Quality Improvement Program database (NSQIP). Patients were considered to have a positive history for bleeding history based on self-reported medical history of bleeding disorders, high-risk medication use, chronic steroid use, disseminated cancer, and renal or liver disease. The study included 11,804 patients. Sixty percent of patients underwent PT and aPTT testing and 90 % had preoperative platelet count. While 4 % had at least one abnormal result, less than 1 % had a severely abnormal result. Given the large sample size, it is unsurprising that each of the abnormal laboratory values was statistically associated with a variety of outcome measures including mortality, transfusion, and return to the OR. However, all coagulation measures had low sensitivity (<0.2) for the outcome measures. A positive clinical history was associated with a 3.5-fold increasing the likelihood of one or more abnormal coagulation tests, and the likelihood of detecting the various clinical outcomes was similar with history vs. one or more abnormal coagulation tests. Concerningly, even when history and abnormal laboratory assessment were combined, only about 1/3 of patients with the outcomes of interest were identified. The authors concluded that there was "limited or absent benefit from routine or standing preoperative hemostatic screening." They further estimated that limiting testing to those with an abnormal history would save $82 million annually in the United States (2012 dollars) [40].

As noted above, Factor XIII plays an important role in the stabilization phase of clot formation, being essential for cross-linking of the fibrin to create a stable polymer. Gerlach and colleagues assessed Factor XIII levels preoperatively in 910 patients undergoing cranial neurosurgery in addition to PT, aPTT, and fibrinogen. In 4.3 % there was a postoperative hemorrhage requiring surgical intervention. Preoperative Factor XIII and Fibrinogen levels were correlated with hemorrhage, whereas PT and aPTT were not. Specifically, patients with Factor XIII levels less than 80 % had a fourfold increase in risk of hematoma [41]. However these study results have not been reproduced [42]. Additionally, Adelman et al. studied 290 patients undergoing craniotomy with a 2.4 % rate of severe bleeding requiring reoperation. No differences in preoperative Factor XIII were seen between the groups, nor were differences in PT, PTT, or platelet count. A fibrinogen level of <200 mg/dl was associated with a tenfold increase in the odds of postoperative hemorrhage, and had a sensitivity of 86 % and specificity of 62 % [43].

Evaluating pediatric patients undergoing craniofacial reconstruction, Genecov et al. retrospectively assessed 168 patients. All had a normal PT, but 6 (3.6 %) had an abnormal PTT and were found to have Factor XI deficiencies (3pts), von Willebrand+low FXII (1 patient), and circulating inhibitors (2 patients) [44].

Karger and colleagues assessed the role of Platelet Function Analysis, specifically the PFA-100, in 93 patients undergoing craniotomy for mass lesion. Patients with abnormally elevated closure times were administered DDAVP. Surgical outcomes were compared to a retrospective cohort and were found to be similar with no reduction in bleeding events in the screened and treated group vs. historical controls. The authors concluded that routine screening and treatment was unnecessary [18].

Patients undergoing epilepsy surgery would appear to have a number of treatment-specific risk factors for hemorrhage. Valproic acid, a common anticonvulsant, has been demonstrated to produce both platelet and coagulation pathway dysfunction, although the clinical importance of these findings has been debated. The ketogenic diet has been reported to induce platelet aggregation deficiencies. Pacione et al. prospectively evaluated 39 children undergoing epilepsy surgery with an extensive battery of laboratory testing through a hematology clinic that included von Willebrand antigen, ristocetin cofactor testing (as part of a vWD work-up), factor VIII assay, and platelet aggregation tests. Fifteen children had Tuberous Sclerosis (TS). Twenty-five percent of patients had abnormal platelet function or a coagulation panel abnormality. One third of children with TS were affected, all with platelet abnormalities. Two of these five children had a negative clinical history screen and one developed a subdural hematoma, despite preoperative platelet transfusion. Twenty percent of children without TS were affected with all suffering coagulation abnormalities. Three of these had negative history, but two had minor enough abnormalities that no treatment was prescribed and no bleeding complications occurred. The authors suggest that children with TS undergoing epilepsy surgery may be at increased risk for hemorrhage and may benefit from more extensive preoperative testing [45].

As noted above, the platelet inhibitor clopidogrel plays an important role in preventing ischemic complications after neuroendovascular procedures. Kashiwazaki and colleagues prospectively evaluated 66 Asian patients undergoing carotid stenting and intracranial stent/coiling procedures, who were all receiving both aspirin and clopidogrel preoperatively. Prior to the procedure, platelet function was assessed using the VerifyNow P2Y12 assay. Based on ROC curve analysis, response to clopidogrel therapy was considered subtherapeutic, when the percent inhibition was <25 % (19 patients), adequate when between 25 % and 75 % (32 patients), and supratherapeutic when >75 % (15 patients). The rates of ischemic complications in the three groups were 37 %, 19 %, and 0 % while the rates of bleeding complications were 0 %, 6 %, and 40 % respectively. All ischemic complications were abnormalities on postprocedure diffusion-weighted imaging and did not appear to have a clinical correlation. Bleeding complications were groin hematomas in six patients, optic disc hemorrhage, and epistaxis [46].

Putting It All Together

Preoperative assessment for bleeding risk should be based primarily on history and physical exam including the identification of medications that increase bleeding risk. Laboratory tests, such as PT/PTT and Platelet Count or other more specific tests, can be reserved for situations in which there are concerning features by history or exam, although given the lack of prospective evidence specific to neurosurgery, the practice of routine laboratory assessment cannot be completely excluded for neurosurgical procedures, particularly where there is limited opportunity to identify and manage hemorrhage, such as in ventriculostomy or deep brain electrode placement. Patients presenting with hemorrhagic events, either spontaneous or traumatic, should be considered at high risk for coagulopathy and assessed accordingly. Preoperative consultation with a hematologist is appropriate in the setting of either a worrisome clinical or laboratory assessment.

References

1. Davie E, Ratnoff O. Waterfall sequence for intrinsic blood clotting. Science. 1964;145:1310–2.
2. Macfarlane R. An enzyme cascade in the blood clotting mechanism, and its function as a biochemical amplifier. Nature. 1964;202:498–9.
3. Achneck HE, et al. Pathophysiology of bleeding and clotting in the cardiac surgery patient: from vascular endothelium to circulatory assist device surface. Circulation. 2010;122(20):2068–77.
4. Palta S, Saroa R, Palta A. Overview of the coagulation system. Indian J Anaesth. 2014;58(5):515–23.
5. Thiruvenkatarajan V, Pruett A, Adhikary SD. Coagu lation testing in the perioperative period. Indian J Anaesth. 2014;58(5):565–72.
6. De Caterina R, et al. General mechanisms of coagulation and targets of anticoagulants (Section I). Position paper of the ESC Working Group on Thrombosis—task force on anticoagulants in heart disease. Thromb Haemost. 2013;109(4):569–79.
7. Chee YL, et al. Guidelines on the assessment of bleeding risk prior to surgery or invasive procedures. British Committee for Standards in Haematology. Br J Haematol. 2008;140(5):496–504.
8. Cosmi B, et al. Assessment of the risk of bleeding in patients undergoing surgery or invasive procedures: Guidelines of the Italian Society for Haemostasis and Thrombosis (SISET). Thromb Res. 2009;124(5):e6–12.
9. Bonhomme F, et al. Pre-interventional haemostatic assessment: Guidelines from the French Society of Anaesthesia and Intensive Care. Eur J Anaesthesiol. 2013;30(4):142–62.
10. Zwisser B. Preoperative evaluation of adult patients prior to elective, non-cardiac surgery. Joint recommendations of German Society of Anesthesiology and Intensive Care Medicine, German Society of Surgery and German Society of Internal Medicine. Urologe. 2011;50(9):1169–82.
11. Serafini G, et al. Preoperative evaluation in infants and children: recommendations of the Italian Society of Pediatric and Neonatal Anesthesia and Intensive Care (SARNePI). Minerva Anestesiol. 2014;80(4):461–9.
12. Committee on Standards and Practice Parameters, et al. Practice advisory for preanesthesia evaluation: an updated report by the American Society of Anesthesiologists Task Force on Preanesthesia Evaluation. Anesthesiology. 2012;116(3):522–38.
13. Guay J, et al. Ability of hemostatic assessment to detect bleeding disorders and to predict abnormal surgical blood loss in children: a systematic review and meta-analysis. Paediatr Anaesth. 2015;25(12):1216–26.
14. Burk CD, et al. Preoperative history and coagulation screening in children undergoing tonsillectomy. Pediatrics. 1992;89(4 Pt 2):691–5.
15. Rapaport SI. Preoperative hemostatic evaluation: which tests, if any? Blood. 1983;61(2):229–31.
16. Samama CM, et al. Perioperative platelet transfusion: recommendations of the Agence Francaise de Securite Sanitaire des Produits de Sante (AFSSaPS) 2003. Can J Anaesth. 2005;52(1):30–7.
17. Greinacher A. Clinical Practice. Heparin-induced thrombocytopenia. N Engl J Med. 2015;373(3):252–61.
18. Karger R, et al. The Platelet Function Analyzer (PFA-100) as a screening tool in neurosurgery. ISRN Hematol. 2012;2012:839242.
19. Kimpton G, Dabbous B, Leach P. New oral anticoagulant and antiplatelet agents for neurosurgeons. Br J Neurosurg. 2015;29(5):614–21.
20. Lordkipanidze M, et al. Assessment of VerifyNow P2Y12 assay accuracy in evaluating clopidogrel-induced platelet inhibition. Ther Drug Monit. 2008;30(3):372–8.
21. Swank RL, Prichard KH. The screen-filtration pressure method for detecting particular matter in fluid. Ann N Y Acad Sci. 1969;158:753–60.
22. Poller L. International Normalized Ratios (INR): the first 20 years. J Thromb Haemost. 2004;2(6):849–60.
23. Matevosyan K, et al. Coagulation factor levels in neurosurgical patients with mild prolongation of prothrombin time: effect on plasma transfusion therapy. J Neurosurg. 2011;114(1):3–7.
24. West KL, Adamson C, Hoffman M. Prophylactic correction of the international normalized ratio in neurosurgery: a brief review of a brief literature. J Neurosurg. 2011;114(1):9–18.
25. Peterson P, et al. The preoperative bleeding time test lacks clinical benefit: College of American Pathologists' and American Society of Clinical Pathologists' position article. Arch Surg. 1998;133(2):134–9.
26. Trapani L. Thromboelastography: current applications, future directions. Open J Anesthesiol. 2013;3:23–7.
27. Windelov NA, et al. The prognostic value of thrombelastography in identifying neurosurgical patients with worse prognosis. Blood Coagul Fibrinolysis. 2011;22(5):416–9.
28. McTaggart RA, et al. Use of thromboelastography to tailor dual-antiplatelet therapy in patients undergoing treatment of intracranial aneurysms with the Pipeline embolization device. J Neurointerv Surg. 2015;7(6):425–30.

29. McDonald MM et al. Thrombelastography does not predict clinical response to rtPA for acute ischemic stroke. J Thromb Thrombolysis. 2015 [Epub ahead of print].
30. van Ryn J, Baruch L, Clemens A. Interpretation of point-of-care INR results in patients treated with dabigatran. Am J Med. 2012;125(4):417–20.
31. Cuker A, et al. Laboratory measurement of the anticoagulant activity of the non-vitamin K oral anticoagulants. J Am Coll Cardiol. 2014;64(11):1128–39.
32. Neyens R, et al. Dabigatran-associated subdural hemorrhage: using thromboelastography (TEG((R))) to guide decision-making. J Thromb Thrombolysis. 2014;37(2):80–3.
33. Sandset PM, Francis C, Key N. Guidelines of the Italian Society for Haemostasis and Thrombosis (SISET). Thromb Res. 2009;124(5):515.
34. Houry S, et al. A prospective multicenter evaluation of preoperative hemostatic screening tests. The French Associations for Surgical Research. Am J Surg. 1995;170(1):19–23.
35. Gabriel P, Mazoit X, Ecoffey C. Relationship between clinical history, coagulation tests, and perioperative bleeding during tonsillectomies in pediatrics. J Clin Anesth. 2000;12(4):288–91.
36. Biss TT, et al. Quantitation of bleeding symptoms in children with von Willebrand disease: use of a standardized pediatric bleeding questionnaire. J Thromb Haemost. 2010;8(5):950–6.
37. Laine C, Williams SV, Wilson JF. In the clinic. Preoperative evaluation. Ann Intern Med. 2009;151(1):ITC1–15. quiz ITC16.
38. Schramm B, et al. Coagulation studies in preoperative neurosurgical patients. Anaesth Intensive Care. 2001;29(4):388–92.
39. Dutzmann S, et al. On the value of routine prothrombin time screening in elective neurosurgical procedures. Neurosurg Focus. 2012;33(5):E9.
40. Seicean A, et al. Use and utility of preoperative hemostatic screening and patient history in adult neurosurgical patients. J Neurosurg. 2012;116(5):1097–105.
41. Gerlach R, et al. Increased risk for postoperative hemorrhage after intracranial surgery in patients with decreased factor XIII activity: implications of a prospective study. Stroke. 2002;33(6):1618–23.
42. Idris Z, et al. Association of perioperative factor XIII activity levels and other haemostatic markers with the risk of postoperative intracranial haematoma in a selected cohort of neurosurgical patients. Acta Neurochir (Wien). 2012;154(5):887–93. discussion 893–4.
43. Adelmann D, et al. Fibrinogen but not factor XIII deficiency is associated with bleeding after craniotomy. Br J Anaesth. 2014;113(4):628–33.
44. Genecov DG, et al. Preoperative screening for coagulopathy using prothrombin time and partial thromboplastin time in patients requiring primary cranial vault remodeling. Plast Reconstr Surg. 2005;116(2):389–94.
45. Pacione D, et al. Coagulation abnormalities in children undergoing epilepsy surgery. J Neurosurg Pediatr. 2011;7(6):654–9.
46. Kashiwazaki D, et al. The roles and issues of P2Y12 percent inhibition assessed by VerifyNow assay for patients undergoing neurointervention: a prospective study. J Stroke Cerebrovasc Dis. 2014;23(7):1830–6.

Safe Strategies for Gradual Suspension and Reinstitution of Anticoagulation to Permit Elective Surgery

22

Christopher Roark

Introduction

Neurosurgeons are performing more elective operations on patients taking anticoagulants. The reasons for this are multifactorial, but include advancing population age with more comorbid disease, newer anticoagulants and the continued expansion of the indications for older drugs such as aspirin and warfarin, as well as a larger breadth of treatment options for various neurosurgical conditions.

The suspension of anticoagulation before elective surgery—and its subsequent reinstitution—is a source of great debate in neurosurgery. This involves a delicate balance that takes into account the daily risk of thromboembolism—stroke, deep venous thrombosis (DVT), pulmonary embolism (PE)—versus the potentially severe consequences of a postoperative hematoma in the central nervous system (CNS). This debate is further intensified by the general lack of high-quality evidence regarding the risks and benefits of chemical anticoagulation in neurosurgical patients. There are high-quality data supporting its use in other surgical specialties, in addition to the wealth of data regarding the use and management of oral and parenteral anticoagulants in "medical patients".

Neurosurgical patients often harbor disease processes that increase the risk of venous thromboembolism (i.e. CNS malignancy, hemiparesis from stroke, morbid obesity, and HTN), and this coupled with a pre-existing reason for systemic anticoagulation raises the stakes even higher. Additionally, the treatment of conditions such as atrial fibrillation (AF) has improved in modern times, and patients are living more productive lives with this condition—which, as an example, may lead to injury or degeneration and the need for spine surgery.

The field of iatrogenic anticoagulation has changed significantly with the recent emergence of a new generation of oral anticoagulants. The evidence continues to point to the overall improved safety—with comparable or improved efficacy—of these medications. The significant caveat to the rapid increase in utilization of these medications lies in the fact that these medications currently have no reliable antidote. That is, their effect is not easily or quickly mitigated in the circumstance of life-threatening bleeding.

The mounting evidence of safety from well-done randomized controlled trials (RCTs) is in stark contrast to the anecdotal experience of neurosurgeons caring for patients on one of these "new drugs" with a significant hemorrhage that is functionally untreatable in many cases. As stated previously, neurosurgical patients can—in many

C. Roark, M.D. (✉)
Department of Neurosurgery, University of Colorado, 12631 E. 17th Ave., C307, Aurora, CO 80045, USA
e-mail: christopher.roark@ucdenver.edu

C.M. Loftus (ed.), *Anticoagulation and Hemostasis in Neurosurgery*,
DOI 10.1007/978-3-319-27327-3_22

instances—already carry diagnoses that require anticoagulation. A common neurosurgical comorbidity for this is malignant glioma. In a study by Semrad et al., the rate of VTE was seven times that of the general population.{Semrad:2007eo}

Regarding direct thrombin inhibitors, there is much anxiety among neurosurgeons due to the current inability to reverse these drugs in the case of severe life-threatening bleeding (i.e. intracranial hemorrhage). Multiple large randomized controlled trials have demonstrated statistically equivalent—if not lower—rates of ischemic stroke and VTE events with these new drugs, as compared with warfarin, with a lower side effect profile. That side effect profile includes a lower risk of intracranial hemorrhage. Studies have also failed to demonstrate an increase in mortality from intracranial hemorrhage due to these medications. While many neurosurgeons have already cared for a patient presenting with an ICH on a new oral anticoagulant, what they are unable to visualize are the patients who are spared from hemorrhage because of the improved safety of newer oral anticoagulants.

The goal of this chapter is not to address neurosurgical emergencies, but rather to give an overview and recommendations regarding the management of the patient on chronic anticoagulant therapy that is in need of an elective neurosurgical operation.

We will begin with the risks and benefits of gradual suspension of individual medications, followed by a discussion of their reinstatement during the postoperative period. Inherent in the discussion of suspension is a further elucidation of the risks for the patient who requires chronic anticoagulation, but cannot receive it due to the proximity of an invasive procedure.

Preoperative Suspension of Anticoagulants—What Is the Risk?

Suspension of anticoagulation for an elective neurosurgical procedure involves exposing the patient to a period of risk due to a "relative hypercoagulable" state in order that their blood clotting cascades are functioning normally on the day of surgery. We use this term "relative" because these patients have a condition that requires therapeutic anticoagulation to prevent thromboembolic events. We will begin by reviewing the thromboembolic risk in common conditions seen by neurosurgeons—if left untreated.

Atrial Fibrillation (AF)

The chief hazard of AF is stroke, the risk of which is increased four- to five-fold compared with patients not in AF. Because of its high prevalence in advanced age, AF assumes great importance as a risk factor for stroke and by the ninth decade becomes a dominant factor. The attributable risk for stroke associated with AF increases steeply from 1.5 % at age 50–59 years to 23.5 % at age 80–89 years.{Kannel:1998ws}

Patients with non-valvular atrial fibrillation have an approximately 4.5 % rate of stroke per year without treatment.{Investigators:1994vd} This yields an approximately 0.01 % daily risk of stroke with untreated atrial fibrillation. There is no current evidence that surgery itself increases the risk of *arterial* embolism in patients with atrial fibrillation or prosthetic heart valves. An extrapolation of this daily risk would lead to a baseline 0.1 % risk of stroke for every 10 days that a patient with AF is "untreated" for perioperative purposes. However, it must be stated that evidence in the literature exists to support the fact that surgery and anesthesia (including non-neurosurgical and non-cardiac procedures) is an independent risk factor for stroke in patients who do not carry a diagnosis of AF.{Wong:2000vd}{Urbanek:2014bt} This risk is well-documented in the first 30 postoperative days, and may extend beyond this period to at least 90 days.{Urbanek:2014bt}

Known risk factors for stroke in atrial fibrillation have been validated in the widely used $CHADS_2$ score{Lip:2010io, NavarBoggan:2015bs}, as well as the updated CHA_2DS_2-VASc score{Lip:2010ioa}, which is the current recommended scoring system for the risk and treatment of thromboembolic complications in patients with non-valvular atrial fibrillation. {January:2014gm} These include history of CHF, HTN, age>75 years, diabetes mellitus, any history of prior ischemic stroke, TIA, or systemic embolic events. Patients with a $CHADS_2$ score ≥ 2 have an annual stroke risk of 4 %, and warfarin has been shown to decrease hospitalization for stroke, MI, or hemorrhage. Patients with a higher $CHADS_2$ or CHA_2DS_2-VASc score would be at a higher interval risk during cessation of anticoagulation.

Prosthetic Heart Valves

In patients with mechanical heart valves, the thromboembolism risk is roughly 8 % if they are given no anticoagulants, which have been shown to decrease this risk by 75 %.{Jafri:2004ht} This risk is adjusted based on the type and location of the valve—with mitral and older valves having higher risks of thromboembolic complications than a newer valve or aortic location. It is common to stop warfarin 5 days before elective procedures, but if the INR is maintained at a level of 3.0 or greater—as is the case in most situations involving mechanical heart valves—this window may need to be extended. This prolongs the period during which a patient who needs intensive anticoagulant therapy is "sub-therapeutic".{Jaffer:2003iw}

The Patient with a History of Cryptogenic Stroke

The standard medical treatment for secondary prevention in patients with cryptogenic stroke is antiplatelet therapy. Recurrent stroke was seen in 6.8 % of patients in the medical arm of a recent RCT comparing PFO closure with medical management in patients with stroke of unknown origin and a documented PFO during work-up.{Carroll:2013cz}{Mattle:2013cu}{Tai:2014bz} Many of these patients will present with a current prescription for aspirin, possibly in conjunction with clopidogrel or another glycoprotein IIb/IIIa inhibitor.

Guidelines from the Medical Literature

The most recent guidelines document from the American College of Chest Physicians (ACCP) regarding perioperative management of anticoagulant and antiplatelet drugs has no direct references to neurosurgical patients. This stems from the previously discussed paucity of RCTs in neurosurgical patients regarding chemical VTE prophylaxis as well as the fact that neurosurgical patients—due to a perceived risk of hemorrhage—were left out of most of the major trials involving perioperative use of anticoagulants.{Douketis:2012ja} In fact, searching this 2012 paper for the word "neuro" returns only three results: a single mention of neurologic deficits after CABG in patients as it relates to ASA usage, and two instances from a single citation in the bibliography. Clearly, the management of these drugs must be carefully considered, and extrapolations from more generalized recommendations are required.

Bridging Therapy

Further nuance arises in the choice for or against postoperative bridging. While there is no disputing the fact that warfarin must be stopped before elective operations, considerable variability and uncertainty exists in regards to the decision of "to bridge or not to bridge" these patients with heparin (either unfractionated or low molecular weight) during the perioperative period. The ACCP guidelines{Douketis:2012ja} recommend bridging therapy in patients with "a mechanical heart valve, atrial fibrillation, or VTE at high risk for thromboembolism". This is qualified, however with the following statement: "Patients who place a higher value on avoiding perioperative bleeding than on avoiding perioperative thromboembolism are likely to decline heparin bridging."{Douketis:2012ja} The British Committee for Standards in Haematology attribute a classification of "high-risk" to any patient with AF and a prior stroke or TIA. In these patients, bridging is recommended during warfarin cessation.{vanVeen:2015dd}{Keeling: 2011gk}

In most elective situations, neurosurgery is not a contraindication for preoperative bridging with unfractionated (UF) or low molecular weight heparin (LMWH). Current recommendations are to stop UF 4–6 h before surgery and LMWH 24 h before surgery{Douketis:2012ja}. This is important as a patient on a LMWH bridge must be told not to administer the last dose of this medication the night before surgery—which could lead to a dose within 12 h of a "first start" procedure.

Neurosurgical patients who are deemed to be at a low risk of a perioperative hemorrhage, such as the patient undergoing a minimally invasive spine procedure, would be a better candidate for bridging therapy than the patient with an incompletely resected vascular tumor, or a large craniotomy. Neurosurgical postoperative hemorrhage rates are typically quoted to be around 1 %. {Palmer:1994tu, Kalfas:1988vf} An important point should be made regarding postoperative bridging. The issue must not be confused with postoperative use of "prophylactic" doses of UF or LMWHs. Bridging therapy often involves therapeutic doses of these medications, to a level that is consistent with the antithrombotic effects of warfarin. Therefore, the initiation of full bridging therapy must not commence before the neurosurgeon is comfortable with a full anticoagulant effect being in force. A middle ground may be forged with lower doses of UF or LMWH, but an anticoagulant effect is still present and evidence for this practice in patients requiring long-term anticoagulant therapy is lacking. The same guidelines recommend withholding bridging therapy for 48–72 h after undergoing "high-bleeding-risk surgery".{Douketis:2012ja} Neurosurgical procedures may not have a higher risk of postoperative bleeding, but postoperative bleeding represents *a higher risk* to these patients as a result of the disastrous effects of even small-volume hematomas in critical areas of the neuraxis.

Antiplatelet Therapy

Aspirin is associated with platelet inhibition within 60 min of administration{Awtry:2000ux} and the effect is irreversible for the life of the exposed platelets. This owes to their inability to generate new cyclooxygenase (COX). The average platelet lifespan is 10 days. Estimates are that approximately 10 % of platelet function is recovered per day after cessation of ASA.{Awtry:2000ux} Some investigators have demonstrated that normal levels of hemostasis may be possible with only 20 % of platelets being functional.{Bradlow:1982wh, Patrono:1985uj} While this may imply that 2 days of cessation would be adequate for surgical hemostasis, there is clinical evidence that bleeding complications are increased in patients who are continued on aspirin during cardiac and non-cardiac procedures.{Palmer:1994tu, Burger:2005bn, Alghamdi:2007hn} This risk was increased 1.5 times in the study by Burger and this was significant for patients undergoing intracranial surgery. {Burger:2005bn}

Current recommendation after coronary stent placement is for uninterrupted dual antiplatelet therapy for 6 weeks after placement of a bare metal stent (BS), and 6 months after placement of a drug-eluting stent (DES). Truly elective neurosurgical procedures should not be performed during this time as even a brief interruption of these agents involves a significant risk of in-stent thrombosis or acute coronary syndrome.

A study by Burger et al. in 2005 looked specifically at the risk of thrombotic events after cessation of low-dose aspirin therapy as well as concomitant bleeding risks when this drug was continued during the procedure. Acute cerebral events occurred on average 14 days after withdrawal of aspirin, while the average time between aspirin cessation and acute coronary syndrome was only 8.5 days in this study.{Burger:2005bn} This is weighed against studies of postoperative neurosurgical hematomas in which the most common risk factor was administration of aspirin or NSAIDs.{Palmer:1994tu}

Daily Risk of Venous Thromboembolism (VTE)

The risk of recurrent VTE drops rapidly over the first 3 months after an initial VTE event. {Jafri:2004ht} The rate is roughly 40 % in the first month after an initial event—without anticoagulation—but drops to 10 % within 2 months. {Jafri:2004ht} Oral anticoagulation can decrease this risk by 80 %. This is, again, a situation where the benefits of any elective surgical procedure need to be substantial in order to counterbalance the significantly elevated risk of recurrent VTE. This increase in the risk of VTE is independent of the fact that both hospitalization and a surgical procedure are independent risk factors for development of a VTE in patients with no such history.

Reinstitution of Anticoagulant Therapy After Neurosurgical Procedures

The primary concern with reinstitution of anticoagulants after neurosurgical procedures involves postoperative hemorrhage at the operative site and wound healing complications that can delay other treatments (e.g. adjuvant radiation therapy for malignant brain tumors).

Hemorrhage Risk

High-quality studies are lacking in regards to the risks of hemorrhage with reinitiation of chronic anticoagulant therapy after elective (or urgent) neurosurgical procedures. There have been multiple small RCTs investigating the use of chemical VTE prophylaxis after neurosurgical procedures. Various anticoagulants—including unfractionated and low molecular weight heparins—have demonstrated a reduction in VTE risk with use of these medications, however, there was an increase seen in clinically significant hemorrhages despite the small sizes of the studies and their being underpowered to detect an increase in hemorrhage risk. A single study of patients undergoing craniotomy who were randomized to preoperative enoxaparin versus placebo was stopped on interim analysis due to a higher rate of hemorrhage in the enoxaparin arm.{Dickinson:1998wy} The applicability of such studies to the question of when to restart chronic anticoagulation is limited, as these were studies using prophylactic doses of, primarily, heparins (unfractionated and low-molecular weight). The dosing of heparins are different when the intent is full anticoagulation, and there are several classes of drugs that are not typically used for prophylaxis, but rather, treatment of the hypercoagulable state.

Recommendations

Informed Consent

Reasonable strategies for cessation of anticoagulants for the purposes of elective neurosurgical procedures would begin with a full discussion with the individual patient of the risks surrounding the cessation and reinstitution of their particular medication. This discussion should be tailored to the patients' specific drug and underlying diagnosis. A clear understanding of the expected benefits of surgery, as well as the risks during this period is of paramount importance. Issues of perioperative ischemic (stroke, TIA, VTE) as well as postoperative hemorrhagic events (hematoma, wound healing issues, infection, and delay in adjuvant therapy) must be carefully balanced.

There should be no hesitation in conferring with physicians from the various specialties that prescribe these anticoagulant drugs, especially colleagues from cardiology and hematology.

Cessation of Warfarin

Chest guidelines from 2004 recommend various schedules for warfarin cessation and reinitiation in the perioperative period. The variability involves the use or omission of bridging therapy and the duration of cessation postoperatively. The 2014 Chest guidelines for the treatment of patients with atrial fibrillation recommend the use of bridging therapy in patient with AF and a mechanical heart valve requiring interruption of warfarin (or new anticoagulants) for surgical procedures.{January:2014gm} It must be reinforced that these recommendations are not specific to neurosurgical patients. The authors of these guidelines merely state that a "normal INR" is important at the time of neurosurgical procedures and that reinstitution of anticoagulation may need to be delayed in the postoperative period out of concern for surgical site hematoma formation. {January:2014gm}

The effective half-life of warfarin ranges 20 to 60 h with an average of 40 h. General recommendations include cessation of warfarin between 3 and 7 days preoperatively. The INR should be checked the morning of the procedure to confirm that it is in the normal range. The length of warfarin cessation should be informed by the underlying reason for its prescription and intensity of therapy. Patients with mechanical heart valves are at an inherently higher risk of thromboembolism than are patients with atrial fibrillation, however warfarin may need to be held for a longer duration to allow its effects to fully reverse and strong consideration should be given to bridging these patients with a low molecular weight heparin.

Reinstitution of Warfarin

The anticoagulant effect of warfarin is not immediate. Additionally, there is an early time window during which warfarin appears to exert a procoagulant effect. This is mediated by a rapid decrease in protein C levels—outpacing the diminution of factors II and X during the initial 48 h of warfarin administration.{Harrison:1997wc} This precipitous drop counterbalances the drop in factor VII levels that lead to the INR prolongation.{Harrison:1997wc}

This change in the coagulation cascade—and the potential for a transient period of relative hypercoagulability—underlies the recommendation for initial use of heparin or LMWHs during institution of warfarin therapy. Other surgical specialties have utilized this delayed efficacy and commenced warfarin therapy on the day of surgery.{Rokito:1996ti} There is no evidence that this strategy is either safe or effective for neurosurgical patients. Neurosurgical patients are felt to be at a higher risk for VTE events for multiple reasons relating to their underlying disease. These include, but are not limited to, conditions such as spinal cord injury, hemiplegia, brain tumors, subarachnoid hemorrhage, and trauma. Most neurosurgical centers do not advocate—owing to the dearth of evidence—use of chemical prophylaxis in the immediate postoperative period.

Given the requirement for bridging chemical prophylaxis, warfarin should be resumed postoperatively when the neurosurgeon has weighed the risks and benefits of an immediate anticoagulant effect (owing to the immediate effects of heparin or LMWHs used in bridging). This will be dictated, once again, by the balance between the underlying reason for chronic anticoagulation and the perceived risk of hemorrhage. While this judgment is variable, very rarely is full anticoagulation started within 24 h of a neurosurgical procedure. Patients with mechanical heart valves should resume their anticoagulation regimen earlier than a patient with paroxysmal atrial fibrillation or DVT, owing to the higher thromboembolic risk associated with this condition.

Cessation of Antiplatelet Agents

Patients with drug-eluting stents (DES) are at a high risk of stent thrombosis, and the factor most closely associated with this event is the cessation of dual antiplatelet therapy.{Abualsaud:2010 cm, Chassot:2007gk, Burger:2005bn} Guidelines for the perioperative management of antiplatelet agents stress the need for continuation of dual antiplatelet therapy whenever possible to reduce the incidence of in-stent thrombosis. It should be noted, however, that intracranial and intraspinal surgery are singled out—along with posterior chamber ocular surgery—as procedures at a high enough risk of bleeding that warrant the cessation of antiplatelet therapy.{Abualsaud:2010 cm}

Additional factors that can coexist between these populations—patients with cardiac stents and the need for neurosurgical procedures—include diabetes mellitus and malignancy, both of which are "patient" risk factors for in-stent thrombosis. The mainstay of prevention of in-stent thrombosis is the uninterrupted use of dual antiplatelet therapy with aspirin and thienopyridines (clopidogrel, ticlopidine, and prasugrel) for a minimum of 6—and ideally 12 months after stent placement. Any truly elective neurosurgical procedure should be delayed until after this window has passed. There are very few situations where neurosurgeons do not stop all antiplatelet agents before elective procedures, with carotid endarterectomy being a notable exception.

ASA and thienopyridines must be stopped well enough in advance of elective neurosurgical procedures to allow their irreversible effect on platelet function to diminish. Studies have demonstrated complete recovery of platelet function seven days after discontinuation of clopidogrel. {KamPCA:2003cv, Weber:2001wv}

Reinstitution of Antiplatelet Agents

ASA and thienopyridines exhibit an antiplatelet effect within hours of administration, if given in a loading dose. As an example, maximal inhibition of platelet aggregation is seen between 2 and 6 h after an oral load of clopidogrel (375–500 mg). This same effect takes 3–7 days of the standard daily clopidogrel dose (75 mg).{KamPCA: 2003cv} A gradual antiplatelet effect, therefore, is achieved with reinstitution of daily clopidogrel dosing without an oral load. It should be noted that while this make some sense as a "middle ground" for neurosurgeons there is no high-level evidence that such a practice is either safe or effective. The only known reversal mechanism for these drugs is platelet transfusion—which carries well-documented risks. Some advocate the use of DDAVP to improve platelet function in cases of emergency,{Korinth:2006kl, Korinth: 2007bk} but its use in neurosurgery is not well-studied.

Cessation of New Oral Anticoagulants

There are three FDA-approved Factor Xa inhibitors on the market—rivaroxaban, apixaban, and most recently edoxaban. These join dabigatran, a direct thrombin inhibitor, as the new generation of oral anticoagulants indicated for treatment of patients with atrial fibrillation. The most common of these, currently, is dabigatran. The half-life and clearance of this drug is highly dependent on the patient's renal function. With the understanding that neurosurgical patients should have normal clotting function before elective surgery, it is reasonable to stop dabigatran 2–4 days before the scheduled operation. Impaired renal function should cause this time interval to be extended. {vanRyn:2010wu}

A consensus statement on the use of rivaroxaban suggests that the last dose be 24 h or more before surgery.{Turpie:2012wf} This stems from the short half-life of the drug (5–13 h depending on age and renal function). Apixaban and edoxaban have similar half-lives to dabigatran (9–14 h for apixaban and 9–11 h for edoxaban) {Cabral:2013ic}, and would therefore require the same interval of cessation before elective surgical procedures for normal clotting to be expected (Table 22.1).

Table 22.1 Pharmacodynamic properties of direct oral anticoagulants compared with warfarin. Adapted from information contained in {Cabral:2013ic, Wang:2014cb}

	Half-life	Peak action (Tmax)	Time to reach full steady state	Time for anticoagulant effect to reverse (five half-lives)[a]
Warfarin	20–60 h	72–120 h	1 week or longer	8.3 days
Dabigatran	12–17 h	1.25–3 h	2 days	3 days
Rivaroxaban	5–9 h	2–4 h	2 days	1.5 days
Apixaban	9–14 h	1–4 h	2 days	2.4 days
Edoxaban	9–11 h	1–2 h	2 days	2.1 days

[a](Average of half-life range × 5)/24

Reinstitution of New Oral Anticoagulants

These drugs are becoming more widely utilized due to their mild side effect profile and the elimination of the intensive laboratory monitoring required of patients on warfarin. The reason for unease among the neurosurgical community is the currently irreversible nature of these medications. While intracranial hemorrhage may be significantly lower with these newer agents, the outcome for that patient can be severe disability or death with no acceptable treatment options.

Rivaroxaban has a rapid onset and short half-life. The peak plasma concentration is achieved within 2–4 h after a single dose, which is similar to the onset of LMWHs. Institution of this medication should not begin until the judgment of the neurosurgeon is that bleeding risk is low enough to commit to full anticoagulation. The current recommendation for emergency reversal is with PCC as this was shown to completely reverse the effects of rivaroxaban in healthy subjects{Eerenberg:2011cn}, with or without activated charcoal if the last oral dose was within 8 h.{Wang:2014cb} Dialysis is not an option with rivaroxaban or apixaban, as it is with dabigatran, owing to the high plasma protein binding of these drugs.

Apixaban reaches a maximum plasma concentration in an average of 3 h after administration of a 20 mg dose.{Frost:2015iz} The concentration and effect of drug was noted to be slightly higher in older patients, which is of importance given its indication for prevention of VTE after orthopedic surgery and stroke in nonvalvular atrial fibrillation. The half-life, route of excretion, and use in renally impaired patients are similar to that of rivaroxaban. As with all Factor Xa inhibitors, there is no direct antidote, and minimal evidence-based experience with reversing this agent. Activated charcoal is advocated by some, if the need for emergent reversal (hemorrhage) occurs within 3 h of the last dose. {Wang:2014cb}

Dabigatran is the only direct thrombin inhibitor on the market in the United States that is used for long-term anticoagulation. Bivalirudin is a direct thrombin inhibitor that is typically used during interventional procedures in patients who are allergic to heparin. Dabigatran has a rapid onset in action that is correlated with a rapid rise in its plasma levels. The maximal anticoagulant effect is achieved in 2–3 h with half-life measured at 14–17 h in patients with normal renal function.{vanRyn:2010wu}{Eerenberg:2011cn} Dabigatran plasma levels will accumulate in patients with renal failure, and its excretion rate is prolonged in patients with moderate or severe kidney disease.{vanRyn:2010wu}

Its use has been increasing rapidly since trials such as RE-COVER{Schulman:2009is}—comparing warfarin with dabigatran—demonstrated no difference in recurrent VTE or death with an improved side effect and safety profile. Specifically, they demonstrated a 3.2 % absolute risk reduction for overall bleeding events in the group receiving dabigatran. A randomized crossover trial of dabigatran and rivaroxaban demonstrated the ineffectiveness of PCC in improving partial thromboplastin time (PTT), prothrombin time (PT), and ecarin clotting time (ECT) in patients taking dabigatran.{Eerenberg:2011cn} The only documented way to definitively reverse dabigatran is with hemodialysis. This is of obvious concern to neurosurgeons who may need to perform an emergency surgical procedure, but that is outside the scope of this chapter. The irreversibility of dabigatran is pertinent here in regards to its reinstitution after elective procedures, as a surgical site hematoma would be extremely difficult—if not impossible—to treat urgently at that point.

Given the short half-life of dabigatran, similar to the factor Xa inhibitors, it does not need to be held preoperatively as long as warfarin.

Conclusions

The process of safely suspending and reinstituting chronic anticoagulants in the perioperative period for a neurosurgical procedure involves several key decision points. The initial decision in this process is determining that the potential benefits of the proposed procedure outweigh the risks of a pause in chronic anticoagulation. This involves considering the underlying medical condition of the patient, with special attention to the reason for chronic anticoagulation and the risks attendant with suspension of anticoagulation.

There is very little high-quality literature regarding any of these medications that has included neurosurgical patients. Recommendations and considerations are extrapolated from the data of other specialties and this will inevitably result in practices that are highly tailored to the individual patient with a large amount of institutional, regional, and national variability. Patients and families will have an easier time accepting this if the issues surrounding chronic anticoagulation and elective surgery are clearly explained to them during discussions surrounding the overall risk/benefit ratio of any proposed procedure. This issue should be a primary discussion point during the informed consent process for chronically anticoagulated patients, not included merely as an afterthought.

Summary Considerations

- For patients on warfarin:
  - A preoperative use of a LMWH bridge may be beneficial in patients with prosthetic heart valves (especially older, mechanical, and mitral valves) and atrial fibrillation with a history of cardioembolic stroke or TIA.
  - Check an INR preoperatively to assure that lab values have completely normalized after warfarin suspension.
  - Postoperative bridging with LMWH or heparin (heparin has higher bleeding events but its effect is reversible with protamine) when reinstituting warfarin therapy due to the transient hypercoagulable state seen with this drug is important.
- For patients on antiplatelet agents with a history of coronary stents:
  - Discuss the need for any elective case with the patient's cardiologist and be certain that the type of coronary stent (bare metal versus drug-eluting) is known as this affects the duration of uninterrupted antiplatelet therapy that is recommended.
  - Do not perform elective neurosurgical cases during the first 6–12 months (institution and local practices may vary) after placement of drug-eluting stents as dual antiplatelet therapy is vital to preventing in-stent thrombosis.
  - All antiplatelets (including ASA) should be discontinued before performing intracranial or intraspinal procedures.
  - Antiplatelet therapy should be resumed as soon as the neurosurgeon feels the chances of a hematoma or wound-healing complication are low, with the knowledge that platelet transfusion is currently the only way to acutely restore adequate platelet function in patients taking these agents.
- For the patient on a new oral anticoagulant:
  - While short half-lives of these drugs may allow for later suspension and obviate the need for bridging therapy, consultation with the specialist prescribing the medication for that patient is important as the clearance of these drugs is dependent on a variety of patient-specific factors, including, but not limited to, age and renal function.
  - The full anticoagulant effect is achieved within hours of administration and acute reversal of these effects is not often easily facilitated—if it is possible at all. This must be taken into account when reinstituting these drugs in the postoperative period.
- In situations where anticoagulation is required earlier than it is felt safe to reinstitute an oral anticoagulant, consideration may be given to short-term use of LMWH (reversible with platelet transfusion) or heparin (reversible with protamine administration).

References

1. Abualsaud AO, Eisenberg MJ. Perioperative management of patients with drug-eluting stents. J Am Coll Cardiol Intv. 2010;3:131–42.
2. Alghamdi AA, Moussa F, Fremes SE. Does the use of preoperative aspirin increase the risk of bleeding in patients undergoing coronary artery bypass grafting

surgery? Systematic review and meta-analysis. J Card Surg. 2007;22:247–56.
3. Awtry EH, Loscalzo J. Aspirin. Circulation. 2000;101:1206–18.
4. Bradlow BA, Chetty N. Dosage frequency for suppression of platelet function by low dose aspirin therapy. Thromb Res. 1982;27:99–110.
5. Burger W, Chemnitius JM, Kneissl GD, Rucker G. Low-dose aspirin for secondary cardiovascular prevention - cardiovascular risks after its perioperative withdrawal versus bleeding risks with its continuation - review and meta-analysis. J Intern Med. 2005;257:399–414.
6. Cabral KP. Pharmacology of the new target-specific oral anticoagulants. J Thromb Thrombolysis. 2013;36:133–40.
7. Carroll JD, Saver JL, Thaler DE, Smalling RW, Berry S, MacDonald LA, et al. Closure of patent foramen ovale versus medical therapy after cryptogenic stroke. N Engl J Med. 2013;368:1092–100.
8. Chassot P-G, Delabays A, Spahn DR. Perioperative antiplatelet therapy: the case for continuing therapy in patients at risk of myocardial infarction. Br J Anaesth. 2007;99:316–28.
9. Dickinson LD, Miller LD, Patel CP, Gupta SK. Enoxaparin increases the incidence of postoperative intracranial hemorrhage when initiated preoperatively for deep venous thrombosis prophylaxis in patients with brain tumors. Neurosurgery. 1998;43:1074–81.
10. Douketis JD, Spyropoulos AC, Spencer FA, Mayr M, Jaffer AK, Eckman MH, et al. Perioperative management of antithrombotic therapy: antithrombotic therapy and prevention of thrombosis, 9th ed: American College of Chest Physicians evidence-based clinical practice guidelines. Chest. 2012;141:e326S–50.
11. Eerenberg ES, Kamphuisen PW, Sijpkens MK, Meijers JC, Buller HR, Levi M. Reversal of rivaroxaban and dabigatran by prothrombin complex concentrate: a randomized, placebo-controlled, crossover study in healthy subjects. Circulation. 2011;124:1573–9.
12. Frost CE, Song Y, Shenker A, Wang J, Barrett YC, Schuster A, et al. Effects of age and sex on the single-dose pharmacokinetics and pharmacodynamics of apixaban. Clin Pharmacokinet. 2015;54:1–12.
13. Harrison L, Johnston M, Massicotte MP, Crowther M, Moffat K, Hirsh J. Comparison of 5-mg and 10-mg loading doses in initiation of warfarin therapy. Ann Intern Med. 1997;126:133–6.
14. Investigators AF. Risk factors for stroke and efficacy of antithrombotic therapy in atrial fibrillation. Analysis of pooled data from five randomized controlled trials. Arch Intern Med. 1994;154:1449–57.
15. Jaffer AK, Brotman DJ, Chukwumerije N. When patients on warfarin need surgery. Cleve Clin J Med. 2003;70:973–84.
16. Jafri SM. Periprocedural thromboprophylaxis in patients receiving chronic anticoagulation therapy. Am Heart J. 2004;147:3–15.
17. January CT, Wann LS, Alpert JS, Calkins H, Cigarroa JE, Cleveland JC, et al. 2014 AHA/ACC/HRS guideline for the management of patients with atrial fibrillation: executive summary: a report of the American College of Cardiology/American Heart Association Task Force on practice guidelines and the heart rhythm society. Circulation. 2014;130:2071–104.
18. Kalfas IH, Little JR. Postoperative hemorrhage: a survey of 4992 intracranial procedures. Neurosurgery. 1988;23:343–7.
19. Kam PCA, Nethery CM. The thienopyridine derivatives (platelet adenosine diphosphate receptor antagonists), pharmacology and clinical developments. Anaesthesia. 2003;58:28–35.
20. Kannel WB, Wolf PA, Benjamin EJ, Levy D. Prevalence, incidence, prognosis, and predisposing conditions for atrial fibrillation: population-based estimates. Am J Cardiol. 1998;82:2N–9.
21. Keeling D, Baglin T, Tait C, Watson H, Perry D, Baglin C, et al. Guidelines on oral anticoagulation with warfarin - fourth edition. Br J Haematol. 2011;154:311–24.
22. Korinth MC. Low-dose aspirin before intracranial surgery results of a survey among neurosurgeons in Germany. Acta Neurochir. 2006;148:1189–96. discussion 1196.
23. Korinth MC, Gilsbach JM, Weinzierl MR. Low-dose aspirin before spinal surgery: results of a survey among neurosurgeons in Germany. Eur Spine J. 2007;16:365–72.
24. Lip GYH, Nieuwlaat R, Pisters R, Lane DA, Crijns HJGM. Refining clinical risk stratification for predicting stroke and thromboembolism in atrial fibrillation using a novel risk factor-based approach: the euro heart survey on atrial fibrillation. Chest. 2010;137:263–72.
25. Lip GYH, Nieuwlaat R, Pisters R, Lane DA, Crijns HJGM. Refining clinical risk stratification for predicting stroke and thromboembolism in atrial fibrillation using a novel risk factor-based approach: the euro heart survey on atrial fibrillation. Chest. 2010;137:263–72.
26. Mattle HP, Mono M-L. Closure of a patent foramen ovale with a device does not offer a greater benefit than medical therapy alone for the prevention of recurrent cerebrovascular events. Evid Based Med. 2013;18:34–5.
27. Navar-Boggan AM, Rymer JA, Piccini JP, Shatila W, Ring L, Stafford JA, et al. Accuracy and validation of an automated electronic algorithm to identify patients with atrial fibrillation at risk for stroke. Am Heart J. 2015;169:39–44.e2.
28. Palmer JD, Palmer JD, Sparrow OC, Sparrow OC, Iannotti F, Iannotti F. Postoperative hematoma: a 5-year survey and identification of avoidable risk factors. Neurosurgery. 1994;35:1061.
29. Patrono C, Ciabattoni G, Patrignani P, Pugliese F, Filabozzi P, Catella F, et al. Clinical pharmacology of platelet cyclooxygenase inhibition. Circulation. 1985;72:1177–84.

30. Rokito SE, Schwartz MC, Neuwirth MG. Deep vein thrombosis after major reconstructive spinal surgery. Spine. 1996;21:853–8. discussion 859.
31. Schulman S, Kearon C, Kakkar AK, Mismetti P, Schellong S, Eriksson H, et al. Dabigatran versus warfarin in the treatment of acute venous thromboembolism. N Engl J Med. 2009;361:2342–52.
32. Semrad TJ, O'Donnell R, Wun T, Chew H, Harvey D, Zhou H, et al. Epidemiology of venous thromboembolism in 9489 patients with malignant glioma. J Neurosurg. 2007;106:601–8.
33. Tai WA, Albers GW. Secondary prevention of atherothrombotic or cryptogenic stroke. Circulation. 2014;129:527–31.
34. Turpie A, Kreutz R, Llau J, Norrving B, Haas S. Management consensus guidance for the use of rivaroxaban-an oral, direct factor Xa inhibitor. Thromb Haemost. 2012;108(5):876–86.
35. Urbanek C, Palm F, Buggle F, Wolf J, Safer A, Becher H, et al. Recent surgery or invasive procedures and the risk of stroke. Cerebrovasc Dis. 2014;38:370–6.
36. van Ryn J, Stangier J, Haertter S, Liesenfeld KH, Wienen W, Feuring M, et al. Dabigatran etexilate-a novel, reversible, oral direct thrombin inhibitor: interpretation of coagulation assays and reversal of anticoagulant activity. Thromb Haemost. 2010;103(6): 1116–27.
37. van Veen JJ, Makris M. Management of peri-operative anti-thrombotic therapy. Anaesthesia. 2015;70 Suppl 1:58–67. e21–3.
38. Wang Y, Bajorek B. New oral anticoagulants in practice: pharmacological and practical considerations. Am J Cardiovasc Drugs. 2014;14:175–89.
39. Weber AA, Braun M, Hohlfeld T, Schwippert B, Tschöpe D, Schrör K. Recovery of platelet function after discontinuation of clopidogrel treatment in healthy volunteers. Br J Clin Pharmacol. 2001;52: 333–6.
40. Wong GY, Warner DO, Schroeder DR, Offord KP, Warner MA, Maxson PM, et al. Risk of surgery and anesthesia for ischemic stroke. Anesthesiology. 2000;92:425–32.

Spontaneous Intracerebral Hemorrhage Due to Coagulation Disorders

23

W. Caleb Rutledge, S. Andrew Josephson, and Michael T. Lawton

Introduction

Intracerebral hemorrhage (ICH) has an incidence of 24.6 cases per 100,000 person-years and is associated with both early mortality and long-term morbidity. Mortality at 1 month is 40 %, and only 12–39 % of patients achieve long-term functional independence following ICH [1]. While the incidence of ICH is decreasing in high-income countries, there has been a substantial rise in low- and middle-income countries, accounting for a 47 % increase in ICH, and a 20 % increase in mortality worldwide; this translates into a 14 % increase in disability-adjusted life years (DALYs) lost [2].

While hypertension and cerebral amyloid angiopathy are the most common causes of primary ICH, patients with coagulation disorders, particularly those taking oral anticoagulants, are at risk of developing lobar ICH which, compared with hypertension, features larger hematoma volumes, more frequent hematoma expansion, and worse outcomes (Figs. 23.1 and 23.2) [3–11]. Mortality at 1 month exceeds 50 % for patients with oral anticoagulant-associated ICH, likely driven in part to hematoma expansion following the initial hemorrhage [12, 13]. While the use of oral anticoagulants is increasing due to a higher prevalence of cardiovascular diseases such as atrial fibrillation [14–16], consensus about how to manage this serious complication is lacking [17, 18].

Antiplatelets, thrombolytic therapy, and oral anticoagulants (including vitamin K antagonists, direct thrombin and factor Xa inhibitors) may all contribute to ICH. Less common risk factors are acquired or congenital platelet and factor deficiencies, such as thrombocytopenia and hemophilia. This chapter focuses on coagulation disorders contributing to ICH and management of patients with ICH and abnormal coagulation.

Antiplatelets and Oral Anticoagulants

Antiplatelets, like aspirin, clopidogrel, and dipyridamole, vitamin K antagonists, direct thrombin inhibitors, and factor Xa inhibitors all increase the risk of ICH. Patients taking aspirin or other

W.C. Rutledge, M.D. • M.T. Lawton, M.D. (✉)
Department of Neurological Surgery, University of California, San Francisco, 505 Parnassus Avenue, San Francisco, CA 94143, USA
e-mail: Michael.Lawton@ucsf.edu

S.A. Josephson, M.D.
Department of Neurology, University of California, San Francisco, 505 Parnassus Avenue, San Francisco, CA 94143, USA

C.M. Loftus (ed.), *Anticoagulation and Hemostasis in Neurosurgery*, DOI 10.1007/978-3-319-27327-3_23

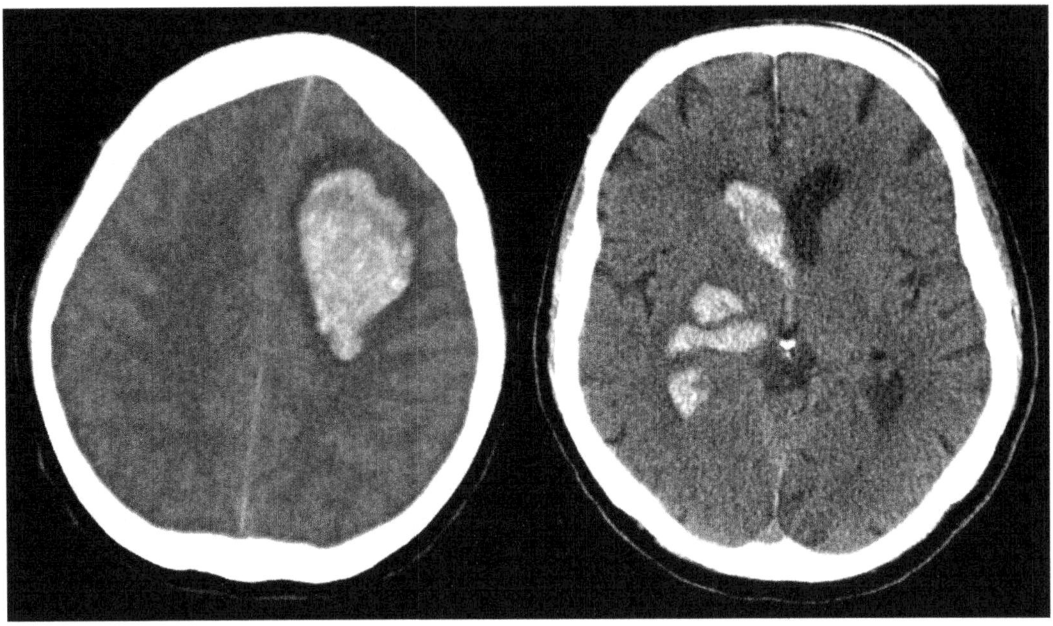

Fig. 23.1 Non-contrast CT showing right basal ganglia (*right*) and lobar ICH (*left*). Hypertension is commonly associated with deep hemorrhage, while lobar hemorrhage is associated with cerebral angiopathy. ICH associated with hemostatic abnormalities is disproportionately lobar

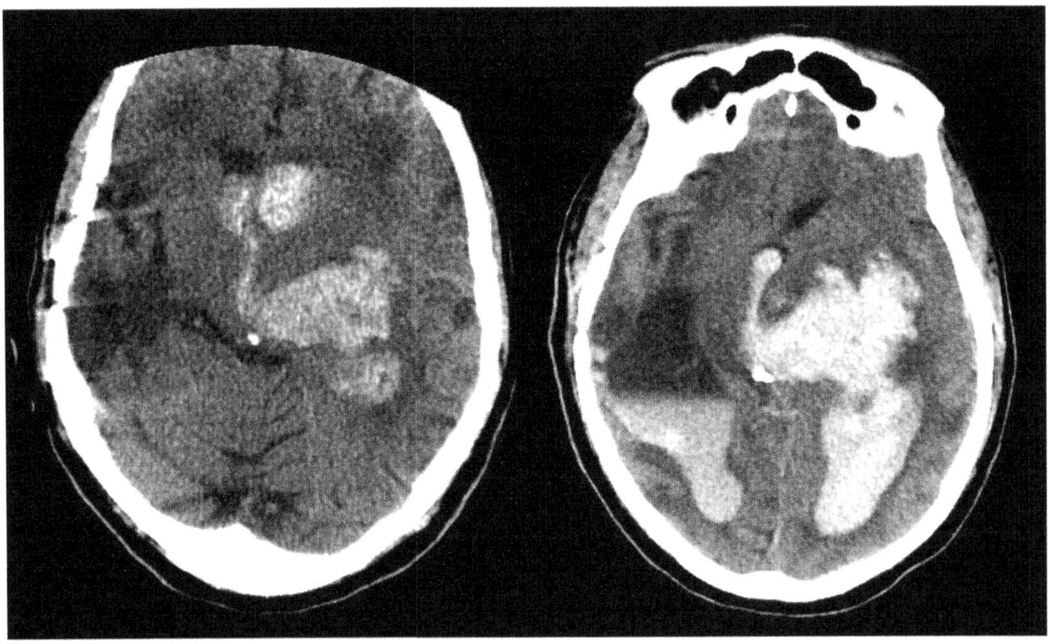

Fig. 23.2 Non-contrast CT demonstrating basal ganglia ICH with intraventricular extension (*left*) in patient with INR of 1.7. Repeat non-contrast CT (*right*) showing hematoma expansion. The patient received 6 units of FFP over approximately 6 h before correction of INR to 1.4

antiplatelets have a small increased risk of ICH, while patients on warfarin are at highest risk [6, 19]. Direct thrombin and factor Xa inhibitors have a significantly lower risk of ICH compared to warfarin, but their risk still far exceeds that associated with antiplatelet medications [20–24].

Antiplatelet-Associated ICH

Aspirin irreversibly inactivates the enzyme cyclooxygenase (COX), inhibiting production of prostaglandin and thromboxane and the aggregation of platelets. Other antiplatelet medications such as clopidogrel inhibit glycoprotein IIb/IIIa, similarly inhibiting platelet aggregation. While some observational studies have found an association between aspirin and worse outcomes, including mortality at 30 days [25–27], others have found no relationship between antiplatelets and the volume of ICH on baseline CT, hematoma expansion, or outcomes [28–30]. Although patients taking aspirin or other antiplatelets have some increased risk of ICH, the benefits of these medications, including prevention of myocardial infarction and ischemic stroke, far outweigh the risks of ICH.

Oral Anticoagulant-Associated ICH

Unlike antiplatelets, oral anticoagulants are clearly associated with a much higher risk of ICH. Anticoagulants are used to treat a variety of common medical conditions including deep venous thrombosis, pulmonary embolism, and atrial fibrillation [14–16]. The vitamin K antagonist warfarin is the most widely used anticoagulant, however novel oral anticoagulants such as dabigatran (Pradaxa), rivaroxaban (Xarelto), and apixaban (Eliquis) are being used with increasing frequency [21, 22, 24].

Vitamin K Antagonists

Warfarin is the most widely used vitamin K antagonist and its mechanism of action involves inhibiting hepatic formation of vitamin K-dependent clotting factors, including factors II, VII, IX, and X as well as protein C and S, ultimately resulting in decreased fibrin production. Warfarin has a narrow therapeutic window and despite frequent drug monitoring, sub-therapeutic and supra-therapeutic levels are common. Patients taking warfarin have a two- to fivefold increased risk of ICH that is level dependent [6, 11]. The intensity of anticoagulation is a strong predictor of ICH volume and hematoma expansion [4, 8]. Warfarin-associated ICH has been associated with large hematoma volumes, hematoma expansion, and mortality [5, 12, 31]. ICH accounts for 90 % of the deaths from hemorrhagic complications of warfarin [13].

Direct Thrombin and Factor Xa Inhibitors

Novel oral anticoagulants such as dabigatran, rivaroxaban, and apixaban, are United States Food and Drug Administration (FDA) approved for the prevention of stroke in patients with nonvalvular atrial fibrillation [21, 22, 24]. These agents have a wider therapeutic window and do not require monitoring like warfarin. Dabigatran is a direct thrombin antagonist and inhibits the conversion of fibrinogen to fibrin. Rivaroxaban and apixaban are antagonists of factor Xa and inhibit conversion of prothrombin to thrombin. Both direct thrombin inhibitors and factor Xa inhibitors have a lower incidence of ICH compared to warfarin [20–22, 24]. In a study comparing ICH in patients taking rivaroxaban and those taking warfarin, patients on rivaroxaban had smaller hematoma volumes, less hematoma expansion, and more favorable outcomes. Similarly, in a study comparing dabigatran to warfarin, the rate of hemorrhagic stroke was 0.38 % per year in patients on warfarin compared with 0.12 % per year with 110 mg of dabigatran ($P<0.001$) or 0.10 % per year with 150 mg of dabigatran ($P<0.001$) [21]. However, unlike warfarin the novel anticoagulants have no specific antidotes, leading to difficulties with management when ICH does occur with these agents.

Hemophilia and Other Congenital and Acquired Coagulation Disorders

ICH is a serious complication for patients with hemophilia and an important cause of morbidity and mortality in this population. It has a prevalence and incidence as high as 12 % and 2 % per year, respectively [32, 33]. Von Willebrand factor (vWF) deficiency, congenital afibrinogenemia, and factor deficiencies including V, VII, and XIII are other congenital disorders that increase the risk of ICH.

Management of ICH due to Coagulation Disorders

Current management of ICH associated with coagulation disorders is aimed at reducing hematoma expansion by rapidly reversing coagulopathy and controlling blood pressure. However, quality, high-level evidence supporting these strategies from randomized controlled trials is lacking.

All anticoagulant and antiplatelet drugs should be discontinued immediately following ICH. While reversal of coagulopathy has not been shown to improve outcomes, current guidelines recommend rapid reversal of coagulopathy to an international normalized ratio (INR) less than 1.4 to prevent further bleeding and hematoma expansion (see below).

Elevated blood pressure after ICH is associated with hematoma enlargement and poor outcomes [34–38]. The INTERACT and INTERACT-2 trials showed intensive blood pressure reduction attenuates hematoma growth after acute ICH and targeting a SBP <140 may be superior to higher targets; however, this more aggressive strategy did not result in a significant reduction in the rate of death or disability [39–42].

More recent evidence suggests reversal of coagulopathy combined with intensive reduction of blood pressure improves clinical outcomes specifically among patients with anticoagulant-associated ICH. Patients with oral anticoagulant-associated ICH who had an INR less than 1.3 and a systolic blood pressure less than 160 within 4 h had lower rates of hematoma enlargement and decreased in-hospital mortality compared with those who did not [43].

Options to Reverse Coagulopathy

Options for reversal of coagulopathy in warfarin-associated ICH include vitamin K, fresh-frozen plasma (FFP), prothrombin complex concentrates (PCC), and recombinant activated factor 7 (rFVIIa). For patients taking heparin, intravenous protamine sulfate is the reversal agent of choice.

Patients with antiplatelet-associated traumatic and spontaneous ICH are often given platelet transfusions to replace non-functional thrombocytes; however, there are few studies and no high-quality evidence that platelet transfusions prevent hematoma expansion or improve outcomes [44, 45].

Vitamin K fully reverses warfarin-induced anticoagulation, but its effect may be delayed up to 24 h. Current recommendations are to administer intravenous vitamin K while replacing vitamin K-dependent factors with FFP or PCCs [17].

FFP is widely available and inexpensive relative to other reversal agents, however the number of units required depends on the extent of INR prolongation, and large volumes are often required. FFP is also associated with a substantial time delay to INR normalization due in part to delays in cross-matching and thawing the drug, risking hematoma expansion [46].

In contrast to FFP, PCCs can be administered faster than FFP and require less volume of infusion [47]. In April of 2013, the FDAs approved a 4-factor PCC (Kcentra) for reversal of ICH associated with vitamin K antagonists. While PCCs have some advantages over FFP, there is no evidence that their use reduces hematoma expansion or improves clinical outcomes. Ongoing randomized controlled trials are comparing FFP with PCCs.

Recombinant human coagulation Factor VIIa (NovoSeven) is a hemostatic agent approved for hemophilia that binds to tissue factor and activates platelets, increasing local thrombin generation and promoting clot formation. rVIIa rapidly decreases the INR in patients taking warfarin and significantly reduces hematoma expansion after ICH, but has not been associated with improvement in clinical outcomes, including mortality, modified Rankin Scare (mRS) score, or Glasgow Outcome Scale (GOS-E) score. rVIIa also increases the risk of arterial thromboembolic events [48–52].

While direct thrombin and Factor Xa inhibitors are associated with a lower incidence of ICH, there are currently no direct antidotes or reversal agents for these drugs. Prothrombin complex concentrates are typically used, based on preclinical data [53]. A number of agents are in development to rapidly reverse these agents.

Hemophiliac patients with life-threatening ICH are treated with infusions of deficient coagulation factors, including von Willebrand factor and factor VIII [54, 55]. Patients with inhibitors often require rVIIa. Prophylaxis may also reduce the likelihood of ICH occurrence [56].

Surgery for Anticoagulant-Associated ICH

Large randomized clinical trials comparing surgery to medical therapy among patients with spontaneous ICH have not shown differences in outcomes. In the first International Surgical Trial in Intracerebral Haemorrhage (STICH), comparing surgery to medical therapy, patients randomized to surgery, who underwent hematoma evacuation within 24 h, demonstrated no difference in outcome at 6 months [57]. Other studies have suggested early surgery may improve outcomes [58]; however, in a second randomized trial (STITCH II), comparing early surgery (within 12 h of randomization) to medical therapy, there was again no difference found in outcomes at 6 months. Patients with superficial ICH without intraventricular extension may benefit from early surgery [59]. Patients with ICH associated with oral anticoagulants were excluded from these studies, as were cerebellar hemorrhages.

Resumption of Anticoagulants

Whether to resume anticoagulation in survivors of anticoagulant-associated ICH remains controversial. Observational studies suggest the risk of recurrent ICH is low and most experts recommend resumption following a variable delay [60–62]. In a recent study, there were significantly fewer ischemic complications among patients who resumed oral anticoagulants after ICH compared to patients who did not and no significant difference in hemorrhage rates. There was a mortality benefit for patients with atrial fibrillation who resumed their anticoagulants [43].

Conclusions

Spontaneous ICH due to hemostatic abnormalities is fatal in approximately 50 % of cases. Patients on oral anticoagulants have larger hematomas and greater mortality compared to patients without coagulopathy. The management of patients with ICH and hemostatic abnormalities is controversial, particularly in regards to correction of coagulopathy. The 2014 European Stroke Organization (ESO) guidelines do not make strong recommendations about how, when, and for whom to normalize coagulation, as "no moderate- to high-quality evidence supports the use of acute hemostatic therapies… benefit from prevention of hematoma expansion [seems] to be counterbalanced by thromboembolic complications with no overall benefit" [18]. Current guidelines from the American Heart Association/American Stroke Association (AHA/ASA) recommend therapy to replace vitamin K-dependent factors and correction of the INR as rapidly as possible despite Level C evidence (very limited populations evaluation, only expert opinion, case studies, or standard of care) [17]. Intensive blood pressure reduction along with rapid reversal of coagulopathy may prevent hematoma expansion and improve outcomes.

References

1. van Asch CJ, Luitse MJ, Rinkel GJ, van der Tweel I, Algra A, Klijn CJ. Incidence, case fatality, and functional outcome of intracerebral haemorrhage over time, according to age, sex, and ethnic origin: a systematic review and meta-analysis. Lancet Neurol. 2010;9:167–76.
2. Krishnamurthi RV, Feigin VL, Forouzanfar MH, Mensah GA, Connor M, Bennett DA, et al. Global and regional burden of first-ever ischaemic and haemorrhagic stroke during 1990–2010: findings from the Global Burden of Disease Study 2010. Lancet Glob Health. 2013;1:e259–81.
3. Falcone GJ, Biffi A, Brouwers HB, Anderson CD, Battey TW, Ayres AM, et al. Predictors of hematoma volume in deep and lobar supratentorial intracerebral hemorrhage. JAMA Neurol. 2013;70:988–94.
4. Fang MC, Chang Y, Hylek EM, Rosand J, Greenberg SM, Go AS, et al. Advanced age, anticoagulation intensity, and risk for intracranial hemorrhage among patients taking warfarin for atrial fibrillation. Ann Intern Med. 2004;141:745–52.

5. Flaherty ML, Tao H, Haverbusch M, Sekar P, Kleindorfer D, Kissela B, et al. Warfarin use leads to larger intracerebral hematomas. Neurology. 2008;71: 1084–9.
6. Garcia-Rodriguez LA, Gaist D, Morton J, Cookson C, Gonzalez-Perez A. Antithrombotic drugs and risk of hemorrhagic stroke in the general population. Neurology. 2013;81:566–74.
7. Horstmann S, Rizos T, Lauseker M, Mohlenbruch M, Jenetzky E, Hacke W, et al. Intracerebral hemorrhage during anticoagulation with vitamin K antagonists: a consecutive observational study. J Neurol. 2013;260: 2046–51.
8. Hylek EM, Go AS, Chang Y, Jensvold NG, Henault LE, Selby JV, et al. Effect of intensity of oral anticoagulation on stroke severity and mortality in atrial fibrillation. N Engl J Med. 2003;349:1019–26.
9. Maas MB, Rosenberg NF, Kosteva AR, Prabhakaran S, Naidech AM. Coagulopathy disproportionately predisposes to lobar intracerebral hemorrhage. Neurocrit Care. 2013;18:166–9.
10. Pezzini A, Grassi M, Paciaroni M, Zini A, Silvestrelli G, Del Zotto E, et al. Antithrombotic medications and the etiology of intracerebral hemorrhage: MUCH-Italy. Neurology. 2014;82:529–35.
11. Rosand J, Eckman MH, Knudsen KA, Singer DE, Greenberg SM. The effect of warfarin and intensity of anticoagulation on outcome of intracerebral hemorrhage. Arch Intern Med. 2004;164:880–4.
12. Cucchiara B, Messe S, Sansing L, Kasner S, Lyden P. Hematoma growth in oral anticoagulant related intracerebral hemorrhage. Stroke. 2008;39:2993–6.
13. Fang MC, Go AS, Chang Y, Hylek EM, Henault LE, Jensvold NG, et al. Death and disability from warfarin-associated intracranial and extracranial hemorrhages. Am J Med. 2007;120:700–5.
14. Go AS, Hylek EM, Phillips KA, Chang Y, Henault LE, Selby JV, et al. Prevalence of diagnosed atrial fibrillation in adults: national implications for rhythm management and stroke prevention: the AnTicoagulation and Risk Factors in Atrial Fibrillation (ATRIA) Study. JAMA. 2001;285:2370–5.
15. Lovelock CE, Molyneux AJ, Rothwell PM. Change in incidence and aetiology of intracerebral haemorrhage in Oxfordshire, UK, between 1981 and 2006: a population-based study. Lancet Neurol. 2007;6: 487–93.
16. Patel NJ, Deshmukh A, Pant S, Singh V, Patel N, Arora S, et al. Contemporary trends of hospitalization for atrial fibrillation in the United States, 2000 through 2010: implications for healthcare planning. Circulation. 2014;129:2371–9.
17. Morgenstern LB, Hemphill 3rd JC, Anderson C, Becker K, Broderick JP, Connolly Jr ES, et al. Guidelines for the management of spontaneous intracerebral hemorrhage: a guideline for healthcare professionals from the American Heart Association/ American Stroke Association. Stroke. 2010;41: 2108–29.
18. Steiner T, Al-Shahi Salman R, Beer R, Christensen H, Cordonnier C, Csiba L, et al. European Stroke Organisation (ESO) guidelines for the management of spontaneous intracerebral hemorrhage. Int J Stroke. 2014;9:840–55.
19. He J, Whelton PK, Vu B, Klag MJ. Aspirin and risk of hemorrhagic stroke: a meta-analysis of randomized controlled trials. JAMA. 1998;280:1930–5.
20. Cameron C, Coyle D, Richter T, Kelly S, Gauthier K, Steiner S, et al. Systematic review and network meta-analysis comparing antithrombotic agents for the prevention of stroke and major bleeding in patients with atrial fibrillation. BMJ Open. 2014;4:e004301.
21. Connolly SJ, Ezekowitz MD, Yusuf S, Eikelboom J, Oldgren J, Parekh A, et al. Dabigatran versus warfarin in patients with atrial fibrillation. N Engl J Med. 2009;361:1139–51.
22. Granger CB, Alexander JH, McMurray JJ, Lopes RD, Hylek EM, Hanna M, et al. Apixaban versus warfarin in patients with atrial fibrillation. N Engl J Med. 2011;365:981–92.
23. Hagii J, Tomita H, Metoki N, Saito S, Shiroto H, Hitomi H, et al. Characteristics of intracerebral hemorrhage during rivaroxaban treatment: comparison with those during warfarin. Stroke. 2014;45: 2805–7.
24. Patel MR, Mahaffey KW, Garg J, Pan G, Singer DE, Hacke W, et al. Rivaroxaban versus warfarin in nonvalvular atrial fibrillation. N Engl J Med. 2011;365:883–91.
25. Roquer J, Rodriguez Campello A, Gomis M, Ois A, Puente V, Munteis E. Previous antiplatelet therapy is an independent predictor of 30-day mortality after spontaneous supratentorial intracerebral hemorrhage. J Neurol. 2005;252:412–6.
26. Thompson BB, Bejot Y, Caso V, Castillo J, Christensen H, Flaherty ML, et al. Prior antiplatelet therapy and outcome following intracerebral hemorrhage: a systematic review. Neurology. 2010;75:1333–42.
27. Toyoda K, Okada Y, Minematsu K, Kamouchi M, Fujimoto S, Ibayashi S, et al. Antiplatelet therapy contributes to acute deterioration of intracerebral hemorrhage. Neurology. 2005;65:1000–4.
28. Caso V, Paciaroni M, Venti M, Alberti A, Palmerini F, Milia P, et al. Effect of on-admission antiplatelet treatment on patients with cerebral hemorrhage. Cerebrovasc Dis. 2007;24:215–8.
29. Foerch C, Sitzer M, Steinmetz H, Neumann-Haefelin T. Pretreatment with antiplatelet agents is not independently associated with unfavorable outcome in intracerebral hemorrhage. Stroke. 2006;37:2165–7.
30. Sansing LH, Messe SR, Cucchiara BL, Cohen SN, Lyden PD, Kasner SE. Prior antiplatelet use does not affect hemorrhage growth or outcome after ICH. Neurology. 2009;72:1397–402.
31. Dowlatshahi D, Butcher KS, Asdaghi N, Nahirniak S, Bernbaum ML, Giulivi A, et al. Poor prognosis in warfarin-associated intracranial hemorrhage despite anticoagulation reversal. Stroke. 2012;43:1812–7.

32. Klinge J, Auberger K, Auerswald G, Brackmann HH, Mauz-Korholz C, Kreuz W. Prevalence and outcome of intracranial haemorrhage in haemophiliacs—a survey of the paediatric group of the German Society of Thrombosis and Haemostasis (GTH). Eur J Pediatr. 1999;158 Suppl 3:S162–5.
33. Nelson Jr MD, Maeder MA, Usner D, Mitchell WG, Fenstermacher MJ, Wilson DA, et al. Prevalence and incidence of intracranial haemorrhage in a population of children with haemophilia. The Hemophilia Growth and Development Study. Haemophilia. 1999;5:306–12.
34. Fogelholm R, Avikainen S, Murros K. Prognostic value and determinants of first-day mean arterial pressure in spontaneous supratentorial intracerebral hemorrhage. Stroke. 1997;28:1396–400.
35. Ohwaki K, Yano E, Nagashima H, Hirata M, Nakagomi T, Tamura A. Blood pressure management in acute intracerebral hemorrhage: relationship between elevated blood pressure and hematoma enlargement. Stroke. 2004;35:1364–7.
36. Okumura K, Ohya Y, Maehara A, Wakugami K, Iseki K, Takishita S. Effects of blood pressure levels on case fatality after acute stroke. J Hypertens. 2005;23:1217–23.
37. Vemmos KN, Tsivgoulis G, Spengos K, Zakopoulos N, Synetos A, Manios E, et al. U-shaped relationship between mortality and admission blood pressure in patients with acute stroke. J Intern Med. 2004;255:257–65.
38. Zhang Y, Reilly KH, Tong W, Xu T, Chen J, Bazzano LA, et al. Blood pressure and clinical outcome among patients with acute stroke in Inner Mongolia, China. J Hypertens. 2008;26:1446–52.
39. Anderson CS, Heeley E, Huang Y, Wang J, Stapf C, Delcourt C, et al. Rapid blood-pressure lowering in patients with acute intracerebral hemorrhage. N Engl J Med. 2013;368:2355–65.
40. Anderson CS, Huang Y, Arima H, Heeley E, Skulina C, Parsons MW, et al. Effects of early intensive blood pressure-lowering treatment on the growth of hematoma and perihematomal edema in acute intracerebral hemorrhage: the Intensive Blood Pressure Reduction in Acute Cerebral Haemorrhage Trial (INTERACT). Stroke. 2010;41:307–12.
41. Anderson CS, Huang Y, Wang JG, Arima H, Neal B, Peng B, et al. Intensive blood pressure reduction in acute cerebral haemorrhage trial (INTERACT): a randomised pilot trial. Lancet Neurol. 2008;7:391–9.
42. Arima H, Anderson CS, Wang JG, Huang Y, Heeley E, Neal B, et al. Lower treatment blood pressure is associated with greatest reduction in hematoma growth after acute intracerebral hemorrhage. Hypertension. 2010;56:852–8.
43. Kuramatsu JB, Gerner ST, Schellinger PD, Glahn J, Endres M, Sobesky J, et al. Anticoagulant reversal, blood pressure levels, and anticoagulant resumption in patients with anticoagulation-related intracerebral hemorrhage. JAMA. 2015;313:824–36.
44. Campbell PG, Sen A, Yadla S, Jabbour P, Jallo J. Emergency reversal of antiplatelet agents in patients presenting with an intracranial hemorrhage: a clinical review. World Neurosurg. 2010;74:279–85.
45. Joseph B, Pandit V, Sadoun M, Larkins CG, Kulvatunyou N, Tang A, et al. A prospective evaluation of platelet function in patients on antiplatelet therapy with traumatic intracranial hemorrhage. J Trauma Acute Care Surg. 2013;75:990–4.
46. Lee SB, Manno EM, Layton KF, Wijdicks EF. Progression of warfarin-associated intracerebral hemorrhage after INR normalization with FFP. Neurology. 2006;67:1272–4.
47. Fredriksson K, Norrving B, Stromblad LG. Emergency reversal of anticoagulation after intracerebral hemorrhage. Stroke. 1992;23:972–7.
48. Al-Shahi Salman R. Haemostatic drug therapies for acute spontaneous intracerebral haemorrhage. Cochrane Database Syst Rev. 2009:CD005951.
49. Diringer MN, Skolnick BE, Mayer SA, Steiner T, Davis SM, Brun NC, et al. Thromboembolic events with recombinant activated factor VII in spontaneous intracerebral hemorrhage: results from the Factor Seven for Acute Hemorrhagic Stroke (FAST) trial. Stroke. 2010;41:48–53.
50. Robinson MT, Rabinstein AA, Meschia JF, Freeman WD. Safety of recombinant activated factor VII in patients with warfarin-associated hemorrhages of the central nervous system. Stroke. 2010;41:1459–63.
51. Yank V, Tuohy CV, Logan AC, Bravata DM, Staudenmayer K, Eisenhut R, et al. Systematic review: benefits and harms of in-hospital use of recombinant factor VIIa for off-label indications. Ann Intern Med. 2011;154:529–40.
52. Yuan ZH, Jiang JK, Huang WD, Pan J, Zhu JY, Wang JZ. A meta-analysis of the efficacy and safety of recombinant activated factor VII for patients with acute intracerebral hemorrhage without hemophilia. J Clin Neurosci. 2010;17:685–93.
53. Steiner T, Bohm M, Dichgans M, Diener HC, Ell C, Endres M, et al. Recommendations for the emergency management of complications associated with the new direct oral anticoagulants (DOACs), apixaban, dabigatran and rivaroxaban. Clin Res Cardiol. 2013;102:399–412.
54. Daniele F, Rossi V, Santoro C. Effective management of intracranial haemorrhage with continuous infusion of highly purified von Willebrand factor/factor VIII complex concentrate in an adult with severe haemophilia A. Blood Transfus. 2011;9:472–4.
55. McMillan CW, Webster WP, Roberts HR, Blythe WB. Continuous intravenous infusion of factor VIII in classic haemophilia. Br J Haematol. 1970;18:659–67.
56. Witmer C, Presley R, Kulkarni R, Soucie JM, Manno CS, Raffini L. Associations between intracranial haemorrhage and prescribed prophylaxis in a large cohort of haemophilia patients in the United States. Br J Haematol. 2011;152:211–6.

57. Mendelow AD, Gregson BA, Fernandes HM, Murray GD, Teasdale GM, Hope DT, et al. Early surgery versus initial conservative treatment in patients with spontaneous supratentorial intracerebral haematomas in the International Surgical Trial in Intracerebral Haemorrhage (STICH): a randomised trial. Lancet. 2005;365:387–97.
58. Gregson BA, Broderick JP, Auer LM, Batjer H, Chen XC, Juvela S, et al. Individual patient data subgroup meta-analysis of surgery for spontaneous supratentorial intracerebral hemorrhage. Stroke. 2012;43:1496–504.
59. Mendelow AD, Gregson BA, Rowan EN, Murray GD, Gholkar A, Mitchell PM. Early surgery versus initial conservative treatment in patients with spontaneous supratentorial lobar intracerebral haematomas (STICH II): a randomised trial. Lancet. 2013;382: 397–408.
60. Biffi A, Halpin A, Towfighi A, Gilson A, Busl K, Rost N, et al. Aspirin and recurrent intracerebral hemorrhage in cerebral amyloid angiopathy. Neurology. 2010;75:693–8.
61. Claassen DO, Kazemi N, Zubkov AY, Wijdicks EF, Rabinstein AA. Restarting anticoagulation therapy after warfarin-associated intracerebral hemorrhage. Arch Neurol. 2008;65:1313–8.
62. Flynn RW, MacDonald TM, Murray GD, MacWalter RS, Doney AS. Prescribing antiplatelet medicine and subsequent events after intracerebral hemorrhage. Stroke. 2010;41:2606–11.

Prophylactic Screening for Venous Thromboembolism in Neurosurgical Patients

24

Michael J. Schneck

Venous thromboembolism (VTE) is a term that typically encompasses pulmonary embolism (PE) or venous thrombosis of the extremities. VTE may also occur in the central nervous system as cerebral venous sinus thrombosis (CVST) or in the abdominal and pelvic veins. Diagnosis of CVST represents a unique challenge outside the framework of this chapter.

Deep venous thromboses (DVT) or superficial venous thromboses (SVT) consist of either partial or total occlusions of draining veins of the upper or lower extremities. SVT and DVT may result in thrombophlebitis with fever, local erythema, or leg swelling. Additionally, early identification of extremity thrombosis is important because of the potential for propagation of emboli to the pulmonary circulation with resultant PE increasing the risk of hypoxia, right heart strain, and death.

DVT is the primary cause of PE [1, 2]. Even clinically asymptomatic DVT is associated with increased PE-related death with fatality rates ranging from 13 % to 15 % [2–4]. Distal (calf vein) DVT has a lower fatality rate compared with proximal lower extremity DVT, but approximately 25 % of patients with distal DVT have concomitant proximal DVT or PE, with 40–50 % risk of calf vein thromboses extending to proximal leg veins [2, 3, 5, 6]. Upper extremity DVT, typically the result of peripherally inserted central catheters (PICC) and central venous lines, occurs less frequently than lower extremity DVT but with a 36 % PE rate that is higher than the PE rate associated with lower extremity DVT [7]. Upper extremity DVT is being increasingly recognized; one series reported that one-fourth of all patients screened for DVT had an upper extremity thrombus [8]. In these patients, cancer and/or presence of an indwelling PICC were the major risk factors for DVT [8].

DVT mortality related to subsequent PE ranges from 10 % to 25 % and up to three-quarters of untreated PE patients will die within the first week of symptom onset [2, 9]. Approximately 25 % of PE patients die suddenly, and long-term survival of PE patients is approximately 71 % [4]. Identification of VTE risk in high-risk neurosurgical patients is therefore critical for reduction of postoperative morbidity and mortality and understanding the inherent VTE risk is therefore necessary in determining the benefit of VTE screening.

VTE screening is a complicated task because patients may not have obvious clinical symptoms or signs. For)DVT, the clinical examination may

M.J. Schneck, M.D. (✉)
Department of Neurology, Loyola University Chicago, Stritch School of Medicine, Maguire Building, Suite 2700, 2160 South First Avenue, Maywood, IL 60153, USA

Department of Neurosurgery, Loyola University Chicago, Stritch School of Medicine, Maguire Building, Suite 2700, 2160 South First Avenue, Maywood, IL 60153, USA
e-mail: mschneck@lumc.edu

C.M. Loftus (ed.), *Anticoagulation and Hemostasis in Neurosurgery*, DOI 10.1007/978-3-319-27327-3_24

be highly variable, and the clinical presentation of an acute painful, enlarged, swollen, and erythematous extremity only occurs in about one-half of patients [9]. A Homan's sign, in which there is pain in the calf with rapid dorsiflexion of the patient's foot with the knee in extension, is very unreliable with accuracy of this sign being less than 50 % for patients with confirmed DVT [10]. Additionally, DVT semiology may be confused with other co-morbid conditions such as painful symptoms that might be wrongly attributed to neuropathy, or lower extremity edema associated with cardiac disease or limb paralysis.

Similarly, the classical PE presentations of pleuritic chest pain, variable degrees of shortness of breath, and/or cardiac arrhythmias are not sufficiently pathognomonic to serve as valid diagnostic criteria. For patients with PE, close to half may be clinically without overt symptoms; for example, a PE may have been discovered as an incidental part of an evaluation in which a DVT was first discovered or incidental to an evaluation for pulmonary neoplasm [2]. Clinical VTE prediction tools such as Well's criteria for DVT or PE are of limited utility in hospitalized neurosurgical patients, the majority of who, by definition, are at high risk [11–16]. Table 24.1 lists the main clinical risk factors for hospitalized neurosurgical patients.

Arterial blood gas (ABG) and electrocardiogram may be suggestive tests for PE. Electrocardiographic (ECG) findings may reflect

Table 24.1 VTE risk factors

Age > 60 years
Cancer (increased risk with chemotherapy)
Central lines or PICC lines
Family history of DVT or PE
History of heart disease
History of prior DVT or PE
Major trauma
Nephrotic syndrome
Oral contraceptive or hormone replacement therapy
Prolonged motor weakness (especially of lower extremity(ies))
Surgery (see text)
Stroke (hemorrhagic or ischemic)
Thrombophilias (acquired or inherited)

acute pulmonary hypertension but are insufficient to conclusively make a PE diagnosis. ECG findings in PE patients may include sinus tachycardia (44 %), right ventricular strain (34 %), right axis deviation (16 %), right bundle branch block (18 %), right axial enlargement (9 %), and atrial tachycardia (8 %). Upwards of 50 % of patients have non-specific ST segment or T wave changes and the classic finding of a deep S wave in lead I, Q wave in lead III, and inverted T wave in lead III, is seen only 20 % of patients. Eighteen percent of PE patients will have a completely normal ECG [17].

Echocardiographic signs of increased pulmonary arterial resurges may suggest but are not definitive for PE either. McConnell's sign, which reflects right heart strain, is an echo finding that may lead to the diagnosis of otherwise unsuspected moderate to large PE [18].

The d-dimer test is the serum assay most often used to evaluate patients with possible VTE. An elevated d-dimer may suggest possible VTE but is of limited utility in most neurosurgical patients because elevated d-dimer levels may also occur in the context of the perioperative setting, recent trauma, acute vascular events (myocardial infarction (MI) or stroke), and in the context of underlying malignancy or autoimmune states. The d-dimer test is mainly useful as a VTE exclusion criterion [12–15]. In the outpatient setting, a negative d-dimer has a negative predictive value of 99 % whereas false-positive d-dimer assays are common in hospitalized patients [13, 19, 20].

In screening for DVT or PE, imaging becomes necessary for a conclusive diagnosis. Contrast venography of the extremities, for DVT diagnosis, or pulmonary catheter directed angiography, for PE diagnosis, are the definitive diagnostic procedures but the invasive risk and cost associated with these procedures has limited their use to those patients in which intravascular thrombolysis is being considered. In the extremities, duplex ultrasound is the mainstay for DVT diagnosis, whereas chest computerized tomographic angiography (CTA) or ventilation/perfusion (V/Q) imaging are used for PE diagnosis [1, 21].

Venous ultrasonography of the extremities has the advantage of being non-invasive, portable,

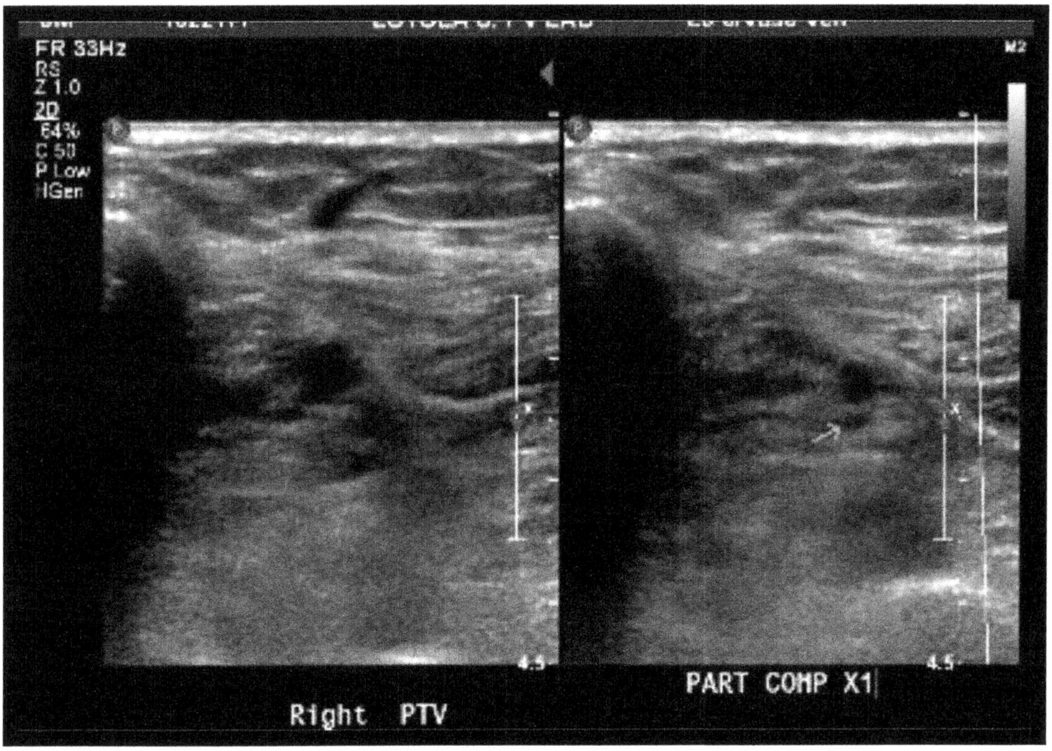

Fig. 24.1 Lower extremity venous duplex ultrasound demonstrating evidence of an acute deep venous thrombosis of the posterior tibial vein

and easily repeated, but it is operator dependent, and provides limited visualization of clot in the pelvic and iliac veins (see Fig. 24.1). Lower extremity venous ultrasonography has sensitivities of 89–96 % and specificities 96–100 % for clinically significant DVT, though for distal lower extremity (calf) vein thrombosis, sensitivities are only 75 % [1, 3, 20, 22, 23]. For imaging of the iliac and pelvic veins, magnetic resonance imaging (MRI) becomes necessary and may be more sensitive than ultrasound in imaging of calf vein thrombosis. MRI has a sensitivity of 91.5 % for lower extremity DVT in comparison with the gold standard of contrast venography [24]. By comparison to MRI, ultrasound has a sensitivity of 93.5 % and CT venography has a sensitivity of 89–100 % [21, 24].

For the diagnosis of PE there are two major options: spiral CT angiography (CTA) and ventilation/perfusion (V/Q) scanning [25, 26]. A normal V/Q scan excludes PE with high sensitivity and specificity, and a high probability V/Q scan had a 95 % positive predictive value in patients deemed at high PE risk [25]. Unfortunately, V/Q scans, using standard techniques, are frequently non-diagnostic in patients with intermediate to high pre-test probability. In one series, high probability V/Q scans were reported in just 41 % of patients with angiographic proven PE [27]. Thus, spiral CTA has become a preferred test compared to VQ scans except for those patients with contrast dye allergies or impaired renal function. CTA has a sensitivity of 99 % and a specificity of 95 % in comparison to catheter-based pulmonary angiography [26] (see Fig. 24.2).

Other testing considerations in VTE screening include serum markers for hypercoaguable states. These include the hereditary and acquired thrombophilias: activated protein C resistance, factor V Leiden mutation, prothrombin G20210A mutation, antiphospholipid antibodies, lupus anticoagulant, elevated factor VIII levels, protein C or protein S deficiency, hyperhomocysteinemia, dysfibrinogenemia, antithrombin deficiency, and

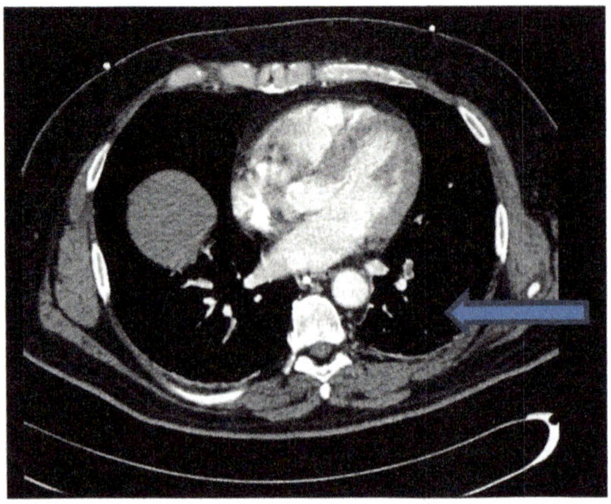

Fig. 24.2 CT angiogram of the pulmonary vessels demonstrating acute pulmonary emboli in the segmental arteries of the left lower lobe (see *arrow*)

heparin-induced thrombocytopenia [1, 28–35]. Factor V Leiden and prothrombin G20210A mutations are the two hereditary thrombophilia markers most strongly associated with increased VTE risk [28–30, 33, 35]. Factor V Leiden prevalence is approximately 5 %, and prothrombin G20210A mutation prevalence is approximately 2 %, in white patients though these markers are less common in African-Americans and Asians [28, 33–35]. While the VTE risk is significant, heterozygous carriers of each mutation alone do not have an increased risk compared to non-carriers [33]. Double heterozygous carriers of factor V Leiden and the prothrombin G20210A mutation have a 20-fold increased VTE risk and homozygous factor V Leiden carriers have an 80-fold increased VTE risk. Antiphospholipid (APL) antibodies are the most common acquired thrombophilia marker and, in the presence of concomitant lupus anticoagulants, VTE risk is elevated but the degree of that risk is ill defined. For recurrent VTE the risk in patients with APL antibodies, off warfarin, is 1.53 and with concomitant lupus anticoagulants, the risk is 2.83 [36]. Routine preoperative screening for thrombophilias is not recommended for clinically asymptomatic patients with no prior medical VTE history, or family history of thrombophilia [34, 35]. At least in one series of patients with spinal cord injury, there was no specific association between spinal cord injury, thrombophilia, and VTE [37].

Indications for VTE screening are based on an awareness of the underlying risk rates. In the outpatient or emergency department settings, clinical prediction scores may have some utility but the standard clinical prediction scores for hospitalized patients are little better than chance in predicting DVT [38]. Hospitalized patients, however, have a significant VTE risk with estimated hospital VTE prevalence of 10–40 % in moderate-risk patients and upwards of 80 % among high-risk patients with the risk particularly high in patients with neurologic or neurosurgical diseases [2]. DVT prevalence ranges from 15 % to 40 % in neurosurgical patients and 20 % to 40 % in stroke patients. DVT incidence approaches 50 % in neurosurgical patients and PE incidence is estimated at 1.5–5 % with an associated PE mortality of 9–59 % in neurosurgical patients [1, 39]. Risk factors for VTE in these patients include concomitant stroke, spinal cord injury, brain neoplasms, degree and duration of immobility, and the type and length of the surgical procedure. Other factors include ventilator dependence, chronic steroid use, and sepsis [1, 15, 40–45]. The estimated 30-day postoperative VTE rate, derived from a large administrative database of neurosurgical patients, was 1.7 %; with DVT frequency of 1.3 % and PE frequency of 0.6 % [15]. In that series, cranial surgeries were associated with greater VTE risk than spine surgeries. For elective neurosurgical and spine procedures, the risk of DVT is lower, particularly if patients receive pharmacologic prophylaxis, with an estimated DVT rate in elective cases of 1.09 % and PE rate of 0.06 % [46].

The Scoliosis Research Society reported the 2004–2007 VTE complication rates for lumbar microdiscectomy, anterior cervical discectomy and fusion, and lumbar spinal stenosis decompression. The DVT rate was 1.18/1000, and the PE rate was 1.38/1000 cases with a mortality rate of 0.34/1000 cases. Type of surgery defined VTE risk with rates being lowest for lumbar microdiscectomy, and highest for spine tumor surgeries [47]. VTE risk is also increased for patients undergoing combined anterior and posterior procedures versus posterior spine procedures alone [48]. A study of the United States (US) Nationwide

Inpatient Sample (NIS) database from 2002 to 2009, of 273,396 cervical procedures, reported that posterior cervical fusions were associated with the highest incidence and anterior cervical fusions were associated with the lowest incidence of DVT and PE ($P < 0.0005$) [49].

Spinal cord injury patients have rates estimated at upwards of 60–80 % [1, 42]. VTE risk for patients with spinal cord injury is highest in the initial 3 months post injury with one large Taiwanese longitudinal cohort study reporting hazard ratios of 16.9 for DVT and 3.6 for PE [50]. Risks were higher for older patients. The DVT risk was highest for patients with cervical spine injury and the PE risk was highest for patients with thoracic cord injuries [50]. Another series of 18,302 patients with spinal cord injury entered into the National Trauma Data Bank (for 2007–2008) reported a 4.3 % VTE rate [51]. This study also reported that spinal cord level was an independent VTE risk factor along with older age, higher Injury Severity Score, being male, traumatic brain injury, and chest trauma. The highest VTE rate (6.3 %) occurred in patients with T1-6 spine injury. Patients with C1-4 injury had VTE rates of 3.4 % whereas patients with lumbar injury had VTE rates of 3.2 %. A large California administrative hospital discharge database of 267,743 trauma patients admitted with traumatic pelvic fractures, vertebral fractures, and spinal cord injuries, found that 3.97 % developed VTE [52]. Patients with vertebral fractures were less likely to develop VTE as compared with patients with associated pelvic fractures (hazard ratio (HR) 0.85) but patients with spinal cord injury were more likely to develop VTE (HR 3.17). As with the other series, patients in the California database with cervical (HR 1.49) or thoracic (HR 1.87) spinal cord injuries had an increased VTE risk as compared with patients with lumbar spine trauma.

The DVT rate has been reported to range from 40 % to 80 % for patients with major head trauma though that rate is estimated at only 25 %, among patients with isolated head injuries [1, 41, 42]. Factors associated with increased VTE risk in patients with head trauma include: subarachnoid hemorrhage (SAH), associated lower extremity injury, higher injury severity scores, and older age [42, 45].

VTE rates are increased in neurosurgical patients with cancer. In general, neoplasms are associated with increased VTE risk but this is especially true for patients with central nervous system (CNS) tumors [40, 53]. DVT is actually the most common postoperative adverse event in patients undergoing craniotomy for brain tumors with a reported incidence ranging from 3 % to 26 % [54].

Patients with intracranial tumors appear to have a higher VTE rate than patients with spinal cord tumors [55]. Symptomatic VTE prevalence rates are estimated at up to 30 % of all patients with intracranial neoplasms [56]. This VTE risk is attributed to tumor-induced hypercoaguable states that may be particularly prevalent in patients with astrocytoma [40]. In a California registry of 9489 cases of hospitalized patients with malignant glioma, the cumulative 2-year incidence of VTE was 7.5 % with over half of those diagnosed within 60 days of the initial surgery. VTE in these patients was associated with an increased mortality risk (HR 1.3) [53]. Factors associated with increased VTE risk included higher-grade tumors, older age, multiple medical co-morbidities, worse functional capacity (assessed by Karnofsky Performance Scale scores), and presence of a motor deficit [53, 57]. Patients with astrocytoma and associated VTE have a 30 % increased risk of death within 2 years [1]. Even for other CNS tumor types, there is an increased though lesser VTE risk. Thus, in one series of 834 patients who had craniotomies for meningioma, 6.8 % had significant medical complications, and clinically symptomatic VTE comprised 0.8 % of all complications [58].

For ischemic stroke, the estimated DVT prevalence rate was 0.8 % and the PE rate was 0.3 % [59]. The risk in stroke patients is related to immobility as well as increased hypercoagulability. Clinical risk predictors cannot distinguish between those immobile stroke patients at low versus high risk of DVT [60]. Without medical prophylactic therapies, 75 % of stroke patients may get a DVT, and upward of 25 % of early post-stroke deaths may be the result of a PE. PE-related deaths typically occur within the first 4 weeks post hemorrhagic or ischemic stroke [61–63]. The VTE rate for hemorrhagic stroke is approximately 65 % higher than for ischemic stroke [64]. The DVT rate among 7651 patients, who underwent aneurysm clipping from the NIS database for the years 2005 through 2009 (48.1 % of whom had unruptured aneurysms and 51.9 % with SAH), was 0.6 % for patients with unruptured aneurysms and 2.8 % for patients with SAH; the PE rate was 2 % for unruptured aneurysm patients and 2.7 % for SAH patients [65]. A smaller study suggested there was no association for VTE risk with coiling versus clipping in SAH patients [66]. For patients with SAH, DVT rates were increased with higher aneurysmal grades, prolonged intensive care unit (ICU) duration, and increased total hospital duration [67]. Smoking and African American race/ethnicity were other predictors for DVT risk in SAH patients [66].

Given the generally higher VTE risk in neurosurgical patients, screening ultrasound for clinically asymptomatic VTE would seem logical—but current ACP guidelines do not support routine screening for DVT despite observations that patients in neuro-critical care units are at particular risk for DVT and PE [2, 12, 41, 68–72]. Screening ultrasonography can result in overutilization of hospital resources [16]. Furthermore, hospitals with more aggressive screening protocols may actually undergo penalties via administrative scorecards that suggest a higher VTE rate, even though this reflects ascertainment biases [16, 72–75]. The wide variability in opinions about DVT screening and lack of uniform reporting standards has profound implications in comparing VTE rates at different institutions [73–76]. Those who argue against screening acknowledge possible improvements in outcomes associated with screening protocols but claim that screening is less necessary if all eligible patients are treated with aggressive mechanical and chemoprophylaxis. Even with appropriate prophylaxis, however, the DVT rate remains high and while chemical prophylaxis can significantly reduce)DVT risk, there are specific predictive factors that would exclude patients from the discovery of otherwise asymptomatic DVT in high-risk neurosurgical or trauma patients [16, 72–75].

In support of screening protocols for cerebrovascular patients, the Prevention of Venous Thromboembolism after Acute Ischaemic Stroke (PREVAIL) Study found a prevalence of close to 50 % in stroke patients with limited mobility screened for asymptomatic DVT [62]. In one study of early versus late DVT, where stroke patients were screened with duplex ultrasound at Day 3 and Day 9, the DVT rate was 8 %; 83 % of DVT were discovered by Day 3 and just 3 % more were discovered by Day 9 [76]. These stroke patients with DVT, identified by screening ultrasound, had a significantly increased mortality risk with a 3-month mortality odds ratio of 12.4 [75]. Additionally, for SAH patients, the DVT frequency for symptomatic patients who underwent surveillance ultrasound was 24 %.

The main rationale for DVT screening in these high-risk asymptomatic patients is prevention of subsequent PE. Overall, the VTE rate in neurosurgical patients screened weekly or biweekly with lower extremity venous ultrasound was approximately 7.5–10 % [68, 69]. The risk of PE subsequent to DVT in asymptomatic patients appears to be much lower than for PE subsequent to symptomatic DVT.

In one of the screening studies, the DVT rate was 9 % in neurosurgical patients screened biweekly with lower extremity ultrasound on pharmacologic prophylaxis [68]. In that study, however, only 94 of 2638 patients had signs of a possible PE and only 22 of those patients (0.8 %) had CTA confirmed PE raising questions about the cost-effectiveness of DVT screening. Still, even with a lower PE rate, screening may indeed be cost-effective. Malhotra et al. suggested that for trauma patients who underwent twice-weekly surveillance, the DVT rate did increase (2.8 % with a screening protocol versus 1.3 % prior to screening implementation) but that PE rates with the surveillance protocol declined from 1.5 % prior to screening to 0.7 % using the screening DVT protocol [72]. Significantly, this was a cost-effective approach, because the authors calculated the incremental costs gained based on Quality Adjusted Life Years (QALY) and estimated a favorable cost of 18,661 to $48,821 per QALY.

Table 24.2 Key points and suggested screening recommendations

1.	Do not rely on Well's criteria or other clinical prediction scores in assessment of VTE risk in hospitalized neurosurgical patients
2.	Do not perform thrombophilia screening unless patients have a prior history of unprovoked VTE ("provoked VTE" might include prior history of VTE during trauma, prolonged immobility, or presence of malignancy)
3.	Consider screening lower extremity ultrasound at least once in the first week for high-risk immobile patients in the neuro-ICU (*not supported in ACCP guidelines but reasonable based on available data)
4.	Maintain a low threshold for early diagnostic testing (extremity ultrasound, chest CTA, or V/Q scanning) with any unexplained extremity swelling, fever, tachycardia, tachypnea, or hypoxia

In conclusion, a low threshold in postoperative neurosurgical patients for considering VTE is essential as the clinical presentation of DVT or PE may be subtle. Recognition of VTE risk factors is a crucial aspect for reduction of neurosurgical morbidity and mortality. While the screening of asymptomatic patients with neurosurgical disease remains controversial, it may be appropriate in those at particularly high risk such as patients with traumatic spinal cord injury, stroke, or recurrent malignant central nervous system neoplasms. Table **24.2** lists some suggested recommendations derived from current guidelines and tailored for the neurosurgical population based on the data reviewed in this chapter. The benefit of early VTE identification has to be tempered by the risk of anticoagulation in otherwise clinically asymptomatic postoperative neurosurgical patients.

References

1. Browd SR, Ragel BT, Davis GE, et al. Prophylaxis for deep venous thrombosis in neurosurgery: a review of the literature. Neurosurg Focus. 2004;17(4):E1.
2. Geerts WH, Bergqvist D, Pineo GF, et al. Prevention of venous thromboembolism: American College of Chest Physicians evidence-based clinical practice guidelines (8th edition). Chest. 2008;133(6 Suppl):381S–453.
3. Giannoukas AD, Labropoulos N, Burke P, et al. Calf deep venous thrombosis: a review of the literature. Eur J Vasc Endovasc Surg. 1995;10(4):398–404.
4. Heit JA, Silberstein MD, Mohr DN, et al. Predictors of survival after deep vein thrombosis and pulmonary embolism. A population-based, cohort study. Arch Intern Med. 1999;159(5):445–53.
5. Decousus H, Quéré' I, Presles E, et al. Superficial venous thrombosis and venous thromboembolism: a large prospective epidemiologic study. Ann Intern Med. 2010;152(4):218–24.
6. Lautz TB, Abbas F, Walsh SJ, et al. Isolated gastrocnemius and soleal vein thrombosis: should these patients receive therapeutic anticoagulation? Ann Surg. 2010;251(4):735–42.
7. Hingorani A, Ascher E, Hanson J, et al. Upper extremity versus lower extremity deep venous thrombosis. Am J Surg. 1997;174(2):214–7.
8. Lee JA, Zierler BK, Zierler RE. Risk factors and clinical outcomes upper extremity deep venous thrombosis. Vasc Endovascular Surg. 2012;46(2):139–44.
9. Danish SF, Burnett MG, Stein SC. Prophylaxis for deep venous thrombosis in patients with craniotomies: a review. Neurosurg Focus. 2004;17(4):E2.
10. Urbano FL. Homans' sign in the diagnosis of deep venous thrombosis. Hosp Physician. 2001;37:22–4.
11. Wells PS, Anderson DR, Bormanis J, et al. Value of assessment of pretest probability of deep-vein thrombosis in clinical management. Lancet. 1997; 350(9094):1795–8.
12. Bates SM, Gaesehke R, Stevens SM, et al. Diagnosis of DVT: Antithrombotic therapy and prevention of thrombosis, 9th ed: American College of Chest Physicians Evidence Based Guidelines. Chest. 2012;141(2 Suppl):e351S–418S.
13. Wells PS, Anderson DR, Rodger M, et al. Excluding pulmonary embolism at the bedside without diagnostic imaging: management of patients with suspected pulmonary embolism presenting to the emergency department by using a simple clinical model and d-dimer. Ann Intern Med. 2001;135(2):98–107.
14. Wells PS, Anderson DR, Roder M, et al. Evaluation of D-dimer in the diagnosis of suspected deep-vein thrombosis. N Engl J Med. 2003;349(13):1227–35.
15. Rolston JD, Han SJ, Bloch O, et al. What clinical factors predict the incidence of deep venous thrombosis and pulmonary embolism in neurosurgical patients? J Neurosurg. 2014;121:908–18.
16. Dermody M, Alessi-Chinetti J, Iafrati MD, Estes JM. The utility of screening for deep venous thrombosis in asymptomatic, non-ambulatory neurosurgical patients. J Vasc Surg. 2011;53(5):1309–15.
17. Burns E, Goebel. The ECG in pulmonary embolism. http://lifeinthefastlane.com/ecg-library/pulmonary-embolism. 2015
18. Torbicki A. Echocardiographic diagnosis of pulmonary embolism: a rise and fall of McConnell sign? Eur J Echocardiogr. 2005;6(1):2–3.
19. Thachil J, Fitzmaurice DA, Toh CH. Appropriate use of D-dimer in hospital patients. Am J Med. 2010;123(1):17–9.
20. Dhall SS, Hadley MN, Aarabi B, et al. Deep Venous thrombosis and thromboembolism in patients with

cervical spinal cord injuries. Neurosurgery. 2013; 72(1):244–54.
21. Miller JC, Lee SI. Radiology rounds: diagnosis of lower extremity deep vein thrombosis. www.mghradrounds.org/index.php?src=gendocs&link=2005_may. 2005.
22. Taniguchi S, Fukuda I, Daitoku K, et al. Prevalence of venous thromboembolism in neurosurgical patients. Heart Vessels. 2009;24(6):425–8.
23. Stein PD, Chenevert TL, Fowler SE, et al. Gadolinium-enhanced magnetic resonance angiography for pulmonary embolism: a multicenter prospective study (PIOPED III). Ann Intern Med. 2010;152(7):434–43.
24. Sampson FC, Goodacre SW, Thomas SM, van Beek EJ. The accuracy of MRI in diagnosis of suspected deep vein thrombosis: systematic review and meta-analysis. Eur Radiol. 2007;17(1):175–81.
25. PIOPED Investigators. Value of the ventilation/perfusion scan in acute pulmonary embolism: results of the prospective investigation of pulmonary embolism diagnosis (PIOPED). JAMA. 1990;263(20):2753–9.
26. Coche EE, Hamoir XL, Hammer FD, et al. Using dual-detector helical CT angiography to detect deep venous thrombosis in patients with suspicion of pulmonary embolism: diagnostic value and additional findings. AJR Am J Roentgenol. 2001;176(4): 1035–9.
27. Kearon C, Kahn SR, Agnelli G, et al. Antithrombotic therapy for venous thromboembolic disease: American College of Chest Physicians evidence-based clinical practice guidelines (8th edition). Chest. 2008;133(6 suppl):454S–545.
28. Rees DC, Cox M, Clegg JB. World distribution of factor V Leiden. Lancet. 1995;346:1133–4.
29. Rosendaal FR, Koster T, Vandenbroucke JP, et al. High risk of thrombosis in patients homozygous for factor V Leiden (activated protein C resistance). Blood. 1995;85:1584–608.
30. Rosendaal FR, Doggen CJM, Zivelin A, et al. Geographic distribution of the 20210G to A prothrombin variant. Thromb Haemost. 1998;79:706–9.
31. Wahl DG, Guillemin F, de Maistre E, et al. Meta-analysis of the risk of venous thrombosis in patients with antiphospholipid antibodies without underlying autoimmune disease or previous thrombosis. Lupus. 1998;7:15–22.
32. Runchey SS, Folsom AR, Tsa MY, et al. Anticardiolipin antibodies as a risk factor for venous thromboembolism in a population-based prospective study. Br J Haematol. 2002;119:1005–10.
33. Lijfering WM, Middeldorp S, Veeger NJ, et al. Risk of recurrent venous thrombosis in homozygous carriers and double heterozygous carriers of factor V Leiden and prothrombin G20210A. Circulation. 2010;121(15):1706–12.
34. De Stefano V, Rossi E. Testing for inherited thrombophilia and consequences for antithrombotic prophylaxis in patients with venous thromboembolism and their relatives. Thromb Haemost. 2013;110(4): 697–705.
35. Martinelli I, De Stefano V, Mannucci PM. Inherited risk factors for venous thromboembolism. Nat Rev Cardiol. 2014;11(3):140–5.
36. Garcia D, Akl EA, Carr RA, Kearon C. Antiphospholipid antibodies and the risk of recurrence after a first episode of venous thromboembolism: a systematic review. Blood. 2013;122(5):817–82.
37. de Campos Guerra JC, Mourao MA, Franca CN, et al. Impact of coagulation in the development of thromboembolic events in patients with spinal cord injury. Spinal Cord. 2014;52(4):327–32.
38. Silveira PC, Ip IK, Goldhaber SZ, et al. Performance of Wells score for deep vein thrombosis in the inpatient setting. JAMA Intern Med. 2015;175(7):1112–7. doi:10.1001/jamainternmed.2015.1687.
39. Auguste KI, Quiñones-Hinojosa A, Berger MS. Efficacy of mechanical prophylaxis for venous thromboembolism in patients with brain tumors. Neurosurg Focus. 2004;17(4):E3.
40. Hamilton MG, Hull RD, Pineo GF. Venous thromboembolism in neurosurgery and neurology patients: a review. Neurosurgery. 1994;34(2):280–96.
41. Rogers FB, Cipolle MD, Velmahos G, et al. Practice management guidelines for the prevention of venous thromboembolism in trauma patients: the EAST practice management guidelines work group. J Trauma. 2002;53(1):142–64.
42. Sharma OP, Oswanski MF, Joseph RJ, et al. Venous thromboembolism in trauma patients. Am Surg. 2007;73(11):1173–80.
43. Ageno W, Agnelli G, Checchia G, et al. Prevention of venous thromboembolism in immobilized neurological patients: Guidelines of the Italian Society for Haemostasis and Thrombosis (SISET). Thromb Res. 2009;124(5):e26–31.
44. Carlile M, Nicewander D, Yablon SA, et al. Prophylaxis for venous thromboembolism during rehabilitations for traumatic brain injury: a multicenter observational study. J Trauma. 2010;68(4):916–23.
45. Ekeh AP, Dominguez KM, Markert RJ, McCarthy MC. Incidence and risk factors for deep venous thrombosis after moderate and severe brain injury. J Trauma. 2010;68(4):912–5.
46. Sansone JM, del Rio AM, Anderson PA. The prevalence of and specific risk factors for venous thromboembolic disease following elective spine surgery. J Bone Joint Surg Am. 2010;92(2):304–13.
47. Smith JS, Fu K-M, Polly Jr DW, et al. Complication rates of three common spine procedures and rates of thromboembolism following spine surgery based on 108419 procedures. A report from the Scoliosis Research Society Morbidity and Mortality Committee. Spine. 2010;35(24):2140–9.
48. Ozturk C, Ganiyusufoglu K, Alanay A, et al. Efficacy of prophylactic placement of inferior vena cava filter in patients undergoing spinal surgery. Spine. 2010;35(20):1893–6.
49. Oglesby M, Fineberg SJ, Patel AA, et al. The incidence and mortality of thromboembolic events in cervical spine surgery. Spine. 2013;38(9):E521–7.

50. Chung WS, Lin CL, Chang SN, et al. Increased risk of deep vein thrombosis and pulmonary thromboembolism in patients with spinal cord injury: a nationwide cohort prospective study. Thromb Res. 2014;133(4):579–84.
51. Maung AA, Schuster KM, Kaplan LJ, et al. Risk of venous thromboembolism after spinal cord injury: not all levels are the same. J Trauma. 2011;71(5c):1241–5.
52. Godat LN, Kobayashi L, Chang DC, Coimbra R. Can we ever stop worrying about venous thromboembolism after trauma?. J Trauma Acute Care Surg. 2013;78(3):475–80.
53. Semrad TJ, O'Donnell R, Wun T, et al. Epidemiology of venous thromboembolism in 9489 patients with malignant glioma. J Neurosurg. 2007;106(4):601–8.
54. Wong JM, Panchmatia JR, Ziewacz JE, et al. Patterns in neurosurgical adverse events: intracranial neoplasm surgery. Neurosurg Focus. 2012;33(5):E16.
55. Smith SF, Simpson JM, Sekhon LH. Prophylaxis for deep venous thrombosis in neurosurgical oncology: review of 2799 admissions over a 9-year period. Neurosurg Focus. 2004;17(4):E4.
56. Perry JR, Julian JA, Lapierre NJ, et al. PRODIGE: a randomized placebo-controlled trial of dalteparin low molecular weight heparin thromboprophylaxis in patients with newly diagnosed malignant glioma. J Thromb Haemost. 2010;8:1959–65.
57. Chaichana KL, Pendleton C, Jackson C, et al. Deep venous thrombosis and pulmonary embolisms in adult patients undergoing craniotomy for brain tumors. Neurol Res. 2013;35(2):206–11.
58. Sughrue ME, Rutkowski M, Shangari G, et al. Risk factors for the development of serious medical complications after resection of meningioma. J Neurosurg. 2011;114(3):695.
59. Tong X, Kuklina EV, Gillespie C, George MG. Medical complications among hospitalizations for ischemic stroke in the Unites States from 1998 to 2007. Stroke. 2010;41:980–6.
60. Dennis M, Sandercock P, Reid J, et al. for the CLOTS trials collaboration. Can clinical features distinguish between immobile patients with stroke at high and low risk of deep vein thrombosis? Statistical modeling based on the CLOTS trials cohorts. J Neurol Neurosurg Psychiatry. 2011;82:1067–73.
61. Kelly J, Rudd A, Lewis R, Hunt BJ. Venous thromboembolism after acute stroke. Stroke. 2001;32(1):262–7.
62. Sherman DG, Albers GW, Bladin C, et al. The efficacy and safety of enoxaparin versus unfractionated heparin for the prevention of venous thromboembolism after acute ischaemic stroke (PREVAIL Study): an open-label randomised comparison. Lancet. 2007;369(9570):1347–55.
63. Kase CS, Albers GW, Bladin C, et al. Neurological outcomes in patients with ischemic stroke receiving enoxaparin or heparin for venous thromboembolism prophylaxis: subanalysis of the Prevention of VTE after Acute Ischemic Stroke with LMWH (PREVAIL) study. Stroke. 2009;40(11):3532–40.
64. Skaf E, Stein PD, Beemath A, et al. Venous thromboembolism in patients with ischemic and hemorrhagic stroke. Am J Cardiol. 2005;96(12):1731–3.
65. Bekelis K, Missios S, MacKenzie TA, et al. Predicting inpatient complications from cerebral aneurysm clipping. The Nationwide Inpatient Sample 2005–2009. J Neurosurg. 2014;120(3):591–8.
66. Serrone JC, Wash EM, Hartings JA, et al. Venous thromboembolism in subarachnoid hemorrhage. World Neurosurg. 2013;80(6):859–63.
67. Ray WZ, Strom RG, Blackburn SL, et al. Incidence of deep venous thrombosis after subarachnoid hemorrhage. J Neurosurg. 2009;110(5):1010–4.
68. Khaldi A, Halo N, Schneck MJ, Origitano TC. Deep venous thrombosis and pulmonary embolism in a neurosurgical population. J Neurosurg. 2011;114:40–6.
69. Henwood PC, Kennedy TM, Thomson L, et al. The incidence of deep vein thrombosis detected by routine surveillance ultrasound in neurosurgery patients receiving dual modality prophylaxis. J Thromb Thrombolysis. 2011;32(2):29–214.
70. Raslan AM, Fields JD, Bhardwaj A. Prophylaxis for venous thrombo-embolism in neurocritical care: a critical appraisal. Neurocrit Care. 2010;12:297–309.
71. Patel AP, Koltz MT, Sansur CA, et al. An analysis of deep vein thrombosis in 1277 consecutive neurosurgical patients undergoing routine weekly ultrasonography. J Neurosurg. 2013;118(3):505–9.
72. Malhotra AK, Goldberg SR, McLay L, et al. DVT surveillance program in the ICU: analysis of cost-effectiveness. PLoS One. 2014;9(9):e106793.
73. De Martino RR, Beck AW, Edwards MS, et al. Impact of screening versus symptomatic measurement of deep vein thrombosis in a national quality improvement registry. J Vasc Surg. 2012;56:1045–51.
74. Wakefield TW, Birkmeyer JD. Regarding "Impact of screening versus symptomatic measurement of deep vein thrombosis in a national quality improvement registry". J Vasc Surg. 2013;57(1):301–1.
75. Haut ER, Schneider EB, Patel A, et al. Duplex ultrasound screening for deep vein thrombosis in asymptomatic trauma patients: a survey of individual trauma surgeon opinions and current trauma center practices. J Trauma. 2011;70(1):27–33.
76. Bembenek J, Karlinski M, Kobayahsi A, Czlowkowska A. Early stroke related deep venous thrombosis: risk factors and influence of outcome. J Thromb Thrombolysis. 2011;32(1):96–102.

Venous Thromboembolism Prophylaxis in Neurosurgery

25

Vikram C. Prabhu

Introduction

Deep vein thrombosis (DVT) is the formation of a blood clot or blood clots within the deep veins of the upper or lower extremities or the pelvic veins; dislodgement of all or a portion of the clot with migration to the pulmonary vasculature results in the syndrome of pulmonary embolism (PE). Venous thromboembolism (VTE) is a more encompassing term now used to collectively refer to the syndromes of DVT and PE [1–3]. Extremity DVT classically presents as a painful, swollen, and erythematous limb, while PE usually manifests with shortness of breath, pleuritic chest pain, and tachycardia [1, 4, 5]. It is a health problem that affects a significant portion of hospitalized or infirm individuals, particularly those with neurological conditions or undergoing surgical procedures; healthy adults are also at risk for VTE [1, 2, 6–18]. Venous thromboembolism is the third most common vascular disease after myocardial infarction and ischemic stroke; it adds a significant expense to an already overburdened health-care system, and the prevention of VTE is a metric that hospitals and individual physicians are increasingly assessed upon [1–3, 7–15, 19–21]. And the extent of the problem may yet be underestimated; neither of the clinical syndromes described above is *sine qua non*; silent DVT or PE without overt clinical signs is relatively common and a more insidious threat that can frequently result in sudden death [2, 6, 7, 10, 14, 15].

The occurrence of VTE adds morbidity and mortality, extends the length of stay in intensive care units and general floor beds, and necessitates diagnostic testing and therapeutic interventions [22]. Neurosurgical patients or those admitted with neurological diseases are considered at moderate to high risk for VTE; this is the most frequent systemic complication in these patients [2, 8, 10, 12, 13, 15, 17–20, 22]. The risk is further increased in those with a brain tumor, traumatic brain injury, ischemic or hemorrhagic stroke, a paralyzed or weak extremity, or in the first week after a surgical procedure [1, 2, 8, 11, 13, 16, 17, 19, 22–27].

Prophylactic measures against VTE can have a significant impact on reducing the incidence and associated morbidity and mortality [1, 3, 6, 7, 9, 10, 14, 17–19]. They are generally divided into mechanical and pharmacological modalities and both are effective; however, while the former is largely without risk, the latter is associated with the risk of fresh or worsening cranial or spinal hemorrhage precluding its ubiquitous implementation [6, 28]. With appropriate prophylaxis,

V.C. Prabhu, M.D., M.S., F.A.C.S., F.A.A.N.S. (✉)
Department of Neurological Surgery, Loyola University Medical Center/Stritch School of Medicine, Maywood, IL, USA
e-mail: VPrabhu@lumc.edu

C.M. Loftus (ed.), *Anticoagulation and Hemostasis in Neurosurgery*,
DOI 10.1007/978-3-319-27327-3_25

VTE can be prevented or largely reduced. In fact, a common cause of VTE is simply not administering appropriate prophylaxis or not doing so for adequate duration [6, 22, 29]. A more nuanced approach to the problem of VTE in neurosurgical patients with identification of high-risk groups that may benefit maximally from prophylactic measures is prudent to avoid complications [1, 2, 16–18, 26].

Pathophysiology of VTE

Under natural conditions, the vascular endothelium maintains a vasodilatory and fibrinolytic state in which coagulation, platelet activation and aggregation, and inflammation and leukocyte activation are inhibited [30]. This occurs through a variety of local mechanisms, production of thrombomodulin and activation of protein C, expression of heparan sulfate and dermatan sulfate, expression of tissue factor (TF) pathway inhibitor, production of tissue plasminogen activator (tPA) and urokinase-type plasminogen activator, and elaboration of nitrous oxide, prostacyclin, and interleukin-10 [31]. Three major intravascular anticoagulant pathways (the heparin–antithrombin, protein C anticoagulant, and TF inhibitor pathways) exist that use these mechanisms to maintain an antithrombotic state. By contrast, conditions such as immobility, malignancy, trauma, surgery, or sepsis create an intravascular environment that favors thrombus formation by actively countering the above mechanisms and inhibiting the anticoagulant pathways and releasing factors that activate platelets, promote inflammation, and favor vasoconstriction [8, 9, 30, 31]. Rudolph Virchow's prescient analysis of the causes of VTE dates back to 1856 and remains relevant today [30, 31]. He postulated that intravascular thrombosis was the result of changes in a triad of factors: the inner vessel wall, composition of blood, and blood flow velocity and pattern [21, 30, 31]. Modern science has built on that. Prolonged stasis in a vein, particularly in the recesses of the valves, causes lowered local oxygen tension leading to the upregulation of stress response proinflammatory genes including hypoxia-inducible factor 1-alpha and P-selectin; this leads to platelet activation and recruitment of microparticles and immune-modulatory cells such as monocytes and granulocytes that express TF and initiate the extrinsic coagulation pathway [21, 30–32]. Inorganic polyphosphates released by activated platelets and factors released by the immune-modulatory cells also activate factor XII triggering the intrinsic coagulation pathway [21]. Thus, intrinsic intravascular factors under certain conditions trigger both coagulation pathways initiating the formation of a thrombus without any injury or violation of the vessel wall [21, 30–32]. These factors are even more implicated in VTE formation in large vessels (arterial or venous) where the ratio of blood to endothelial cell surface components is less than that seen in smaller capillary or venule beds; the greater the exposure of the endothelial cell surface to circulating anticoagulants, the less the risk of VTE [30]. In fact, most proximal vein DVT form de novo in major veins rather than propagating or extending from calf veins [14].

Venous valves play a critical role in maintaining blood flow in the extremities, particularly the legs [8, 21, 30, 31]. They are also prone to decay or dysfunction and become a site for stasis and hypoxia leading to a local hypercoagulable microenvironment with upregulation of procoagulant proteins and downregulation of anticoagulant proteins; in effect, they become the nidus for thrombus formation and subsequent propagation of the clot, and hypoxic changes can even be seen in as little as 2 h of immobility [8, 21, 30, 31]. Venous blood clots are composed of successive layer of fibrin, platelets, red blood cells, and leukocytes [30, 32]. The role of platelets in the formation of venous thrombi was not recognized until recently [33]. It is now postulated that not only are platelets important activators of the intrinsic and extrinsic coagulation pathways leading to intravascular thrombosis, but they may also be the link between chronic conditions such as obesity and the occurrence of VTE [21]. Microparticles are submicron vesicles shed from the surface of intravascular cells, in particular platelets that express TF essential in the initiation of the extrinsic coagulation pathway. They may be mediators of VTE in patients undergoing surgery, following trauma, during pregnancy and delivery, or in malignant states [21]. Surgery causes direct damage to veins but also elicits an inflammatory response and the release of procoagulants into the bloodstream patients [1, 8–10, 22, 30]. Pregnancy (all trimesters) and postpartum and the use of oral contraceptives and estrogen-hormone replacement therapy also have a prothrombotic effect increasing the risk of VTE [13, 19, 21, 30].

Changes in intravascular physiology observed with age provide an excellent window into the process of VTE: increase in procoagulant levels without a concomitant increase in natural anticoagulant (like protein C) levels, increase in body mass, decrease in activity, and an increase in frequency of infections, and systemic comorbidities make older patients more susceptible to VTE [14, 30]. An increase in intravascular thrombosis markers such as D-dimer and prothrombin fragment 1–2 and inflammatory markers such as interleukin-6 and C-reactive protein is seen in elderly patients [30]. Malignancy is also more common in older individuals and is another reason for the greater incidence of VTE in that age group.

Malignant tumors shed membrane particles that express TF, and the membrane lipids on tumor cells serve to augment the coagulation response [13, 21, 30, 34]. The relationship of VTE and malignant glioma is unique and well described. Plasmin inhibition, thromboplastin release, and increased procoagulant activity and platelet aggregation are some of the mechanisms that predispose brain tumor patients to VTE [14, 34, 35]. At surgery, intraluminal thrombosis is commonly seen in malignant gliomas, especially GBM. This is due to a combination of factors: slow and abnormal blood flow, distorted vessel lumen, increased interstitial pressure, and an imbalance in favor of procoagulant proteins. Histologically, zones of necrosis are seen in GBM that express hypoxia-inducible factor-1 and that may be the result of intravascular thrombosis within tumor vessels. Cells in the pseudopalisading belt that surrounds the necrotic zone secrete pro-angiogenic factors that promote microvascular proliferation and express higher levels of TF via induction of the transcription factor early growth response protein-1 [36]. The loss of phosphatase and tensin homolog (PTEN), overexpression or mutations of epidermal growth factor receptor (EGFR), and VEGF overexpression are hallmarks of primary glioblastoma that are more common in elderly individuals; these have been shown to further upregulate TF expression. Other malignant glioma pathways such as Ras/MEK/ERK and PI3K/Akt/mTOR modulate TF expression as well, particularly under hypoxic conditions [36]. Some of the chemotherapy agents used to treat malignant gliomas such as bevacizumab, a monoclonal antibody against VEGF that is used to treat recurrent malignant gliomas, may also contribute to changes in the vasculture and endothelium. The sum total of these processes is a prothrombotic environment that favors intravascular thrombosis [36].

A small percentage of the population harbors one or more of six defined genetic factors that increase the risk of VTE nearly tenfold [6, 14, 21, 30]. These include heterozygous deficiencies of the natural anticoagulants antithrombin, protein C, and protein S and an increase of procoagulants factor V Leiden, prothrombin G20201A, and blood group type non-O [6, 14, 21]. Elevations of factor V Leiden and prothrombin G20201A are more common among Caucasians [21]. Blood group non-O is the most common genetic risk factor for VTE and is seen in all races [21]. The presence of lupus anticoagulant antibodies in the blood also increases the risk of thrombosis by several mechanisms, binding to platelets and endothelium and activating complement eliciting an inflammatory response and inhibiting the protein C pathway [21, 30]. Other conditions that may influence the formation of VTE include myeloproliferative disorders such as polycythemia vera and thrombocytosis or erythrocytosis.

Epidemiology of VTE

The incidence of VTE varies widely as the methods used to detect it are not consistently applied; it is estimated that almost one million persons are affected by VTE in the United States annually and that VTE may be the cause of almost 300,000 deaths [6, 21, 37]. The incidence of VTE is estimated at 2–3/1000 individuals [37]. And the incidence of VTE is even higher in patients who enter a rehabilitation facility, particularly those with a paretic limb and mobility constraints [26, 38]. The influence of age is significant, and the rate of VTE sharply increases after the fourth decade and peaks in the eighth and ninth decades; the incidence among children is estimated at 0.1/1000 compared with 8/1000 among older adults [37]. And the associated morbidity and incidence of PE is also significantly higher in older patients with increased mortality [30].

Gender and racial differences are noted as well; the rates of VTE are slightly higher in men and among African-Americans [17, 19]. Two-thirds of VTE manifest as DVT, while one-thirds present as PE with or without DVT [10, 21, 39]. Most DVT develop in the lower extremities [10, 14]. Infrapopliteal DVT in the calf veins are more common but are less likely to contribute to the development of PE; nonetheless, they do require close follow-up as approximately 15 % will go on to affect more proximal veins, especially in the first 2 weeks following surgery [10, 14]. Upper extremity DVT, particularly in hospitalized patients with central venous access catheters, occur less frequently but are also a concern and may be the source for PE [6, 7].

The Center for Disease Control and Prevention estimates that 10–30 % of patients with VTE will die within a month of the diagnosis, and 33 % of patients will have a recurrence of the VTE within 10 years. Among patients who develop a DVT, 50 % will develop a post-thrombotic syndrome in the affected limb. Proximal above-knee DVT are the source of emboli causing PE in 90 % of cases [7, 14]. Among patients who develop a PE, 25 % will suffer a sudden death as a result of it; 90 % of patients in whom a PE occurs outside a hospital setting die within an hour of the event [1]. Pulmonary embolism is the leading cause of preventable death in hospitalized patients and may account for almost 16 % of all deaths in this group; in addition, mortality rates are highest when VTE occurs in patients with a malignancy [9, 15, 40].

There is absolutely no doubt that prophylaxis against VTE works: the rate of DVT among neurosurgical patients who do not receive DVT prophylaxis can be as high as 50 % [1, 7, 12, 16, 18, 19, 41, 42]; one study reported a 24 % incidence of DVT in the first 17 months following cranial surgery for high-grade gliomas [43]. The rate of PE in neurosurgical patients who do not receive VTE prophylaxis can be as high as 25 %; autopsy studies suggest the rate may actually be higher [7]. On the other hand, with prophylaxis, the incidence of VTE is lower. Black et al. reported a 2.3 % incidence of DVT and 1.8 % incidence of PE in craniotomy patients who receive mechanical VTE prophylaxis [44]. Auguste et al. reported a 2.2 % incidence of DVT and a 1.1 % incidence of PE in glioma patients undergoing motor mapping procedures in which mechanical prophylaxis during surgery was only used on the non-monitored lower extremity [8].

Recent reports provide a reasonable snapshot of the extent of the problem in neurosurgical patients [3, 9, 20, 45]. Kimmell and Jahromi reported a VTE rate of 3.5 % (DVT 2.6 % and PE 1.4 %) among 4844 adult patients who underwent cranial procedures; this data was collated from a national surgical quality database maintained by the American College of Surgeons. Given that the database sampling extended from 2006 to 2010, it is a safe assumption that at the minimum, these patients received mechanical prophylaxis against DVT during surgery and for the next few days following surgery as has been the customary practice for the past decade [8, 14]. Rolston et al. estimated a VTE incidence of 1.7 % among a database sampling of 38,058 neurosurgical cases over a similar time period (2006–2011); DVT occurred in 1.3 % and PE in 0.6 % [45]. Kshettry et al. reported an overall VTE rate of 4.4 % (DVT 3.5 % and PE 1.2 %) among 15,968 patients with aneurysmal SAH; VTE rates were similar in patients who underwent clipping or coiling procedures [19]. The rate of VTE following spine surgery is in the 2–4 % range [9]. Strom and Frempong-Boadu reported a 3.8 % DVT rate in patients undergoing cervical and lumbar laminectomy who received a combination of mechanical and pharmacological prophylaxis [3].

Risk Factors for VTE

Conditions that predispose to VTE may be commonly seen in the general population and in hospitalized patients; prolonged immobility even among healthy travelers, soldiers being evacuated from faraway battlefields who may be immobilized for many hours on long flights, pelvic or lower extremity fractures, use of oral contraceptives, pregnancy, smoking, obesity or increased body mass index, heart failure, sleep apnea, acute infections or sepsis, lupus anticoagulant antibodies, and chronic inflammatory states such as rheumatoid arthritis have all been implicated in the predisposition to VTE [6, 19, 21, 23, 25, 26]. In addition to these, neurosurgical patients have unique characteristics that make them even more susceptible to VTE [1, 2, 6, 8, 9, 13, 14, 22]. Head trauma or spinal cord injury, ischemic or hemorrhagic stroke, and benign or malignant tumors are major risks [1, 2, 7, 11, 16, 26]. Others risk factors include pre- or postoperative paresis or weakness, active cancer, longer intensive care or general hospital stay, prolonged central venous access, prolonged immobility or delayed ambulation, and the use of corticosteroids or dehydrating agents [2, 7, 9, 10, 13, 16, 18, 35]. Intraoperative factors include ventilation time and duration of surgery, and craniotomy patients may be at higher risk than those undergoing spinal procedures [6–8, 14, 22]. The use of regional anesthesia does not increase the risk of VTE [46].

Patients with brain tumors, particularly malignant gliomas and meningiomas, are uniquely susceptible to VTE; the overall risk of DVT in brain tumor patients is reported to be as high as 45 % [1, 2, 8, 13, 17, 22, 24, 25, 35, 47, 48]. Even patients with pituitary tumors such as ACTH-secreting adenomas and Cushing's disease are at increased risk for VTE [49]. In particular, the presence of extremity paresis, diagnosis of malignant glioma, age >60 years, large tumor size, length of surgery >4 h, the use of corticosteroids and dehydrating agents, and the use of chemotherapy with nitrosureas or cisplatin all increase the risk of VTE in these patients [2, 50]. Ray et al. reported a DVT incidence of 18 % among patients with subarachnoid hemorrhage, and symptomatic PE developed in 2 % despite early initiation of mechanical and pharmacological prophylaxis on admission to the neurosurgical ICU or at least within 24 h of admission [51].

Diagnosis and Surveillance for VTE

Estimates of the incidence of VTE vary; the clinical syndrome is not always overt, and diagnostic tests are not consistently employed. Utilization of diagnostic studies varies tremendously among different neurosurgical units or rehabilitation facilities; those that maintain a high index of suspicion and attentiveness to the problem of VTE may report higher rates simply because they detect the problem better. The mode and use of prophylaxis is not uniform either. But surveillance for VTE allows early detection and institution of treatment to minimize complications [2, 12, 52]. Three tests have proven robust: serum D-dimer assay, Doppler ultrasonography, and multidetector computed tomography (CT) angiography [2, 12, 52]. D-dimer levels can be rapidly assessed in the outpatient or inpatient settings. A low D-dimer assay is very sensitive in ruling out VTE [10]. On the other hand, elevated levels are not specific and may be seen in postoperative patients even in the absence of VTE [10]. However, there may be a difference in physiological elevations of D-dimer and those associated with VTE; 2 mg/l may be a reasonable threshold with values above that indicating the presence of VTE even in postoperative patients [10].

Doppler ultrasonography detects abnormal venous blood flow patterns in the presence of a thrombus; it has a high sensitivity (96 %) and specificity (99 %) in detecting a DVT of the proximal lower extremity particularly in a symptomatic patient [12, 51, 52]. In asymptomatic patients, "silent DVT," the sensitivity of this test is reduced, but it remains highly specific. It has some other limitations; it has a lower sensitivity and specificity for DVT of the calf or upper extremity or pelvic veins and does not reliably distinguish between old and new clots. However, these limitations aside, it is a useful and portable bedside test with excellent availability in practical hospital settings and has largely supplanted other tests for DVT such as impedance plethysmography and contrast venography [12, 52]. Real-time B-mode imaging allows better definition of the venous anatomy and clot structure. Multidetector CT angiography is the test of choice and most commonly used to detect PE, and it has supplanted other traditional tests such as ventilation–perfusion (V/Q) scans and pulmonary angiography [7, 22, 51].

The frequency of testing varies. Patients undergoing routine spine surgery, mobilized within 24 h after surgery, may not warrant any testing or screening for DVT [41]. In patients who have a hospital stay exceeding 3 days, it would seem reasonable to perform routine Doppler ultrasound screening during the first week of hospitalization and then repeating the test in those with clinical suspicion of new DVT or progression of existing DVT [2, 12, 52]. Multidetector CT angiography is usually obtained with clinical suspicion for PE; however, a low threshold of suspicion is helpful in high-risk patients or those with known DVT given the inconsistent or surreptitious nature of clinical PE presentations [7, 22].

Prophylactic Agents Against VTE

Mechanical Prophylaxis

Early ambulation following hospitalization or surgery is the simplest and most effective form of VTE prophylaxis. However, prior to that, measures are employed to reduce the risk of VTE. Regional anesthesia is considered to have less associated DVT risk than general anesthesia and should be considered where appropriate [46, 53]. During surgery or following admission to a neurological or neurosurgical unit, mechanical VTE prophylaxis in the form of graduated compression stockings (CS) and intermittent pneumatic compression (IPC) devices is standard [2, 3, 9, 13, 16, 54]. Graduated CS are elastic, contoured, circumferential leg compression devices that apply pressure in a staggered fashion, greater lower down around the ankles (~18 mmHg) and progressively lesser as one ascends up the thigh (~8 mmHg). Intermittent pneumatic compression devices are comprised of segmental diaphragms wrapped around the leg; a microprocessor directs pressurized air into them in an automated sequential manner producing a cyclical, wave line milking effect to evacuate the blood from the extremity mimicking the action of calf muscles.

Both graduated CS and IPC reduce the cross-sectional area of the limb, decrease venous wall distension and venous stasis, improve venous return from the extremities, and improve venous valve function. They are independently effective and may work synergistically when used together; in fact, most neurosurgical surgeries employ them together [1, 3, 54]. In addition to this mechanical effect, they promote fibrinolysis by increasing the amount of tPA release [1, 8]. This is why they can be effective even when they are applied to just one extremity or applied to the upper extremity [8]. They are simple to use, ubiquitously available, and relatively risk-free. Both graduated CS and IPC have been shown to reduce the incidence of DVT significantly and that of PE to a lesser extent [2, 9, 54, 55]. They are also augmented in their effectiveness when used along with pharmacological prophylaxis in the form of SC UFH or LMWH [1, 3, 7, 56]. Graduated knee or thigh high CS are reported to be equivalent to IPC, but the latter are more commonly used and considered more effective at reducing DVT and PE, even when applied to just one extremity [8]. In a series of patients who underwent motor mapping glioma surgery, where only one lower extremity was targeted with mechanical prophylaxis, no increase in DVT was noted in the contralateral extremity [8]. The use of CS and IPC alone without any pharmacological prophylaxis in patients undergoing routine spinal surgery is also common and reported to be effective in reducing VTE [6, 54].

Contraindications or conditions that preclude the use of CS or IPC are few: morbid obesity, severe dermatitis or skin reactions, gangrene, recent skin grafts, severe ischemic peripheral vascular disease or ulcers, severe lower extremity edema, and leg deformity [57]. Unless specifically contraindicated, mechanical prophylaxis with IPC should be employed universally in all patients [1, 6, 18]. Even patients undergoing cortical mapping procedures may have the IPC placed and used on the limb being tested; the IPC is simply disconnected during the testing portion of the case and then reconnected. Additionally, mechanical devices such as IPC or CS are generally avoided on a limb that has an existing DVT to avoid breaking up the clot and precipitating a PE. Complications of IPC or CS are rare: common peroneal nerve compression or rare instances of allergic reaction to the component materials.

Pharmacological Prophylaxis

Pharmacological agents used for VTE prophylaxis include subcutaneous (SC) low-dose unfractionated heparin (UFH) and low molecular weight heparin (LMWH) [2, 16, 53]. They are effective in combating the intravascular factors that dispose toward a hypercoagulable state and VTE and augment the effectiveness of mechanical prophylaxis agents [9, 23, 46, 53]. Khaldi et al. evaluated 2638 neurosurgical patients over a 3-year span and estimated the risk of DVT with mechanical prophylaxis only to be 16 %; this was reduced to 9 % when mechanical prophylaxis was augmented with pharmacological prophylaxis using twice daily SC UFH (5000 units), a 43 % risk reduction [7].

The routine use of pharmacological prophylaxis is mitigated by concerns that they may increase the risk of intracranial or intraspinal hemorrhage; hence, their use is not universal among neurosurgical patients [1, 14, 58–60]. A survey published in 2003 indicated that 76 % of neurosurgeons in the United States used mechanical prophylaxis only when operating on brain and spine tumors [58]. The risk of hemorrhage or bleeding complications is clear with oral anticoagulants such as Coumadin and dextran, and they are rarely used as primary VTE prophylaxis [53, 61]. However, with SC UFH and LMWH, the evidence suggesting risk of intracranial or spinal hemorrhage is not clear; recent studies refute the notion of increased hemorrhage risk with these agents and suggest that they have an acceptable safety profile [3, 9, 16]. Clearly pharmacological prophylaxis should be avoided in patients with acute intracranial or intraspinal blood or those with hemorrhagic primary brain tumors or with metastatic tumors that have a known propensity to bleed (choriocarcinoma, renal cell carcinoma, melanoma, thyroid cell carcinoma) [2]. Pharmacological VTE prophylaxis should also be used cautiously or not at all in patients with bleeding diatheses such as hemophilia, thrombocytopenia or thrombocythemia, or coagulation disorders, patients who have had recent bleeding problems such as epistaxis or gastrointestinal bleeds, or those who need to undergo lumbar puncture or placement of lumbar subarachnoid drains.

Heparin is a naturally occurring anticoagulant synthesized and secreted by mast cells in the body [14]. It binds to antithrombin III and inactivates factor IIa and Xa, thereby inhibiting thrombus formation [1]. Larger heparin fragments can also bind directly to thrombin inactivating it; this may elevate the partial thromboplastin time [1, 14]. Heparin used for clinical purposes is obtained from animal sources; it is a heterogenous mixture of negatively charged, sulfated glycosaminoglycans administered by SC injection (5000 units) either twice or three times a day [9, 62]. Unfractionated heparin has a short half-life of 1.5 h and variable binding to plasma proteins. It has compared efficacy at VTE prevention as LMWH and may have a less risk of bleeding complications and intracranial hemorrhage [62–65].

Low molecular weight heparins are fragments formed by enzymatic depolymerization of UFH. They have a shorter glycosaminoglycan chain length that prevents them from binding to thrombin; they preferentially inactivate factor Xa [1, 14]. They are as effective as UFH for VTE prophylaxis and have several advantages over unfractionated heparin: greater bioavailability, longer half-life, and a more predictable anticoagulant response [3, 16, 23, 46, 63, 66, 67]. In addition, there is less inhibition of platelet function and lower incidence of heparin-induced thrombocytopenia (HIT) than with UFH, a factor that can be of significant importance in neurosurgical patients [16]. Various formulations of LMWH are available: nadroparin (Fraxiparine), enoxaparin (Lovenox), dalteparin (Fragmin), tinzaparin (Innohep), ardeparin (Normiflo), reviparin (Clivarine), and danaparoid (Orgaran) [2, 16, 46]. They each have different potencies and availability varies. Among these, enoxaparin (Lovenox) is the formulation most commonly used in neurosurgical practices in the United States at a dose of 40 mg once a day or 30 mg twice daily SC [46]. Fondaparinux (Arixtra) is a non-heparin synthetic pentasaccharide that selectively inhibits factor Xa [27]. It has an efficacy that is similar to LMWH and does not carry the risk of thrombocytopenia. It has been studied in hip fracture patients and those undergoing general surgery procedures and found to be effective with an acceptable safety profile; it may be useful in patients with HIT [27, 68].

Heparin-Induced Thrombocytopenia

Heparin-induced thrombocytopenia is the most frequent drug-induced thrombocytopenia [68–70]. It can occur in patients of all ages and as a response to any form of heparin regardless of dose or route of administration. The risk, estimated at 1–5 %, is greater with bovine rather than porcine heparin, with UFH rather than LMW, in postsurgical patients, and with longer duration of heparin administration [69, 70]. Thrombocytopenia results due to the clearance of activated platelets and antibody-coated platelets by the reticuloendothelial system and typically starts 5–14 days after initiation of heparin; although if a patient has circulating antibodies from prior heparin exposure, HIT could be seen more rapidly [69, 70]. Paradoxically, despite thrombocytopenia, bleeding is rare; rather, HIT is strongly associated with thromboembolic complications involving both the arterial and venous systems [69, 70].

There are two distinct forms of HIT: type I and type II. HIT type I is a non-immunologic and occurs due to direct interaction between heparin and circulating platelets causing platelet clumping or sequestration [68–70]. It usually starts 48–72 h after initiation of heparin treatment and is characterized by a mild and transient thrombocytopenia (rarely <100,000/mm^3) that rapidly returns to normal within a few days after the heparin is stopped. It is not associated with an increased risk of thrombosis [69, 70]. Type II HIT, on the other hand, is immune mediated, results in specific antibody formation, and associated with a risk of thrombosis. The main antigen is a complex of heparin and platelet factor 4 (PF4) that is normally found in α-granules of platelets. Heparin's affinity for PF4 varies with different heparin formulations [68–70]. When heparin binds PF4 it becomes immunogenic leading to the generation of heparin–PF4 IgG antibodies (HIT antibodies). These antibodies activate platelets via their FcγIIa receptors causing the release of platelet-derived microparticles and platelet consumption. Platelet-derived microparticles and the antigen–antibody complexes also cause endothelial injury and interact with monocytes leading to TF production activating the coagulation cascade and promoting thrombosis [69].

The risk of thrombosis with HIT is significant. It can take the form of DVT, PE, myocardial infarction, ischemic stroke, or arterial occlusion. Postsurgical patients or those with indwelling central venous catheters are at particular risk for DVT and PE [68–70]. For patients with HIT, the heparin formulation should be immediately discontinued allowing the platelet count to recover. Direct thrombin inhibitors such as lepirudin, argatroban, or bivalirudin are considered; these are anticoagulant medications that do not cause HIT and they are administered intravenously. An alternative agent such as fondaparinux may also be used; the risk of HIT with fondaparinux is very low but not negligible. A transition to coumadin is made only after the platelet counts have recovered; consultation with a hematologist is essential under these circumstances [68–70].

Timing of VTE Prophylaxis

It is postulated that VTE evolves during the prolonged immobilization of a surgical procedure or in patients with impaired mobility following admission to a critical care or other unit; mechanical prophylaxis with graduated CS or IPC is most effective when initiated at that time and should be universally employed unless specifically contraindicated or unfeasible due to physical constraints [9, 16–18, 24]. It would make sense to also initiate pharmacological prophylaxis at that stage; some authors have reported it to be safe [13, 47, 71], but others have reported higher risks of bleeding complications and cautioned against this practice [24, 60, 65].

Initiating SC low-dose UFH (5000 units three times a day; twice a day in patients older than 75 years and weighing less than 50 kg), or LMWH, 24 h following a cranial or spinal surgical procedure or 24 h after a head CT showing stable ICH or ischemic stroke has been shown to be safe and is a reasonable measure which has an additive prophylactic effect to the mechanical devices employed [2, 3, 9, 11, 16]. Even perioperative SC UFH administration is considered safe in patients undergoing cranial procedures [13, 42, 71], but this is not universally employed. Tanveer et al. also reported that initiation of early pharmacological prophylaxis within 24 h of admission did not increase the risk of ICH in patients with external ventricular drains [72]. For patients undergoing deep brain stimulation procedure, Bauman et al. recommended perioperative mechanical prophylaxis with graduated CS and IPC devices supplemented with SC heparin perioperatively [73].

For patients who present with traumatic brain injury, spontaneous intracranial hemorrhage, or ischemic cerebrovascular events, mechanical prophylaxis is standard, and SC UFH or LMWH may be initiated 24 h after a cranial CT documenting stability of any intracranial blood and the absence of new hemorrhage [11, 16]. The PREVAIL (prevention of VTE following acute ischemic stroke with enoxoparin) demonstrated a 43 % risk reduction of VTE with enoxaparin as compared to UFH; symptomatic hemorrhage rate was <1 % although slightly higher in the LMWH group [74]. Recent ACCP guidelines recommend LMWH or UFH for patients with acute ischemic stroke and impaired mobility starting 24 h after the ictus [2, 75]. Special circumstances that warrant withholding pharmacological prophylaxis include the administration of recombinant tPA or thrombolytics or hemorrhagic transformation of an ischemic stroke; a 24 h waiting period following radiographic stability of any intracranial blood would be reasonable before initiating pharmacological prophylaxis [2, 16]. Similarly, in patients who present with aneurysmal subarachnoid hemorrhage, it is prudent to wait until the aneurysm is secured and the intracranial bleeding is stable [2]. The use of antiplatelet agents in patients with ischemic cerebrovascular disease does not preclude the use of SC UFH or LMWH [16].

For patients undergoing routine and elective spinal surgery, intraoperative IPC or CS prophylaxis is mandatory; given the relatively short duration of surgery, early ambulation and discharge, and low incidence of VTE, the use of mechanical prophylaxis alone with uncomplicated elective spine surgery is reasonable and effective in maintaining a low VTE rate [6, 41, 76]. In select patients at high risk for VTE, SC UFH or LMWH can be safely initiated 24–36 h following surgery and reduces the risk of DVT without an increased risk of spinal epidural hematoma formation [3, 6, 9, 41, 77]. With complex and staged spinal procedures, a different approach that avoids pharmacological prophylaxis may be considered; standard mechanical prophylaxis combined with IVC filter placement may be an option to minimize the risk of DVT and PE, respectively, without increasing the risk of bleeding complications [15]. Patients with spinal cord injury are a very high-risk group, and while the risk of VTE in these patients is lifelong, it is most significant in the first 2 weeks following the injury [26]. Enoxaparin is standard of care prophylaxis for all patients with spinal cord injury and should be initiated within 72 h of the injury to minimize the risk of VTE; IVC filters may be considered in select cases of established DVT in which anticoagulant therapy is contraindicated [2, 77].

Continuation of mechanical (IPC or CS) and pharmacological (SC UFH or LMWH) prophylaxis is generally employed for the first 1–2 weeks following surgery or admission or until the patient is fully ambulatory, whichever occurs first [7, 13, 17]. The majority of VTE events occur during this period and would be effectively covered by this regimen. Given the high risk of VTE in brain tumor patients, the option of outpatient prophylaxis with LMWH (dalteparin) was studied. The study was reportedly not completed (or published, except in abstract form) due to unavailability of the study drug. However, among the 186 patients who did get enrolled, some important information was gleaned; while the risk of DVT was slightly higher in the placebo group (17 %) versus the LMWH group (11 %), there was a 5 % annual risk of bleeding in the LMWH group compared to 1 % in the placebo group. An analysis of this study suggested that the routine use of outpatient VTE prophylaxis with LMWH was not advisable [2].

Risk of Hemorrhage with VTE Prophylaxis

The risk of hemorrhage associated with SC low-dose UFH and LMWH has been reviewed extensively [53]. Constantini et al. found no increase in intraoperative bleeding or postoperative bleeding complications among 103 patients who underwent brain tumor surgery and received SC UFH 2 h prior to surgery compared to placebo [78]. Wen and Hall presented data on 2400 craniotomy patients; risk of ICH was 1.2 % in patients receiving low-dose SC UFH and 1.6 % in those who did not receive pharmacological VTE prophylaxis [42]. Raabe et al. reported a 2 % risk of hemorrhage in 1500 patients undergoing craniotomy with LMWH prophylaxis [60]. Gerlach et al. reported a 1.5 % risk of ICH with LMWH (nadroparin) prophylaxis administered 24 h following a craniotomy and a slightly less than 1 % risk using the same regimen with spinal procedures [79, 80]. Khaldi et al. noted no increase in the rate of surgical site or other hemorrhage when subcutaneous heparin was initiated 24 h following a neurosurgical procedure [7]. Chibbaro et al. reported a 1 % rate of significant postoperative hemorrhages following cranial surgery and reported no objective clotting or hematological abnormalities with the use of LMWH (tinzaparin 3500 units daily starting 24 h after surgery); in fact, they doubled the dose of heparin in high-risk patients and began the administration preoperatively [13]. Bauman et al. reported a 3.8 % risk of intracranial hemorrhage with perioperative SC UFH; prior to introduction of this protocol and with mechanical prophylaxis only, they noted an intracranial hemorrhage rate of 0.8 %. However, none of the patients who received SC UFH prophylaxis developed clinically significant VTE while three of the non-SC heparin group developed VTE, of which two were PE [73]. Other groups have demonstrated that LMWH is safe and does not increase bleeding risk when started approximately 24 h following cranial surgery while still being effective at reducing the risk of DVT [81, 82]. Farooqui et al. reported similar results in patients with traumatic brain injury; initiation of SC UFH or LMWH 24 h after a head CT showed stable ICH did not increase the risk of hemorrhage progression while reducing the risk of DVT formation [11]. Hackett et al. noted no increase in risk of hemorrhage with the use of SC UFH or LMWH in ischemic stroke patients; 98 % of the patients received simultaneous antiplatelet agents as well [16].

Recent results using combination (mechanical and pharmacological) prophylaxis with spine surgery have been promising [3, 9]. Strom and Frempong-Boadu reported no postoperative hemorrhages or bleeding complications in 367 patients who underwent cervical and lumbar laminectomy with perioperative mechanical prophylaxis and LMWH administered approximately 24 h following surgery; they concluded that this regimen was effective VTE prophylaxis in this population of patients, and the addition of LMWH 24–36 h after surgery added no increased bleeding risk [3]. Cox et al. reported a 0.4 % rate of symptomatic spinal epidural hematoma formation requiring surgical evacuation in 992 patients who received intraoperative mechanical IPC prophylaxis along with SC UFH (5000 units two or three times a day) administered preoperatively if they were admitted before surgery or immediately postoperatively if the patient was admitted the day of surgery [9]. Goldhaber et al. compared the bleeding risk with UFH against LMWH and were unable to detect a statistical difference; although two patients in the LMWH group suffered major bleeding episodes [63]. Similarly, MacDonald et al. did not note a statistical difference in terms of bleeding risk between unfractionated heparin and LMWH, but two patients in the LMWH group had hemorrhages compared with one in the UFH group [66].

These studies are counterbalanced by concerns that even though a low incidence of bleeding complications is reported, when they do occur, they can have significant neurological consequences and necessitate additional surgery [6]. In the study by Gerlach and colleagues using LMWH prophylaxis 24 h following spine surgery, 13 postoperative hemorrhages occurred in 1954 patients; however, 10 of the 13 patients developed neurological deficits and four were permanent [79]. The risk of intracranial or spinal hemorrhage may be related to the timing of administration; one study that showed increased incidence of intracerebral hemorrhage initiated enoxaparin preoperatively [65]. In a meta-analysis of previous studies using LMWH prophylaxis for VTE, Iorio and Agnelli noted a bleeding risk from 4 to 11 % in the LMWH group compared with a risk of 1–7 % in the control group that did not receive LMWH prophylaxis; the risk of major ICH was 2.2–2.6 % in the former group and 0.8–2.6 % in the control group [67]. Danish et al. used a decision analytic modeling process and noted that VTE risk reduction gained by adding pharmacological prophylaxis with UFH or LMWH to standard mechanical prophylaxis in neurosurgical patients was outweighed by the risk of ICH; this was especially true with LMWH. They advocated mechanical prophylaxis only for patients undergoing craniotomy procedures [83]. Epstein performed an extensive review on the topic of VTE in neurosurgical patients in 2005 and concluded that mechanical prophylaxis alone had a significant impact in reducing the incidence of VTE with both cranial and spinal procedures [6]. Based on her review of the existing literature at the time, she further concluded that the addition of low-dose SC UFH or LMWH increased the risk of postoperative hematoma in neurosurgery patients [6].

Treatment of Established VTE

Prevention of recurrent VTE is also a priority in terms of prophylaxis; a prior history of VTE is highly predictive of a postoperative DVT [17]. One in five patients who suffer a DVT will have a recurrence within 5 years, and the risk of recurrent DVT increases with each episode [84]. Factors that contribute to recurrent DVT include the presence of cancer or malignancy, repeat surgical procedures, and an inadequate length or course of anticoagulant treatment [6, 84, 85]. The standard treatment of established above-knee or pelvic DVT, or PE, is anticoagulation therapy for 3–6 months [15]. With therapeutic anticoagulation, up to 85 % of DVT of thrombosed veins will recanalize [86]. Patients with below-knee DVT require no treatment other than careful follow-up with compression ultrasonography; however anticoagulation may be considered in patients who have risk factors such as active cancer or those who are hospitalized. The incidence of PE in these patients is 7 % [86]. Most practitioners do not use mechanical devices such as IPC or CS on a limb that has an existing DVT to avoid breaking up the clot and precipitating a PE.

Warfarin (coumadin) is a vitamin K antagonist that is orally administered and is approved for the prophylaxis and treatment of VTE. It has a narrow therapeutic index and dosage, and effectiveness varies among individuals based on diet, metabolism, and interaction with other drugs. It can interact with antibiotic and antifungal agents and must be used with caution in patients on antiplatelet agents, anticoagulants, nonsteroidal anti-inflammatory drugs, and serotonin reuptake inhibitors [86]. Regular monitoring of prothrombin time and international normalized ratio (INR) is essential in patients on coumadin as supratherapeutic levels may predispose to cranial or spinal hemorrhage.

With anticoagulation therapy, the risk of bleeding complications in patients who have undergone cranial or spinal procedures or who harbor malignant brain tumors is not insignificant. Additionally, although effective prophylaxis against DVT (mechanical and pharmacological combined) is the best way to prevent PE, some studies do not note a concomitant decrease in the PE rate with these regimens [7, 51]. Additional PE protection strategies may be considered under these circumstances. Inferior vena cava (IVC) filters are small cone-shaped devices that are deployed through the femoral vein and placed in the inferior vena cava just below the kidneys. They are useful devices that can reduce the risk of PE in patients with an established above-knee DVT or patients with below-knee DVT with additional risk factors for clot propagation who are not good candidates for therapeutic systemic anticoagulation or who may have developed a PE despite therapeutic anticoagulation [6, 23]. They are particularly effective in lowering PE rates from established proximal DVT in postsurgical patients and in spinal cord injury patients with paraplegia [87]. However, they have potential risks: they may actually induce a hypercoagulable state and complications such as caval obstruction and lower extremity swelling may occur, and complications with IVC filters may be higher in patients with malignant glioma [2, 88]. Newer filters are known as optional retrievable filters; they can be left in place permanently or used for temporary protection during a period of high VTE risk or until the resolution of a known DVT and then retrieved successfully. However, IVC filter retrieval is not consistently done. The use of IVC filters as prophylaxis against DVT is not recommended; they should be used cautiously and with careful consideration to a specific patient circumstance [88].

Xarelto (rivaroxaban) is a factor Xa inhibitor that indirectly inhibits platelet aggregation induced by thrombin; it does not have a direct effect on platelet aggregation by itself. It is administered orally in a fixed dose and has a rapid onset of action in 2–4 h, a wide therapeutic window, minimal drug interactions, and requires no blood monitoring. It is FDA approved for the treatment of atrial fibrillation, DVT and PE, for reducing the risk of recurrent DVT or PE, and for prophylaxis against DVT and PE in patients undergoing hip and knee replacement surgery [31, 89]. It is associated with an increased bleeding risk and spinal or epidural hematoma in patients receiving spinal anesthesia, and premature discontinuation may increase the risk of thrombosis [89]. There is no reversal agent for rivaroxaban; if bleeding complications occur, it is stopped and mechanical compression employed.

Pradaxa (dabigatran) is a thrombin inhibitor that is administered orally in a fixed dose; has a rapid onset of action in 2–4 h, a wide therapeutic window, and minimal drug interactions; and requires no blood monitoring. It is FDA approved to treat DVT and PE in patients who have received parental anticoagulation for 5–10 days and also to reduce the risk of recurrent DVT and PE. It should not be used in patients with a creatine clearance <50 ml/min or patients on prostaglandin-p inhibitors. It is also associated with an increased bleeding risk and spinal or epidural hematoma in patients receiving spinal anesthesia, and premature discontinuation may increase the risk of thrombosis [89]. There is no reversal agent for dabigatran; if bleeding complications occur, it is stopped and mechanical compression employed.

Recommendations for VTE Prophylaxis in Neurosurgery Patients

The complexity of neurosurgical practice necessitates a careful approach to VTE and precludes absolute guidelines. Familiarity with the pathophysiology and extent of the problem, understanding the prophylactic measures and their risks and benefits, and an individualized approach tailored to patient-specific circumstances are prudent. Some general cues are available and can be useful with the decision-making process:

1. Graduated CS and IPC devices provide excellent prophylaxis for almost every neurosurgical patient with minimal risk and should be ubiquitously employed. They are most effective when used on both lower extremities during surgery and for at least 1 week following surgery or until the patient is ambulatory.
2. Pharmacological prophylaxis augments the effectiveness of mechanical prophylaxis and

should be considered in patients at higher risk for VTE. It is in the form of SC UFH or LMWH and may be safely initiated 24 h following an uncomplicated cranial or spinal neurosurgical procedure if indicated.

3. For patients who present with traumatic brain injury, spontaneous intracranial hemorrhage, or ischemic cerebrovascular events, mechanical prophylaxis is standard and SC UFH or LMWH may be initiated 24 h after a cranial CT documenting stability of any intracranial blood and the absence of new hemorrhage. In patients with aneurysmal SAH, securing the aneurysm prior to initiating pharmacological prophylaxis is a prudent measure. There does not appear to be an increased risk of ICH with the use of SC UFH or LMWH in patients with external ventricular drains.
4. For patients undergoing elective spinal surgery, intraoperative CS and IPC prophylaxis is mandatory. The addition of pharmacological prophylaxis is not mandatory; however, in select high-risk patients, SC UFH or LMWH can be safely initiated 24 h following surgery.
5. With complex and staged spinal procedures, standard mechanical prophylaxis (CS and IPC) combined with IVC filter placement may be an option.
6. Patients with established DVT in proximal leg veins who are not candidates for anticoagulant therapy or who have progression of DVT despite anticoagulant therapy may be considered for IVC filter placement; retrievable filters are an option in these cases.
7. Inferior vena cava filters in and of themselves are not standard prophylaxis against VTE.
8. Coumadin or intravenous heparin or dextran infusion is not used for primary VTE prophylaxis.
9. D-dimer levels may be used for surveillance for DVT but false-positive elevations may occur.
10. In admitted patients, weekly or biweekly ultrasound examination of the lower extremities, and similar evaluation of the upper extremities if indicated, is reasonable surveillance for DVT. Multidetector CT angiography is optimal to detect PE.
11. Clinical signs of DVT and PE may not always be present and a high index of suspicion helps detect occult VTE.
12. For patients with HIT, the heparin formulation should be immediately discontinued, and an alternative agent such as fondaparinux or a direct-thrombin inhibitor may be considered; it is transitioned to coumadin after the platelet counts have recovered. Consultation with a hematologist is essential under these circumstances.

References

1. Browd SR, Ragel BT, Davis GE, Scott AM, Skalabrin EJ, Couldwell WT. Prophylaxis for deep venous thrombosis in neurosurgery: a review of the literature. Neurosurg Focus. 2004;17(4):E1.
2. Raslan AM, Fields JD, Bhardwaj A. Prophylaxis for venous thrombo-embolism in neurocritical care: a critical appraisal. Neurocrit Care. 2010;12(2):297–309.
3. Strom RG, Frempong-Boadu AK. Low-molecular-weight heparin prophylaxis 24 to 36 hours after degenerative spine surgery: risk of hemorrhage and venous thromboembolism. Spine (Phila Pa 1976). 2013;38(23):E1498–502.
4. Bounameaux H, Perrier A, Righini M. Diagnosis of venous thromboembolism: an update. Vasc Med. 2010;15(5):399–406.
5. Schulte LM, O'Brien JR, Bean MC, Pierce TP, Yu WD, Meals C. Deep vein thrombosis and pulmonary embolism after spine surgery: incidence and patient risk factors. Am J Orthop (Belle Mead NJ). 2013; 42(6):267–70.
6. Epstein NE. A review of the risks and benefits of differing prophylaxis regimens for the treatment of deep venous thrombosis and pulmonary embolism in neurosurgery. Surg Neurol. 2005;64(4):295–301. discussion 302.
7. Khaldi A, Helo N, Schneck MJ, Origitano TC. Venous thromboembolism: deep venous thrombosis and pulmonary embolism in a neurosurgical population. J Neurosurg. 2011;114(1):40–6.
8. Auguste KI, Quinones-Hinojosa A, Gadkary C, Zada G, Lamborn KR, Berger MS. Incidence of venous thromboembolism in patients undergoing craniotomy and motor mapping for glioma without intraoperative mechanical prophylaxis to the contralateral leg. J Neurosurg. 2003;99(4):680–4.
9. Cox JB, Weaver KJ, Neal DW, Jacob RP, Hoh DJ. Decreased incidence of venous thromboembolism

after spine surgery with early multimodal prophylaxis: clinical article. J Neurosurg Spine. 2014;21(4):677–84.
10. Prell J, Rachinger J, Smaczny R, et al. D-dimer plasma level: a reliable marker for venous thromboembolism after elective craniotomy. J Neurosurg. 2013;119(5):1340–6.
11. Farooqui A, Hiser B, Barnes SL, Litofsky NS. Safety and efficacy of early thromboembolism chemoprophylaxis after intracranial hemorrhage from traumatic brain injury. J Neurosurg. 2013;119(6):1576–82.
12. Patel AP, Koltz MT, Sansur CA, Gulati M, Hamilton DK. An analysis of deep vein thrombosis in 1277 consecutive neurosurgical patients undergoing routine weekly ultrasonography. J Neurosurg. 2013;118(3):505–9.
13. Chibbaro S, Tacconi L. Safety of deep venous thrombosis prophylaxis with low-molecular-weight heparin in brain surgery. Prospective study on 746 patients. Surg Neurol. 2008;70(2):117–21. discussion 121.
14. Danish SF, Burnett MG, Stein SC. Prophylaxis for deep venous thrombosis in patients with craniotomies: a review. Neurosurg Focus. 2004;17(4):E2.
15. Rosner MK, Kuklo TR, Tawk R, Moquin R, Ondra SL. Prophylactic placement of an inferior vena cava filter in high-risk patients undergoing spinal reconstruction. Neurosurg Focus. 2004;17(4):E6.
16. Hackett CT, Ramanathan RS, Malhotra K, et al. Safety of venous thromboembolism prophylaxis with fondaparinux in ischemic stroke. Thromb Res. 2015;135(2):249–54.
17. Smith TR, Nanney III AD, Lall RR, et al. Development of venous thromboembolism (VTE) in patients undergoing surgery for brain tumors: results from a single center over a 10 year period. J Clin Neurosci. 2015;22(3):519–25.
18. Schneck MJ. Venous thromboembolism in neurologic disease. Handb Clin Neurol. 2014;119:289–304.
19. Kshettry VR, Rosenbaum BP, Seicean A, Kelly ML, Schiltz NK, Weil RJ. Incidence and risk factors associated with in-hospital venous thromboembolism after aneurysmal subarachnoid hemorrhage. J Clin Neurosci. 2014;21(2):282–6.
20. Kimmell KT, Walter KA. Risk factors for venous thromboembolism in patients undergoing craniotomy for neoplastic disease. J Neurooncol. 2014;120(3):567–73.
21. Reitsma PH, Versteeg HH, Middeldorp S. Mechanistic view of risk factors for venous thromboembolism. Arterioscler Thromb Vasc Biol. 2012;32(3):563–8.
22. Smith SF, Simpson JM, Sekhon LH. Prophylaxis for deep venous thrombosis in neurosurgical oncology: review of 2779 admissions over a 9-year period. Neurosurg Focus. 2004;17(4):E4.
23. Phelan HA. Venous thromboembolism after traumatic brain injury. Semin Thromb Hemost. 2013;39(5):541–8.
24. Salmaggi A, Simonetti G, Trevisan E, et al. Perioperative thromboprophylaxis in patients with craniotomy for brain tumours: a systematic review. J Neurooncol. 2013;113(2):293–303.
25. Hoefnagel D, Kwee LE, van Putten EH, Kros JM, Dirven CM, Dammers R. The incidence of postoperative thromboembolic complications following surgical resection of intracranial meningioma. A retrospective study of a large single center patient cohort. Clin Neurol Neurosurg. 2014;123:150–4.
26. Chung SB, Lee SH, Kim ES, Eoh W. Incidence of deep vein thrombosis after spinal cord injury: a prospective study in 37 consecutive patients with traumatic or nontraumatic spinal cord injury treated by mechanical prophylaxis. J Trauma. 2011;71(4):867–70. discussion 870–1.
27. Toker S, Hak DJ, Morgan SJ. Deep vein thrombosis prophylaxis in trauma patients. Thrombosis. 2011;2011:505373.
28. Gnanalingham KK, Holland JP. Attitudes to the use of prophylaxis for thrombo-embolism in neurosurgical patients. J Clin Neurosci. 2003;10(4):467–9.
29. Bryson DJ, Uzoigwe CE, Braybrooke J. Thromboprophylaxis in spinal surgery: a survey. J Orthop Surg Res. 2012;7:14. doi:10.1186/1749-799X-7-14.
30. Esmon CT. Basic mechanisms and pathogenesis of venous thrombosis. Blood Rev. 2009;23(5):225–9.
31. Wakefield TW, Myers DD, Henke PK. Mechanisms of venous thrombosis and resolution. Arterioscler Thromb Vasc Biol. 2008;28(3):387–91.
32. Bovill EG, van der Vliet A. Venous valvular stasis-associated hypoxia and thrombosis: what is the link? Annu Rev Physiol. 2011;73:527–45.
33. Vanschoonbeek K, Feijge MA, Van Kampen RJ, et al. Initiating and potentiating role of platelets in tissue factor-induced thrombin generation in the presence of plasma: subject-dependent variation in thrombogram characteristics. J Thromb Haemost. 2004;2(3):476–84.
34. Bick RL. Cancer-associated thrombosis. N Engl J Med. 2003;349(2):109–11.
35. Sawaya RE, Ligon BL. Thromboembolic complications associated with brain tumors. J Neurooncol. 1994;22(2):173–81.
36. Jenkins EO, Schiff D, Mackman N, Key NS. Venous thromboembolism in malignant gliomas. J Thromb Haemost. 2010;8(2):221–7.
37. Naess IA, Christiansen SC, Romundstad P, Cannegieter SC, Rosendaal FR, Hammerstrom J. Incidence and mortality of venous thrombosis: a population-based study. J Thromb Haemost. 2007;5(4):692–9.
38. Kelly BM, Yoder BM, Tang CT, Wakefield TW. Venous thromboembolic events in the rehabilitation setting. PM R. 2010;2(7):647–63.
39. Wong JM, Panchmatia JR, Ziewacz JE, et al. Patterns in neurosurgical adverse events: intracranial neoplasm surgery. Neurosurg Focus. 2012;33(5):E16.
40. Geerts WH, Bergqvist D, Pineo GF, et al. Prevention of venous thromboembolism: American College of Chest Physicians evidence-based clinical practice

guidelines (8th edition). Chest. 2008;133(6 Suppl):381S–453.
41. Glotzbecker MP, Bono CM, Wood KB, Harris MB. Thromboembolic disease in spinal surgery: a systematic review. Spine (Phila Pa 1976). 2009;34(3): 291–303.
42. Wen DY, Hall WA. Complications of subcutaneous low-dose heparin therapy in neurosurgical patients. Surg Neurol. 1998;50(6):521–5.
43. Brandes AA, Scelzi E, Salmistraro G, et al. Incidence of risk of thromboembolism during treatment high-grade gliomas: a prospective study. Eur J Cancer. 1997;33(10):1592–6.
44. Black PM, Baker MF, Snook CP. Experience with external pneumatic calf compression in neurology and neurosurgery. Neurosurgery. 1986;18(4):440–4.
45. Rolston JD, Han SJ, Bloch O, Parsa AT. What clinical factors predict the incidence of deep venous thrombosis and pulmonary embolism in neurosurgical patients? J Neurosurg. 2014;121(4):908–18.
46. Holley AB, Petteys S, Mitchell JD, et al. Venous thromboembolism prophylaxis for patients receiving regional anesthesia following injury in Iraq and Afghanistan. J Trauma Acute Care Surg. 2014;76(1): 152–9.
47. Eisenring CV, Neidert MC, Sabanes Bove D, Held L, Sarnthein J, Krayenbuhl N. Reduction of thromboembolic events in meningioma surgery: a cohort study of 724 consecutive patients. PLoS One. 2013;8(11): e79170.
48. Levi AD, Wallace MC, Bernstein M, Walters BC. Venous thromboembolism after brain tumor surgery: a retrospective review. Neurosurgery. 1991;28(6): 859–63.
49. Barbot M, Daidone V, Zilio M, et al. Perioperative thromboprophylaxis in Cushing's disease: what we did and what we are doing? Pituitary. 2015;18(4): 487–93.
50. Muchmore JH, Dunlap JN, Culicchia F, Kerstein MD. Deep vein thrombophlebitis and pulmonary embolism in patients with malignant gliomas. South Med J. 1989;82(11):1352–6.
51. Ray WZ, Strom RG, Blackburn SL, Ashley WW, Sicard GA, Rich KM. Incidence of deep venous thrombosis after subarachnoid hemorrhage. J Neurosurg. 2009;110(5):1010–4.
52. Henwood PC, Kennedy TM, Thomson L, et al. The incidence of deep vein thrombosis detected by routine surveillance ultrasound in neurosurgery patients receiving dual modality prophylaxis. J Thromb Thrombolysis. 2011;32(2):209–14.
53. Roderick P, Ferris G, Wilson K, et al. Towards evidence-based guidelines for the prevention of venous thromboembolism: systematic reviews of mechanical methods, oral anticoagulation, dextran and regional anaesthesia as thromboprophylaxis. Health Technol Assess. 2005;9(49):iii–iv, ix–x, 1–78.
54. Papadimitriou K, Amin AG, Kretzer RM, et al. Thromboembolic events and spinal surgery. J Clin Neurosci. 2012;19(12):1617–21.
55. Vanek VW. Meta-analysis of effectiveness of intermittent pneumatic compression devices with a comparison of thigh-high to knee-high sleeves. Am Surg. 1998;64(11):1050–8.
56. Frim DM, Barker II FG, Poletti CE, Hamilton AJ. Postoperative low-dose heparin decreases thromboembolic complications in neurosurgical patients. Neurosurgery. 1992;30(6):830–2. discussion 832–3.
57. Jeffery PC, Nicolaides AN. Graduated compression stockings in the prevention of postoperative deep vein thrombosis. Br J Surg. 1990;77(4):380–3.
58. Carman TL, Kanner AA, Barnett GH, Deitcher SR. Prevention of thromboembolism after neurosurgery for brain and spinal tumors. South Med J. 2003; 96(1):17–22.
59. Collen JF, Jackson JL, Shorr AF, Moores LK. Prevention of venous thromboembolism in neurosurgery: a metaanalysis. Chest. 2008;134(2):237–49.
60. Raabe A, Gerlach R, Zimmermann M, Seifert V. The risk of haemorrhage associated with early postoperative heparin administration after intracranial surgery. Acta Neurochir (Wien). 2001;143(1):1–7.
61. Schaible KL, Smith LJ, Fessler RG, Rachlin JR, Brown FD, Mullan S. Evaluation of the risks of anticoagulation therapy following experimental craniotomy in the rat. J Neurosurg. 1985;63(6):959–62.
62. Misra M, Roitberg B, Ebersole K, Charbel FT. Prevention of pulmonary embolism by combined modalities of thromboprophylaxis and intensive surveillance protocol. Neurosurgery. 2004;54(5):1099–102. discussion 1102–3.
63. Goldhaber SZ, Dunn K, Gerhard-Herman M, Park JK, Black PM. Low rate of venous thromboembolism after craniotomy for brain tumor using multimodality prophylaxis. Chest. 2002;122(6):1933–7.
64. McLeod RS, Geerts WH, Sniderman KW, et al. Subcutaneous heparin versus low-molecular-weight heparin as thromboprophylaxis in patients undergoing colorectal surgery: results of the Canadian colorectal DVT prophylaxis trial: a randomized, double-blind trial. Ann Surg. 2001;233(3):438–44.
65. Dickinson LD, Miller LD, Patel CP, Gupta SK. Enoxaparin increases the incidence of postoperative intracranial hemorrhage when initiated preoperatively for deep venous thrombosis prophylaxis in patients with brain tumors. Neurosurgery. 1998; 43(5):1074–81.
66. Macdonald RL, Amidei C, Baron J, et al. Randomized, pilot study of intermittent pneumatic compression devices plus dalteparin versus intermittent pneumatic compression devices plus heparin for prevention of venous thromboembolism in patients undergoing craniotomy. Surg Neurol. 2003;59(5):363–72. discussion 372–4.
67. Iorio A, Agnelli G. Low-molecular-weight and unfractionated heparin for prevention of venous thromboembolism in neurosurgery: a meta-analysis. Arch Intern Med. 2000;160(15):2327–32.
68. Baroletti SA, Goldhaber SZ. Heparin-induced thrombocytopenia. Circulation. 2006;114(8):e355–6.

69. Ahmed I, Majeed A, Powell R. Heparin induced thrombocytopenia: diagnosis and management update. Postgrad Med J. 2007;83(983):575–82.
70. Linkins LA. Heparin induced thrombocytopenia. BMJ. 2015;350:g7566.
71. Macdonald RL, Amidei C, Lin G, et al. Safety of perioperative subcutaneous heparin for prophylaxis of venous thromboembolism in patients undergoing craniotomy. Neurosurgery. 1999;45(2):245–51. discussion 251–2.
72. Tanweer O, Boah A, Huang PP. Risks for hemorrhagic complications after placement of external ventricular drains with early chemical prophylaxis against venous thromboembolisms. J Neurosurg. 2013;119(5): 1309–13.
73. Bauman JA, Church E, Halpern CH, et al. Subcutaneous heparin for prophylaxis of venous thromboembolism in deep brain stimulation surgery: evidence from a decision analysis. Neurosurgery. 2009;65(2):276–80. discussion 280.
74. Sherman DG, Albers GW, Bladin C, et al. The efficacy and safety of enoxaparin versus unfractionated heparin for the prevention of venous thromboembolism after acute ischaemic stroke (PREVAIL study): an open-label randomised comparison. Lancet. 2007; 369(9570):1347–55.
75. Adams Jr HP, del Zoppo G, Alberts MJ, et al. Guidelines for the early management of adults with ischemic stroke: a guideline from the American Heart Association/American Stroke Association Stroke Council, Clinical Cardiology Council, Cardiovascular Radiology and Intervention Council, and the atherosclerotic peripheral vascular disease and quality of care outcomes in research interdisciplinary working groups: The American Academy of Neurology Affirms the value of this guideline as an educational tool for neurologists. Stroke. 2007;38(5): 1655–711.
76. Schuster JM, Fischer D, Dettori JR. Is chemical antithrombotic prophylaxis effective in elective thoracolumbar spine surgery? Results of a systematic review. Evid Based Spine Care J. 2010;1(2):40–5.
77. Christie S, Thibault-Halman G, Casha S. Acute pharmacological DVT prophylaxis after spinal cord injury. J Neurotrauma. 2011;28(8):1509–14.
78. Constantini S, Kornowski R, Pomeranz S, Rappaport ZH. Thromboembolic phenomena in neurosurgical patients operated upon for primary and metastatic brain tumors. Acta Neurochir (Wien). 1991;109(3–4): 93–7.
79. Gerlach R, Raabe A, Beck J, Woszczyk A, Seifert V. Postoperative nadroparin administration for prophylaxis of thromboembolic events is not associated with an increased risk of hemorrhage after spinal surgery. Eur Spine J. 2004;13(1):9–13.
80. Gerlach R, Scheuer T, Beck J, Woszczyk A, Seifert V, Raabe A. Risk of postoperative hemorrhage after intracranial surgery after early nadroparin administration: results of a prospective study. Neurosurgery. 2003;53(5):1028–34. discussion 1034–5.
81. Agnelli G, Sonaglia F. Prevention of venous thromboembolism in high risk patients. Haematologica. 1997; 82(4):496–502.
82. Norwood SH, McAuley CE, Berne JD, et al. Prospective evaluation of the safety of enoxaparin prophylaxis for venous thromboembolism in patients with intracranial hemorrhagic injuries. Arch Surg. 2002;137(6):696–701. discussion 701–2.
83. Danish SF, Burnett MG, Ong JG, Sonnad SS, Maloney-Wilensky E, Stein SC. Prophylaxis for deep venous thrombosis in craniotomy patients: a decision analysis. Neurosurgery. 2005;56(6):1286–92. discussion 1292–4.
84. Hansson PO, Sorbo J, Eriksson H. Recurrent venous thromboembolism after deep vein thrombosis: incidence and risk factors. Arch Intern Med. 2000;160(6): 769–74.
85. Swann KW, Black PM. Deep vein thrombosis and pulmonary emboli in neurosurgical patients: a review. J Neurosurg. 1984;61(6):1055–62.
86. Gillet JL, Perrin MR, Allaert FA. Short-term and mid-term outcome of isolated symptomatic muscular calf vein thrombosis. J Vasc Surg. 2007;46(3):513–9. discussion 519.
87. Wilson JT, Rogers FB, Wald SL, Shackford SR, Ricci MA. Prophylactic vena cava filter insertion in patients with traumatic spinal cord injury: preliminary results. Neurosurgery. 1994;35(2):234–9. discussion 239.
88. Gorman PH, Qadri SF, Rao-Patel A. Prophylactic inferior vena cava (IVC) filter placement may increase the relative risk of deep venous thrombosis after acute spinal cord injury. J Trauma. 2009;66(3): 707–12.
89. Cabral KP, Ansell JE. The role of factor Xa inhibitors in venous thromboembolism treatment. Vasc Health Risk Manag. 2015;11:117–23.

Can Patients with Known Intracranial and Intraspinal Vascular Lesions Be Anticoagulated?

26

Christopher P. Robinson, Michael Star, and José Biller

Introduction

Known intracranial and intraspinal vascular lesions are a particularly difficult problem to manage due to their wide range in behavior, from the completely benign to the emergently malignant. That, along with the relative rarity of most of the lesions, makes it challenging to develop any evidence-based guidelines for their direct management, not to mention the management of secondary issues that arise, or unrelated medical issues whose treatment could have a major repercussion on the stability of a given lesion.

It is with this understanding that we humbly attempt to address the balance of risk and benefit in the rapidly growing body of patients requiring anticoagulant therapy for, among many other conditions, non-valvular atrial fibrillation (NVAF), mechanical heart valve prosthesis (MHVP), and pulmonary embolism (PE) and who have a known intracranial or intraspinal vascular lesion. This has become an increasingly vital issue to address as, in today's world of "defensive medicine," many clinicians unfamiliar with the very complex literature on both of these topics might incorrectly assume that the risk of initiating anticoagulant therapy in a patient with any intracranial or intraspinal lesion poses too great of risk of hemorrhage.

We set out to provide a very rough roadmap for these difficult to manage patients with full knowledge that there are few or no clinical studies to rely on. Instead, we provide a review of the studied natural history of each of the major types of intracranial and intraspinal lesions, focusing on the risk of hemorrhage associated with each lesion and clinical factors that need to be taken into account that significantly alter the risk of hemorrhage. It cannot be stressed enough that each patient is different and requires unique consideration of all possible variables, of which we only cover the most notable. We also review the benefits and risks associated with major indications for anticoagulant therapy, focusing on the absolute risk reduction (ARR) associated with anticoagulant therapy in each indication. Finally, taking into account the significant increase in mortality associated with patients suffering from intracranial bleeding while being treated with anticoagulant therapy, we propose a very crude system of comparing the known yearly risk of hemorrhage of a given lesion with the known yearly reduction in either mortality or severe morbidity associated with anticoagulant therapy in a given indication. As we will be relying on so-called "expert opinion" in piecing together

C.P. Robinson, D.O., M.S. • M. Star, M.D. (✉)
J. Biller, M.D., F.A.C.P., F.A.A.N.
Department of Neurology, Stritch School of Medicine, Loyola University Chicago, 2160 S. First Avenue, Maywood, IL, USA
e-mail: Michael.j.star@gmail.com

C.M. Loftus (ed.), *Anticoagulation and Hemostasis in Neurosurgery*,
DOI 10.1007/978-3-319-27327-3_26

these recommendations, the level of evidence according to the Center for Evidence-Based Guidelines is Level E, at best, and the class/strength of the recommendations is Class IIb [1].

Brain Arteriovenous Malformations

Brain arteriovenous malformations (AVMs) are lesions with a direct connection between one or more arteries to one or more draining veins with no intervening capillary bed. They are made up of three parts: arterial feeders, nidus, and venous outflow. They are congenital lesions thought to be due an incomplete resorption of vascular anastomoses in early embryogenesis, though some believe they continue to form after birth [2]. Brain AVMs are the most common intracranial vascular malformation [3, 4]. Symptomatic brain AVMs usually present before 40 years of age and have roughly similar gender prevalence. Symptomatic and incidentally discovered lesions are usually found alone, unless associated with an underlying genetic disorder such as hereditary hemorrhagic telangiectasia (HHT) and the Wyburn–Mason syndrome [5]. Up to 22 % of AVMs are associated with intracranial aneurysms, which affect either the arterial feeders or are within the nidus (intranidal aneurysms). Vein of Galen aneurysmal malformations are AVMs of the choroidal system that drain into the vein of Galen forerunner, not to be confused with an AVM with venous drainage into an already formed and dilated vein of Galen, termed a false vein of Galen malformation [6]. As a rule, vein of Galen aneurysmal malformations are symptomatic and treated with embolization at a young age, with 74 % of patients continuing on with a normal neurological outcome [6].

There is low sensitivity for detection of AVMs on non-contrast head CT and contrast enhancement can sometimes outline the lesion. MRI is much more sensitive, demonstrating flow voids and hemosiderin deposition on T1 and T2 sequences. The prevalence of gradient echo (GRE) sequences has provided even higher sensitivity for the hemosiderin deposition that is often found surrounding an AVM. MR angiography (MRA) can demonstrate further information regarding feeding and draining vessels, but the gold standard remains catheter angiography. The Spetzler–Martin grading system (Table 26.1) was developed to determine the safety of surgical excision of the lesion and is based on size (either <3 cm, 3–6 cm, >6 cm), venous drainage (superficial or deep), and eloquence of the AVM location. While there is much literature on both surgical and endovascular treatment of these lesions, the recent "A Randomised trial of Unruptured Brain Arteriovenous malformations" (ARUBA) trial has called into question their safety over standard medical management of the unruptured brain AVM [7].

Table 26.1 Classification scales for AVMs and DAVFs

Classification of intracranial vascular lesions	
AVMs	
Spetzler–Martin Grading Scale [111]	Maximum diameter – <3 cm, 1 point – 3–6 cm, 2 points – >6 cm, 3 points Location – Noneloquent cortex tissue, 0 points – In or adjacent to eloquent cortex tissue, 1 point Venous drainage – Superficial only, 0 points – Deep, 1 point
DAVFs	
Borden classification [33]	1: Venous drainage directly into dural venous sinus or meningeal vein 2: Venous drainage into dural venous sinus with CVR 3: Venous drainage directly into subarachnoid veins (CVR only)
Cognard classification [34]	I: Venous drainage into dural venous sinus with antegrade flow IIa: Venous drainage into dural venous sinus with retrograde flow IIb: Venous drainage into dural venous sinus with antegrade flow and CVR IIa+b: Venous drainage into dural venous sinus with retrograde flow and CVR III: Venous drainage directly into subarachnoid veins (CVR only) IV: Type III with venous ectasias of the draining subarachnoid veins

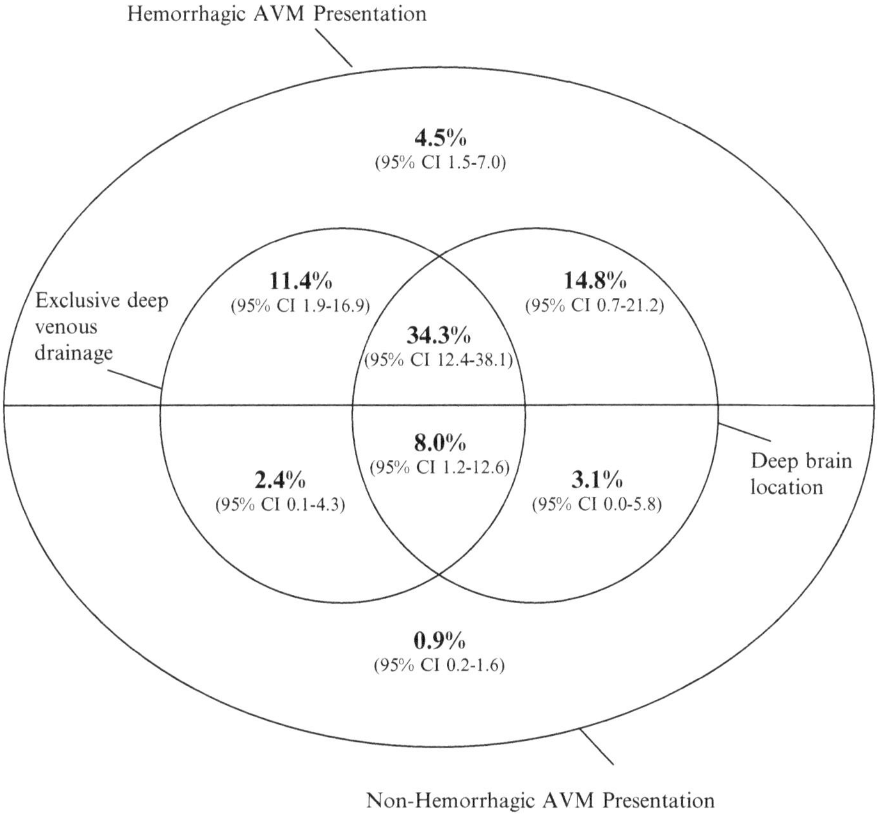

Fig. 26.1 Hemorrhagic risk based on three factors of an untreated AVM: previous hemorrhage, deep venous drainage, and deep brain location [13]

Intracranial AVMs are more commonly discovered due to symptoms compared to all other vascular lesions, and account for 1–2 % of all strokes [8, 9]. In the Scottish Intracranial Vascular Malformation Study (SIVMS), 79 % of the AVMs reported were from symptomatic lesions [4]. Many natural history studies have demonstrated that, among all AVMs, there is a 2–3 % annual risk of hemorrhage. However, these numbers can be misleading, as there are factors that are associated with significantly higher and lower risks of hemorrhage. For example, a meta-analysis of AVM natural history studies demonstrated that the annual hemorrhage rate for an unruptured AVM is 2.2 % versus the annual hemorrhage rate for a previously ruptured AVM of 4.5 % [10]. The other risk factors associated with subsequent hemorrhage were initial hemorrhagic presentation, deep AVM location, exclusive deep venous drainage, and associated intracranial aneurysm [10–13]. One natural history study proposed a risk model based on the presence or absence of the three risk factors found significant in their study (Fig. 26.1). There are many concerns, however, that all studies of AVM natural history have an inherent selection bias, as the most aggressive lesions are rarely included in these studies, either because the presenting episode is fatal or the lesion is necessarily operated upon. Also of note is the relatively low level of morbidity associated with AVM bleeding compared to other causes of intracranial hemorrhage, with studies reporting a rate as high as 61 % of AVM hemorrhages presented with an National Institute of Health Stroke Scale (NIHSS) of either 0 or 1 and up to 68 % with a follow-up modified Rankin Score (mRS) of 0–2 [14]. AVM-related parenchymatous hemorrhages were prognostically worse than AVM-related non-parenchymatous hemorrhages, though they still have improved outcomes compared to non-AVM-related parenchymatous hemorrhages [14]. This is consistent across most studies, with a meta-analysis demonstrating that around 80 % of patients with AVM-related hemorrhages have good long-term functional outcome compared to only about 40 % of patients with non-AVM-related hemorrhages [15].

Despite their relatively high incidence, there have been no studies directly studying the effect of antithrombotic therapy on the subsequent hemorrhage rate of AVMs. There have been two surveys of patients with HHT receiving either antiplatelets or anticoagulants, with no reports of intracranial hemorrhage in either report [16, 17]. As has been noted with cavernous malformations (CMs) and intracranial aneurysms (see below), there is no reason to believe that anticoagulant therapy increases the rate of hemorrhage of an unruptured AVM, though it is safe to assume that patient outcomes will be worse if an AVM ruptures while on anticoagulation.

Cavernous Malformations

CMs are well-circumscribed lesions with tightly packed, sinusoidal low-flow vascular channels without intervening parenchyma. Grossly, they appear multilobulated and purple, as a small mulberry. They have a crude detection rate of 0.56 per 100,000 adults per year [4], occur equally in men and women, and the mean age at presentation is 30 [18]. Though they were long thought to be congenital, they may also be secondary to radiation therapy, trauma, and viral infections [19]. CMs are usually solitary, though when there are multiple lesions, it is usually due to an underlying genetic disorder, which can be seen in approximately 19 % of patients [18], though is seen at higher rates in patients of Latin-American origin [19]. Mutations in three genes, CCM1 (KRIT1), CCM2 (MGC4607), and CCM3 (PDCD10), have been implicated in the majority of hereditary forms of CM, though the exact mechanism of action of these genes is unknown [20]. MRI is very sensitive at detecting CMs, demonstrating the classic "popcorn-like" lesion on GRE and susceptibility-weighted imaging. Due to their low-flow nature, the lesions are angiographically occult. CMs are associated with developmental venous anomalies (DVAs) in 9 % of cases as well, and some theorize that these CMs are formed as a result of venous outflow restriction through the DVAs [18]. The clinical presentation of CMs can vary. Approximately 10 % of lesions are discovered incidentally [18], but some screening studies have suggested the number may be as high as 40 % [20]. In a meta-analysis of natural history studies of CMs, the most common clinical presentation was noted to be a seizure (37 %), followed closely by hemorrhage (36 %) and headache (23 %) [18]. Prognosis after a clinical event in CMs is good: approximately 1/3 of patients have resolution of symptoms, 1/3 improve, and 1/3 suffer permanent sequelae, with no significant difference between hemorrhagic and nonhemorrhagic lesions, deep and superficial lesions, and supratentorial and infratentorial lesions [21].

The reported hemorrhage rate of CMs has varied from study to study, ranging from 1.6 % per lesion-year to 3.1 % per patient-year, with an average of 2.4 % per patient-year [21–24]. This wide range is likely due to issues ranging from the broad range of definitions of the word "hemorrhage" to whether the hemorrhage rate was reported in patient-years or lesion-years. The average annual hemorrhage rate for all lesions across multiple studies was determined to be 0.7 % per lesion-year. In patients with multiple lesions, the average hemorrhage rate is 5.1 % per patient-year, though only 0.8 % when calculated by lesion-year [18]. It is true across most of the literature that neither CM size nor the presence of multiple lesions increased the risk of hemorrhage. A few larger studies reported an increased risk of hemorrhage associated with female gender [22, 23, 25] and prior hemorrhage [21, 24, 25]. The rate of rebleeding has been reported as low as 3.1 % per lesion-year [21] and as high as 22.9 % per lesion-year [25].

Though previous reviews and case studies have recommended against anticoagulation in patients with CMs [26–28], there is only one study that reports a systematic study of patients with CM receiving anticoagulation. In that study, five patients receiving anticoagulant therapy were studied for a total of 56.4 patient-years, during which none had any hemorrhage [29]. *These results suggest that patients with CMs on anticoagulants are at least at no higher risk of hemorrhage compared to those not on anticoagulation.* Another study of patients receiving low molecular weight heparin postoperatively noted that nine patients had a CM, none of whom suffered any hemorrhagic complication [30].

Dural Arteriovenous Fistulas (DAVFs)

DAVFs, also known as dural AVMs, are vascular lesions involving the intracranial venous sinuses. Grossly, they are made up of feeding arteries that can be both cerebral and extracranial and a nidus connecting to a cerebral venous sinus. They are rare lesions, with a crude detection rate of 0.16 per 100,000 adults per year in the SIVMS study [4]. They are often acquired, formed secondary to a venous drainage obstruction, including cerebral venous thrombosis, as well as secondary to trauma, surgery, and congenital factors [31]. MRI scans can detect the surrounding dilated veins and feeding arteries, but are not as sensitive as MR angiography, which can incorrectly characterize the lesions as a venous thrombosis [36]. Catheter angiography is the gold-standard for diagnosis of possible lesions [32]. DAVFs are graded by the Borden [33] and Cognard [34] grading scales based primarily on the venous drainage (Table 26.1), with higher ratings correlating with more clinically aggressive lesions. The patients' presenting symptoms and signs are usually directly related to the anatomical location and nature of the lesion. For example, lesions that involve the superior sagittal sinus (SSS) are more likely to cause an increase in global venous pressure, which leads to raised intracranial pressure (ICP), papilledema, and headaches. Alternatively, lesions affecting the transverse sinus can cause an increase in local venous pressure, with more localized neurological deficits, including pulsatile tinnitus. Lesion embolization is currently recommended as the treatment for more aggressive lesions, specifically Borden 2 or 3 lesions [35].

As higher grade lesions are very likely to bleed and there is strong evidence for endovascular or surgical treatment [31, 35, 36], there is little published on the natural history of these lesions. Brown et al. [32] studied the course of 52 patients treated conservatively, and noted a 1.8 % risk of hemorrhage per patient-year. Patients with lesions of the petrosal and straight sinuses, along with those with a venous varix on a draining vein, had an increased risk of hemorrhage. Other studies noted that drainage via leptomeningeal veins, drainage via the vein of Galen, tentorial, middle cranial fossa, and orbital lesions were noted to be associated with an aggressive clinical course, whereas drainage via the transverse sinuses, sigmoid sinuses, and cavernous sinus were less aggressive [9, 31].

Developmental Venous Anomalies (DVAs)

DVAs, also known as venous malformations and previously as venous angiomas, are abnormally enlarged venous channels with normal intervening neural parenchyma. Importantly, the lesions act as functional, draining veins, as opposed to other intracranial vascular lesions. The lesions are thought to be quite common, noted in one study to be present in 2.6 % of all autopsies [112]. DVAs are commonly discovered incidentally on either a contrast-enhanced CT head or MRI of the brain, which demonstrate a large draining vein and flow void, respectively, sometimes with the classic "caput medusae" pattern due to smaller veins converging in centrifugal fashion toward the DVA [9, 37].

The lesions are rarely symptomatic, though they are occasionally associated with seizures, motor and sensory changes, and trigeminal neuralgia [37]. While DVAs were thought to rarely present with intracranial hemorrhage and seizures, it is now believed that those were more likely due to associated CMs, as the observed hemorrhage rate is estimated well below 1 % [38]. There are cases reported of thrombosed DVAs that caused both hemorrhagic and ischemic infarction; the recommended treatment in these cases, assuming a similar pathophysiology to cerebral venous thrombosis, is anticoagulation [37].

Unruptured Intracranial Aneurysm

Intracranial aneurysms, including traumatic, saccular, fusiform, atherosclerotic, and oncotic aneurysms, are outpouchings of the arterial blood supply that are known to be susceptible to rupture causing subarachnoid hemorrhage (SAH) or other types of intracranial bleeding. Based on a systematic review of many prospective and retrospective studies, including ones based on autopsy studies and imaging studies, there is approximately a 2 % prevalence rate of all intracranial aneurysms [39]. The lesions are detected by both MRA and intracranial CT angiography (CTA). Approximately 85 % of aneurysms are found in the anterior circulation, with common sites including the internal carotid artery (ICA) posterior communicating artery junction (PComm aneurysm), the anterior communicating artery to anterior cerebral artery junction, and the middle cerebral artery (MCA) branch points [40]. The occurrence of intracranial saccular aneurysms is increased in disorders such as autosomal dominant polycystic kidney disease (ADPKD), multiple endocrine neoplasia type I, HHT, Ehlers–Danlos syndrome type IV, Marfan's syndrome, COL4A1, COL4A2, and neurofibromatosis type I, and has higher rates of detection in those with a family member with a known aneurysm and with increasing age [40, 41].

The rate of rupture of detected intracranial aneurysms varies according to size, location, and risk factors. A large meta-analysis of natural histories of unruptured aneurysms found that the risk factors of: age older than 60, female gender, and Japanese or Finnish descent were all statistically significant risk factors, with relative risks of 2.0, 1.6, and 3.4, respectively [42]. Due to the varying nature of reporting statistics in many studies, an annual rate of hemorrhage per patient year is difficult to compute for a meta-analysis. The overall risk of rupture of untreated aneurysms is 1.2 %

Table 26.2 Risk factors for rupture of intracranial unruptured aneurysms

	Relative risk (95 % CI)
Age >60 years old	2.0 (1.1–3.7)
Female gender	1.6 (1.1–2.4)
Japanese or Finnish Population	3.4 (2.6–4.4)
Posterior circulation	2.5 (1.6–4.1)
Size	
5–10 mm	2.3 (1.0–5.2)
>10 mm	2.9 (1.5–5.7)
>15 mm	11.9 (5.5–25.8)

Based on results from Wermer et al. [42]

Table 26.3 Cumulative 5-year rupture rate

Unruptured aneurysm risk			
	Carotid (%)	Anterior circulation (%)	Posterior circulation (%)
7–12 mm	0	2.6	14.5
13–24 mm	3.0	14.5	18.4
>24 mm	6.4	40	50

Anterior circulation includes the anterior communicating or anterior cerebral arteries, internal carotid artery, and middle cerebral artery. Posterior circulation includes aneurysms involving the vertebrobasilar artery, posterior cerebral arterial system, or the posterior communicating artery. Based on table from Wiebers et al. [43]

per patient year [42]. The relative risk of various risk factors is noted in Table 26.2. Another perspective is noted in a table from Wiebers et al. [43] who calculated the cumulative 5 year risk of rupture for lesions of various sizes and location (Table 26.3). It is important to note that smaller aneurysms (<5 mm) in the anterior circulation are not even calculated in this table, as their annual rate of rupture may be well below 1 %.

The safety of using anticoagulants in patients harboring intracranial aneurysms has not been studied extensively. One retrospective study followed 42 patients with intracranial aneurysms taking anticoagulation for a total of 57 patient-years [44]. *The study resulted in no aneurysmal SAH, which suggests that the rate of rupture for patients with an intracranial aneurysm receiving anticoagulant therapy is no higher than in patients with an intracranial aneurysm not receiving anticoagulation* [44]. Another retrospective study noted that the mortality in patients with aneurysmal SAH on oral anticoagulation was

9/15 patients (60 %) compared to 38/126 patients (30 %) with aneurysmal SAH not on anticoagulation [45]. *While the study does not have statistical power, it suggests that there may be a twofold increase in mortality for patients with known intracranial aneurysm on an anticoagulant* [45].

Capillary Telangiectasias

Noted to be mildly enlarged ectatic capillaries on pathological examination, capillary telangiectasias are usually associated with other vascular malformations. These lesions are MRI, CT, and angiographically occult, noted to often be found in the posterior fossa or spinal cord, are unlikely to cause any symptoms, and are a common incidental discovery at necropsy [9, 46]. When associated with CMs, they should be treated the same as CMs in isolation [47].

Intracranial Arteriopathies

Intracranial arteriopathies include lesions such as intracranial dissections and moyamoya disease.

Intracranial artery dissections (IADs) can present either as SAH or as brain ischemia. A SAH occurs when the dissection is caused due to a tear between the media and the adventitia or due to a transmural dissection, and it is occlusive when the tear is between the elastica interna and the media [48]. While relatively rare in Caucasian populations, they are more common than extracranial cervicocephalic artery dissections in East Asian populations [49]. There has been increasing ability to diagnose IADs with noninvasive imaging such as MRI/MRA and CT/CTA, though the gold standard remains digital subtraction angiography [50]. There is, however, difficulty in diagnosing IADs due to their protean nature, with imaging features that can include the double lumen sign, the pearl-and-string sign, contrast media stasis, irregular stenosis (string sign), tapered occlusion, and focal fusiform dilatation [50]. Treatment of unruptured IADs is controversial, with some studies recommending anticoagulation for stroke prevention [49, 50], some reporting the relative safety of anticoagulation in these lesions [48], and some who continue to question whether it is safe [51].

Moyamoya disease is defined as stenosis or occlusion of the distal ICA or proximal MCA/ACA causing the formation of a network of very fine vasculature near the circle of Willis without any predisposing factors, such as Down syndrome, radiation exposure, and neurofibromatosis type 1 [52]. Those with a predisposing factor are called moyamoya syndrome [53]. The disease is relatively common in Japan, with a prevalence of 3.16 per 100,000 people there, and only 10 % of that in Europe [52]. Moyamoya disease has a bimodal distribution of the age of presentation, with younger patients presenting usually with ischemic strokes and older patients presenting with hemorrhagic strokes. Recently, moyamoya syndrome has been described in cohorts with X-linked genetic mutations causing loss of expression of BRCC3 and MTCP1 genes [54, 55]. Intracerebral hemorrhage in patients with moyamoya occurs either due to rupture of the moyamoya vessels or rupture of an associated saccular aneurysm and occurs in about 20 % of all patients presenting in Japan [56]. In a Japanese cohort of hemorrhagic type moyamoya, the rebleeding rate is 7.09 % per patient year [56]. However, a US cohort with more ethnic diversity not only focusing on rebleeding noted a hemorrhage rate of 1.7 % per year [57]. *Due to the increased risk of emboli forming at areas of arterial stenosis, patients are routinely treated with antiplatelet medications, though rarely anticoagulant therapy due to concern for hemorrhage* [53]. Revascularization surgery, both direct and indirect, is increasingly viewed as primary treatment for moyamoya disease pediatric patients [58].

Spinal Cord Vascular Malformations

Vascular malformations of the spinal cord are rare comprising 5–9 % of all central nervous system (CNS) malformations. The first documented classification system of such lesions is traced to Virchow in 1865, who described them as vascular neoplasms [59]. With the advances in pathologic

Table 26.4 Spinal vascular malformation classifications

Spinal cord vascular malformations: classification schemes		
Kendall and Logue (1977) [61]	Spetzler classification (2002) [62]	Jahan and Viñuela classification (2002) [60]
Type I—Direct AVF	*Neoplastic vascular lesions*	*Arteriovenous malformations*
Ia—single radiculomedullary feeder	Hemangioblastoma	*Dural AVF*
Ib—≥2 radiculomedullary feeders	Cavernous malformation	*Epidural AVF*
Type II—Glomus AVM	*Spinal aneurysms*	*Cavernous malformation*
Intramedullary AVM	*Arteriovenous malformations*	*Complex vascular malformations*
Type III—Juvenile AVM	Extradural-Intradural	*Pial AVF*
Intramedullary and extramedullary AVM	Intradural	Type I
Type IV—Pial AVF	Intramedullary	Small fistula
IVa	Compact	Type II
Small, single AV shunts fed by a single artery	Diffuse	Large fistula
IVb	Conus Medullaris	Type III
Several feeding arteries that drain directly into dilated veins	*Arteriovenous fistulas*	Giant fistula
IVc	Extradural	
Giant shunts fed by dilated arteries draining into a giant perimedullary vein	Intradural ventral	
	Small shunt	
	Medium shunt	
	Large shunt	
	Intradural dorsal	
	Single feeder	
	Multiple feeders	

AVF arteriovenous fistula, *AVM* arteriovenous malformation

and radiologic techniques, other cohorts have created their own unique classification systems [60–62] (Table 26.4). Though several schemata for identifying such lesions exist today, no uniform system has yet been widely adopted. For the purpose of this text, spinal cord vascular malformations are divided into five pathologic categories:

- Arteriovenous malformations (AVMs)
- Dural arteriovenous fistulas (dAVFs)
- Pial arteriovenous fistulas (pAVFs)
- Epidural arteriovenous fistulas (eAVFs)
- Cavernous malformations (CMs)

Spinal cord AVM's are rare and constitute 2–4 % of all spinal vascular malformations [63]. These lesions can be extradural, intradural-extramedullary, or intramedullary. The dAVF's are by far the most common vascular malformations of the spinal cord making up 70–80% of spinal vascular malformations [64]. Most lesions arise in the thoracolumbar region, with cervical malformations being far less common. pAVF's which differ from dAVF's due to paraspinal venous drainage are also rare and constitute 3–5 % of all vascular malformations [65]. The eAVF's usually arise as a sequelae of a metameric syndrome such as Klippel–Trenaunay Syndrome or Parkes–Weber Syndrome, which are also associated with lymphatic, bone, and skin malformations. They typically comprise 1–3 % of all spinal malformations. CMs of the spinal cord are 5–7 % of spinal cord vascular malformations, can be multifocal, and affect all parts of the neuraxis [66].

Despite being pathologically distinct entities, each of the vascular malformations of the spinal cord may have similar clinical presentations and pathophysiology. Symptomatic patients may present with localized back pain, myelopathy, radiculomyelopathy, sensory disturbances, motor disturbances, and bowel or bladder dysfunction [67]. Such symptoms result from distortion of normal functional anatomy leading to associated mass effect, venous hypertension, arterial steal, and hemorrhage.

Of importance, spinal cord hemorrhage due to vascular malformation is a greatly underrecognized etiology. Such pathology, when combined with other comorbidities, carries an increased risk of bleeding and long term neurologic disability.

Spinal Cord Hemorrhage from Vascular Malformations

Spinal canal hemorrhage is a serious complication of spinal vascular malformations and produces a variety of neurologic symptoms (Table 26.5). A variety of hemorrhage subtypes may occur including epidural hemorrhage (EDH), subdural hemorrhage (SDH), subarachnoid hemorrhage (SAH), and hematomyelia. Spinal AVM's have the highest spontaneous hemorrhage rates with a prevalence of 50 %, with greater risk occurring in intramedullary lesions compared to extradural lesions [68]. Another key factor in determining spontaneous hemorrhage rates in spinal AVMs is the venous drainage pattern. The presence of one draining vein, severely impaired venous drainage, or deep venous drainage greatly increases the risk of hemorrhage [69].

In comparison, AVFs have a decreased likelihood of spontaneous hemorrhage. The risk of hemorrhage in dAVF's is largely dependent on anatomic location. With dAVF's confined to the thoracic and lumbar regions, the hemorrhage rate is 0–1 % [68]. In contrast, when dAVF's are located in the cervical region, the spontaneous hemorrhage rate is far greater at 45 % [68, 70, 71]. With respect to pAVF's, where a perimedullary drainage pattern has been confirmed via angiography, the hemorrhage rate ranges from 30 to 32 % [68]. The eAVF's carry a 15–17 % overall risk of hemorrhage and depend largely on etiology and other comorbidities including anticoagulation [72]. The vast difference in hemorrhage rates between categorical AVFs relates to anatomic variance and localization. Associated risk factors include perimedullary venous drainage, intracranial venous drainage, and venous drainage into a varix.

CMs of the spinal cord are a distinct entity with characteristics separate from intracranial lesions. The annual risk of symptomatic hemorrhage from a CM of the spinal cord is 4.5 % per person/year [73]. Following initial hemorrhage, intramedullary lesions have a disproportionately high re-hemorrhage risk of 66 % per patient year [73]. This risk highlights the need for surgical intervention following initial presentation to deter further decompensation. Symptomatic hemorrhage from spinal CMs present uniquely when compared to other vascular malformations of the spinal cord. Four distinct subtypes of hemorrhage exist, each with its own unique characteristics [73] (Table 26.6). An associated risk factor for increased hemorrhage rates appears to be the presence of a high cervical lesion [73].

Bleeding Complications in the Neuraxis with Target Specific Anticoagulation

Millions of patients worldwide suffer from conditions requiring long term anticoagulation including atrial fibrillation, venous thromboembolism, and mechanical valve prosthesis. To date, no studies have shown that anticoagulation

Table 26.5 Presence (+) or absence (–) of symptoms in major spinal cord hemorrhage disorders

Symptomatology of spinal canal hemorrhages						
	Back or neck pain with or without radicular pain	Headache	Meningismus	Motor deficit	Sensory deficit	Sphincter dysfunction
Epidural	+	–	–	+	+	+
Subdural	+	–	–	+	+	+
SAH	+	+	+	+/–	+/–	+/–
Hematomyelia	+	–	–	+	+	+

Table 26.6 Hemorrhage subtypes in spinal CMs

Type I	Type II	Type III	Type IV
Isolated, relapsing episodes of neurologic decline	Slow, progressive neurologic decline	Acutely symptomatic with rapid decline	Acutely symptomatic with gradual decline

Adapted from Sandalcioglu et al.

increases the risk of spontaneous spinal hemorrhage from known, previously unruptured central nervous system (CNS) vascular malformations. However, it is vital that clinicians have a firm knowledge of the risks associated with anticoagulation, and those that may be potentiated in the presence of an underlying intracranial or spinal cord vascular malformation.

The use of anticoagulation in modern medicine has advanced disease targeted therapy by improving outcomes and decreasing mortality. Its use is seen in a wide array of clinical scenarios including myocardial infarction, atrial fibrillation, PE, venous thrombosis, intracardiac thrombus, cardiac valve replacement, and arterial dissection. Along with the benefits sustained from such intervention, the associated side effects have serious implications that may alter functionality. Amongst the greatest concern for neurologic specialists is CNS hemorrhage.

Unfractionated heparin and low-molecular weight heparins have long been used as initial or bridging therapy to oral anticoagulation in specific conditions. The overall risk of major bleeding is comparable between unfractionated heparin and low-molecular weight heparins at 0–2 %, and dependent on disease pathology, dose of medication, and length of treatment [74]. *The only study quantifying intracerebral hemorrhage (ICH) risk with heparin use was in the International Stroke Trial which showed that heparin doses >5000 units twice daily carried a 3.1 % risk of ICH compared to 0.6 % risk with placebo* [75].

The oral anticoagulants include vitamin K antagonists (VKAs) and the newer target specific novel anticoagulants (NOACs). VKAs have been the standard of care when treating thromboembolic states. In association with the benefit that has been shown with their use, the complication of major bleeding has a major effect on patient selection and overall outcome. Major bleeding rates associated with the use of VKAs range from 1.5 to 5.2 % per year [76]. Of those bleeding episodes, intracranial hemorrhage is the most devastating, with an 8.7 % frequency and a mortality of 46–55 % [77]. The frequency of VKA related spinal canal hemorrhage is not addressed in the literature.

However, over the past decade, the introduction of factor Xa and direct thrombin inhibitors (NOACs) has changed the landscape of oral anticoagulation in the treatment of NVAF and venous thromboembolism (VTE). *When compared to VKA's in NVAF, the NOACs are both noninferior and have less major bleeding.* In a meta-analysis comparing major bleeding rates between VKAs and NOACs, the overall rate was 4.64 % and 4 % respectively, with an intracranial bleeding risk of 1.08 % with VKAs and 0.51 % with NOACs [76]. The frequency of NOAC related spinal hemorrhage is not addressed in the literature. Given the positive results and increased safety profiles, more patients today are being prescribed NOAC's than in the past.

Anticoagulation in Specific Prothrombotic States

Prevention of VTE

VTE is an important and modifiable risk factor that leads to increased morbidity and mortality in a large subset of patients. Without appropriate intervention, the incidence of deep vein thrombosis (DVT) in the acute care setting ranges from 10 to 40 % [78]. These adverse events can lead to fatal complications including PE and increase the excess cost burden on health care. With the advent of thromboprophylaxis and subsequent clinical trials, there is no question that treatment with unfractionated heparin (UFH) or low-molecular weight heparin (LMWH) significantly reduces the risk of DVT and PE [78]. Additionally, studies have shown that DVT prophylaxis reduces the risk of adverse events and lowers overall costs [79]. In a review of associated complications, meta-analyses showed little to no overall increase in clinically relevant bleeding, providing an appropriate benefit-to-risk ratio with treatment [78, 80]. With respect to neurosurgical patients, current evidence based guidelines recommend the routine use of thromboprophylaxis in combination with pneumatic compression devices, providing an overall relative risk reduction of 68 % of thromboembolic events [81, 82].

Proximal Lower Extremity DVT

Proximal lower extremity DVT is a life-threatening condition that requires prompt diagnosis and treatment. Over 90 % of all PE result from proximal DVT, significantly increasing patient mortality. The mainstay of therapy for acute upper and lower extremity DVT is therapeutic anticoagulation. In one of the only randomized trials comparing anticoagulation to placebo for treatment of VTE, there was a significant reduction in mortality in the anticoagulated population from 5/19 (26 %) to zero [83]. Further uncontrolled studies have also corroborated this evidence [84]. The current evidence based guidelines for treatment of proximal DVT recommend the initial use of intravenous UFH, LMWH, or fondaparinux with concurrent warfarin administration to a target INR goal of 2–3 [85]. In patients with a history of first unprovoked DVT, long term oral anticoagulation with warfarin should be continued for a time period of 3 months. In patients with a history of recurrent unprovoked DVT, long term anticoagulation with warfarin should be continued for 3–6 months [85]. In patients with recurrent DVT and history of a hypercoagulable state, anticoagulation with warfarin should be continued indefinitely [85]. Though it is not currently recommended in the guidelines, the use of NOACs in the treatment of VTE is supported by a meta-analysis demonstrating equal efficacy and lower bleeding rates compared to warfarin [86]. The overall risk of clinically significant bleeding events with such associated therapies ranges from 1 to 5 %.

Distal Lower Extremity DVT

Distal lower extremity (LE) DVT carries a lower risk when compared to proximal sources for extension and subsequent thromboembolism. Natural history studies suggest that when untreated, only 15 % of distal DVTs will extend into the proximal veins, and if no extension has occurred by 2 weeks, progression is unlikely [87]. The current recommendations in the treatment of acute distal LE DVT are based on the risk factors for extension. These factors include multiple vein involvement, >5 cm in length, >7 mm in diameter, active malignancy, history of VTE, inpatient status, positive D-dimer, and no reversible provoking factors [87]. In patients with high risk for extension, controlled trials demonstrated that initial treatment with UFH followed by 3 months of warfarin prevented DVT extension and recurrent VTE [88]. Current evidence suggests that all patients with acute lower extremity DVT displaying high risk characteristics should receive anticoagulation for a 3 month time period.

Upper Extremity DVT

DVT of the upper extremity (UE) is categorically divided into two distinct groups; primary (unprovoked) and secondary (provoked). The secondary group accounts for 75 % of all UE DVT's, and common etiologies include central venous catheterization, malignancy, and pacemakers. UE DVT can lead to serious complications including PE (5 %), recurrent DVT (8 %), and post-thrombotic syndrome (20 %) [89]. The general consensus on treatment of UE DVT follows the recommendations for distal LE DVT. In cases of provoked pathology, such stimulus should be removed and the patient placed on 3 months of oral anticoagulation [85]. In cases of unprovoked pathology, those patients who demonstrate high risk characteristics should receive 3 months of oral anticoagulation [85].

Pulmonary Embolism

PE has long been recognized as a significant complication in the acute care setting. It is estimated that 90 % of all PEs can be attributed to VTE, and if left untreated, carries a mortality risk of 30 % [90]. In those populations who receive therapeutic anticoagulation as treatment, the 3 month mortality risk can be as high as 17 % [91]. Although several therapeutic advances, including thromboprophylaxis have been made, mortality and antemortem diagnosis of PE have remained

Table 26.7 Classification of atrial fibrillation based on types and duration

Classification of atrial fibrillation	
Types	Episode duration
Valvular AF	*Paroxysmal*
• Rheumatic heart disease	• AF that terminates spontaneously within 7 days
• Mechanical heart valve	
• Bioprosthetic heart valve	
• Mitral valve repair	*Persistent*
• Aortic valve repair	• AF that is sustained >7 days
Non-valvular AF	*Longstanding*
• Absence of all valvular etiologies	• AF that is sustained >12 months
	Permanent
	• AF with multiple failed attempts to restore sinus rhythm

AF arterial fibrillation
Adapted from January et al.

relatively constant for the past 40 years [92]. The mortality associated with PE is not only attributed to hemodynamic compromise, but with other comorbidities including cardiopulmonary disease, cancer, and VTE recurrence. The current evidence based recommendations for the treatment of PE are based largely in part on the data from DVT trials. It is recommended that both parenteral anticoagulation with IV UFH and warfarin be initiated with a long term oral anticoagulation goal of 3–12 months [85]. There is currently only weak evidence to suggest that therapy with warfarin is superior to the NOACs. In the case of vena caval filters, it should be noted, that there is no evidence base for primary prevention of PE. The only studies in which filters provided effective reduction of PE were those in which filters were combined with anticoagulation [85]. The clinically significant bleeding risks in the treatment of PE are similar to those associated with the treatment of DVT.

Atrial Fibrillation

Atrial fibrillation is the most common cardiac arrhythmia in the general population affecting one in four individuals over the age of 40 [93]. Its classification is described based upon the presence or absence of valvular disease and independently upon episode duration [94] (Table 26.7). Valvular and NVAF are well-defined independent risk factors for stroke, with a 20-fold and 5-fold increase respectively [95]. Such risks necessitate the use of long term anticoagulation to prevent thromboembolism. For the purpose of this section, we will only further discuss NVAF, as those with valvular disease fall under the scope of MHVP (mechanical heart valve prosthesis). Several randomized controlled trials comparing warfarin to placebo in NVAF demonstrated that treatment with anticoagulation decreases the risk of nonfatal stroke by 67 % and overall stroke mortality by 25 % [96]. There was also a decrease in mortality from 53/1000 deaths to 38/1000 deaths per year, which is an ARR in mortality of 2.5 % [96]. The ARR of all ischemic strokes was 6.3 % for patients with Congestive heart failure, Hypertension, Age more than 75 years old, Diabetes, and Stroke or TIA ($CHADS_2$) score >2 [96]. Newer studies comparing warfarin to NOACs in the treatment of NVAF have shown NOACs to be noninferior and with less serious bleeding complications [94]. Ultimately, the decision to start therapy with long term anticoagulation depends on careful assessment of multiple factors including comorbidities, patient population, and yearly stroke risk. The most validated and widely used risk stratification tools for such assessments are the $CHADS_2$ and Congestive heart failure, Hypertension, Age more than 75 years old, Diabetes, Stroke or TIA, Vascular disease, and Sex categories (CHA_2DS_2-VASc) scores (Table 26.8). The current evidence based

Table 26.8 Stroke incidence in patients with atrial fibrillation based on the $CHADS_2$ and CHA_2DS_2-VASc scores

Risk stratification of yearly stroke incidence							
$CHADS_2$				CHA_2DS_2-VASc			
Risk factors	Points	$CHADS_2$ score	Stroke risk (%/year)	Risk factors	Points	CHA_2DS_2-VASc score	Stroke risk (%/year)
Congestive heart failure	1	0	1.9	Congestive heart failure	1	0	0
Hypertension	1	1	2.8	Hypertension	1	1	1.3
Age ≥75	1	2	4.0	Age ≥75	2	2	2.2
Diabetes	1	3	5.9	Diabetes	1	3	3.2
Stroke/TIA	2	4	8.5	Stroke/TIA	2	4	4.0
		5	12.5	Vascular disease	1	5	6.7
		6	18.2	Age 65–74	1	6	9.8
				Female gender	1	7	9.6
						8	6.7
						9	15.2

Vascular disease refers to myocardial infarction, peripheral artery disease, or aortic plaque. Table adopted from You et al.

guidelines for NVAF recommends that patients with a CHA_2DS_2-VASc score of >2 be started on long term oral anticoagulation with either VKAs or NOACs [94]. The risk for serious bleeding complications associated with various oral anticoagulation ranges from 1 to 5 %, with VKAs having a slightly higher risk than the NOACs.

Mechanical Heart Valvular Prosthesis

Patients with MHVP are commonly encountered in clinical practice. With advances in cardiothoracic surgery, more and more patients are undergoing valvular interventions. The use of mechanical aortic and mitral valve prosthesis requires the initiation of long term anticoagulation due to their thrombogenic nature. The most widely accepted study by Baudet et al. showed a yearly thromboembolism risk of 22 % with mitral valves and 12 % with aortic valves without antithrombotic prophylaxis [97]. Additionally, the study showed that with anticoagulation, the estimated yearly risk of thromboembolism was 2.2 % with mitral valve and 1.1 % with aortic valve replacements [97]. Further studies examined the need for targeted INR therapy in the 2.5–3.5 range. They found no significant difference in thromboembolic rates with aortic valves when compared to the standard INR goal of 2.0–3.0. Alternatively, patients with mitral valves fared better with a higher INR goal, showing a decrease in yearly stroke risk from 3.9 to 2.8 % [98]. *The current evidence based guidelines for long term anticoagulation in mechanical valve replacement is treatment with warfarin to an INR goal of 2.0–3.0 with aortic valves, and an INR goal of 2.5–3.5 with mitral valves* [99]. The use of target specific anticoagulation with dabigatran was also studied in these groups, but the study was terminated early due to adverse bleeding events [100]. The annual risk of hemorrhage in the aortic valvular group is 2.8 % compared to 3.8 % in the mitral valvular group [99].

Non ST-Segment Myocardial Infarction (NSTEMI)

NSTEMI is a common condition that requires prompt diagnosis and adequate medical therapy. The overall incidence of NSTEMI in the Western world has remained relatively constant over the past 15 years at 150/100,000 person-years [101]. Without efficient recognition of such condition, patients are at high risk for poor outcomes including 2–4 % risk of death and 10–12 % risk of myocardial infarction in the first 30 days [102].

Theroux et al. conducted the only study comparing aspirin, UFH, and combination therapy in the treatment of unstable angina and NSTEMI, finding that MI occurred in 3.3 %, 1.6 %, and 0.9 % of patients respectively [103]. Pooled analysis of all studies comparing combination therapy to aspirin showed a 53 % relative risk reduction of early death and myocardial infarction, from 6.2 to 3.3 % early death and mortality [104]. Current evidence based guidelines in the treatment of NSTEMI recommend prompt initiation of both aspirin and intravenous UFH, followed by prompt percutaneous coronary intervention [105]. The risk of serious clinical bleeding events with combination aspirin and IV UFH is 3.3 % [103]. To date, there is no evidence to support the use or oral anticoagulants in the acute management of such patient populations.

Acute Limb Ischemia

Acute limb ischemia is a condition resulting from acute arterial occlusion of an extremity. The most frequent causes of such are thrombosis and embolism. Eighty percent of all emboli are cardioembolic, with the remaining cases occurring due to hypercoagulability, large vessel thromboembolism, and paradoxical venous embolism [106]. Irrespective of cause, patients typically receive anticoagulation as initial therapy, followed by thrombolysis or surgical intervention. Although anticoagulation is an accepted form of intervention, there are no randomized controlled trials proving its efficacy to date [106]. Additionally, a meta-analysis comparing outcomes between thrombolysis and surgery showed no effect on amputation rates or death in the thrombolysis group, with an increased risk of stroke and major bleeding [107]. *The current evidence based guidelines in the management of acute limb ischemia recommend initiation of intravenous UFH, followed by surgical intervention over thrombolysis if necessary* [106]. The complication rate of serious bleeding ranges between 0 and 2 % and increases following surgical intervention.

Thrombophilias

Thrombophilias, which include antiphospholipid antibody syndrome (APAS), factor V Leiden mutation, protein S deficiency, protein C deficiency, prothrombin 20210A mutation, hyperhomocysteinemia, and antithrombin deficiency, are genetic and acquired disorders that predispose patients to VTE. *The decision to start indefinite anticoagulant therapy is made in cases where there are two or more spontaneous events, one spontaneous life-threatening event, or one spontaneous event associated with the riskier APAS and antithrombin deficiency* [108]. The relative risk of recurrent VTE ranges for the various disorders from 1.4 in Factor V Leiden mutation and prothrombin 20210A gene mutation to as high as nine in APLA syndrome, which can translate to a risk of recurrence of up to 67 % per year [109]. One case–control study demonstrated a 15 % mortality rate at 4 years in patients with VTE diagnosed with APLA syndrome versus 6 % in patients with VTE without APAS [110].

Risk Stratification of Vascular Lesions for Possible Anticoagulation

The decision to recommend anticoagulation in a given prothrombotic situation with a known intracranial or spinal vascular lesion can be a challenging decision, especially given past attitudes that most intracranial vascular lesions were contraindications for anticoagulation. However, a careful analysis of the existing data demonstrates that not all vascular lesions are created alike, and the benefits and risks of each patient's situation should be carefully weighed before a decision is reached. For example, consider a patient with a brain AVM with a non-hemorrhagic presentation who is also noted to have non-valvular atrial fibrillation with a CHADS2 score of 3. Without considering any other factors, one could note that the risk of hemorrhage in this type of lesion is 0.9 % per year, and that any bleeding event while on anticoagulation will likely be

Table 26.9 Lesions in each column can be considered reasonably safe to anticoagulate in situations in that correspond to a similar or higher benefit from anticoagulant therapy

High-risk lesions	Medium-risk lesions	Low-risk lesions
Intracranial: • Unruptured intracranial aneurysms that are: – Giant (>15 mm) – Combination of other significant risk factors • AVM with hemorrhagic presentation • Deep, deep-draining AVMs with non-hemorrhagic presentation • CMs with previous hemorrhage • Multiple CMs • Moyamoya disease, hemorrhagic type Spinal: • Cervical dAVF • pAVF • eAVF • AVMs	Intracranial • Unruptured intracranial aneurysm that are: – Posterior circulation – Japanese or Finnish patient – Patient over 60 years old – Female patient • Solitary CMs • Dural AV fistulas • AVMs with non-hemorrhagic presentation • Moyamoya disease, non-hemorrhagic type Spinal: • Lumbar dAVF • Thoracic dAVF	• Unruptured intracranial aneurysms <5 mm • Capillary telangiectasias • Intracranial artery dissections • DVAs

For example, a medium risk lesion should at least be considered for anticoagulant therapy in cases (in Table 26.6) where there is either a large benefit or medium benefit, and should probably not be considered in cases of low benefit

significantly worse, if not fatal, compared to not being on anticoagulation. One must also consider that treating the patient's atrial fibrillation with an anticoagulant will decrease his mortality from stroke from 5.3 to 2.8 %, an absolute reduction in mortality of 2.5 %. In this example, the absolute risk reduction of fatal stroke by 2.5 % strongly outweighs the 0.9 % risk of hemorrhage the AVM carries. However, one must also note the location of the AVM, and other risk factors. If, for example, the AVM is located in the basal ganglia and drains to the deep venous system, it would then carry a risk of hemorrhage of 8.0 % per year, which would tip the balance of benefit and risk to make anticoagulation unwise.

Table 26.10 Relative benefit conferred by anticoagulant therapy in various conditions

Large benefit of anticoagulation	Medium benefit of anticoagulation	Mild benefit of anticoagulation
• PE • NSTEMI • Limb ischemia • Mechanical valve replacement	• Nonvalvular atrial fibrillation (NVAF) • DVT treatment (lower extremity and upper extremity)	• None

Patients suffering from disorders in the "large benefit" column should be strongly considered for anticoagulant therapy unless they have a lesion with very high likelihood of rupture. Patients with disorders in the "medium benefit" category should be more carefully considered for anticoagulant therapy, as the benefit conferred is more likely to be close to or less than the risk of hemorrhage

While it is not possible to compare every permutation of every vascular lesion to every indication for anticoagulation, we have set up Tables* 26.9 *and* 26.10 *to help guide the clinician with starting the decision-making process about various lesions. The tables are arranged into high-risk, medium risk, and low risk lesions (Table* 26.9*) along with pathology with demonstrated large benefit of anticoagulation (>10 % absolute risk reduction of major event or mortality), medium benefit of anticoagulation (1–10 % absolute risk reduction of major event or mortality), and low benefit of anticoagulation (<1 % absolute risk reduction) (Table* 26.10*).

Due to the wide spectrum of clinical presentation of most CNS vascular lesions, it is of utmost importance to reiterate the large magnitude of difference various clinical risk factors make in the risk of bleeding. The clinician must account for these clinical factors during their decision making process in these patients, as no two lesions are created equal.

References

1. Phillips B, Ball C, Sackett D, Badenoch D, Straus S, Haynes B. Oxford Centre for Evidence-based Medicine-levels of evidence (March 2009). Centre for Evidence Based Medicine Web site. 1998.
2. Lasjaunias P. A revised concept of the congenital nature of cerebral arteriovenous malformations. Interv Neuroradiol. 1997;3(4):275–81.
3. Brown Jr RD, Wiebers DO, Torner JC, O'Fallon WM. Incidence and prevalence of intracranial vascular malformations in Olmsted county, Minnesota, 1965 to 1992. Neurology. 1996;46(4):949–52.
4. Al-Shahi R, Bhattacharya JJ, Currie DG, et al. Prospective, population-based detection of intracranial vascular malformations in adults: the Scottish intracranial vascular malformation study (SIVMS). Stroke. 2003;34(5):1163–9.
5. Wyburn-Mason R. Arteriovenous aneurysm of midbrain and retina, facial naevi and mental changes. Brain. 1943;66(3):163–203.
6. Lasjaunias PL, Chng SM, Sachet M, Alvarez H, Rodesch G, Garcia-Monaco R. The management of vein of galen aneurysmal malformations. Neurosurgery. 2006;59(5 Suppl 3):S184–94. discussion S3–13.
7. Mohr J, Parides MK, Stapf C, et al. Medical management with or without interventional therapy for unruptured brain arteriovenous malformations (ARUBA): a multicentre, non-blinded, randomised trial. Lancet. 2014;383(9917):614–21.
8. Duong D, Hartmann A, Isaacson S, et al. Arteriovenous malformations of the brain in adults. N Engl J Med. 1999;340(23):1812–8.
9. Brown RD, Flemming KD, Meyer FB, Cloft HJ, Pollock BE, Link MJ. Natural history, evaluation, and management of intracranial vascular malformations. Mayo Clin Proc. 2005;80(2):269–81.
10. Gross BA, Du R. Natural history of cerebral arteriovenous malformations: a meta-analysis: clinical article. J Neurosurg. 2013;118(2):437–43.
11. da Costa L, Wallace MC, Ter Brugge KG, O'Kelly C, Willinsky RA, Tymianski M. The natural history and predictive features of hemorrhage from brain arteriovenous malformations. Stroke. 2009;40(1):100–5.
12. Yamada S, Takagi Y, Nozaki K, Kikuta K, Hashimoto N. Risk factors for subsequent hemorrhage in patients with cerebral arteriovenous malformations. J Neurosurg. 2007;107(5):965–72.
13. Stapf C, Mast H, Sciacca RR, et al. Predictors of hemorrhage in patients with untreated brain arteriovenous malformation. Neurology. 2006;66(9):1350–5.
14. Choi JH, Mast H, Sciacca RR, et al. Clinical outcome after first and recurrent hemorrhage in patients with untreated brain arteriovenous malformation. Stroke. 2006;37(5):1243–7.
15. Hartmann A, Mast H, Mohr JP, et al. Morbidity of intracranial hemorrhage in patients with cerebral arteriovenous malformation. Stroke. 1998;29(5):931–4.
16. Edwards CP, Shehata N, Faughnan ME. Hereditary hemorrhagic telangiectasia patients can tolerate anticoagulation. Ann Hematol. 2012;91(12):1959–68.
17. Devlin HL, Hosman AE, Shovlin CL. Antiplatelet and anticoagulant agents in hereditary hemorrhagic telangiectasia. N Engl J Med. 2013;368(9):876–8.
18. Gross BA, Lin N, Du R, Day AL. The natural history of intracranial cavernous malformations. Neurosurg Focus. 2011;30(6):E24.
19. Ramirez-Zamora A, Biller J. Brainstem cavernous malformations: a review with two case reports. Arq Neuropsiquiatr. 2009;67(3B):917–21.
20. Batra S, Lin D, Recinos PF, Zhang J, Rigamonti D. Cavernous malformations: natural history, diagnosis and treatment. Nat Rev Neurol. 2009;5(12):659–70.
21. Porter PJ, Willinsky RA, Harper W, Wallace MC. Cerebral cavernous malformations: natural history and prognosis after clinical deterioration with or without hemorrhage. J Neurosurg. 1997;87(2):190–7.
22. Robinson JR, Awad IA, Little JR. Natural history of the cavernous angioma. J Neurosurg. 1991;75(5):709–14.
23. Moriarity JL, Wetzel M, Clatterbuck RE, et al. The natural history of cavernous malformations: a prospective study of 68 patients. Neurosurgery. 1999;44(6):1166–71.
24. Kondziolka D, Lunsford LD, Kestle JR. The natural history of cerebral cavernous malformations. J Neurosurg. 1995;83(5):820–4.
25. Aiba T, Tanaka R, Koike T, Kameyama S, Takeda N, Komata T. Natural history of intracranial cavernous malformations. J Neurosurg. 1995;83(1):56–9.
26. Haasdijk RA, Cheng C, Maat-Kievit AJ, Duckers HJ. Cerebral cavernous malformations: from molecular pathogenesis to genetic counselling and clinical management. Eur J Hum Genet. 2012;20(2):134–40.
27. Labauge P, Denier C, Bergametti F, Tournier-Lasserve E. Genetics of cavernous angiomas. Lancet Neurol. 2007;6(3):237–44.
28. Pozzati E, Zucchelli M, Marliani AF, Riccioli LA. Bleeding of a familial cerebral cavernous malformation after prophylactic anticoagulation therapy: case report. Neurosurg Focus. 2006;21(1):1–3.
29. Schneble HM, Soumare A, Herve D, et al. Antithrombotic therapy and bleeding risk in a prospective cohort study of patients with cerebral cavernous malformations. Stroke. 2012;43(12):3196–9.
30. Chibbaro S, Tacconi L. Safety of deep venous thrombosis prophylaxis with low-molecular-weight heparin in brain surgery. prospective study on 746 patients. Surg Neurol. 2008;70(2):117–21.
31. Awad IA, Little JR, Akrawi WP, Ahl J. Intracranial dural arteriovenous malformations: factors predisposing to an aggressive neurological course. J Neurosurg. 1990;72(6):839–50.

32. Brown Jr RD, Wiebers DO, Nichols DA. Intracranial dural arteriovenous fistulae: angiographic predictors of intracranial hemorrhage and clinical outcome in nonsurgical patients. J Neurosurg. 1994;81(4):531–8.
33. Borden JA, Wu JK, Shucart WA. A proposed classification for spinal and cranial dural arteriovenous fistulous malformations and implications for treatment. J Neurosurg. 1995;82(2):166–79.
34. Cognard C, Gobin YP, Pierot L, et al. Cerebral dural arteriovenous fistulas: clinical and angiographic correlation with a revised classification of venous drainage. Radiology. 1995;194(3):671–80.
35. van Dijk JM, ter Brugge KG, Willinsky RA, Wallace MC. Clinical course of cranial dural arteriovenous fistulas with long-term persistent cortical venous reflux. Stroke. 2002;33(5):1233–6.
36. Simon S, Yao T, Ulm AJ, Rosenbaum BP, Mericle RA. Dural arteriovenous fistulas masquerading as dural sinus thrombosis. J Neurosurg. 2009;110(3):514–7.
37. San Millán Ruíz D, Yilmaz H, Gailloud P. Cerebral developmental venous anomalies: current concepts. Ann Neurol. 2009;66(3):271–83.
38. Hon JM, Bhattacharya JJ, Counsell CE, et al. The presentation and clinical course of intracranial developmental venous anomalies in adults: a systematic review and prospective, population-based study. Stroke. 2009;40(6):1980–5.
39. Rinkel GJ, Djibuti M, Algra A, van Gijn J. Prevalence and risk of rupture of intracranial aneurysms: a systematic review. Stroke. 1998;29(1):251–6.
40. Brown Jr RD, Broderick JP. Unruptured intracranial aneurysms: epidemiology, natural history, management options, and familial screening. Lancet Neurol. 2014;13(4):393–404.
41. Gunda B, Mine M, Kovács T, et al. COL4A2 mutation causing adult onset recurrent intracerebral hemorrhage and leukoencephalopathy. J Neurol. 2014;261(3):500–3.
42. Wermer MJ, van der Schaaf IC, Algra A, Rinkel GJ. Risk of rupture of unruptured intracranial aneurysms in relation to patient and aneurysm characteristics: an updated meta-analysis. Stroke. 2007;38(4):1404–10.
43. Wiebers DO, International Study of Unruptured Intracranial Aneurysms Investigators. Unruptured intracranial aneurysms: natural history, clinical outcome, and risks of surgical and endovascular treatment. Lancet. 2003;362(9378):103–10.
44. Tarlov N, Norbash AM, Nguyen TN. The safety of anticoagulation in patients with intracranial aneurysms. J Neurointerv Surg. 2013;5(5):405–9.
45. Rinkel GJ, Prins NE, Algra A. Outcome of aneurysmal subarachnoid hemorrhage in patients on anticoagulant treatment. Stroke. 1997;28(1):6–9.
46. McCormick WF, Hardman JM, Boulter TR. Vascular malformations ("angiomas") of the brain, with special reference to those occurring in the posterior fossa. J Neurosurg. 1968;28(3):241–51.
47. Awad IA, Robinson Jr JR, Mohanty S, Estes ML. Mixed vascular malformations of the brain: clinical and pathogenetic considerations. Neurosurgery. 1993;33(2):179–88.
48. Metso TM, Metso AJ, Helenius J, et al. Prognosis and safety of anticoagulation in intracranial artery dissections in adults. Stroke. 2007;38(6):1837–42.
49. Kim BM, Kim SH, Kim DI, et al. Outcomes and prognostic factors of intracranial unruptured vertebrobasilar artery dissection. Neurology. 2011;76(20):1735–41.
50. Sikkema T, Uyttenboogaart M, Eshghi O, et al. Intracranial artery dissection. Eur J Neurol. 2014;21(6):820–6.
51. Arnold M, Bousser MG, Baumgartner RW. Prognosis and safety of anticoagulation in intracranial artery dissections in adults. Stroke. 2007;38(11):e140. author reply e141.
52. Kuroda S, Houkin K. Moyamoya disease: current concepts and future perspectives. Lancet Neurol. 2008;7(11):1056–66.
53. Scott RM, Smith ER. Moyamoya disease and moyamoya syndrome. N Engl J Med. 2009;360(12):1226–37.
54. Miskinyte S, Butler MG, Hervé D, et al. Loss of BRCC3 deubiquitinating enzyme leads to abnormal angiogenesis and is associated with syndromic moyamoya. Am J Human Genet. 2011;88(6):718–28.
55. Herve D, Touraine P, Verloes A, et al. A hereditary moyamoya syndrome with multisystemic manifestations. Neurology. 2010;75(3):259–64.
56. Kobayashi E, Saeki N, Oishi H, Hirai S, Yamaura A. Long-term natural history of hemorrhagic type moyamoya disease in 42 patients. J Neurosurg. 2000;93(6):976–80.
57. Gross BA, Du R. The natural history of moyamoya in a North American adult cohort. J Clin Neurosci. 2013;20(1):44–8.
58. Fung LW, Thompson D, Ganesan V. Revascularisation surgery for paediatric moyamoya: a review of the literature. Childs Nerv Syst. 2005;21(5):358–64.
59. Virchow RLK. Die krankhaften geschwülste, vol. 2. Berlin: A. Hirschwald; 1865.
60. Jahan R, Vinuela F. Vascular anatomy, pathophysiology, and classification of vascular malformations of the spinal cord. Semin Cerebrovasc Dis Stroke. 2002;2(3):186–200.
61. Kendall B, Logue V. Spinal epidural angiomatous malformations draining into intrathecal veins. Neuroradiology. 1977;13(4):181–9.
62. Spetzler RF, Detwiler PW, Riina HA, Porter RW. Modified classification of spinal cord vascular lesions. J Neurosurg Spine. 2002;96(2):145–56.
63. Aminoff MJ. Spinal angiomas. Oxford: Wiley-Blackwell; 1976.
64. Thron AK, Rossberg C. Vascular anatomy of the spinal cord: neuroradiological investigations and clinical syndromes. New York: Springer Science & Business Media; 1988.

65. Gueguen B, Merland JJ, Riche MC, Rey A. Vascular malformations of the spinal cord: intrathecal perimedullary arteriovenous fistulas fed by medullary arteries. Neurology. 1987;37(6):969–79.
66. Spetzger U, Gilsbach J, Bertalanffy H. Cavernous angiomas of the spinal cord clinical presentation, surgical strategy, and postoperative results. Acta Neurochir. 1995;134(3–4):200–6.
67. Saladino A, Atkinson JL, Rabinstein AA, et al. Surgical treatment of spinal dural arteriovenous fistulae: a consecutive series of 154 patients. Neurosurgery. 2010;67(5):1350–7. discussion 1357–8.
68. Rosenblum B, Oldfield EH, Doppman JL, Di Chiro G. Spinal arteriovenous malformations: a comparison of dural arteriovenous fistulas and intradural AVM's in 81 patients. J Neurosurg. 1987;67(6): 795–802.
69. Miyasaka Y, Yada K, Ohwada T, Kitahara T, Kurata A, Irikura K. An analysis of the venous drainage system as a factor in hemorrhage from arteriovenous malformations. J Neurosurg. 1992;76(2):239–43.
70. Aviv RI, Shad A, Tomlinson G, et al. Cervical dural arteriovenous fistulae manifesting as subarachnoid hemorrhage: report of two cases and literature review. AJNR Am J Neuroradiol. 2004;25(5):854–8.
71. Narisawa A, Endo T, Sato K, Watanabe M, Takahashi A, Tominaga T. Spinal dural arteriovenous shunt presenting with intramedullary hemorrhage: case report. J Neurosurg Spine. 2014;20(3):322–6.
72. Liu Z, Jiao Q, Xu J, Wang X, Li S, You C. Spontaneous spinal epidural hematoma: analysis of 23 cases. Surg Neurol. 2008;69(3):253–60.
73. Sandalcioglu IE, Wiedemayer H, Gasser T, Asgari S, Engelhorn T, Stolke D. Intramedullary spinal cord cavernous malformations: clinical features and risk of hemorrhage. Neurosurg Rev. 2003;26(4):253–6.
74. Schulman S, Beyth RJ, Kearon C, Levine MN. Hemorrhagic complications of anticoagulant and thrombolytic treatment: American College of Chest Physicians evidence-based clinical practice guidelines. Chest. 2008;133(6 Suppl):257S–98.
75. International Stroke Trial Collaborative Group. The International Stroke Trial (IST): a randomised trial of aspirin, subcutaneous heparin, both, or neither among 19 435 patients with acute ischaemic stroke. Lancet. 1997;349(9065):1569–81.
76. Chai-Adisaksopha C, Crowther M, Isayama T, Lim W. The impact of bleeding complications in patients receiving target-specific oral anticoagulants: a systematic review and meta-analysis. Blood. 2014;124(15):2450–8.
77. Fang MC, Go AS, Chang Y, et al. Death and disability from warfarin-associated intracranial and extracranial hemorrhages. Am J Med. 2007;120(8):700–5.
78. Kahn SR, Lim W, Dunn AS, et al. Prevention of VTE in nonsurgical patients: antithrombotic therapy and prevention of thrombosis: American College of Chest Physicians evidence-based clinical practice guidelines. Chest. 2012;141(2 suppl):e195S–226.
79. Avorn J, Winkelmayer WC. Comparing the costs, risks, and benefits of competing strategies for the primary prevention of venous thromboembolism. Circulation. 2004;110(24 Suppl 1):IV25–32.
80. Koch A, Ziegler S, Breitschwerdt H, Victor N. Low molecular weight heparin and unfractionated heparin in thrombosis prophylaxis: meta-analysis based on original patient data. Thromb Res. 2001;102(4):295–309.
81. Gould MK, Garcia DA, Wren SM, et al. Prevention of VTE in nonorthopedic surgical patients: antithrombotic therapy and prevention of thrombosis: American College of Chest Physicians evidence-based clinical practice guidelines. Chest. 2012;141(2 suppl):e227S–77.
82. Iorio A, Agnelli G. Low-molecular-weight and unfractionated heparin for prevention of venous thromboembolism in neurosurgery: a meta-analysis. Arch Intern Med. 2000;160(15):2327–32.
83. Barritt D, Jordan S. Anticoagulant drugs in the treatment of pulmonary embolism: a controlled trial. Lancet. 1960;275(7138):1309–12.
84. Kernohan R, Todd C. Heparin therapy in thromboembolic disease. Lancet. 1966;287(7438):621–3.
85. Kearon C, Akl EA, Comerota AJ, et al. Antithrombotic therapy for VTE disease: antithrombotic therapy and prevention of thrombosis: American College of Chest Physicians evidence-based clinical practice guidelines. Chest. 2012;141(2 suppl):e419S–94.
86. Hulle T, Kooiman J, Exter P, et al. Effectiveness and safety of novel oral anticoagulants as compared with vitamin K antagonists in the treatment of acute symptomatic venous thromboembolism: a systematic review and meta-analysis. J Thromb Haemost. 2014;12(3):320–8.
87. Kearon C. Natural history of venous thromboembolism. Circulation. 2003;107(23 Suppl 1):I22–30.
88. Lagerstedt C, Fagher B, Olsson C, Öqvist B, Albrechtsson U. Need for long-term anticoagulant treatment in symptomatic calf-vein thrombosis. Lancet. 1985;326(8454):515–8.
89. Flinterman L, Van Der Meer F, Rosendaal F, Doggen C. Current perspective of venous thrombosis in the upper extremity. J Thromb Haemost. 2008;6(8): 1262–6.
90. Carson JL, Kelley MA, Duff A, et al. The clinical course of pulmonary embolism. N Engl J Med. 1992;326(19):1240–5.
91. Goldhaber SZ, Visani L, De Rosa M. Acute pulmonary embolism: clinical outcomes in the international cooperative pulmonary embolism registry (ICOPER). Lancet. 1999;353(9162):1386–9.
92. Stein PD, Henry JW. Prevalence of acute pulmonary embolism among patients in a general hospital and at autopsy. Chest. 1995;108(4):978–81.
93. Lloyd-Jones DM, Wang TJ, Leip EP, et al. Lifetime risk for development of atrial fibrillation: the Framingham Heart Study. Circulation. 2004;110(9): 1042–6.

94. January CT, Wann LS, Alpert JS, et al. 2014 AHA/ACC/HRS guideline for the management of patients with atrial fibrillation: a report of the American College of Cardiology/American Heart Association Task Force on Practice Guidelines and the Heart Rhythm Society. J Am Coll Cardiol. 2014;64(21):e1–76.
95. Wolf PA, Abbott RD, Kannel WB. Atrial fibrillation as an independent risk factor for stroke: the Framingham Study. Stroke. 1991;22(8):983–8.
96. You JJ, Singer DE, Howard PA, et al. Antithrombotic therapy for atrial fibrillation: antithrombotic therapy and prevention of thrombosis: American College of Chest Physicians evidence-based clinical practice guidelines. Chest. 2012;141(2 suppl):e531S–75.
97. Baudet EM, Puel V, McBride JT, et al. Long-term results of valve replacement with the St. Jude medical prosthesis. J Thorac Cardiovasc Surg. 1995;109(5):858–70.
98. Hering D, Piper C, Bergemann R, et al. Thromboembolic and bleeding complications following St. Jude medical valve replacement: results of the German experience with low-intensity anticoagulation study. Chest. 2005;127(1):53–9.
99. Whitlock RP, Sun JC, Fremes SE, et al. Antithrombotic and thrombolytic therapy for valvular disease: antithrombotic therapy and prevention of thrombosis: American College of Chest Physicians evidence-based clinical practice guidelines. Chest. 2012;141(2 suppl):e576S–600.
100. Eikelboom JW, Connolly SJ, Brueckmann M, et al. Dabigatran versus warfarin in patients with mechanical heart valves. N Engl J Med. 2013;369(13):1206–14.
101. Yeh RW, Sidney S, Chandra M, et al. Population trends in the incidence and outcomes of acute myocardial infarction. N Engl J Med. 2010;362(23):2155–65.
102. Savonitto S, Ardissino D, Granger CB, et al. Prognostic value of the admission electrocardiogram in acute coronary syndromes. JAMA. 1999;281(8):707–13.
103. Théroux P, Ouimet H, McCans J, et al. Aspirin, heparin, or both to treat acute unstable angina. N Engl J Med. 1988;319(17):1105–11.
104. Eikelboom JW, Anand SS, Malmberg K, et al. Unfractionated heparin and low-molecular-weight heparin in acute coronary syndrome without ST elevation: a meta-analysis. Lancet. 2000;355(9219):1936–42.
105. Harrington RA, Becker RC, Cannon CP, et al. Antithrombotic therapy for non-ST-segment elevation acute coronary syndromes: American College of Chest Physicians evidence-based clinical practice guidelines. Chest. 2008;133(6 suppl):670S–707.
106. Alonso-Coello P, Bellmunt S, McGorrian C, et al. Antithrombotic therapy in peripheral artery disease: antithrombotic therapy and prevention of thrombosis: American College of Chest Physicians evidence-based clinical practice guidelines. Chest. 2012;141(2 suppl):e669S–90.
107. Berridge DC, Kessel DO, Robertson I. Surgery versus thrombolysis for initial management of acute limb ischaemia. Cochrane Database Syst Rev. 2002;6, CD002784.
108. Bauer KA. The thrombophilias: well-defined risk factors with uncertain therapeutic implications. Ann Intern Med. 2001;135(5):367–73.
109. Lim W, Crowther MA, Eikelboom JW. Management of antiphospholipid antibody syndrome: a systematic review. JAMA. 2006;295(9):1050–7.
110. Schulman S, Svenungsson E, Granqvist S. Anticardiolipin antibodies predict early recurrence of thromboembolism and death among patients with venous thromboembolism following anticoagulant therapy. Am J Med. 1998;104(4):332–8.
111. Spetzler RF, Martin NA. A proposed grading system for arteriovenous malformations. J Neurosurg. 1986;65(4):476–83.
112. Sarwar M, McCormick W. Intracerebral venous angioma. Case report and review. Arch Neurol. 1978;35:323–5.

27 Intrathecal Access and Devices in Patients on Antiplatelet or Anticoagulant Therapy

Kevin N. Swong, Drew A. Spencer, and Christopher M. Loftus

Introduction

External ventricular drain (EVD) placement for cerebrospinal fluid (CSF) drainage is a well-established tool in the neurosurgeon's armamentarium. It was initially described in 1977 as a life saving measure. Over the years, it has undergone progressive refinement, with the modern practice of placement at Kocher's point implemented in 1894 [1]. The role for EVD placement has expanded to include management of elevated intracranial pressure (ICP), subarachnoid hemorrhage, traumatic brain injury, hydrocephalus, CSF fistula, and intraventricular hemorrhage (IVH) in addition to analysis of the CSF profile [2–5]. Other forms of CSF diversion, such as lumbar puncture (LP), lumbar drain (LD), or ventriculoperitoneal shunt (VPS) are also commonly used and can also diagnose or treat a variety of conditions such as meningitis, CSF fistula, normal pressure hydrocephalus (NPH), and pseudotumor cerebri [2, 6, 7]. EVD and LP/drainage have persisted in clinical practice based on their safety profile and efficacy. Special consideration must be given, however, when these procedures are enacted in patients on preprocedural antiplatelet or anticoagulant medications. This is an ever-growing population, and the current chapter will attempt to review the existing data guiding management of these complex situations.

K.N. Swong (✉) • D.A. Spencer • C.M. Loftus
Department of Neurosurgery, Loyola University
Stritch School of Medicine, Maywood, IL 60153, USA
e-mail: KSWONG@lumc.edu

EVD

EVD placement is not without risks which include infection, hemorrhage, aneurysm formation, or seizures. Maniker et al. found that the overall incidence of intracranial hemorrhage (ICH) after EVD placement was up to 33 %, however, only 2.5 % of the patients suffered a neurologic compromise or required surgical intervention after placement of the EVD [8]. The only factor that was a significant predictor of hemorrhage was a history of cerebrovascular disease. There was also a larger intraparenchymal hemorrhage (IPH) in patients with hypertensive hemorrhages due to hypertension compared to patients with post aneurysmal SAH [8]. Hemorrhages were also felt to be more likely in cases of multiple attempts or manipulating the catheter after it was inserted [9]. It is therefore reasonable to conclude that the benefit of EVD placement, when indicated, outweighs the risk of symptomatic hemorrhage.

The neurosurgical patient population is ever increasing in complexity, with a growing proportion of patients requiring antiplatelet or anticoagulant therapy for other medical conditions

C.M. Loftus (ed.), *Anticoagulation and Hemostasis in Neurosurgery*,
DOI 10.1007/978-3-319-27327-3_27

[10]. Despite the increasing frequency with which the population is on antiplatelet or anticoagulant therapy, there remain no prospective, high-level data to compare the safety of CSF diversion with or without the use of these medications. A small case series by Kung et al. demonstrated that the incidence of radiographic hemorrhages on dual antiplatelet therapy is similar to those seen in patients without antiplatelet therapy; however, they had a higher rate of symptomatic hemorrhages. Additionally, the responsible lesion in aneurysmal SAH is increasingly being treated with endovascular intervention, frequently requiring the use of single or dual antiplatelet therapy based on coil and/or stent placement [11]. This scenario represents the most extensive area of study and source of data, comparing patients who undergo EVD placement either with or without antiplatelet or anticoagulant therapy [12, 13].

There are many conflicting reports regarding EVD associated hemorrhages after endovascular intervention in the literature, and the safety with which a catheter may be placed after antiplatelet therapy has been initiated. A higher rate of hemorrhage is possible when an EVD is placed after an endovascular intervention has taken place; however, there is no significant difference in the rate of symptomatic hemorrhages even when an EVD is placed after an endovascular procedure has been completed that requires antiplatelet therapy [14, 15]. Furthermore, many have reported that there is no increase in the incidence of hemorrhage requiring surgical intervention [12, 13, 16]. Accounting for these facts, the safest practice is to place an EVD prior to any intervention when possible. Even though placing an EVD prior to an endovascular intervention is not exempt from risk—including delayed hemorrhage after the procedure—the rate of hemorrhage appears similar to that seen when EVDs are placed in patients not on antiplatelet or anticoagulant agents. *It is therefore recommended to place an EVD prior to any endovascular treatment, especially in cases where there is a high suspicion that antiplatelet agents will be required postoperatively.*

As a significant cohort of SAH patients acutely requiring CSF drainage will develop long-term hydrocephalus, it is prudent to know the risks incurred with VPS placement in patients on antiplatelet or anticoagulant medications as well. Shunt dependence is a possibility in patients with other pathology as well, extending the relevance of this discussion. There are a number of retrospective studies that have investigated the safety of VPS placement while on antiplatelet therapy. There does not appear to be a significantly increased risk of *symptomatic* intracranial hemorrhage for VPS placed in patients on dual antiplatelet therapy, even though the rate of hemorrhage formation is higher when compared to patients not receiving dual antiplatelet therapy [17]. Studies regarding anticoagulant medications are lacking, likely due to the fact that they are almost universally held prior to the operation. The duration of interruption of therapy is agent dependent, with two half-lives being the almost universal recommendation in addition to normalization of measurable lab values when relevant [18].

On the authors' service, it is common to place an EVD if there is concern for developing hydrocephalus before an endovascular intervention is undertaken, which has a hemorrhage rate similar to those reported in the literature without endovascular intervention or antiplatelet use. In situations where heparin has been given, but no long-acting anticoagulation has been started, an activated partial thromboplastin time (aPTT) is drawn and the EVD is inserted once the aPTT is normal, if time allows. If the aPTT is elevated, and the patient requires more urgent treatment, then the heparin is reversed with protamine sulfate before the procedure begins. If an EVD must be placed after an endovascular intervention is performed while on antiplatelet agents, we typically do not reverse the antiplatelet effects of the medication, and only use a single agent when possible. If an EVD must be placed for any other etiology in patients on antiplatelet or anticoagulant agents, the clinical scenario dictates pretreatment. With the exception of impending neurological collapse, appropriate reversal therapy is instituted followed by prompt drain placement. Reversal strategies include platelet or fresh frozen plasma transfusion, activated Factor VII, or prothrombin complex concentrates. Coagulation parameters are then closely monitored and repeat therapy administered as clinically dictated. Our current practice is to proceed with VPS placement after 1 week without antiplatelet therapy. If there is dual antiplatelet therapy, and the patient is able to withhold their medication for 2 weeks, then clopidogrel is held for 10 days and aspirin is held for 1 week. Both agents are resumed on post op day number three, based on previously published results and experiences [18]. *Anticoagulant medications are held for 5 days preoperatively or acutely reversed if indicated. Resumption of therapy is tailored to the patient and preference of the surgeon.*

LP or LD Placement

Literature guidance for LD placement or LP in patients on antiplatelet or anticoagulant medications is even sparser than that addressing EVDs. Most of the existing literature comes from studies in regional anesthesia via LP and epidural catheters, with the consensus being that postprocedural spinal hematomas are exceedingly rare (1 in 10,000) [19–22]. Similar to ventricular drain placement, procedural risks such as multiple attempts, traumatic placement, and aberrant anatomy are independent risk factors for hemorrhage that represent additive hazards in the face of antiplatelet or anticoagulant therapy [23]. There is no definitive increased risk from antiplatelet therapy alone [18]. *Anticoagulant therapy, however, definitively increases the spinal hemorrhage risk and demands interruption of therapy both pre- (2+ half-lives) and postprocedure (4–12 h)* [18, 24, 25]. While the overall complication rate is low, often times LP or LD placement is a less urgent intervention than an EVD, and therefore it is usually reasonable to wait a period of time before performing the procedure. In cases where time is of the essence, the risks of reversing an antiplatelet agent must be weighed against the benefit of the procedure. However, extrapolating the data on EVD and VPS to LD and LP shunt, it can be reasoned that there is also no increased risk from LP shunt placement on an antiplatelet agent if it must be performed [12, 13, 26]. Limited documentation supports this, with an even rarer incidence of hemorrhagic complications requiring surgical intervention [19, 20].

Again, at the authors' institution, current practice is to proceed immediately with an LP or LD if the patient is only on a single antiplatelet agent. If there is dual antiplatelet therapy, and they are able to withhold their medication for 2 weeks, then clopidogrel is held for 10 days and aspirin is held for 1 week. Both agents are resumed on post op day number three. Platelet transfusion is utilized when the procedure must be done emergently. Anticoagulant medications are routinely held for several days (3–5, agent dependent) before the procedure, with only rare circumstances requiring urgent reversal—usually those where LP is the only definitive mode of diagnosis and delay in therapy can be life threatening (meningitis, SAH). It is not our policy to proceed with LP or LD on anticoagulated patients without a preprocedure reversal strategy. Resumption of therapy is variable as described for EVD management.

Restarting Antiplatelet and Anticoagulant Medication

Resumption of antiplatelet and anticoagulant medications is a crucial component in the management of patients with multiple comorbidities. Regarding the placement and management of intrathecal catheters, there are two patient populations to consider: those on preexisting therapy for cardiac or cerebrovascular risks, and those who require it after percutaneous intervention to treat intracranial circulatory disorders. In both scenarios, clinicians must weigh the risk of thrombosis against that of hemorrhage in neurologically susceptible patients.

In patients on preprocedural antiplatelet or anticoagulant medications, standard practices are quite variable—similar to the practices previously discussed for drain placement. Some authors have advocated for periprocedural continuation of antiplatelet therapy and have cited a low incidence of untoward events [13, 15, 27]. The primary pathology, including rehemorrhage risk and the potential need for operative intervention, must be considered as well. The decision of when to resume therapy frequently requires multidisciplinary collaboration with cardiology, stroke/vascular neurology, or both. Ultimately, the treating neurosurgeon must decide when it is safe to resume therapy. Before or after drain removal, and how long to wait after drain removal are the two primary dilemmas. There is a glaring lack of evidence for either, *the only undisputed risk being that of hemorrhage after drain removal in patients on therapeutic anticoagulation with any agent* [18]. Given the potential consequences, the only prudent recommendation is to withhold antiplatelet therapy at least 1 day and as long as 1 week after drain removal. Extenuating circumstances (e.g., cardiac stent<3 months postplacement), however, often force the clinician's hand by demanding immediate postprocedure or postoperative resumption of therapy [18]. Anticoagulant medications allow a different approach based on their onset of action. They can frequently be restarted within a few hours of a procedure when the clinical condition dictates (mechanical heart valve, acute DVT/PE, etc.) with close clinical surveillance until a therapeutic level is achieved. The absolute length of time to delay therapy after intervention is agent dependent, with at least one half or one full half-life being the recommended time for most agents [18].

With the continued evolution of endovascular therapy, many more patients now undergo stent-assisted procedures that require antiplatelet therapy after intervention [11]. The most common indications for endovascular intervention (SAH, IPH, IVH) are also common indications for ventricular drain placement. *A decision point arises when these patients no longer require ventricular drainage. Others have reported their experiences both of devastating results as well as uncomplicated drain removal in patients on antiplatelet therapy, with the literature overall favoring the latter outcome* [12, 13, 15, 18, 28]. *Some clinicians, including at our institution, have removed catheters after either interruption of therapy or platelet transfusion in high risk patients. Comparable to other conditions discussed elsewhere in this text, no consensus exists regarding when it is safe to resume antiplatelet therapy after drain removal.* Multiple factors must be considered—including elective versus ruptured aneurysm repair, vasospasm and other vascular injuries, and patient comorbidities—when restarting postprocedural or post-drain removal antiplatelet therapy and deciding between aggressive (hours) and conservative (days to weeks) resumption schedules. In this patient population, management of anticoagulant therapy should follow the guidelines previously delineated for similar scenarios.

Conclusion

Patients requiring CSF sampling or drainage typically harbor serious pathology and require aggressive management. Posthemorrhagic or infectious hydrocephalus, meningitis, CSF leak, and NPH are just a few of the conditions requiring CSF analysis or continuous drainage. As with most other medical and surgical conditions, these events are more likely to occur in the aged or ill, those with more comorbidities and therefore a higher likelihood of antiplatelet or anticoagulant medication use. When these patients present with intracranial or other processes prompting intrathecal access, there is an increased, though undefined, risk of periprocedural hemorrhage. Documented rates are highly variable (5–30 %), as are their clinical consequences [11, 12, 15, 19]. There is even less evidence and published opinion regarding the appropriate management of antiplatelet and anticoagulant medications as well their pharmacologic effect—when to reverse, how to reverse and the duration of reversal. Ensuring patient safety often becomes a multidisciplinary endeavor, and one highly reliant on expert opinion.

When access of the intrathecal space is required despite abnormal coagulation parameters, the current evidence suggests an uncertain rate of clinically relevant complications. Many authors to date have referenced low power, retrospective studies citing low rates of hemorrhagic events, but with inherent variability preventing any consequential conclusions [13, 15].

Many prior evaluations have found a propensity for small hemorrhages in these scenarios. In an otherwise healthy patient, a small hemorrhage may be well tolerated. A patient with an acute neurological injury represents an entirely different challenge, with poor reserve to overcome a second insult. This principle underlies the importance of careful clinical planning and decision making in this patient population. As treatment of previously devastating injuries (SAH, IPH, acute hydrocephalus) continues to improve, clinicians need to be aware of the peripheral risk factors for continued progress.

We err on the side of caution, patient safety, and patient welfare, as described. Whenever possible, in the brain or lumbar spine, we insert, maintain, and remove CSF diversion devices in the absence of systemic antiplatelet or anticoagulant drugs unless there is a compelling, essentially life threatening, need to proceed with such therapy in place.

References

1. Srinivasan VM, O'Neill BR, Jho D, Whiting DM, Oh MY. The history of external ventricular drainage. J Neurosurg. 2014;120(1):228–36.
2. Lundberg N. Continuous recording and control of ventricular fluid pressure in neurosurgical practice. Acta Psychiatr Scand Suppl. 1960;36(149):1–193.
3. Kusske JA, Turner PT, Ojemann GA, Harris AB. Ventriculostomy for the treatment of acute hydrocephalus following subarachnoid hemorrhage. J Neurosurg. 1973;38(5):591–5.
4. Becker DP, Miller JD, Ward JD, Greenberg RP, Young HF, Sakalas R. The outcome from severe head injury with early diagnosis and intensive management. J Neurosurg. 1977;47(4):491–502.
5. Aschoff A, Kremer P, Hashemi B, Kunze S. The scientific history of hydrocephalus and its treatment. Neurosurg Rev. 1999;22(2–3):67–93. discussion 4–5.
6. Kramer SC, Gorich J, Rilinger N, et al. Interventional treatment of hemorrhages in advanced cervical carcinoma. Radiologe. 1999;39(9):795–8.
7. Golz L, Ruppert FH, Meier U, Lemcke J. Outcome of modern shunt therapy in patients with idiopathic normal pressure hydrocephalus 6 years postoperatively. J Neurosurg. 2014;121(4):771–5.
8. Maniker AH, Vaynman AY, Karimi RJ, Sabit AO, Holland B. Hemorrhagic complications of external ventricular drainage. Neurosurgery. 2006;59(4 Suppl 2):ONS419–24; discussion ONS24–5.
9. Ross IB, Dhillon GS. Ventriculostomy-related cerebral hemorrhages after endovascular aneurysm treatment. AJNR Am J Neuroradiol. 2003;24(8):1528–31.
10. Labuz-Roszak B, Pierzchala K, Skrzypek M, Swiech M, Machowska-Majchrzak A. Oral anticoagulant and antiplatelet drugs used in prevention of cardiovascular events in elderly people in Poland. BMC Cardiovasc Disord. 2012;12:98.
11. Kung DK, Policeni BA, Capuano AW, et al. Risk of ventriculostomy-related hemorrhage in patients with acutely ruptured aneurysms treated using stent-assisted coiling. J Neurosurg. 2011;114(4):1021–7.
12. Bruder M, Schuss P, Konczalla J, et al. Ventriculostomy related hemorrhage after treatment of acutely ruptured aneurysms: the influence of anticoagulation and antiplatelet treatment. World Neurosurg. 2015;84:1653–9.
13. Scholz C, Hubbe U, Deininger M, Deininger MH. Hemorrhage rates of external ventricular drain (EVD), intracranial pressure gauge (ICP) or combined EVD and ICP gauge placement within 48 h of endovascular coil embolization of cerebral aneurysms. Clin Neurol Neurosurg. 2013;115(8):1399–402.
14. Zhu X. The hemorrhage risk of prophylactic external ventricular drain insertion in aneurysmal subarachnoid hemorrhage patients requiring endovascular aneurysm treatment: a systematic review and meta-analysis. J Neurosurg Sci. 2015.
15. Hoh BL, Nogueira RG, Ledezma CJ, Pryor JC, Ogilvy CS. Safety of heparinization for cerebral aneurysm coiling soon after external ventriculostomy drain placement. Neurosurgery. 2005;57(5):845–9. discussion 845–9.
16. Sims-Williams HP, Weinberg D, Jadun CK, Brydon HL. Ventriculostomy associated haemorrhage: a complication of anti-platelet therapy during coiling. Br J Neurosurg. 2014;28(6):782–4.
17. Mahaney KB, Chalouhi N, Viljoen S, et al. Risk of hemorrhagic complication associated with ventriculoperitoneal shunt placement in aneurysmal subarachnoid hemorrhage patients on dual antiplatelet therapy. J Neurosurg. 2013;119(4):937–42.
18. Gogarten W, Vandermeulen E, Van Aken H, et al. Regional anaesthesia and antithrombotic agents: recommendations of the European Society of Anaesthesiology. Eur J Anaesthesiol. 2010;27(12): 999–1015.
19. Horlocker TT, Wedel DJ, Schroeder DR, et al. Preoperative antiplatelet therapy does not increase the risk of spinal hematoma associated with regional anesthesia. Anesth Analg. 1995;80(2):303–9.
20. van Veen JJ, Nokes TJ, Makris M. The risk of spinal haematoma following neuraxial anaesthesia or lumbar puncture in thrombocytopenic individuals. Br J Haematol. 2010;148(1):15–25.
21. Gustafsson H, Rutberg H, Bengtsson M. Spinal haematoma following epidural analgesia. Report of a patient with ankylosing spondylitis and a bleeding diathesis. Anaesthesia. 1988;43(3):220–2.

22. Wang US, Ju CI, Kim SW, Kim SH. Spontaneous concomitant intracranial and spinal subdural hematomas in association with anticoagulation therapy. J Korean Neurosurg Soc. 2012;51(4):237–9.
23. Rocchi R, Lombardi C, Marradi I, Di Paolo M, Cerase A. Intracranial and intraspinal hemorrhage following spinal anesthesia. Neurol Sci. 2009;30(5):393–6.
24. Godet G, Goarin JP, Fléron MH, Bertrand M, Kieffer E, Coriat P. Subdural haemorrhage following lumbar spinal drainage during repair of thoraco-abdominal aneurysm. Ann Fr Anesth Reanim. 2003;22(4):353–8.
25. Castillo JM, Afanador HF, Manjarrez E, Morales XA. Non-traumatic spontaneous spinal subdural hematoma in a patient with non-valvular atrial fibrillation during treatment with rivaroxaban. Am J Case Rep. 2015;16:377–81.
26. Møller A, Bjerrum OW, Afshari A. Haemostasis and safety measures before lumbar puncture in the haematology ward: the Danish routines. Acta Haematol. 2015;133(1):108–12.
27. Tamura Y, Yamada Y, Tucker A, et al. Endoscopic surgery for hemorrhagic pineal cyst following antiplatelet therapy: case report. Neurol Med Chir (Tokyo). 2013;53(9):625–9.
28. Sweeney JM, Vasan R, van Loveren HR, Youssef AS, Agazzi S. Catheter fixation and ligation: a simple technique for ventriculostomy management following endovascular stenting. J Neurosurg. 2013;118(5):1009–13.

Is It Safe to Shunt Anticoagulated NPH Patients?

28

Eric W. Sankey, C. Rory Goodwin, Ignacio Jusue-Torres, and Daniele Rigamonti

Introduction

Normal pressure hydrocephalus (NPH) is a common and treatable neurological disorder that often results in progressive gait impairment, urinary incontinence, and dementia in the context of ventricular enlargement with normal cerebrospinal fluid (CSF) opening pressure on lumbar puncture and absence of papilledema [1, 2]. NPH may be idiopathic or secondary to traumatic brain injury, subarachnoid hemorrhage, tumor, infection, or surgical complication [3]. While secondary NPH can occur at any age, idiopathic NPH (iNPH) typically affects individuals in their 60s and 70s [4]. Epidemiological data regarding NPH remains limited; however, based on studies from Scandinavia and Japan, the estimated incidence of NPH ranges from 5.5 to 120/100,000 persons per year, in patients above 70 years of age [5, 6]. According to five community-based studies, the overall prevalence of iNPH ranges from 0.12 % to 2.9 %, with a prevalence as high as 5.9 % in patients above 80 years of age [7].

CSF diversion is warranted in the majority of patients with symptomatic NPH and results in clinical improvement in up to 80–90 % of individuals [2]. As such, CSF shunting is the most commonly employed treatment for the long-term management of NPH. However, like all surgical interventions, CSF shunting carries a risk of both intraoperative and postoperative complications. Immediate complications include parenchymal injury and/or intracranial hemorrhage during catheter placement, and delayed complications include shunt obstruction, infection, subdural hygroma or hematoma, and shunt migration [8, 9]. Complications from hematologic causes can be particularly devastating in this group, given the aforementioned potential surgical complications and intrinsic or extrinsic patient-specific factors that can increase risk. iNPH typically occurs in the elderly and common cardiovascular comorbidities associated with thrombosis in this age group are prevalent, including: atrial fibrillation, valvular disease, ischemic heart disease, and deep venous thrombosis (DVT). Likewise, Krauss et al. reported a significant association between NPH and diabetes mellitus ($P<0.015$), as well as cardiac ($P<0.001$), cerebral arteriosclerotic ($P=0.007$), and other arteriosclerotic diseases ($P=0.001$) [10]. Similarly, Eide and

E.W. Sankey, B.S. • C.R. Goodwin, M.D., Ph.D.
I. Jusue-Torres, M.D.
D. Rigamonti, M.D., F.A.C.S., F.A.H.A. (✉)
Department of Neurosurgery, The Johns Hopkins Hospital, 600 North Wolfe Street, Phipps 126, Baltimore, MD, USA
e-mail: DR@jhmi.edu

C.M. Loftus (ed.), *Anticoagulation and Hemostasis in Neurosurgery*,
DOI 10.1007/978-3-319-27327-3_28

Pripp found a significantly increased prevalence of diabetes mellitus and cardiovascular diseases, such as arterial hypertension (males), angina pectoris (females and males), and cardiac infarction (males) in iNPH patients compared to healthy controls [11]. Patients with these cardiovascular diseases are commonly prescribed antithrombotic therapy (i.e., anticoagulant and/or antiplatelet) to reduce the risk of stroke. Moreover, long-term daily use of aspirin or anticoagulants is recommended for diabetic patients unless otherwise contraindicated, due to an increased risk of developing arterial disease (e.g., coronary artery, cerebrovascular and peripheral arterial disease) [12]. As such, many NPH patients presenting for shunt placement may have a history of long-term antithrombotic therapy.

Long-term anticoagulation is often considered to be a relative contraindication to shunt surgery for patients with NPH given serious concerns regarding the increased risk of anticoagulant-associated bleeding in the elderly, particularly with regard to immediate intracranial hemorrhage (ICH) or delayed subdural hematoma (SDH) during or after CSF shunting [13]. Furthermore, elderly patients often have additional concomitant physical and medical issues necessitating the use of multiple medications, such as antiplatelet drugs, that increase the interactions and risks associated with anticoagulant therapy. According to the National Center for Health Statistics' *Health, United States, 2013* report, 47.5 % of adults aged 65 and over were taking at least five or more drugs simultaneously between 2007 and 2010. Therefore, a careful assessment of the overall risk-benefit ratio associated with CSF shunting in anticoagulated NPH patients must be employed. While few studies have objectively explored the outcomes after shunt placement in anticoagulated NPH patients, the results of our previous study demonstrated that patients on long-term anticoagulant therapy using warfarin can be safely and effectively evaluated and treated for NPH [3].

In this chapter, we discuss the risks associated with CSF shunting in anticoagulated NPH patients, and review the evidence on management strategies to reduce the risk of hematologic morbidity related to CSF diversion in these patients.

Common Anticoagulants Encountered in the NPH Population

Diseases associated with thrombosis are more common in the elderly population, including those with NPH. Appropriate antithrombotic therapy effectively reduces morbidity and mortality due to stroke and thromboembolism, and is therefore warranted for many elderly patients. According to the National Center for Health Statistics' *Health, United States, 2013* report, 18.1 % of adults 65 years and older were using one or more anticoagulant and/or antiplatelet medication between 2007 and 2010, increased from 9.1 % between 1999 and 2002. Commonly used antithrombotic agents in this age group include: warfarin, heparin, direct factor Xa inhibitors (e.g., Rivaroxaban), direct thrombin inhibitors (e.g., Dabigatran), aspirin, and clopidogrel. Each agent has unique applications and risks that must be individually considered when encountering an anticoagulated NPH patient who presents for CSF shunting. However, an individual discussion surrounding the unique aspects of particular antithrombotic therapies is beyond the scope of this chapter, and consultation with a hematologist and/or cardiologist is encouraged prior to shunt placement.

Diagnostic Protocol for Patients on Anticoagulants

The efficacy of CSF shunting in patients with suspected NPH varies widely in the literature, with rates of clinical improvement ranging from 24 % to greater than 96 %; however, in appropriately selected patients, shunt insertion can result in significant improvement in the majority of patients with NPH, with low iatrogenic morbidity and mortality [14]. As such, several imaging techniques and invasive procedures, ranging from CSF drainage, to continuous intracranial pressure monitoring, to hydrodynamic study methods, can be utilized to improve diagnostic evaluation and predict response to CSF shunting [15]. Despite their utility, invasive diagnostic procedures carry a low, but important, risk of hemorrhagic complications, particularly in patients receiving antithrombotic therapy [16–18].

Gait impairment is the most common and often is the presenting symptom in patients with NPH [19]. The Timed Up and Go (TUG) and Tinetti Performance Oriented Mobility Assessment are often utilized to reliably and accurately measure functional outcomes related to gait [20]. In addition to monitoring gait outcomes after shunting, these assessments are valuable tools that can be used to assess falling risk in anticoagulated NPH patients, potentially predicting the risk of traumatic intracranial hemorrhage. More robust studies evaluating the ability of these noninvasive tests to predict the risk of a fall-related intracranial hemorrhage could be useful in stratifying patients that would benefit from increased prophylactic measures, irrespective of their NPH status.

Lumbar drainage, whether through a large volume tap or continuous drainage, can be used to determine whether a patient is likely to respond to CSF shunting. This modality is one of the preferred diagnostic interventions of choice used to assist surgeons in the evaluation of the risk-benefit ratio associated with shunt placement in NPH patients. However, it is important to note that in patients on concomitant anticoagulation therapy, anticoagulant-associated bleeding can occur due to lumbar puncture itself. While rare, hemorrhagic complications including epidural, subdural, and subarachnoid hemorrhage are serious potential side effects of lumbar puncture [21, 22]. For example, in 2004, Samdani et al. reported a case of a 34-year-old man, with a history of daily aspirin use for back pain, who experienced a subdural hematoma after diagnostic lumbar puncture [23]. Likewise, Paal et al. reported a case of spinal subarachnoid hemorrhage caused by diagnostic lumbar puncture in a 51-year-old patient on a daily combined regimen of aspirin and clopidogrel [24]. In 2005, Burger et al. performed a meta-analysis of randomized controlled trials regarding the discontinuation of aspirin prior to diagnostic or therapeutic interventions and, based on the evidence, concluded that aspirin should only be discontinued in cases where its continued use would be associated with a higher risk of mortality than the increased risk of vascular accident without it [25]. Likewise, the risk for hemorrhage after lumbar puncture is increased in patients using anticoagulants such warfarin, low molecular weight heparins, and direct factor Xa and thrombin inhibitors [18].

Intracranial pressure (ICP) monitoring may also be employed during the evaluation and treatment of NPH. In 2010, Eide et al. reported that improvement after surgery can be anticipated in 90 % of iNPH patients with abnormal ICP pulsatility, compared to 10 % of patients with normal ICP pulsatility, highlighting the utility of this invasive procedure in the diagnosis of NPH [26]. While the authors reported a low complication rate related to ICP monitoring, with no reports of hemorrhagic complication [26], other studies have reported low, but significant rates of intracranial hemorrhage associated with ICP monitoring via the gold standard procedure of external ventricular drain (EVD) placement. The rate of hemorrhagic complication associated with EVDs ranges from 0 % to 15 %, with two (0.6 %) deaths occurring in Karkala et al.'s study of the safety and accuracy of bedside EVD placement [17]. Of note, the rate of hemorrhage associated with EVD placement estimated in these studies is likely higher than in the general NPH population given the fact that the majority of patients had an EVD placed for emergent circumstances, such as subarachnoid hemorrhage, intracranial hemorrhage, and intraventricular hemorrhage in Karkala et al.'s study, while diagnostic EVD placement for NPH is generally an elective procedure. Therefore, complete reversal of anticoagulation in patients on antithrombotic therapy in these studies may not have been possible. Although the factors of this study do not match the NPH population, given the increased risk of bleeding in anticoagulated NPH patients, careful evaluation for evidence of potential hemorrhagic complication should be performed in patients who undergo diagnostic ICP monitoring.

Preoperative Anticoagulation Management Strategy: Complication Avoidance and Preoperative Considerations

Studies regarding perioperative management of anticoagulation in neurosurgical patients remain limited [27], particularly regarding shunt placement for NPH. Currently, there is no consensus on the most appropriate perioperative anticoagulation regimen in elective and emergent intracranial shunt surgery. As a result, surgeons often base their perioperative anticoagulation management strategy upon anecdotal observations and personal professional experiences [28]. To complicate matters further, the majority of neurosurgical procedures are considered to be high risk for perioperative bleeding and thrombosis [29–31]. For example, Hamilton et al. reported postoperative DVTs in >25 % of non-anticoagulated patients who underwent craniotomies [32]. Furthermore, temporary cessation of long-term anticoagulation exposes patients to an increased risk of thrombotic complications [30, 33, 34]. Conversely, continuation or early postoperative resumption of therapeutic anticoagulation increases the risk of postoperative hemorrhagic complications [28, 30, 34–37]. Several factors associated with a patients' risk of thrombotic and bleeding complications include: the primary indication for long-term anticoagulation, type and duration of anticoagulant therapy, the patients' baseline bleeding and thrombotic risks, urgency of surgery, duration of perioperative anticoagulant cessation, and whether partial or complete reversal of anticoagulation is achieved [31, 38–40]. Therefore, a meticulous balance between the opposing thrombotic and bleeding risks is crucial for safe and effective management of patients who undergo shunt placement for the management of NPH.

Given the unique considerations above, we recommend perioperative consultation with a hematologist and/or cardiologist in anticoagulated NPH patients undergoing shunt surgery. Due to the high risk of bleeding associated with intracranial procedures [29, 30, 41, 42], the majority of anticoagulated NPH patients require temporary interruption of therapy prior to shunt surgery. While long-term cessation of antithrombotic therapy is associated with a substantially increased risk of thrombotic complication in patients who require antithrombotic therapy, temporary cessation of therapy can be generally considered safe.

For patients on warfarin, Goodwin et al. proposed a perioperative anticoagulation management strategy, in which anticoagulation should be stopped at least 5–7 days before invasive diagnostic procedures or surgery to allow adequate time for their INR to normalize (Fig. 28.1) [3]. In patients whose INR remains above 1.5, oral phytonadione (vitamin K) may be used the day prior to surgery to reach normal levels. In patients considered too high risk for thromboembolism with complete cessation of anticoagulant therapy, bridging to intravenous (IV) unfractionated heparin (UFH), or therapeutic doses of subcutaneous (SQ) low molecular weight heparin (LMWH) can be utilized. Patients who may not be amenable to cessation of anticoagulation include those with a mechanical heart valve, history of atrial fibrillation, or recent venothromboembolism (<6 months). Bridging should be performed 36–48 h after the last dose of warfarin. The appropriate dose of anticoagulant used for bridging is dependent on the patient's individual risk of thrombosis and bleeding, weight, and renal function. In an effort to reduce the risk of perioperative bleeding, bridging therapy should be stopped at least 24 h prior to surgery in patients receiving SQ LMWH, or 4–6 h prior to surgery if the patient is receiving IV UFH. The decision to bridge anticoagulation in patients who are determined to be at a moderate- to low-risk level for thromboembolism can be left to the discretion of the surgical and/or hematology/cardiology team. Furthermore, patients considered to be at a very low risk for thromboembolism, such as patients with bileaflet aortic valve prosthesis without atrial fibrillation or other risk factors for stroke, CHADS2 score of 0–2 without a history of prior stroke or transient ischemic attack or >12 months since their last and no other thromboembolic risk factors [42], should not be bridged prior to surgery [31]. Patient-specific factors such as medication adherence, comprehension, and ability to comply with the management plan should also be considered when deciding to bridge AC prior to surgery, particularly in NPH patients with significant dementia.

In our practice, we suspend the use of aspirin and other antiplatelet agents at least 7–14 days prior to surgery in order to reduce the risk of hemorrhagic complications. This time frame is recommended based on the fact that many antiplatelet agents, such as aspirin, are irreversible inhibitors and platelet formation takes at least

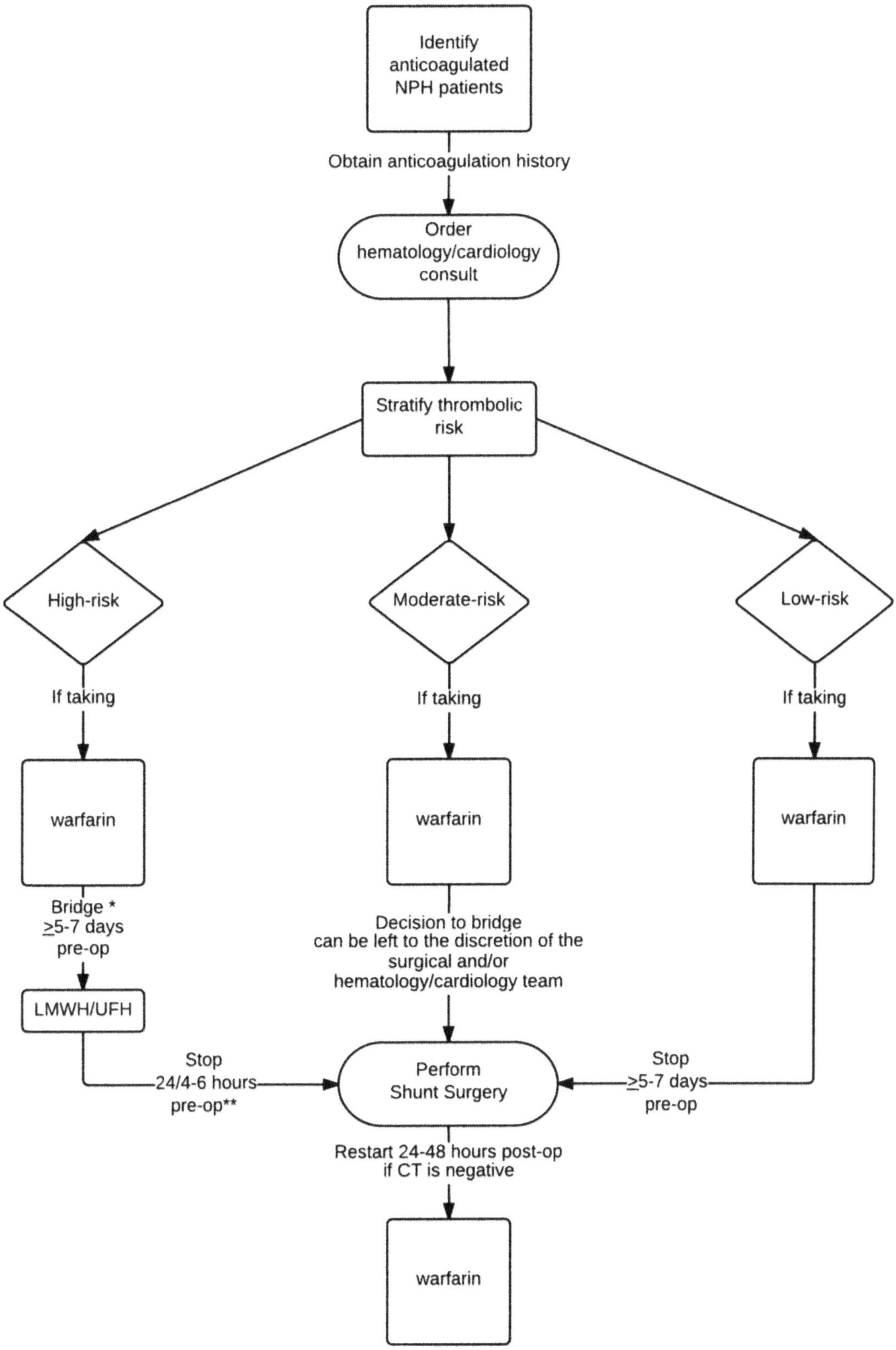

Fig. 28.1 A proposed algorithm for perioperative management of NPH patients on warfarin therapy. Abbreviations: *NPH* normal pressure hydrocephalus, *UFH* unfractionated heparin, *LMWH* low molecular weight heparin. *Bridging therapy refers to stopping warfarin and transitioning to intravenous UFH or subcutaneous LMWH. **AC is stopped at least 24 h prior to surgery in patients receiving LMWH, or 4–6 h if UFH is used

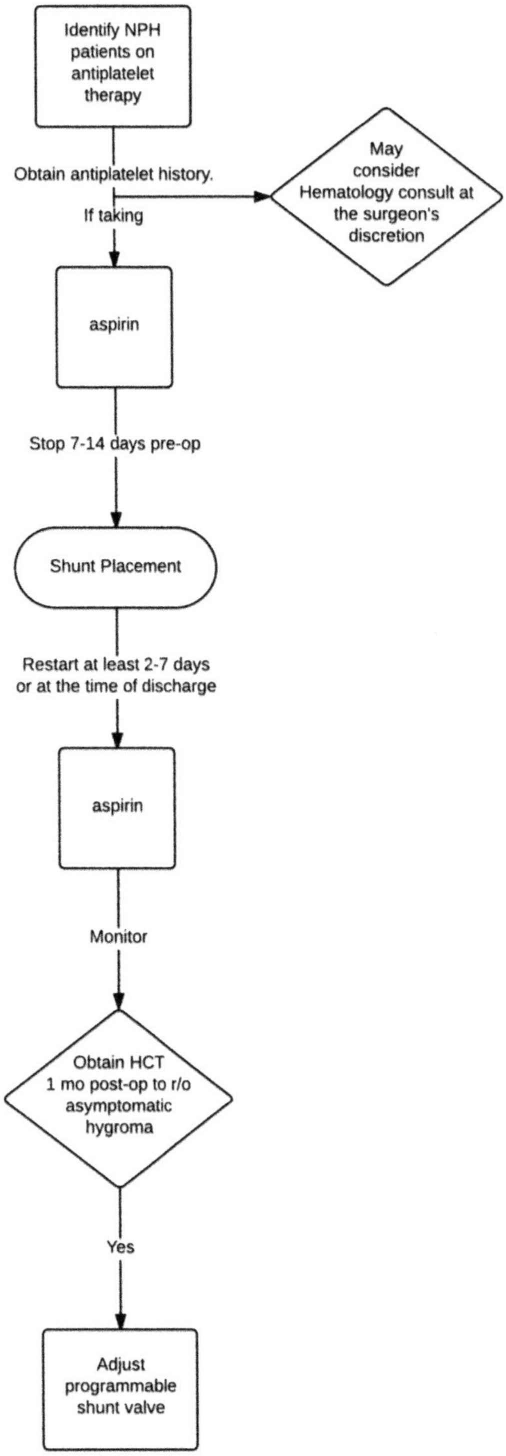

Fig. 28.2 A proposed algorithm for perioperative management of NPH patients on aspirin therapy. Adapted from Birkeland P, Lauritsen J, Poulsen FR. Aspirin is associated with an increased risk of subdural hematoma in normal pressure hydrocephalus patients following shunt implantation. J Neurosurg. 2015;123:423–6. Abbreviations: *NPH* normal pressure hydrocephalus, *HCT* head computed tomography, *r/o* rule out

5–7 days to replenish the available pool for clotting. Birkeland et al. also recommended the same timeline for cessation of antiplatelet therapy in their analysis of 35 patients receiving aspirin therapy in their study regarding the risk of subdural hematoma associated with shunt placement in patients with NPH (Fig. 28.2) [43].

The above approach should only be considered as a guideline for anticoagulated NPH patients, and is not a substitute for clinician judgment regarding perioperative anticoagulation in this challenging patient population. Likewise, newer antithrombotic therapies may require different perioperative management; therefore, consultation with a hematologist and/or cardiologist is encouraged. In all NPH patients receiving antithrombotic therapy, the INR, aPTT, and/or bleeding time should be measured in order to confirm that they are within the normal range prior to surgery. Placement of an IVC filter prior to shunt surgery can also be considered in patients at a particularly high risk for thromboembolism.

Surgical Considerations and Potential Intraoperative Complications

Aside from the general risks associated with performing a craniotomy or burr hole in an anticoagulated NPH patient, unique risks associated with shunt placement should also be considered. For example, incision of the pia mater prior to insertion of the shunt catheter is essential to avoid a subdural hematoma caused by unintentional stretching and tearing of the bridging veins from pushing the brain away from the overlying dura with catheter insertion. Image guidance may also improve the accuracy of ventricular shunt catheter placement, and avoid parenchymal injury and hemorrhagic complication due to multiple passes particularly in the hands of less experienced surgeons who do not commonly perform the procedure [44, 45]. In addition, an adjustable shunt valve with an anti-siphon device should be utilized to allow gradual adjustment of the pressure setting in order to lower the risk of subdural hygroma or hematoma postoperatively [46], particularly in anticoagulated NPH patients. In their randomized prospective study of 96 patients with NPH, Boon et al. found an increased risk of subdural effusions in patients receiving a low pressure shunt system (71 %) compared to a medium pressure system (34 %) [47]. However, a recent randomized controlled trial in iNPH patients found that gradual lowering of an adjustable shunt valve setting to a mean of 7 cm H_2O resulted in a similar rate of shunt complications and overdrainage, when compared to a fixed valve setting of 13 cm H_2O [48]. Of note, the use of perioperative antithrombotic therapy was similar between groups; though, anticoagulant medication was discontinued at least 1 week prior to shunt surgery in all patients in their study.

Postoperative Anticoagulation Management Strategy—Complication Avoidance and Postoperative Consideration

A head CT (HCT) should be performed within 24 h after shunt placement in anticoagulated NPH patients to assess for early, postoperative hemorrhagic complications (Figs. 28.3 and 28.4). If there is no radiographic or clinical evidence of hemorrhage, antithrombotic therapy can be restarted within an appropriate time frame as deemed by the management team. However, if a clinical or radiographic bleed is identified, antithrombotic therapy should be held until serial imaging shows resolution (in low-risk patients) or stability (in high-risk patients) of the hemorrhage. Also, the patient should be carefully evaluated for evidence of thrombotic complications secondary to temporary cessation of antithrombotic therapy.

Long-acting warfarin therapy may be subsequently restarted 24–48 h postoperatively if the postoperative CT is negative, or as soon as it is considered safe by the multidisciplinary team. Of note, in our previous study, warfarin therapy was restarted 3–5 days after surgery or at the time of discharge [3]; however, based on recent evidence, the American College of Chest Physicians (ACCP) guidelines recommends earlier resumption of warfarin after surgery [42]. However, in their 2013 New England Journal of Medicine review, Baron et al. deemed all neurosurgical procedures as high risk of hemorrhagic complication [31]. The authors also stated that due to the fact that resumption of warfarin therapy takes several days to achieve full anticoagulation, it can typically be restarted the evening of postoperative day 1, "unless there is a substantial risk of delayed bleeding or unless reoperation is anticipated" [31].

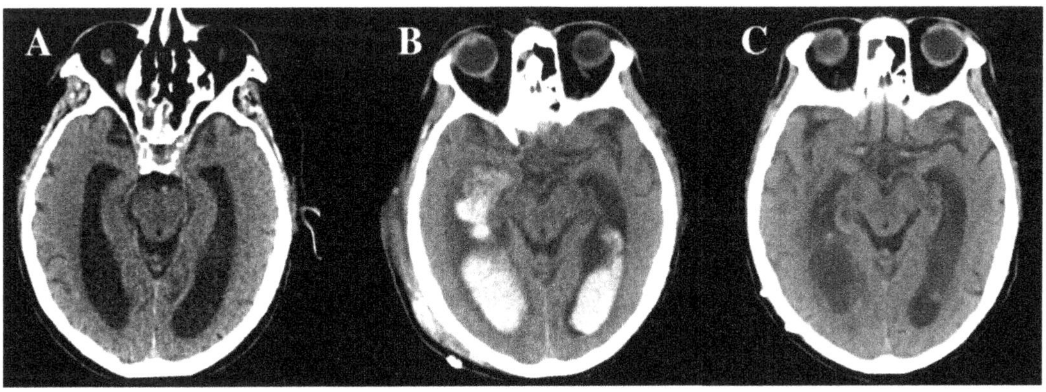

Fig. 28.3 Non-contrast axial head CT depicting preoperative (**a**), post-hemorrhage (**b**), and post-resolution (**c**) images in an 80-year-old male on long-term coumadin therapy prior to shunt placement for NPH. (On postoperative day 1, the patient experienced a large intraventricular hemorrhage bilaterally, involving the occipital horns and a small intraparenchymal hemorrhage around the catheter. The hemorrhage completely resolved 2 months postoperatively)

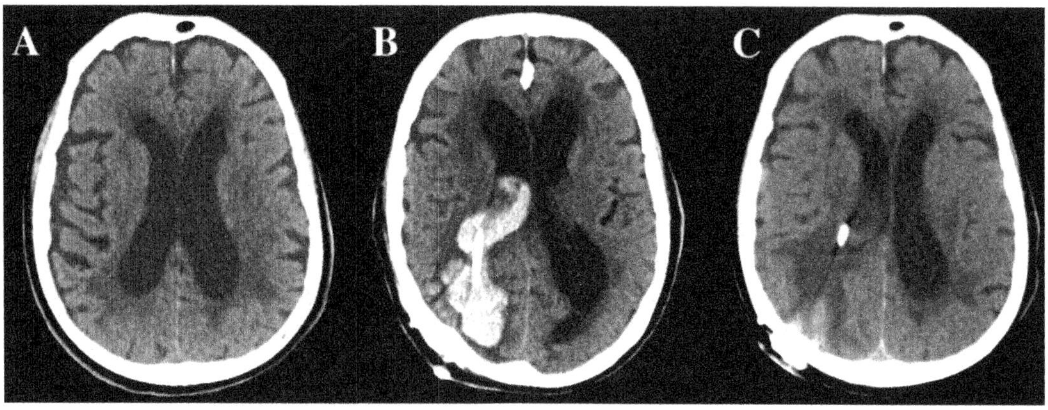

Fig. 28.4 Non-contrast axial head CT depicting preoperative (**a**), post-hemorrhage (**b**), and last follow-up (**c**) images in an 85-year-old male on high-dose (325 mg daily) aspirin therapy prior to shunt placement for NPH. (On postoperative day 5, the patient experienced a large intraparenchymal hemorrhage along the course of the right posterior parietal approach ventricular shunt catheter extending into the right lateral ventricle. The hemorrhage continued to gradually evolve, with extension into the intraventricular system, until the patient's death 1 month postoperatively)

Due to the higher risk of significant morbidity and mortality associated with intracranial hemorrhage, and need for emergent surgical intervention if substantial bleeding is encountered, further studies are needed to substantiate this recommendation and to determine whether restarting warfarin 24 h postoperatively is safe after neurosurgical procedures and in the NPH population. Furthermore, caution should be taken in this particular population due to their increased gait instability and higher fall risk. Importantly, it may take >48 h after resumption of warfarin to reach a partial response (INR >1.5). In patients taking LMWH or UFH, anticoagulation can be resumed 24–72 h postoperatively, or after adequate hemostasis has been achieved. Based on the 2012 ACCP guidelines, antiplatelet therapy may be resumed 24–48 h after surgery [40]; however, based on the increased risk described above, most neurosurgeons prefer to wait at least 7 days for the resumption of aspirin therapy or 1–2 months for clopidogrel.

After restarting antithrombotic therapy, additional cranial imaging can be obtained after one to two doses of the medication to determine if a hemorrhagic event has occurred. If bleeding is identified, serial imaging should be performed until the bleed is stable to assess for progression/regression, as mentioned above. Surgical versus medical management with blood products is determined based on the extent and location of the bleed ± neurologic symptomatology. If no evidence of bleeding is observed, anticoagulant therapy can be continued. Additional imaging should be obtained if there is new onset of neurologic deficits or worsening of symptoms (i.e., headache). Imaging may also be obtained if anticoagulation becomes supratherapeutic and the patient is at substantial risk for hemorrhage that would necessitate immediate and complete interruption of therapy versus gradual dosing adjustment.

In the outpatient setting, gradual lowering of the pressure setting should be performed over time until maximum symptomatic improvement is achieved, without the onset of low pressure symptomatology [3].

Postoperative Complications

The most serious, and deadly, complication associated with antithrombotic therapy is intracranial hemorrhage, most commonly via ICH [49]. According to McGovern et al.'s study, symptomatic ICH was observed in 1.5 % of NPH patients who received a ventriculoperitoneal shunt; however, the effect of antithrombotic therapy was not assessed [50]. Importantly, however, the initial volume and duration of expansion is greater in anticoagulant-associated ICH compared to spontaneous ICH, with a corresponding mortality rate greater than 50 % [51]. Furthermore, warfarin therapy doubles the risk of fatal intracranial hemorrhage, with ICH causing approximately 90 % of permanent morbidity and mortality in patients with bleeding associated with anticoagulation [52, 53]. Likewise, the risk of ICH is increased with the use of aspirin therapy by approximately 40 % [49]. Combined use of warfarin and aspirin likely further increases the risk of hemorrhage than either therapy alone [54], and approximately 20 % of elderly adults are on a combined regimen of anticoagulant-antiplatelet therapy [55]. While newer anticoagulants are associated with a lower risk of intracranial hemorrhage compared to warfarin, as demonstrated by the RE-LY (i.e., dabigatran) [56], ROCKET-AF (i.e., rivaroxaban) [57], and ARISTOTLE (i.e., apixaban) trials [58], caution must be performed due to the lack of available reversal agents for these newer agents.

Common, delayed, postoperative complications after shunt surgery include shunt obstruction, infection, subdural hygroma or hematoma, and shunt migration [8, 9]. Surgical overdrainage of CSF via ventricular shunting, particularly in the upright position, increases the risk of subdural hygroma or hematoma. Overdrainage adversely affects surgical and postoperative clinical outcomes for NPH and, to a lesser degree, generic measures of health-related quality of life [59]. Subdural hematoma occurs after 2–17 % of shunt surgeries for the treatment of NPH [3, 43]. Khan et al. reported eight (5 %) cases of SDH requiring surgical evacuation after shunt placement in patients with iNPH; however, the effect of antithrombotic therapy was not assessed [60]. In their systematic review of the outcome after shunt surgery for iNPH, Toma et al. reported a 6.3 % (range 2–47 %) rate of subdural hematoma (SDH) or hygroma and an ICH or stroke rate of 0.4 % (range 0–18 %) [61]. The effect of antithrombotic therapy was not determined in these cases. Epidural hematoma after CSF shunting is much less common, and almost always develops within the first few hours after surgery; on the other hand, SDH may be either acute or delayed [62]. Similarly, anticoagulation-associated subarachnoid hemorrhage is rare, with Mattle et al. reporting only seven out of 76 cases (9.2 %) of intracranial hemorrhage over a 6-year period [63].

In our previous study of 15 anticoagulated NPH patients who underwent shunt surgery, two (13 %) patients experienced symptomatic, postoperative bleeding complications [3]. One patient, with comorbid cirrhotic hepatitis C, who received bridging therapy with IV UFH, experienced an SDH 13 days after shunt surgery. Subsequently, anticoagulation was stopped immediately until the INR and aPTT normalized, and the shunt was removed 2 days after cessation of anticoagulant therapy. Another patient developed a large abdominal subcutaneous hematoma 5 days after shunt surgery, and required surgical evacuation.

In a recent assessment of the risk of subdural hematoma (SDH) in 80 patients who underwent shunt surgery for NPH, 35 of whom were taking aspirin and 13 who were on combined anticoagulant-antiplatelet therapy, 11 (14 %) cases of symptomatic SDH occurred. All cases of SDH after shunt surgery arose in patients receiving aspirin or clopidogrel, with a hazard ratio of 12.8 (95 % CI 3.1–53) associated with aspirin use (Fig. 28.5). The authors concluded that clopidogrel may pose an even greater risk of postoperative subdural hematoma after shunt surgery [43]. In this study, the authors hypothesized that shunting in NPH patients increases the risk for the brain to collapse, resulting in increased susceptibility to SDH, particularly in patients receiving antiplatelet therapy (e.g., aspirin and/or clopidogrel). Mahaney et al. reported a slightly lower, but significant, rate of postoperative hemorrhage associated with shunt placement in patients on dual antiplatelet therapy with 325 mg acetylsalicylic acid daily and 75 mg clopidogrel daily ($P=0.0075$), with a total of four (10.8 %) cases of intracranial hemorrhage associated with dual antiplatelet therapy [64]. Of note, dual antiplatelet therapy was not stopped prior to shunt placement in any of the patients in their study [64].

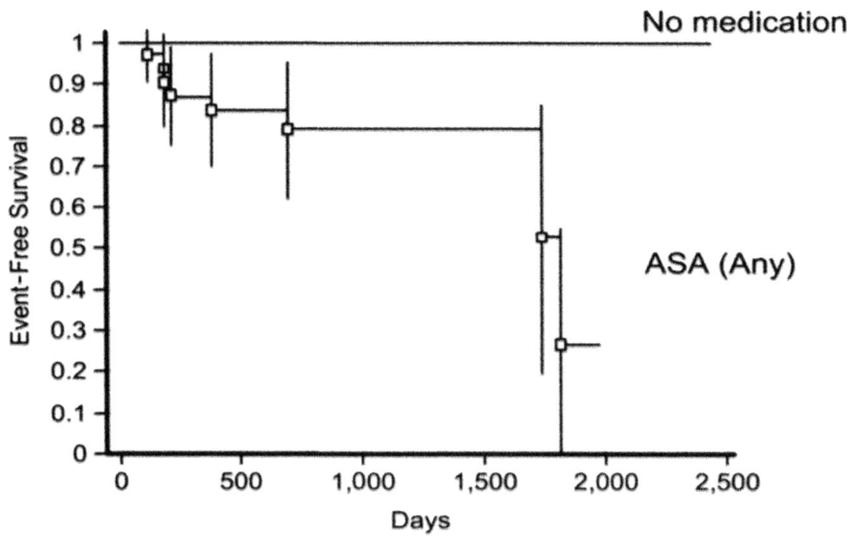

Fig. 28.5 Kaplan-Meier plot of event-free survival in patients on aspirin therapy. Courtesy of Birkeland P, Lauritsen J, Poulsen FR. Aspirin is associated with an increased risk of subdural hematoma in normal-pressure hydrocephalus patients following shunt implantation. J Neurosurg. 2015;123:423–6

Conclusions

Ultimately, patients on long-term antithrombotic therapy can be safely and effectively evaluated and treated for NPH, with the use of appropriate perioperative and postoperative management. While the overall risk of bleeding associated with shunt placement is low, NPH patients receiving antithrombotic therapy are at a significantly increased risk of hemorrhagic complication compared to patients who are not on antithrombotic therapy. Given the advanced age, gait impairment, and dementia associated with NPH, the bleeding and thrombotic risk may be even higher in NPH than the general population receiving antithrombotic therapy. Therefore, consultation with a hematologist and/or cardiologist is warranted in order to determine which patients can safely suspend antithrombotic therapy prior to surgery versus those who require bridging. Operative considerations that can reduce the risk of hemorrhagic complication include incision of the pia mater prior to ventricular catheter insertion, potential use of intraoperative imaging guidance, and placement of and adjustable and gravity-assisted shunt valve to lower the risk of overdrainage. In the outpatient setting, gradual lowering of the pressure setting should be performed over time until a balance is reached between maximum symptomatic improvement and the onset of symptoms suggestive of low intracranial pressure (e.g., orthostatic headache and dizziness). Postoperatively, the time to resumption of antithrombotic therapy depends on the patients' individual risk of thrombosis and bleeding as well as radiographic evaluation for intracranial hemorrhage.

References

1. Adams RD, Fisher CM, Hakim S, Ojemann RG, Sweet WH. Symptomatic occult hydrocephalus with "normal" cerebrospinal-fluid pressure. A treatable syndrome. N Engl J Med. 1965;273:117–26.
2. Hakim S, Adams RD. The special clinical problem of symptomatic hydrocephalus with normal cerebrospinal fluid pressure. Observations on cerebrospinal fluid hydrodynamics. J Neurol Sci. 1965;2(4):307–27.
3. Goodwin CR, Kharkar S, Wang P, Pujari S, Rigamonti D, Williams MA. Evaluation and treatment of patients with suspected normal pressure hydrocephalus on long-term warfarin anticoagulation therapy. Neurosurgery. 2007;60(3):497–501. discussion 502.
4. Black PM, Ojemann RG, Tzouras A. CSF shunts for dementia, incontinence, and gait disturbance. Clin Neurosurg. 1985;32:632–51.

5. Iseki C, Takahashi Y, Wada M, Kawanami T, Adachi M, Kato T. Incidence of idiopathic normal pressure hydrocephalus (iNPH): a 10-year follow-up study of a rural community in Japan. J Neurol Sci. 2014; 339(1–2):108–12.
6. Brean A, Eide PK. Prevalence of probable idiopathic normal pressure hydrocephalus in a Norwegian population. Acta Neurol Scand. 2008;118(1):48–53.
7. Jaraj D, Rabiei K, Marlow T, Jensen C, Skoog I, Wikkelsø C. Prevalence of idiopathic normal-pressure hydrocephalus. Neurology. 2014;82(16):1449–54.
8. Aoki N. Lumboperitoneal shunt: clinical applications, complications, and comparison with ventriculoperitoneal shunt. Neurosurgery. 1990;26(6):998–1003. discussion 1003–4.
9. Samuelson S, Long DM, Chou SN. Subdural hematoma as a complication of shunting procedures for normal pressure hydrocephalus. J Neurosurg. 1972;37(5):548–51.
10. Krauss JK, Regel JP, Vach W, Droste DW, Borremans JJ, Mergner T. Vascular risk factors and arteriosclerotic disease in idiopathic normal-pressure hydrocephalus of the elderly. Stroke. 1996;27(1):24–9.
11. Eide PK, Pripp AH. Increased prevalence of cardiovascular disease in idiopathic normal pressure hydrocephalus patients compared to a population-based cohort from the HUNT3 survey. Fluids Barriers CNS. 2014;11:19.
12. Hager KK, Loprinzi P, Stone D. Implementing diabetes care guidelines in long term care. J Am Med Dir Assoc. 2013;14(11):851.e7–15.
13. Bergsneider M, Black PM, Klinge P, Marmarou A, Relkin N. Surgical management of idiopathic normal-pressure hydrocephalus. Neurosurgery. 2005;57(3 Suppl):S29–39. discussion ii–v.
14. Poca MA, Mataró M, Del Mar Matarín M, Arikan F, Junqué C, Sahuquillo J. Is the placement of shunts in patients with idiopathic normal-pressure hydrocephalus worth the risk? Results of a study based on continuous monitoring of intracranial pressure. J Neurosurg. 2004;100(5):855–66.
15. Pfisterer WK, Aboul-Enein F, Gebhart E, Graf M, Aichholzer M, Mühlbauer M. Continuous intraventricular pressure monitoring for diagnosis of normal-pressure hydrocephalus. Acta Neurochir (Wien). 2007;149(10):983–90. discussion 990.
16. Koskinen LO, Grayson D, Olivecrona M. The complications and the position of the Codman MicroSensor™ ICP device: an analysis of 549 patients and 650 sensors. Acta Neurochir (Wien). 2013;155(11):2141–8. discussion 2148.
17. Kakarla UK, Kim LJ, Chang SW, Theodore N, Spetzler RF. Safety and accuracy of bedside external ventricular drain placement. Neurosurgery. 2008;63(1 Suppl 1):ONS162–6; discussion ONS166–7.
18. Pitkänen M, Fürster J. Complications caused by lumbar puncture. Duodecim. 2014;130(18):1834–42.
19. Fisher CM. Hydrocephalus as a cause of disturbances of gait in the elderly. Neurology. 1982;32(12): 1358–63.
20. Feick D, Sickmond J, Liu L, et al. Sensitivity and predictive value of occupational and physical therapy assessments in the functional evaluation of patients with suspected normal pressure hydrocephalus. J Rehabil Med. 2008;40(9):715–20.
21. Vos PE, de Boer WA, Wurzer JA, van Gijn J. Subdural hematoma after lumbar puncture: two case reports and review of the literature. Clin Neurol Neurosurg. 1991;93(2):127–32.
22. Hillemacher T, Bleich S, Wiltfang J, Weber M, Kornhuber J, Frieling H. Should aspirin be discontinued for diagnostic lumbar puncture? J Am Geriatr Soc. 2006;54(1):181–2.
23. Samdani A, Garonzik IM, Zahos P. Subdural hematoma after diagnostic lumbar puncture. Am J Emerg Med. 2004;22(4):316–7.
24. Paal P, Putz G, Gruber E, Le GT, Lemberger P. Subarachnoid hemorrhage after lumbar puncture in a patient receiving aspirin and clopidogrel. Anesth Analg. 2006;102(2):644–5.
25. Berger JS, Roncaglioni MC, Avanzini F, Pangrazzi I, Tognoni G, Brown DL. Aspirin for the primary prevention of cardiovascular events in women and men: a sex-specific meta-analysis of randomized controlled trials. JAMA. 2006;295(3):306–13.
26. Eide PK, Sorteberg W. Diagnostic intracranial pressure monitoring and surgical management in idiopathic normal pressure hydrocephalus: a 6-year review of 214 patients. Neurosurgery. 2010;66(1): 80–91.
27. Scheller C, Rachinger J, Strauss C, Alfieri A, Prell J, Koman G. Therapeutic anticoagulation after craniotomies: is the risk for secondary hemorrhage overestimated? J Neurol Surg A Cent Eur Neurosurg. 2014;75(1):2–6.
28. Rachinger JC, Koman G, Scheller C, Prell J, Rampp S, Strauss C. Practice in the perioperative prevention of deep vein thrombosis in German neurosurgical departments: is there a trend towards homogenization? Cent Eur Neurosurg. 2011;72(3):115–9.
29. Zakaryan A. Perioperative management of neurosurgical patients receiving chronic anticoagulation therapy. Front Pharmacol. 2014;5:64.
30. Thachil J, Gatt A, Martlew V. Management of surgical patients receiving anticoagulation and antiplatelet agents. Br J Surg. 2008;95(12):1437–48.
31. Baron TH, Kamath PS, McBane RD. Management of antithrombotic therapy in patients undergoing invasive procedures. N Engl J Med. 2013;368(22): 2113–24.
32. Hamilton MG, Hull RD, Pineo GF. Venous thromboembolism in neurosurgery and neurology patients: a review. Neurosurgery. 1994;34(2):280–96. discussion 296.
33. Schanbacher CF, Bennett RG. Postoperative stroke after stopping warfarin for cutaneous surgery. Dermatol Surg. 2000;26(8):785–9.
34. Lecompte TP. Antithrombotic agents and invasive procedures—hematologist point of view. Thromb Res. 2012;130 Suppl 1:S61–2.

35. Kearon C, Hirsh J. Management of anticoagulation before and after elective surgery. N Engl J Med. 1997;336(21):1506–11.
36. Laohaprasit V, Mayberg MR. Risks of anticoagulation therapy after experimental corticectomy in the rat. Neurosurgery. 1993;32(4):625–8. discussion 628–9.
37. Schaible KL, Smith LJ, Fessler RG, Rachlin JR, Brown FD, Mullan S. Evaluation of the risks of anticoagulation therapy following experimental craniotomy in the rat. J Neurosurg. 1985;63(6):959–62.
38. Grant PJ, Brotman DJ, Jaffer AK. Perioperative anticoagulant management. Anesthesiol Clin. 2009;27(4): 761–77.
39. Douketis JD. Perioperative anticoagulation management in patients who are receiving oral anticoagulant therapy: a practical guide for clinicians. Thromb Res. 2002;108(1):3–13.
40. Gleason LJ, Friedman SM. Preoperative management of anticoagulation and antiplatelet agents. Clin Geriatr Med. 2014;30(2):219–27.
41. Lazio BE, Simard JM. Anticoagulation in neurosurgical patients. Neurosurgery. 1999;45(4):838–47. discussion 847–8.
42. Douketis JD, Spyropoulos AC, Spencer FA, et al. Perioperative management of antithrombotic therapy: Antithrombotic therapy and prevention of thrombosis, 9th ed: American College of Chest Physicians Evidence-Based Clinical Practice Guidelines. Chest. 2012;141(2 Suppl):e326S–50.
43. Birkeland P, Lauritsen J, Poulsen FR. Aspirin is associated with an increased risk of subdural hematoma in normal-pressure hydrocephalus patients following shunt implantation. J Neurosurg. 2015;123:423–6.
44. Kim YB, Lee JW, Lee KS, Lee KC. Image-guided placement of ventricular shunt catheter. J Clin Neurosci. 2006;13(1):50–4.
45. Jakola AS, Reinertsen I, Selbekk T, et al. Three-dimensional ultrasound-guided placement of ventricular catheters. World Neurosurg. 2014;82(3–4): 536.e5–9.
46. Freimann FB, Vajkoczy P, Sprung C. Patients benefit from low-pressure settings enabled by gravitational valves in normal pressure hydrocephalus. Clin Neurol Neurosurg. 2013;115(10):1982–6.
47. Boon AJ, Tans JT, Delwel EJ, et al. Dutch Normal-Pressure Hydrocephalus Study: randomized comparison of low- and medium-pressure shunts. J Neurosurg. 1998;88(3):490–5.
48. Sæhle T, Farahmand D, Eide PK, Tisell M, Wikkelsö C. A randomized controlled dual-center trial on shunt complications in idiopathic normal-pressure hydrocephalus treated with gradually reduced or "fixed" pressure valve settings. J Neurosurg. 2014;121(5): 1257–63.
49. Connolly BJ, Pearce LA, Kurth T, Kase CS, Hart RG. Aspirin therapy and risk of subdural hematoma: meta-analysis of randomized clinical trials. J Stroke Cerebrovasc Dis. 2013;22(4):444–8.
50. McGovern RA, Kelly KM, Chan AK, Morrissey NJ, McKhann GM. Should ventriculoatrial shunting be the procedure of choice for normal-pressure hydrocephalus? J Neurosurg. 2014;120(6):1458–64.
51. El Ahmadieh TY, Aoun SG, Daou MR, et al. New-generation oral anticoagulants for the prevention of stroke: implications for neurosurgery. J Clin Neurosci. 2013;20(10):1350–6.
52. Fang MC, Go AS, Chang Y, et al. Death and disability from warfarin-associated intracranial and extracranial hemorrhages. Am J Med. 2007;120(8):700–5.
53. Rosand J, Eckman MH, Knudsen KA, Singer DE, Greenberg SM. The effect of warfarin and intensity of anticoagulation on outcome of intracerebral hemorrhage. Arch Intern Med. 2004;164(8):880–4.
54. Hart RG, Benavente O, Pearce LA. Increased risk of intracranial hemorrhage when aspirin is combined with warfarin: a meta-analysis and hypothesis. Cerebrovasc Dis. 1999;9(4):215–7.
55. Shireman TI, Howard PA, Kresowik TF, Ellerbeck EF. Combined anticoagulant-antiplatelet use and major bleeding events in elderly atrial fibrillation patients. Stroke. 2004;35(10):2362–7.
56. Connolly SJ, Ezekowitz MD, Yusuf S, et al. Dabigatran versus warfarin in patients with atrial fibrillation. N Engl J Med. 2009;361(12):1139–51.
57. Patel MR, Mahaffey KW, Garg J, et al. Rivaroxaban versus warfarin in nonvalvular atrial fibrillation. N Engl J Med. 2011;365(10):883–91.
58. Granger CB, Alexander JH, McMurray JJ, et al. Apixaban versus warfarin in patients with atrial fibrillation. N Engl J Med. 2011;365(11):981–92.
59. Meier U, Stengel D, Müller C, et al. Predictors of subsequent overdrainage and clinical outcomes after ventriculoperitoneal shunting for idiopathic normal pressure hydrocephalus. Neurosurgery. 2013;73(6):1054–60.
60. Khan QU, Wharen RE, Grewal SS, et al. Overdrainage shunt complications in idiopathic normal-pressure hydrocephalus and lumbar puncture opening pressure. J Neurosurg. 2013;119(6):1498–502.
61. Toma AK, Papadopoulos MC, Stapleton S, Kitchen ND, Watkins LD. Systematic review of the outcome of shunt surgery in idiopathic normal-pressure hydrocephalus. Acta Neurochir (Wien). 2013;155(10): 1977–80.
62. Driesen W, Elies W. Epidural and subdural haematomas as a complication of internal drainage of cerebrospinal fluid in hydrocephalus. Acta Neurochir (Wien). 1974;30(1–2):85–93.
63. Mattle H, Kohler S, Huber P, Rohner M, Steinsiepe KF. Anticoagulation-related intracranial extracerebral haemorrhage. J Neurol Neurosurg Psychiatry. 1989;52(7):829–37.
64. Mahaney KB, Chalouhi N, Viljoen S, et al. Risk of hemorrhagic complication associated with ventriculoperitoneal shunt placement in aneurysmal subarachnoid hemorrhage patients on dual antiplatelet therapy. J Neurosurg. 2013;119(4):937–42.

Surgical Hemostasis in the Era of Anticoagulation: Guidelines and Recommendations Summary

29

Drew A. Spencer, Paul D. Ackerman, Omer Iqbal, and Christopher M. Loftus

Introduction

An aging population and improved management of chronic conditions are at the crux of an issue confronting all surgeons—the increasing use of anticoagulation in older patients more likely to harbor surgical pathology and more susceptible to even trivial trauma when compared to younger cohorts. Cardiac, vascular, and prothrombotic conditions are the primary indications for antiplatelet or anticoagulant therapy, with the specific indications continually expanding. Furthermore, inconveniences and failures in past experience with these agents drives discovery and utilization of new agents, often before a reliable inhibitor or reversal agent exists [1–3]. The inherent risk in this situation is magnified further in neurosurgery due to the complex, unforgiving system involved.

The aging and elderly are uniquely susceptible to devastating complications related to antiplatelet and anticoagulant agents. This population boasts the highest age-specific incidence of traumatic brain injury (TBI), and accounts for 25 % of all trauma-related deaths. Mortality is likely affected in elderly TBI patients on both antiplatelet and anticoagulant agents pre-injury, with a glaring lack of conclusive evidence [4–8]. The deficiency in high-level evidence extends beyond trauma, applying to emergent and elective surgical conditions and in any age group. Overall, current trauma and perioperative practices are largely based on the summation of observational and small cohort studies, with no regimen providing a clear survival benefit [9, 10]. High-level evidence is both lacking and near impossible to obtain, as most properly designed trials would deprive a group of patients of the best currently available care.

The management of trauma and surgical patients on antiplatelet and anticoagulant medications is therefore largely an empirical process. Guidelines regarding reversal are followed without strong evidence of their efficacy in many cases because the risk of proof of principal studies is unrealistic and unacceptable. As such, clinicians must rely on both their knowledge of currently used agents and case-by-case clinical judgment with the goal of successful surgical intervention without hemorrhagic or thrombotic complications. By continuing to track and share not only our successes, but those cases that escape even the most detailed plan, this evidentiary hurdle becomes less significant and patients gain access to care not previously thought possible. Below we will review the available medications and current recommendations for their utilization in neurosurgical patients.

D.A. Spencer • P.D. Ackerman • C.M. Loftus (✉)
Department of Neurosurgery, Loyola University Medical Center
e-mail: cloftus@lumc.edu

O. Iqbal
Department of Pathology, Loyola University Medical Center

C.M. Loftus (ed.), *Anticoagulation and Hemostasis in Neurosurgery*,
DOI 10.1007/978-3-319-27327-3_29

Classes and Mechanisms of Medications Affecting Blood Clotting

The volume of antiplatelet and anticoagulant agents in clinical use continues to expand as we continually seek medications that enact a specific inhibition that is reliable, reversible, and carries a low risk of hemorrhagic complications. Neurosurgeons, while far from the primary prescribers of these agents, must maintain robust knowledge of their indications, mechanisms, and antidotes to safely treat patients in the face of this challenge. It is prudent then to begin with a review of the current classes of agents, indications for their use, and how to negate the therapeutic effect when necessary (Tables 29.1 and 29.2).

Antiplatelet Agents

Antiplatelet agents fall into three main classes—cyclo-oxygenase-1 (COX-1) inhibitors, adenosine diphosphate (ADP) receptor inhibitors, and glycoprotein (GP) IIb/IIIa receptor inhibitors. COX-1 inhibitors, with aspirin as the primary example, irreversibly inhibit the COX-1 enzyme and stop the production of thromboxanes from arachidonic acid—preventing platelet activation, aggregation, and degranulation. Clopidogrel and its homologues inhibit the $P2Y_{12}$ or ADP receptors on the platelet surface. The activated receptor binds fibrin and participates in platelet cross-linking to form a preliminary plug at sites of bleeding. The GPIIb/IIIa inhibitors prevent platelet aggregation by blocking receptor interaction with von Willebrand Factor (vWF) and fibrinogen (Fig. 29.1). Antiplatelet agents target the inciting event in overall clot formation, platelet activation, and plug formation on exposure to damaged tissues. Based on the moieties they interact with (vWF, fibrinogen, etc.), they also have downstream effects on the entire clotting cascade. Both pathways must be considered carefully when deciding on an appropriate reversal strategy, which is discussed later in the chapter.

Anticoagulant Agents

Warfarin, first introduced in 1954, is the most widely known and used anticoagulant in clinical practice. Warfarin inhibits the vitamin K-mediated carboxylation of coagulation factors II, VII, IX, and X (Fig. 29.2). While it effectively regulates blood clotting, warfarin is a labor-intensive medication both for the patient and the physician. Patients are subjected to dietary restraints, activity restrictions, and frequent blood draws for International Normalized Ratio (INR) monitoring. Physicians must consider patient risks, make frequent changes to dosing regimens, and consider other health needs including surgical procedures. Reversal can require days and multiple rounds of fresh frozen plasma (FFP), in a patient population with prevalent cardiac comorbidity [11, 12].

Table 29.1 Classes and mechanisms of currently used antiplatelet agents

Name	Mechanism	Indications
Aspirin	Irreversible COX-1 inhibitor	Cardiac risk factors, PCI
Clopidogrel	P2Y12, ADP receptor inhibitor	MI/stroke prevention, PAD, MI, PCI
Prasugrel	P2Y12, ADP receptor inhibitor	NSTEMI
Ticlopidine	P2Y12, ADP receptor inhibitor	MI/stroke prevention, aspirin intolerance
Ticagrelor	P2Y12, ADP receptor inhibitor	MI/stroke prevention, ACS
Abciximab	Glycoprotein IIb/IIIa receptor antagonist	PCI, diabetes
Eptifibatide	Glycoprotein IIb/IIIa receptor antagonist	Unstable angina, NSTEMI, PCI
Tirofiban	Glycoprotein IIb/IIIa receptor antagonist	Cardiac risk factors, NSTEMI

COX-1 cyclo-oxygenase-1, *ADP* adenosine diphosphate, *PCI* percutaneous coronary intervention, *PAD* peripheral arterial disease, *MI* myocardial infarction, *NSTEMI* non-ST elevation myocardial infarction, *ACS* acute coronary syndrome

Table 29.2 Classes and mechanisms of currently used anticoagulant agents

Name	Mechanism	Indications	Reversal
Warfarin	Vitamin K antagonist	VTE, PE, Afib, mechanical heart valve	First line: Vitamin K, FFP *Can use Factor VIIa, PCC, FEIBA
UFH	Anti-thrombin III activation	ACS, Afib, VTE prophylaxis, DVT/PE, cardiopulmonary bypass, hemodialysis	Protamine sulfate
LMWH	Factor Xa inhibitor	VTE prophylaxis, DVT/PE	Protamine sulfate, FFP
Dabigatran	Direct thrombin inhibitor	NV-Afib, DVT/PE	Factor VIIa, PCC, FEIBA with FFP
Rivaroxaban	Factor Xa inhibitor	NV-Afib, VTE prophylaxis	Factor VIIa, PCC, FEIBA with FFP
Apixaban	Factor Xa inhibitor	NV-Afib, VTE prophylaxis, DVT/PE	Factor VIIa, PCC, FEIBA with FFP
Edoxaban	Factor Xa inhibitor	NV-Afib, DVT/PE	Factor VIIa, PCC, FEIBA with FFP
Fondaparinux	Factor Xa inhibitor	VTE prophylaxis, DVT/PE	Factor VIIa, PCC, FEIBA with FFP

VTE venous thrombo-embolism, *PE* pulmonary embolism, *Afib* atrial fibrillation, *FFP* fresh frozen plasma, *PCC* prothrombin complex concentrate, *FEIBA* factor eight inhibitor bypass activity, *UFH* unfractionated heparin, *ACS* acute coronary syndrome, *DVT* deep venous thrombosis, *LMWH* low molecular weight heparin, *NV-Afib* non-valvular atrial fibrillation

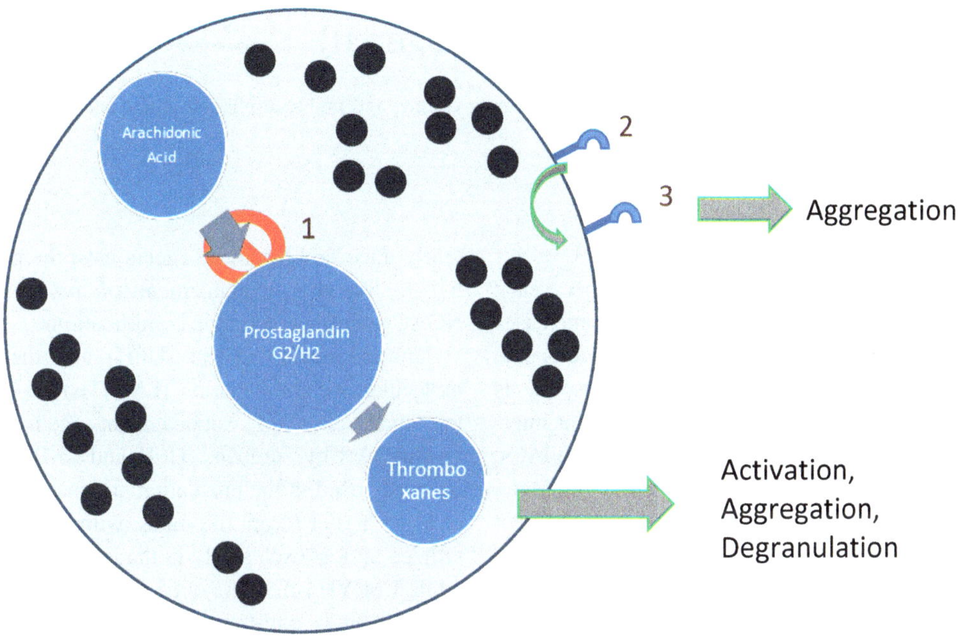

Fig. 29.1 Platelet structure including the receptors and pathways required for activation and normal function, as well as the points of inhibition by current antiplatelet agents

The drawbacks of warfarin have prompted the development of a newer class of drugs, referred to as the Novel Oral Anticoagulants (NOACs). These medications are direct inhibitors of either activated Factor X (Xa) (rivaroxaban, apixaban, and edoxaban) or thrombin (dabigatran). This class is attractive for its relatively short half-life and reliable anticoagulant effect, enabling a quick and reliable onset of action while obviating the need for stringent monitoring [13]. More importantly, patients taking NOACs are increasingly believed to have a lower bleeding risk than

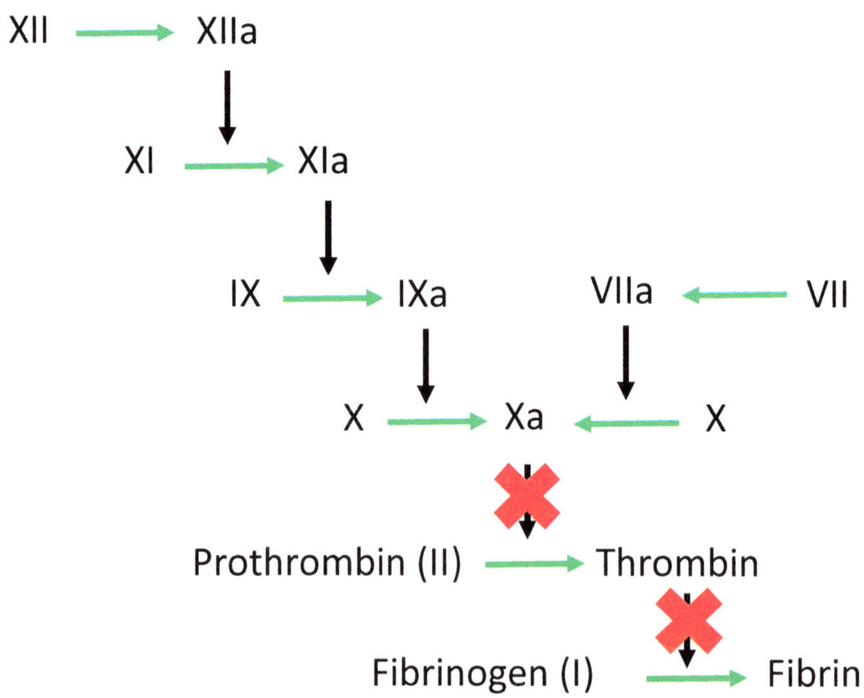

Fig. 29.2 Schematic representation of the normal clotting cascade and points of pharmacologic interruption from currently available agents

those on warfarin (major bleeding 2–3 % per year, intracranial hemorrhage 0.2 % per year), though this data is incomplete and in some cases contradictory [14–16]. The short half-life is also advantageous when rapid return to baseline is required in the case of elective and urgent interventions. The primary limitation of the NOACs, however, is that there is no specific antidote. These agents therefore present a management conundrum in emergent surgical conditions, as reversal is still a process driven by case reports and small cohort experiences [2, 11, 12, 17, 18]. This has prompted the development of some promising new options that are currently progressing toward clinical relevance. Recently discovered antibodies (Idarucizumab (Boehringer Ingelheim®) to reverse dabigatran) and synthetic proteins (andexanet alfa (Portola®) to reverse rivaroxaban, apixaban, edoxaban) have reached advanced phases of clinical development to evaluate their efficacy in reversal of these NOACs [2, 19–21]. Their ultimate role is currently uncertain but these agents have the potential to simplify management of patients on NOACs with hemorrhagic complications.

Unfractionated heparin (UFH) and the low molecular weight heparins (LMWHs) represent the final class of anticoagulant medications encountered by surgeons. UFH and LMWH are primarily used in the prevention and management of acute and/or recent thrombus, with UFH being utilized almost exclusively in the inpatient setting while LMWH offers the option of outpatient use. Heparin binds anti-thrombin III (AT) and augments its activity 1000-fold, effectively catalyzing the inactivation of thrombin and other factors, most notably activated factor X. The LMWHs more directly target activated factor X and less so factor II, with a more predictable effect and less requirement for laboratory monitoring. Heparin-induced thrombocytopenia (HIT) is a potential complication with use of either, though less so with the LMWHs. The only known agent for prompt reversal is protamine sulfate, while Fresh

Frozen Plasma (FFP) has a controversial role if any in this situation [2]. The most recently introduced agent in this class is fondaparinux, a pentasaccharide that binds and activates AT to inhibit the function of factor Xa. Fondaparinux is approved for use mainly in VTE prevention, though this requires caution as there is not currently a definitive reversal agent—with studies utilizing factor VIIa showing only incomplete inactivation [22].

According to current best estimates, the proportion of the population on either antiplatelet (~30 %) or anticoagulant (~3 %) medications is striking and likely to increase [3, 12, 23]. This number in no way accounts for those patients on both medications, a population especially susceptible to hemorrhagic complications in the face of existing comorbidity [14]. Neurosurgeons will continue to be confronted with this issue and will benefit from at least a framework understanding of the mechanisms of these agents.

Emergency Reversal of Antiplatelet and Anticoagulant Agents

Antiplatelet Reversal

Patients with acute, operative pathology frequently require the emergent reversal of antiplatelet agents. Traumatic and other intracranial hemorrhages not requiring an operation are also a relative indication for reversal, with some authors advocating for reversal in all cases [5, 17, 24, 25]. This too remains a point of debate among clinicians though, as some trauma literature opposes platelet transfusion [26]. The only approved mode of reversal when necessary is to transfuse platelets, as most of these agents are irreversible [27]. In high-risk cases, such as expanding intracranial hemorrhage, other adjuncts are sometimes necessary. Concurrent administration of platelets and 0.3 μg/kg DDAVP (1-desamino-8-D-arginine vasopressin) can be used in this case to achieve maximal platelet activation [24, 28]. Some advocate for continued platelet transfusions every 12 h for the first 48 h after the inciting event until physiologic turnover of the platelet pool has occurred [2, 24].

Anticoagulation Reversal

While there are very few established guidelines for the reversal of anticoagulant agents, the available options provide clinicians the luxury of tailoring a regimen to the patient and situation. For years the lone options in anticoagulant reversal were vitamin K administration and replenishing functional coagulation factors via transfusion of FFP. Physicians and surgeons now have multiple options, among them low-volume and specific agents tailored for the precise clotting deficiency created pharmacologically. An additional benefit is that newer reversal agents can near instantaneously overcome the anticoagulant effect, allowing for more timely intervention and improving the potential for better surgical outcomes. These newer agents can and often should be used in conjunction with FFP. The activated factors require an intact pathway of clotting factors with a therefore synergistic effect in restoring coagulant homeostasis [2].

FFP is the oldest reversal agent, in clinical use for nearly 40 years now, and that with which clinicians likely have the most experience. FFP is particularly rich in clotting factors II, V, VII, IX, X, and XI. It is more effective in replacing these factors and overcoming the effects of warfarin and factor X inhibitors than in bleeding due to factor VIII deficiency [29]. Individual factors also have different sensitivities, or minimum levels present for effective clotting [2, 12]. This can account for excessive transfusion volumes needed to reverse a coagulopathy, complicating patient management in those with cardiac comorbidities or multisystem injury after trauma. FFP will continue to be useful in the emergent reversal of coagulopathy, both alone and as complementary therapy to the newer agents that have been introduced recently.

The newer agents available for quick correction of deficiencies in coagulation aim to reconstitute the activated factors at crucial points in the clotting cascade. Activated factor VII restores the catalyst necessary to drive activation of factors V and X, with resultant completion of the clotting cascade. It has a short onset of action but requires concomitant administration of FFP [2, 12, 18]. Prothrombin complex concentrates (PCC) are targeted reversal agents comprised mainly of concentrated factors II, IX, and X with variable amounts of activated factor VII [2, 12, 18]. Standard PCC has a wide spectrum of urgent and emergent applications, while derivatives with high concentrations of activated factor VII (KCentra, CSL Behring, King of Prussia, PA) are most useful in emergent scenarios [10, 14]. Clinical studies have shown these agents to have a reversal time over four times faster than that of FFP, though laboratory monitoring of reversal and the duration of their effect have not been definitively determined. There is likely some variation based on the individual clinical scenario including the agent being reversed. Factor Eight Inhibitor Bypassing Activity (FEIBA) is the final relatively novel agent to be discussed, and it consists of factors II, IX, X (mainly nonactivated), and VIIa (mainly activated) in addition to 1–6 units of FVIII coagulation antigen (FVIIIC:Ag) per ml. Each one of the agents listed above has the advantage of providing concentrated factors, in amounts sufficient to re-establish normal factor function in the clotting cascade. Activated Factor VII, KCentra, PCC, and FEIBA are undoubtedly useful tools in emergent surgical conditions, but much remains to be discovered about their duration of action and how best to supplement their effect until physiologic coagulation parameters are re-established. Concomitant administration of FFP is frequently used and recommended to replenish all clotting factors and avoid a consumptive complication or limitation in reversal [12]. All patients undergoing anticoagulant reversal have a tangible, if undefined, increase in risk of thrombosis in the postoperative period as well [12].

Familiarity with the available agents allows for the concoction of a reasonable and relatively evidence-based reversal plan in nearly all patients encountered, with the understanding that treating physicians must have the flexibility to adjust the plan. *For patients on warfarin*, Vitamin K should be administered in almost all cases as it aids in relatively rapid reversal of INR, within 12–16 h [2]. Intravenous administration is preferred in urgent and emergent cases while oral dosing is acceptable in less critical situations. FFP remains a first-line option for relatively rapid reversal, though factor VIIa and PCCs are increasingly used for more rapid correction and intervention [3, 30]. All patients require careful clinical and laboratory monitoring of hemostasis postoperatively, frequently requiring continued therapy until the aPTT and INR are consistently in the normal range. *Patients on NOACs* represent a less tangible target without clear guidelines in the emergent setting. Many have shared their experience with factor VIIa and PCCs allowing early intervention with a low incidence of hemorrhagic complications [3, 14]. FFP can and often should be co-administered at the discretion of the provider. Ultimately however, case-by-case variation is likely in regard to doses administered and duration of reversal therapy. Just as the direct action of NOACs negates the need for outpatient laboratory monitoring, it has so far escaped objective measures to inform clinicians when a coagulopathy no longer exists.

Reversal of Antiplatelet and Anticoagulant Agents for Elective Surgery

The reversal of antiplatelet and anticoagulant agents for elective surgical procedures is a more methodical, carefully planned process, though not one without inherent risk and the potential for serious complications. Even so, the current risk of both hemorrhagic and thrombotic complications is low, and good outcomes are possible with proper patient selection and judicious resumption of therapy postoperatively.

The safe reversal of antiplatelet agents rarely requires more than holding medication for 5 days preoperatively, enough time for the production of a sufficient pool of functional platelets [2]. *Vitamin K antagonists are also typically held for 5 days pre-op.* At this time point, clinical studies have supported the finding that over 90 % of patients starting at an INR 2.0–3.0 will have an INR under 1.4 [2, 11]. An additional consideration, however and especially with warfarin, is the variability in pharmacokinetics. Diverse factors, including hepatic impairment, medication noncompliance, and dietary changes, can significantly alter metabolism and factor production, necessitating pre-op confirmation of INR. The NOACs, though most difficult in the emergent setting, all have relatively short half-lives and are largely reliable for elective reversal. Renal function is the only major comorbidity to significantly affect clearance. In healthy individuals with a creatinine clearance >50, the clotting cascade returns to normal within 1–2 days. When creatinine clearance is <50, a coagulopathic state can persist for up to 5 days [2, 11, 13].

The general clinical practices described here represent the safest guidelines based on the collaborative efforts of those publishing their experience [1, 2, 17, 24, 25, 31]. The fact remains that high-level clinical studies are lacking, and clinical equipoise likely prevents its pursuit. Clinical judgment plays a still prominent role in deciding what is best for the patient. Avoidance of complications is twofold: simultaneously minimizing both hemorrhagic and thrombotic complications. The latter is as much about pre-op management as it is about prompt and judicious resumption post-op. The schedule for restarting antiplatelet and anticoagulant agents post-op is again one lacking a clear, evidence-based and universal procedure. The current best practice guidelines will be discussed subsequently after current procedures for perioperative bridging of therapy.

Perioperative Bridging of Anticoagulation

In a number of conditions, the risk of thromboembolic events precludes full anticoagulant reversal for more than the immediate perioperative period [32, 33]. This category includes conditions such as mechanical heart valve (mitral = highest risk), A-fib with a $CHADS_2$ score ≥3, VTE within 6 months, VTE with severe thrombophilia, lupus, and anti-thrombin III deficiency. The latter two conditions only meet this requirement when the patient is on anticoagulation therapy prior to the operation. These patients carry a high (10–20 %) risk of thromboembolic events compared to their age-matched counterparts [34]. In emergency scenarios, the risk of devastating insult trumps the possibility of embolic sequelae. However, when considering these patients for elective operations, careful assessment of their risks and the required bridging plan is a detailed endeavor that often requires multidisciplinary collaboration. The first step in this process is to assess whether the operation is imperative. Depending on age and chronicity, VTE may not require lifelong anticoagulation, which advocates for delayed surgery. Similarly, a patient's $CHADS_2$ score may be a fluid entity based on medical and other interventions. Mechanical heart valves and biochemical anomalies, however, are permanent indications for anticoagulation and the potential benefit of surgery must clearly outweigh the potential for complications.

When surgery is deemed necessary, planning and executing an effective bridging plan requires a detailed assessment of a patient's risk of hemorrhage. Despite even the best planning, this patient population carries a significant risk of hemorrhagic complications regardless of whether a bridge is used (5.0 % vs 1.3 %) [34]. *Current opinion holds that patients in all risk groups should stop warfarin 5 days prior to the operation* [32, 33]. *Patients with a low risk of hemorrhage can begin bridging therapy with UFH or LMWH 36 h after the last dose of warfarin. High-risk patients should be kept off of all medications for 48–72 h before starting a similar bridge. Each group receives the last infusion 6 h before surgery, and a half dose is recommended for patients on LMWH.* The preferred bridging agent has long been UFH, though recently LMWH is gaining in popularity due to convenience and decreased overall cost. LMWH can be used safely in the outpatient setting, benefitting patients and providers [33]. When a proper bridge is followed, the rate of perioperative hemorrhage is 5 % or lower [34]. These patients warrant an aggressive nonpharmacologic approach during the anticoagulation holiday period, utilizing all the available clinical options—early ambulation, compression stockings, and sequential compression devices (SCDs).

Postoperative Resumption of Antiplatelet and Anticoagulant Agents

To ensure optimal surgical outcomes, the timing of postoperative resumption of therapy is nearly as important as preoperative interruption of therapy. While there are no set protocols on how and when to reinstitute either antiplatelet or anticoagulant therapy, clinical experience provides some aid in decision-making.

Current practice at the authors' institution varies among providers and the type of operation, but *antiplatelet agents are rarely restarted prior to 5 days post-op*. Even in the context of literature on the topic of this chapter in general, reports and studies addressing antiplatelet resumption are sparse. In regard to neurosurgical, intimately invasive procedures, the risk prior to the fifth post-op day appears significant [35]. Conversely, Ahmed et al. found no significant differences in hemorrhagic or thrombotic complications in craniotomy patients who either stopped aspirin perioperatively or continued to take it up to and through the operation [36]. Another study found no increase in the risk of hemorrhage in transsphenoidal operations for sellar and parasellar lesions [37]. Pending much more study, the only reasonable recommendation is to wait 5 days postoperatively, or until the individual physician feels the risk is acceptable. Trauma represents a completely separate group of patients with no clear recommendation regarding antiplatelet therapy. Our current practice in cases of traumatic intracranial hemorrhage routinely involves holding therapy until outpatient follow-up with repeat imaging, except in rare cases where the thrombotic risk is deemed too great.

Re-instituting anticoagulant therapy differs fundamentally between two main groups: those able to tolerate a perioperative therapeutic holiday and those requiring a bridge. For patients not requiring a bridge, therapy is restarted at the treating physician's discretion. If it must be resumed while in the hospital, warfarin can be started as early as 24 h post-op, and INR monitoring can often be done as an outpatient. In less urgent cases, the prudent option is likely delaying re-institution of therapy until outpatient surgeon follow-up to minimize bleeding risk. When a patient requires bridging, many have shared their experiences and offer a relatively reliable plan of action [32, 33]. In low-risk patients, current recommendations are to restart warfarin 24 h post-op with a UFH or LMWH bridge. The advantage of LMWH is the aforementioned outpatient use without a need for laboratory monitoring, allowing for shorter hospital stays. In patients considered at high risk of hemorrhage, which likely involves a significant portion of neurosurgical patients, current practice is to restart warfarin 48–72 h post-op with a concurrent bridge beginning as soon as possible after surgery, typically at least 6 h post-op.

While appropriate timing of therapy is somewhat ambiguous, clinical experience is more abundant regarding *how to dose anticoagulants* [11, 32, 33, 38]. Traditionally, either the pre-op dose or a gradually escalating warfarin dose has been used until achieving a therapeutic INR. A recent study advocates an initial dose double the patient's maintenance dose, finding that an increased number of patients achieved a therapeutic INR at day 5 over those receiving their maintenance dose (50 % vs. 13 %) [38]. No increase in adverse events was noted despite the rapid increase in INR. When using the NOACs, current evidence supports initiation of the pre-op dose 24–72 h after surgery [13]. In extreme cases involving patients in both bridge and non-bridge situations, anticoagulation can be held for 1–4 weeks post-op, provided the physician and the patient have an open understanding of the inherent thrombotic risk.

DVT Screening and Prophylaxis

Recently developed, standardized assessment tools have improved clinicians' ability to stratify patients' DVT risk and institute appropriate prophylaxis [39]. While the initial patient assessment is still reliant on subjective, patient-initiated information, reliable algorithms are in place to correctly assign importance to all clinical factors. Extremity swelling and pain, as well as dyspnea, tachycardia, tachypnea, or pleuritic pain should always raise suspicion. Symptoms combined with the Wells score [40], a reliable clinical assessment tool introduced in the early 2000s, and in some cases a d-dimer level have proven effective in determining which patients warrant radiologic confirmation of a pathologic thrombosis [40–42]. D-dimer testing alone, and more so in combination with the Wells score, has a high negative predictive value and reliably identifies patients who should undergo further testing. Compression Doppler ultrasound is the gold standard exam for DVT. CT angiogram of the chest is the current standard for PE, with ventilation/perfusion radionuclide scanning as an adjunct when the test is inconclusive or unavailable.

In 2012, the American College of Chest physicians published another clinical tool, the Caprini assessment, the score of which assists in instituting appropriate DVT prophylaxis for each patient based on a litany of clinical factors [43]. Patients are stratified into four different risk groups—very low, low, moderate, and high—with specific prophylactic modalities for each. Patients with a score of 0 are at very low risk and only ambulation is recommended, with a VTE incidence of 0.5 %. A score of 1–2 is low risk, and prophylaxis utilizing ambulation and SCDs results in a VTE incidence of 1.5 %. Patients scoring 3–4 are in the moderate-risk group, for which ambulation, SCDs, and pharmacologic prophylaxis (UFH/LMWH) are recommended with VTE incidence at 3 %. Those patients in the high-risk group have a Caprini score 5 and over, and carry a VTE incidence of 6 %. Prophylaxis for these patients should include all of the above interventions, with compression stockings added as well. Neurosurgery patients are nearly universally considered to be in the high-risk group, with small numbers of patients falling into the low or moderate groups—those undergoing outpatient procedures or only requiring an overnight hospital stay.

Inferior Vena Cava (IVC) Filters

IVC filter placement has increased steadily in recent years likely due to an increase in trained providers and the expansion of relative indications. Standard indications for IVC filter placement include both acute proximal lower extremity DVT and/or PE, with a contraindication for anticoagulation—the most frequently cited reasons being recent surgery or a bleeding diathesis [44]. Other indications include recurrent VTE and VTE through anticoagulant therapy. Medication-related indications apply to patients who have an adverse reaction, are poorly compliant, or represent a fall risk. An expanding area of interest is in IVC filters placed as a prophylactic measure. Patients with a propensity for thrombosis involved in severe trauma (TBI, spinal cord injury, long bone and pelvic fractures) or otherwise expected to require a long course of immobilization have IVC filters placed with some regularity [44, 45]. Recent evaluations also show that up to 20–40 % of IVC filters are placed outside of clear indications, based on clinician judgment and preference [44].

Clinical decision-making is no longer limited to simply placing an IVC filter. Older patients as well as those with a relatively short life expectancy or a lifelong thrombotic risk can still receive the standard, permanent filter. The advent of retrievable IVC filters has provided an effective, nonpermanent option for patients with short-term, reversible conditions requiring PE prevention [46]. The window for removal is 3–18 months after placement, after which scar tissue, remodeling of the vessel wall, and degradation of the filter itself can make retrieval difficult or impossible. When done in the appropriate time period, these filters boast an 80–90 % successful retrieval rate [46]. Retrievable filters remain a topic of debate though, as the indications are open to provider interpretation and they pose a unique set of risks. Case reports additionally describe IVC injury and embolic migration of broken filter tines and hooks as devastating complications from an elective procedure [46]. Most retrievable filters have the versatility to be left permanently when necessary, though data is still being acquired regarding their long-term safety [45]. At the end of the day, there is no class I evidence or tested algorithm that decides who gets a permanent versus retrievable filter, and the involved providers are left to consider which is best for the patient.

Conclusion

Neurosurgical patients harbor some of the most diverse and challenging pathology in all of medicine. When combined with coagulopathy due to any cause, surgeons must proceed with caution in first treating the most direct threat to the patient's well-being. In the case of coagulopathy, clinicians often have to do this without the benefit of established clinical guidelines. Current clinical guidelines exist based on a wide variety of past experiences, but their use requires significant user interpretation and manipulation in response to unique clinical scenarios. Myriad barriers limit the amount of high-level evidence, and accentuate the importance of knowledge of proper coagulation physiology, how it is altered physiologically and chemically, and how to restore function—even temporarily.

Striving for positive outcomes subsequently requires much more than the planning and execution of an operation; it requires detailed knowledge of each patient's unique clinical history. Antiplatelet and anticoagulant medications have profoundly impacted the management of cardiac and thrombotic conditions, and their use is likely to remain stable if not increase in the future. Neurosurgeons then must maintain at least basic knowledge of the agents in clinical practice, how to circumvent their effect when needed, and how to transition patients back to prior management when the operative risk has subsided. This is an undertaking best approached with an eye on previous experience, and a willingness for multidisciplinary collaboration. Further still, all providers have a responsibility to not only consider each situation carefully but to share their experiences with the rest of the community. With a collaborative effort perhaps we can attain the goal of preserving neurological function without devastating thrombotic complications.

References

1. James RF, Palys V, Lomboy JR, Lamm JR, Simon SD. The role of anticoagulants, antiplatelet agents, and their reversal strategies in the management of intracerebral hemorrhage. Neurosurg Focus. 2013;34(5), E6.
2. Levi M, Eerenberg E, Kamphuisen PW. Bleeding risk and reversal strategies for old and new anticoagulants and antiplatelet agents. J Thromb Haemost. 2011;9(9): 1705–12.
3. Goy J, Crowther M. Approaches to diagnosing and managing anticoagulant-related bleeding. Semin Thromb Hemost. 2012;38(7):702–10.
4. Grandhi R, Harrison G, Voronovich Z, Bauer J, Chen SH, Nicholas D, et al. Preinjury warfarin, but not antiplatelet medications, increases mortality in elderly traumatic brain injury patients. J Trauma Acute Care Surg. 2015;78(3):614–21.
5. Cull JD, Sakai LM, Sabir I, Johnson B, Tully A, Nagy K, et al. Outcomes in traumatic brain injury for patients presenting on antiplatelet therapy. Am Surg. 2015;81(2):128–32.
6. Peck KA, Calvo RY, Schechter MS, Sise CB, Kahl JE, Shackford MC, et al. The impact of preinjury anticoagulants and prescription antiplatelet agents on outcomes in older patients with traumatic brain injury. J Trauma Acute Care Surg. 2014;76(2): 431–6.
7. Moussouttas M. Challenges and controversies in the medical management of primary and antithrombotic-related intracerebral hemorrhage. Ther Adv Neurol Disord. 2012;5(1):43–56.
8. Suárez-Pinilla M, Fernández-Rodríguez Á, Benavente-Fernández L, Calleja-Puerta S. Vitamin K antagonist-associated intracerebral hemorrhage: lessons from a devastating disease in the dawn of the new oral anticoagulants. J Stroke Cerebrovasc Dis. 2014;23(4): 732–42.
9. Pakraftar S, Atencio D, English J, Corcos A, Altschuler EM, Stahlfeld K. Dabigatran etixilate and traumatic brain injury: evolving anticoagulants require evolving care plans. World J Clin Cases. 2014;2(8):362–6.
10. Majeed A, Meijer K, Larrazabal R, Arnberg F, Luijckx GJ, Roberts RS, et al. Mortality in vitamin K antagonist-related intracerebral bleeding treated with plasma or 4-factor prothrombin complex concentrate. Thromb Haemost. 2014;111(2):233–9.
11. Yorkgitis BK, Ruggia-Check C, Dujon JE. Antiplatelet and anticoagulation medications and the surgical patient. Am J Surg. 2014;207(1):95–101.
12. McCoy CC, Lawson JH, Shapiro ML. Management of anticoagulation agents in trauma patients. Clin Lab Med. 2014;34(3):563–74.
13. Mavrakanas TA, Samer C, Fontana P, Perrier A. Direct oral anticoagulants: efficacy and safety in patient subgroups. Swiss Med Wkly. 2015;145:w14081.
14. Suryanarayan D, Schulman S. Potential antidotes for reversal of old and new oral anticoagulants. Thromb Res. 2014;133 Suppl 2:S158–66.
15. Fox BD, Kahn SR, Langleben D, Eisenberg MJ, Shimony A. Efficacy and safety of novel oral anticoagulants for treatment of acute venous thromboembolism: direct and adjusted indirect meta-analysis of randomised controlled trials. BMJ. 2012;345:e7498.
16. Chatterjee S, Sardar P, Biondi-Zoccai G, Kumbhani DJ. New oral anticoagulants and the risk of intracranial

hemorrhage: traditional and Bayesian meta-analysis and mixed treatment comparison of randomized trials of new oral anticoagulants in atrial fibrillation. JAMA Neurol. 2013;70(12):1486–90.
17. Gordon JL, Fabian TC, Lee MD, Dugdale M. Anticoagulant and antiplatelet medications encountered in emergency surgery patients: a review of reversal strategies. J Trauma Acute Care Surg. 2013;75(3):475–86.
18. Medow JE, Dierks MR, Williams E, Zacko JC. The emergent reversal of coagulopathies encountered in neurosurgery and neurology: a technical note. Clin Med Res. 2015;13(1):20–31.
19. Lu G, DeGuzman FR, Hollenbach SJ, Karbarz MJ, Abe K, Lee G, et al. A specific antidote for reversal of anticoagulation by direct and indirect inhibitors of coagulation factor Xa. Nat Med. 2013;19(4):446–51.
20. Na SY, Mracsko E, van Ryn J, Veltkamp R. Idarucizumab improves outcome in murine brain hemorrhage related to dabigatran. Ann Neurol. 2015;78:137–41.
21. Glund S, Moschetti V, Norris S, Stangier J, Schmohl M, van Ryn J, et al. A randomised study in healthy volunteers to investigate the safety, tolerability and pharmacokinetics of idarucizumab, a specific antidote to dabigatran. Thromb Haemost. 2015;113(5):943–51.
22. Gerotziafas GT, Depasse F, Chakroun T, Samama MM, Elalamy I. Recombinant factor VIIa partially reverses the inhibitory effect of fondaparinux on thrombin generation after tissue factor activation in platelet rich plasma and whole blood. Thromb Haemost. 2004;91(3):531–7.
23. Labuz-Roszak B, Pierzchala K, Skrzypek M, Swiech M, Machowska-Majchrzak A. Oral anticoagulant and antiplatelet drugs used in prevention of cardiovascular events in elderly people in Poland. BMC Cardiovasc Disord. 2012;12:98.
24. Campbell PG, Sen A, Yadla S, Jabbour P, Jallo J. Emergency reversal of antiplatelet agents in patients presenting with an intracranial hemorrhage: a clinical review. World Neurosurg. 2010;74(2–3):279–85.
25. Campbell PG, Yadla S, Sen AN, Jallo J, Jabbour P. Emergency reversal of clopidogrel in the setting of spontaneous intracerebral hemorrhage. World Neurosurg. 2011;76(1–2):100–4. discussion 59–60.
26. Washington CW, Schuerer DJ, Grubb RL. Platelet transfusion: an unnecessary risk for mild traumatic brain injury patients on antiplatelet therapy. J Trauma. 2011;71(2):358–63.
27. Thiele T, Sümnig A, Hron G, Müller C, Althaus K, Schroeder HW, et al. Platelet transfusion for reversal of dual antiplatelet therapy in patients requiring urgent surgery: a pilot study. J Thromb Haemost. 2012;10(5):968–71.
28. Sarode R. How do I transfuse platelets (PLTs) to reverse anti-PLT drug effect? Transfusion. 2012;52(4):695–701. quiz 694.
29. Agus N, Yilmaz N, Colak A, Liv F. Levels of factor VIII and factor IX in fresh-frozen plasma produced from whole blood stored at 4 degrees C overnight in Turkey. Blood Transfus. 2012;10(2):191–3.
30. Flaherty ML. Anticoagulant-associated intracerebral hemorrhage. Semin Neurol. 2010;30(5):565–72.
31. Hobl EL, Derhaschnig U, Firbas C, Schoergenhofer C, Schwameis M, Jilma B. Reversal strategy in antagonizing the P2Y12-inhibitor ticagrelor. Eur J Clin Invest. 2013;43(12):1258–61.
32. Ortel TL. Perioperative management of patients on chronic antithrombotic therapy. Hematology Am Soc Hematol Educ Program. 2012;2012:529–35.
33. Spyropoulos AC. Bridging therapy and oral anticoagulation: current and future prospects. Curr Opin Hematol. 2010;17(5):444–9.
34. Steinberg BA, Peterson ED, Kim S, Thomas L, Gersh BJ, Fonarow GC, et al. Use and outcomes associated with bridging during anticoagulation interruptions in patients with atrial fibrillation: findings from the Outcomes Registry for Better Informed Treatment of Atrial Fibrillation (ORBIT-AF). Circulation. 2015; 131(5):488–94.
35. Carragee EJ, Golish SR, Scuderi GJ. A case of late epidural hematoma in a patient on clopidogrel therapy postoperatively: when is it safe to resume antiplatelet agents? Spine J. 2011;11(1):e1–4.
36. Rahman M, Donnangelo LL, Neal D, Mogali K, Decker M, Ahmed MM. Effects of perioperative acetyl salicylic acid on clinical outcomes in patients undergoing craniotomy for brain tumor. World Neurosurg. 2015;84(1):41–7.
37. Ogawa Y, Tominaga T. Sellar and parasellar tumor removal without discontinuing antithrombotic therapy. J Neurosurg. 2015;123(3):794–8.
38. Schulman S, Hwang HG, Eikelboom JW, Kearon C, Pai M, Delaney J. Loading dose vs. maintenance dose of warfarin for reinitiation after invasive procedures: a randomized trial. J Thromb Haemost. 2014;12(8): 1254–9.
39. Buesing KL, Mullapudi B, Flowers KA. Deep venous thrombosis and venous thromboembolism prophylaxis. Surg Clin North Am. 2015;95(2):285–300.
40. Wells PS, Anderson DR, Rodger M, Forgie M, Kearon C, Dreyer J, et al. Evaluation of D-dimer in the diagnosis of suspected deep-vein thrombosis. N Engl J Med. 2003;349(13):1227–35.
41. Owaidah T, AlGhasham N, AlGhamdi S, AlKhafaji D, ALAmro B, Zeitouni M, et al. Evaluation of the usefulness of a D dimer test in combination with clinical pretest probability score in the prediction and exclusion of Venous Thromboembolism by medical residents. Thromb J. 2014;12(1):28.
42. Wells PS, Anderson DR, Rodger M, Ginsberg JS, Kearon C, Gent M, et al. Derivation of a simple clinical model to categorize patients probability of pulmonary embolism: increasing the models utility with the SimpliRED D-dimer. Thromb Haemost. 2000;83(3): 416–20.
43. Guyatt GH, Akl EA, Crowther M, Gutterman DD, Schuunemann HJ, American College of Chest

Physicians Antithrombotic Therapy and Prevention of Thrombosis Panel. Executive summary: Antithrombotic therapy and prevention of thrombosis, 9th ed: American College of Chest Physicians Evidence-Based Clinical Practice Guidelines. Chest. 2012;141 (2 Suppl):7S–47.

44. Patel G, Panikkath R, Fenire M, Gadwala S, Nugent K. Indications and appropriateness of inferior vena cava filter placement. Am J Med Sci. 2015;349(3): 212–6.
45. Kaufman JA, Kinney TB, Streiff MB, Sing RF, Proctor MC, Becker D, et al. Guidelines for the use of retrievable and convertible vena cava filters: report from the Society of Interventional Radiology multidisciplinary consensus conference. Surg Obes Relat Dis. 2006;2(2):200–12.
46. Berczi V, Bottomley JR, Thomas SM, Taneja S, Gaines PA, Cleveland TJ. Long-term retrievability of IVC filters: should we abandon permanent devices? Cardiovasc Intervent Radiol. 2007;30(5): 820–7.

Index

C.M. Loftus (ed.), *Anticoagulation and Hemostasis in Neurosurgery*,
DOI 10.1007/978-3-319-27327-3

Lightning Source UK Ltd.
Milton Keynes UK
UKOW07n1306190716

278637UK00003B/55/P

9 783319 273259